NAPLEX® 2017
STRATEGIES, PRACTICE & REVIEW
with 2 Practice Tests

NAPLEX 2017
STRATEGIES, PRACTICE & REVIEW
with 2 Practice Tests

ONLINE + BOOK

Amie D. Brooks, PharmD, FCCP, BCPS, BCACP
Cynthia Sanoski, BS, PharmD, FCCP, BCPS
Emily R. Hajjar, PharmD, BCPS, BCACP, CGP
Brian R. Overholser, PharmD, FCCP

KAPLAN) MEDICAL

Published by Kaplan Publishing, a division of Kaplan, Inc.
750 Third Avenue
New York, NY 10017

Retail ISBN: 978-1-5062-0843-5
10 9 8 7 6 5 4 3 2 1

Course ISBN: 978-1-5062-0887-9
10 9 8 7 6 5 4 3 2 1

Kaplan Publishing books are available at special quantity discounts to use for sales promotions, employee premiums, or educational purposes. For more information or to purchase books, please call the Simon & Schuster special sales department at 866-506-1949.

JUN 21 2017

About the Authors

Amie D. Brooks, PharmD, FCCP, BCPS, BCACP, is an associate professor of pharmacy practice at the St. Louis College of Pharmacy and a clinical pharmacy specialist in ambulatory care at St. Louis County Department of Health. Dr. Brooks is the program director for a PGY1 residency program, a board-certified pharmacotherapy specialist, and a fellow of the American College of Clinical Pharmacy. She received her Doctor of Pharmacy degree from the St. Louis College of Pharmacy and completed her pharmacy residency training at the Jefferson Barracks VA Medical Center in St. Louis, Missouri. Her research interests include clinical pharmacy services, diabetes, resistant hypertension, and collaborative practice.

Cynthia Sanoski, BS, PharmD, FCCP, BCPS, is the chair of the department of pharmacy practice at the Jefferson School of Pharmacy at Thomas Jefferson University. Dr. Sanoski received her Doctor of Pharmacy degree from Ohio State University, and subsequently completed a 2-year fellowship in cardiovascular pharmacotherapy at the University of Illinois at Chicago. She is also a board-certified pharmacotherapy specialist and a fellow of the American College of Clinical Pharmacy. Dr. Sanoski serves as an instructor with Kaplan Medical, teaching NAPLEX review courses for graduating pharmacy students across the country.

Emily Hajjar, PharmD, BCPS, BCACP, CGP, is associate professor in the Jefferson School of Pharmacy at Thomas Jefferson University in Philadelphia, Pennsylvania. Dr. Hajjar earned her PharmD at Duquesne University. She completed a pharmacy practice residency at the University of Rochester Medical Center in Rochester, New York, a geriatric pharmacy specialty residency at the Minneapolis Veteran's Affairs Medical Center, and a geriatric pharmacotherapy-epidemiology fellowship at the University of Minnesota, College of Pharmacy. Dr. Hajjar provides clinical services to the Jefferson Family and Community Medicine Senior Center Practice and the Kimmel Cancer Center Senior Adult Oncology and Outpatient Palliative Care clinics. Her research interests include geriatric pharmacotherapy and polypharmacy.

Brian R. Overholser, PharmD, FCCP, is associate professor of pharmacy practice in the College of Pharmacy at Purdue University and Adjunct Associate Professor in the Division of Clinical Pharmacology at the Indiana University School of Medicine in Indianapolis, Indiana. Dr. Overholser earned his PharmD and conducted his postdoctoral research in pharmacokinetics and pharmacodynamics at Purdue University. His primary teaching responsibilities include courses in pharmacokinetics, pharmacodynamics, and pharmacogenetics at both Purdue and Indiana University. Dr. Overholser's research program is focused on elucidating the pathological regulation that increases the susceptibility of arrhythmias in patients with heart failure.

The authors wish to thank the following test item writers: LeAnn C. Boyd, PharmD, BCPS, CDE; Elizabeth Langan, MD; Amy Egras, PharmD, BCPS; Stacey Thacker, PharmD; and Arneka Tillman, PharmD candidate, Xavier University College of Pharmacy.

The authors also wish to thank the following individuals for serving as expert reviewers: Rebecca Bragg, PharmD, BCPS, Assistant Professor St. Louis College of Pharmacy; and Ashley H. Vincent, PharmD, BCACP, BCPS, Clinical Assistant Professor, Purdue University College of Pharmacy. The authors would also like to acknowledge the contributions of Karen Nagel, BS Pharm, PhD, and Steven T. Boyd, PharmD, BCPS, CDE.

Table of Contents

PART THREE: Pharmaceutical Sciences, Calculations, and Biostatistics Clinical Trial Design

PART FOUR: Resources and Policy

PART FIVE: Practice Test

KAPLAN) MEDICAL

Part One

Overview

How to Use This Book

Congratulations! You've taken the first step to prepare yourself for the NAPLEX®. This book contains the information you want and need to do your best.

The authors are proud to release the 2017 edition of this NAPLEX® review book, which incorporates readers' feedback. The edition has been updated throughout with current drug information and Top 200 drugs as determined by the authors.

REVIEW STRUCTURE

The content of this book is designed to provide a concentrated and concise review of the competency areas tested on the exam. This book is not intended to replace standard textbooks in pharmacy. Rather, it should serve as a primary tool in the weeks and months prior to taking the exam. Since it is not practical to re-read textbooks, you will need a resource that will provide concise, focused review. This book fills that need.

Kaplan suggests that areas in which you feel weakest should be studied first; in this way, you can spend additional review time on difficult concepts.

This book covers all of the areas tested on the NAPLEX® and features an efficient time-management tool to ensure adequate preparation. Each chapter includes a *suggested study time*, prepared by the authors. These are only suggested rates; certainly, the study rate will vary based on your own level of comfort with the subject matter. By gauging yourself, however, you will be able to practice for test day, when your time on the computer will be limited.

The review is arranged by disease states, focusing on the following:

- Definitions of the disease
- Diagnosis
- Signs and symptoms
- Guidelines
- Guidelines summary

- Medication charts
- Storage & administration pearls
- Patient education pearls

Each chapter also contains a few practice questions, allowing you to apply the information you have just reviewed.

PRACTICE TESTS

The NAPLEX® is a computer-adaptive examination consisting of 250 questions. To assist you in preparing for the test-taking experience, this book offers two partial practice examinations with 185 questions each. One practice exam, along with answer explanations, is included in the text of this book. A second test is available online.

Practice Test 1 should be taken prior to the beginning of your study period. Then, use the results to identify areas of strength and weakness and to tailor an individualized study plan. For example, if you score below average on questions related to oncology therapeutics, plan to spend some additional days studying this subject. Likewise, if cardiovascular therapeutics was the area in which you scored the highest, you may want to leave this section for last.

Both practice tests should be taken in quiet areas—dedicate 4 hours and 15 minutes for each test. This time provides the same per-question time allotment on the current 250-question NAPLEX exam. It is advisable to take the practice exam somewhere with limited distractions, such as a library. The goal is to simulate examlike conditions and to obtain data that will help structure an effective study plan.

As you work through the items, pay particular attention to the explanations. Often, studying the explanations is one of the most valuable study resources. Note that for difficult questions, explanations have been provided that explain the reasoning for not choosing the incorrect answer choices. Use this information to understand the rationale behind eliminating each distracter.

Finally, take Practice Test 2 a week or two prior to your exam date. Test 2 should be taken once the majority of your study has been completed. Test 2 is provided as an online companion to this book and also contains a partial exam with 185 unique questions. The time you allow to take this online exam should also be 4 hours and 15 minutes. Our intention—and our hope—is that this book will be an integral part of your preparation for the NAPLEX®.

ACCESS THE ONLINE COMPANION

kaptest.com/booksonline

As owner of this guide, you are entitled to get more practice online. Log on to kaptest.com/booksonline to access the second full-length practice test.

Just as in the book, the 185-question partial practice test includes detailed answer explanations. Access to online NAPLEX® practice material is free of charge to purchasers of this book. You'll be asked for a specific password derived from the text in this book, so have your book handy when you log on.

Best of luck to you on your journey toward a successful career as a pharmacist!

TEST CHANGES OR LATE-BREAKING DEVELOPMENTS

kaptest.com/publishing

The material in this book is up-to-date at the time of publication. However, the NABP® may have instituted changes in the test after this book was published. Be sure to carefully read the materials you receive when you register for the test. If there are any important late-breaking developments—or any changes or corrections to the Kaplan test preparation materials in this book—we will post that information online at kaptest.com/publishing.

Introduction and Test-Taking Strategies

WHAT IS THE NAPLEX®?

NAPLEX stands for North American Pharmacist Licensure Examination. The NAPLEX is issued by the National Association of Boards of Pharmacy (NABP®) and is utilized by the boards of pharmacy as part of their assessment of competence to practice pharmacy. NABP represents each of the 50 states in the United States, the District of Columbia, and the five major U. S. territories. South Africa, New Zealand, Australia, and Canada also utilize the NAPLEX for licensure.

These boards of pharmacy have a mandate to protect the public from unsafe and ineffective pharmacy care, and each board has been given responsibility to regulate the practice of pharmacy in its respective state. In fact, the NAPLEX is often referred to as "The Boards" or "State Boards."

Each state requires applicants to take and pass the NAPLEX in order to obtain a license to practice as a registered pharmacist. The NAPLEX has only one purpose: to determine if it is safe for you to begin practicing as an entry-level pharmacist.

To take the NAPLEX, you must meet the eligibility requirements of the board of pharmacy from which you seek licensure. The board will determine your eligibility in accordance with the jurisdiction's requirements. If you are determined to be eligible, the board will notify NABP of your eligibility. Once that happens, a letter will be issued to you by Pearson VUE, the test administrator, with information about how to schedule your testing appointment.

CONTENT AND STRUCTURE

The NAPLEX is a linear form exam that consists of 250 multiple-choice questions. Of these, 200 questions will be used to calculate your test score. The remaining 50 items serve as experimental questions and do not affect your score.

The NAPLEX is not a test of achievement or intelligence, nor is it designed for pharmacists with years of experience. The questions do not involve high-tech clinical pharmacy or equipment. Note, too, that you will not be tested on all the content you were taught in pharmacy school.

Many of the questions on the NAPLEX are asked in a scenario-based format (i.e., patient profiles with accompanying test questions). To properly analyze and answer the questions, you must refer to the information provided in the patient profile. Other questions are answered solely from the information provided in the question.

The previously popular K-type questions have been phased out of the NAPLEX exam. K-type questions were a frequently used style on previous NAPLEX exams and are still used by many pharmacy schools in the United States. Over the past few years, the number of K questions has been declining on the NAPLEX, and they have now been phased out completely. The newer question formats on the NAPLEX include the following:

(1) multiple choice
(2) multiple response
(3) constructed response
(4) ordered response
(5) hot-spot

Each format is described with examples in the sections that follow. Note that the examples provided are to demonstrate the question structure rather than to stress NAPLEX content.

Multiple-Choice Format

The multiple-choice format has been used historically on the NAPLEX and remains a mainstay of the exam. An example of a multiple-choice question is provided:

Which of the following is most likely a symptom of digoxin overdose and toxicity?

(A) Ototoxicity
(B) Hepatotoxicity
(C) Visual disturbances
(D) Renal failure
(E) Dizziness

Multiple-Response Format

The multiple-response format is likely designed to replace the traditional K-style questions on the NAPLEX. The premise of these questions is very similar to K questions, but more options are available. These can be broken down into a series of true and false statements. The test-taker's goal is to identify all the true statements. An example multiple-response question is provided:

Which of the following could alter a patient's response to warfarin? (Select **ALL** that apply.)

(A) Increased intake of charred meats
(B) New prescription for amiodarone
(C) Increased intake of vitamin D
(D) Acute hepatic failure
(E) New prescription for fexofenadine

Constructed-Response Format

The constructed-response format is simply a fill-in-the-blank style of question. Although the NABP has not given much guidance regarding the use of these questions, the examples they have provided have largely been calculation questions answered to the nearest whole number. In the examples provided by the NABP, the units of the final answer have been stated in the question, as in the constructed-response example here:

The "Sig" for a prednisone prescription is "25 mg today, 10 mg bid for 2 days, 5 mg bid for 3 days, then 5 mg qd for 1 week." How many 5-mg tablets should be dispensed?

(Answer must be numeric; round the final answer to the nearest **WHOLE** number.)

Ordered-Response Format

The ordered-response format is designed for the test taker to assign ranks to an unordered list of options. The NABP has listed a sample question in this format to rank topical corticosteroids from highest to lowest potencies. Another example of an ordered-response question is provided:

Rank the following HMG-CoA reductase inhibitors from highest to lowest potency. (**ALL** options must be used.)

Unordered Options	Ordered Response
Atorvastatin	
Fluvastatin	
Pravastatin	
Rosuvastatin	

Hot-Spot Format

The hot-spot format is designed for the test taker to identify the correct portion of a diagram that is related to the question presented. The NABP NAPLEX-MPJE registration guide presents a sample question in this format. The question displays a diagram of the HIV life cycle and asks the test taker to identify the portion of the life cycle during which maraviroc exerts its mechanism of action. Another example of a hot-spot question is provided here:

> Using the diagram below, identify where on a ventricular action potential ibutilide would exert the greatest effect. (Select the TEXT response, and left-click the mouse. To change your answer, move the cursor, select alternate TEXT response and click.)

HOW IS THE NAPLEX SCORED, AND WHAT SCORE DO YOU NEED TO PASS?

Your NAPLEX score is a scaled score, not a number-correct score or a percentile score. The scoring scale ranges will likely be from 0 to 200 with the minimum passing score likely to be set at 100. At the time of this writing, the NABP hadn't released these exact numbers since the exam implemented these changes in November 2016. The minimum score will likely not represent the number of questions answered correctly or a percentage but will be a scaled score. The algorithms for determining your scaled score are highly confidential and are not released to the public.

Candidates who fail to answer a set limit of questions will not receive any score. Since the computer format requires that you answer every question on the screen, the only way you could answer less than the set limit would be to stop short before the end of the exam. If you complete minimum limit but not the entire exam, you will receive a penalty, and your score will be adjusted to reflect the number of questions that remained unanswered. It is certainly in your best interest to answer all questions presented.

NABP will forward your NAPLEX score to the board of pharmacy from which you are seeking licensure. NABP **does not** provide scores to candidates, and score results **are not** released at the test center.

WHAT IF YOU FAIL THE NAPLEX?

First of all, it's unlikely you will fail. Currently, the passage rate is approximately 93%. Candidates who receive a failing score on the NAPLEX will automatically be provided with a diagnostic report that indicates their relative performance in each major competency area. The board of pharmacy will notify the candidates of the NAPLEX results and diagnostic report.

Strategies for Success

1. There is a timer at the top of the computer screen to help you pace yourself. You can hide it if it distracts you—but since the test is timed, you might find it helpful for pacing. You have **6 hours** to complete all 250 questions. The total appointment time will be for 6.5 hours to give time to read the instructions and sign disclosures.

2. There will be a minimum of 1 break provided during the exam which will not count against your exam time. Make sure to take any available break! You need to rest your brain. Remember there are no bonus points for finishing early.

3. It is possible that questions involving mathematical calculations will be weighted more heavily than other questions. Spend extra time solving them, but try to limit yourself to a maximum of 5 or 6 minutes each, if time is a concern.

4. If a question calls for a calculation or a certain mechanism, scratch a rough image. Having a crude diagram to look at, rather than having to imagine it from the computer screen, will help you to see what you're dealing with. Such notes also often stimulate more recall.

5. Look for key words in questions. Words such as "most likely" may help you eliminate some choices even when you don't have comprehensive recall—the most likely choice is probably the one that is most familiar as you review the choices.

6. You cannot cross off an answer choice and banish it from your sight (it's on a computer screen, after all), so you have to be disciplined about not reconsidering choices you've already eliminated.

NAPLEX REGISTRATION

The NAPLEX is administered year-round on business days. There are several steps in registering for the exam. As of this printing, the fee for the exam is $575. (Also, be sure to check with your local board of pharmacy for its fees.)

- **First Step:**
  - Contact the board of pharmacy in the state in which you want to be licensed. The state board will issue paperwork and instructions that determine your eligibility, and will notify the NABP. You will then be issued an authorization to test (ATT), as well as other documents, including:
    - » Test authorization number
    - » Expiration date
    - » Range of dates during which you can take the NAPLEX
- **Second Step:**
  - Once you receive your authorization packet from the NABP, you can call or register online at Pearson VUE to choose your testing center to schedule your test date. You will need your ATT information to schedule a testing date.
  - For more information about registration, go to:
    - » NABP   http://www.nabp.net
    - » Pearson VUE   http://www.pearsonvue.com/

TAKING THE EXAM

There is no time limit for each individual question; however, you have a total of 6 hours to complete the exam. This does not include the beginning tutorial or any break given.

Remember, every question counts. There is no warm-up time, so it is important for you to be ready to answer questions correctly from the very beginning. Concentration is also key. You need to give your best thinking to each question.

ON THE DAY OF THE EXAM

1. Arrive at the test center at least 30 minutes before your scheduled testing time to allow for check-in. If you arrive late, you may be required to forfeit your appointment. **If you forfeit your appointment, your testing fee will not be refunded.**

2. Bring two forms of identification: a picture ID that includes your signature and a second form of ID. You will be required to show these IDs for entry. Your thumbprint will also be required when you enter the testing room.

3. You will be provided with laminated note boards, which may be replaced as needed during testing. You will not be allowed to take your own scratch paper or pencil into the testing room.

4. An on-screen, five-function calculator can be activated during the test administration for your use. You may also request a hand-held, five-function calculator from the test administrator.

5. The seating time for the exam is 6 hours.

NAPLEX BLUEPRINT

The questions on the NAPLEX involve integrated pharmacy content. The NAPLEX Competency Statements provide a blueprint of the topics covered on the exam. In November 2015, the NABP revised this blueprint and Competency Statements for the NAPLEX. This revision decreased the blueprint to include 2 Competence Areas. Despite the change in the structure of the competency statements, there is not much difference in content between previous years. The new competency statements and blueprint are covered in this review book. Nonetheless, reviewing the subcategories under the two major Competence Areas may assist you in preparation for the exam and these are available through the NABP website listed.

- **Competence Area 1:** Ensure Safe and Effective Pharmacotherapy and Health Outcomes (approximately 67% of exam)

- **Competence Area 2:** Safe and Accurate Preparation, Compounding, Dispensing, and Administration of Medications and Provision of Health Care Products (approximately 33% of exam)

For specific subcategories under each competence area, go to **www.nabp.net**.

TEST-TAKING STRATEGIES

As you review each chapter in this book, it is important to focus on your own areas of weakness. To help you do so, keep the following in mind:

Key Steps toward Preparedness

- Assess your strengths and weaknesses. Review your weakest subjects first. The best way to identify your weaknesses is through practice exams.

- Focus heavily on the Top 200 drugs identified with a star (☆) in the tables throughout the book.

- Practice calculations to increase your confidence.

- Schedule extra time before your testing date to revisit your weaker areas.

- Complete the practice test under real exam conditions.

- Order and complete the Pre-NAPLEX exam, available from NABP.

- When you review the practice exams, make sure you understand why your incorrect answer choices were incorrect.

- Be sure you understand why you missed a question. Did you simply forget a fact? Choose your answer too quickly? Misunderstand the question? Miss an important clue within the question? Finally, do you keep making the same mistakes over and over? If so, it is important to spend more time on those areas.

Guessing

During the exam, there are sure to be some questions that stump you. For those, just narrow down the choices and take your best guess. You don't want to spend too much time analyzing a question you do not know and then run out of time toward the end of the exam. Remember, you cannot simply leave a question blank, so in some shape or form, you'll have to take your best guess.

Keep in mind that 50 experimental questions are not calculated into your score, so if you answer a few questions incorrectly, it's possible that they won't be scored at all.

When you just don't know the answer: narrow the answer choices to two likely choices, then use the "upper, then lower" decision rule to select one of them. This rule means you alternate your guess, using the upper choice the first time you are stuck, then the lower choice the next time you are stuck. This technique helps keep you moving forward.

Positive Attitude

The most important decision you can make in your studying process is to have a positive attitude, especially on test day. Remember this:

- The odds are on your side; around 93% of pharmacy graduates pass the NAPLEX.

- This is a minimal competency exam.

- You spent a minimum of 6 years in school to become a pharmacist. If you did that, you can conquer this exam!

You **are** prepared, and this book is a tool to increase your confidence.

Part Two

Review of Therapeutics

Cardiovascular Disorders

This chapter covers the following topics:

- **Hypertension**
- **Dyslipidemia**
- **Heart failure**
- **Antiarrhythmic drugs**
- **Antithrombotic drugs**
- **Ischemic heart disease**
- **Acute pharmacologic management of UA/NSTEMI and STEMI**
- **Secondary prevention of MI**

 Suggested Study Time: **2.5 hours**

HYPERTENSION

Definitions

Hypertension (HTN) is defined as a systolic blood pressure (SBP) >140 mmHg, a diastolic blood pressure (DBP) >90 mmHg, or any patient requiring antihypertensive therapy. Most patients with HTN have primary (essential) HTN (due to an unknown cause, likely genetic), while less than 10% have secondary HTN (due to chronic kidney disease [CKD], pheochromocytoma, Cushing's syndrome, or medications [nonsteroidal anti-inflammatory drugs (NSAIDs), corticosteroids, cyclosporine, tacrolimus, estrogens, erythropoietin, venlafaxine, sympathomimetics, cocaine]).

Diagnosis

- Average of ≥2 blood pressure (BP) measurements ≥140/90 mmHg

Signs and Symptoms

- Can develop target organ damage with chronic, uncontrolled HTN:
  - Cardiac
    - » Angina, myocardial infarction (MI), history of coronary revascularization (e.g., percutaneous coronary intervention [PCI], coronary artery bypass graft [CABG] surgery), left ventricular hypertrophy (LVH), left ventricular (LV) dysfunction (i.e., heart failure with reduced ejection fraction [HFrEF])
  - Cerebrovascular
    - » Stroke, transient ischemic attack (TIA)
  - Renal
    - » CKD
  - Ophthalmologic
    - » Retinopathy, blindness
  - Vascular
    - » Peripheral arterial disease (PAD)

Guidelines

James PA, Oparil S, Carter BL, et al. 2014 evidence-based guideline for the management of high blood pressure in adults: report from the panel members appointed to the Eighth Joint National Committee (JNC 8). *JAMA* 2014;311:507–520.

Rosendorff C, Lackland DT, Allison M, et al. Treatment of hypertension in patients with coronary artery disease: a scientific statement from the American Heart Association, American College of Cardiology, and American Society of Hypertension. *Circulation* 2015;131:e435-e470.

Kidney Disease: Improving Global Outcomes (KDIGO) Blood Pressure Work Group. KDIGO clinical practice guideline for the management of blood pressure in chronic kidney disease. *Kidney Int Suppl* 2012:337–414.

American Diabetes Association. 8. Cardiovascular disease and risk management. *Diabetes Care* 2016;(39 suppl 1):S60-71.

Guidelines Summary

- General population <60 yr: <140/90 mmHg (JNC 8 guidelines)
- General population ≥60 yr: <150/90 mmHg (JNC 8 guidelines)
- CKD
  - BP goal <140/90 mmHg (JNC 8 guidelines)
  - Urine albumin excretion <30 mg/day: BP goal <140/90 mmHg (KDIGO guidelines)

- Urine albumin excretion ≥30 mg/day: BP goal <130/80 mmHg (KDIGO guidelines)

- Diabetes mellitus (DM)
  - BP goal <140/90 mmHg (JNC 8 guidelines and American Diabetes Association guidelines)

- Patients with coronary artery disease (CAD) for secondary prevention of cardiovascular events:
  - BP goal <140/90 mmHg (American Heart Association/American College of Cardiology/American Society of Hypertension guidelines)

- Lifestyle modifications: weight loss (goal body mass index [BMI] 18.5–24.9 kg/m²), diet rich in fruits, vegetables, and low-fat dairy products with ↓ saturated and total fat, ↓ sodium (Na⁺) intake (≤2.4 g/day), ↑ physical activity (30 minutes most days of the week), moderation of alcohol use (≤1 ounce of ethanol/day), smoking cessation

- Pharmacologic therapy:
  - Initial antihypertensive drug selection (JNC8 guidelines):
    » Nonblack patients (with or without DM): Thiazide diuretic, angiotensin-converting enzyme inhibitor (ACEI), angiotensin II receptor blocker (ARB), and/or calcium channel blocker (CCB)
    » Black patients (with or without DM): Thiazide diuretic and/or CCB
    » CKD (regardless of race or presence of DM): ACEI or ARB (alone or in combination with other drug class)
    » NOTE: β-blockers are no longer considered first-line therapy for patients with HTN without specific comorbidities (see below)
  - Presence of other comorbidities may warrant selection of other agents as first-line antihypertensive therapy (based on guidelines for each of these conditions):
    » HFrEF: Diuretic, ACEI, β-blocker (carvedilol, metoprolol succinate, or bisoprolol), ARB, aldosterone receptor antagonist (ARA), hydralazine/isosorbide dinitrate (for black patients)
    » Post-MI: β-blocker, ACEI (or ARB)
    » High coronary disease risk: ACEI (or ARB), thiazide diuretic, CCB
    » Recurrent stroke prevention: ACEI, diuretic
  - Three approaches for initiation and titration of antihypertensive therapy:
    » Initiate one antihypertensive drug → Titrate to maximum dose to achieve goal BP → If goal BP not achieved, add second antihypertensive drug → Titrate dose of second drug to maximum → If goal BP still not achieved, add third antihypertensive drug
      – Avoid concomitant use of ACEI and ARB
    » Initiate one antihypertensive drug → If goal BP not achieved, add second antihypertensive drug before maximum dose of initial drug achieved → If

goal BP not achieved, titrate doses of both drugs up to maximum → If goal BP still not achieved, add third antihypertensive drug

– Avoid concomitant use of ACEI and ARB

» Initiate two antihypertensive drugs at same time (avoid concomitant use of ACEI and ARB) → If goal BP not achieved, titrate doses of both drugs up to maximum → If goal BP still not achieved, add third antihypertensive drug

– Initial two-drug approach should be considered when: BP >160 mmHg and/or DBP >100 mmHg **OR** SBP is >20 mmHg and/or DBP is >10 mmHg above goal

Diuretics

Generic • Brand • Dose	Contra-indications	Primary Side Effects	Key Monitoring	Pertinent Drug Interactions	Med Pearl
Thiazide Diuretics – inhibit Na$^+$ reabsorption in the distal convoluted tubule					
Chlorothiazide • Diuril • 500–2,000 mg/day Chlorthalidone☆ • Only available generically • 12.5–100 mg/day Hydrochlorothiazide☆ • Microzide • 12.5–50 mg/day Indapamide • Only available generically • 1.25–5 mg/day Metolazone☆ • Zaroxolyn • 2.5–5 mg/day	Sulfa allergy	• Hypokalemia • Hypomagnesemia • Hyponatremia • Hypercalcemia • Hyperglycemia • Hyperuricemia • Photosensitivity	• BP • Electrolytes • Blood urea nitrogen (BUN)/serum creatinine (SCr) • Blood glucose • Uric acid	• May ↑ risk of lithium toxicity • May ↓ effect of antidiabetic agents • NSAIDs ↓ antihypertensive effects	• Often used as first-line therapy for HTN • Synergistic effect with other antihypertensives • Not effective (except metolazone) when creatinine clearance (CrCl) <30 mL/min; use loop diuretics • Have ceiling dose (unlike loop diuretics) • Chlorothiazide also available as injection
Loop Diuretics – inhibit Na$^+$ reabsorption in the ascending limb of loop of Henle (should only be used for HTN in patients with renal impairment [maintain efficacy when CrCl <30 mL/min], severe edema, or HF) (see HF section for further details)					
Potassium-Sparing Diuretics – inhibit Na$^+$ reabsorption in the collecting ducts					
Amiloride • Only available generically • 5–10 mg/day Triamterene • Dyrenium • 50–100 mg/day	• Hyperkalemia • CKD	Hyperkalemia	• BP • Potassium (K$^+$) • BUN/SCr	Use with K$^+$ supplements, ACEIs, ARBs, ARAs, or NSAIDs may ↑ risk of hyperkalemia	• Not used often as monotherapy (weak antihypertensives) • Often used with hydrochlorothiazide to ↓ K$^+$ loss
Combination products: Triamterene/hydrochlorothiazide (Dyazide, Maxzide) Amiloride/hydrochlorothiazide (only available generically)					

Diuretics *(cont'd)*

Generic • Brand • Dose	Contra- indications	Primary Side Effects	Key Monitoring	Pertinent Drug Interactions	Med Pearl
Aldosterone Receptor Antagonists – have similar mechanism of action to K+-sparing diuretics (also block the effects of aldosterone) (not used often for HTN) (see HF section for further details)					
Combination products: Spironolactone/hydrochlorothiazide (Aldactazide)					

β-Blockers

Generic • Brand • Dose	Contra- indications	Primary Side Effects	Key Monitoring	Pertinent Drug Interactions	Med Pearl
Mechanism of action – ↓ cardiac output (CO) by negative inotropic (↓ contractility) and negative chronotropic (↓ heart rate [HR]) effects • Cardioselective – bind more to β_1 than β_2 receptors (at low doses); less likely to cause bronchoconstriction or vasoconstriction at low doses (safer to use in patients with asthma, chronic obstructive pulmonary disease [COPD], PAD, or DM); cardioselectivity may be lost at higher doses 　　– Bisoprolol, atenolol, metoprolol, betaxolol, acebutolol, nebivolol (BAMBAN) • Intrinsic sympathomimetic activity (ISA) – have partial β-receptor agonist activity 　　– Carteolol, acebutolol, pindolol, penbutolol (CAPP) • Lipophilic vs. hydrophilic – lipophilic (propranolol, metoprolol, carvedilol, labetalol, pindolol, nebivolol) more likely to cause central nervous system (CNS) side effects (e.g., depression, fatigue) than hydrophilic (atenolol)					
Cardioselective:					
Acebutolol • Sectral • 200–1,200 mg/day Atenolol☆ • Tenormin • 25–100 mg/day Betaxolol • Only available generically • 5–20 mg/day Bisoprolol • Zebeta • 2.5–20 mg/day Metoprolol☆ • Tartrate: Lopressor (2 × daily), Succinate: Toprol XL (1 × daily) • 25–400 mg/day Nebivolol☆ • Bystolic • 5–40 mg/day	• ≥2nd degree heart block (in absence of pacemaker) • HF (except metoprolol succinate or bisoprolol)	• Bradycardia/heart block • HF exacerbation • Bronchospasm • Cold extremities • Fatigue • ↓ exercise tolerance • Depression • Glucose intolerance • Mask hypoglycemia (in patients with DM)	• BP • HR • S/S of HF • Blood glucose (in patients with DM)	Use with other negative chronotropes (e.g., digoxin, vera-pamil, diltiazem, clonidine, or ivabradine) may ↑ risk of bradycardia	• Abrupt discontinuation may cause angina, MI, or hypertensive emergency; need to taper over 2 wks • Metoprolol tartrate also available as injection

β-Blockers *(cont'd)*

Generic • Brand • Dose	Contra-indications	Primary Side Effects	Key Monitoring	Pertinent Drug Interactions	Med Pearl
Nonselective:					
Carvedilol ☆ • Coreg, Coreg CR • Immediate-release (IR): 12.5–50 mg/day (in two divided doses) • Controlled-release (CR): 20–80 mg/day (1 × daily)	• ≥2nd degree heart block (in absence of pacemaker) • HF (except carvedilol)	Same as with cardioselective β-blockers	Same as with cardioselective β-blockers	Same as with cardioselective β-blockers	• Same as with cardioselective β-blockers • Labetalol and carvedilol also have α_1-blocking properties • Labetalol and propranolol also available as injection
Labetalol • Trandate • 200–2,400 mg/day					
Nadolol • Corgard • 20–320 mg/day					
Pindolol • Only available generically • 5–60 mg/day					
Propranolol ☆ • Inderal, Inderal LA, InnoPran XL • 80–640 mg/day (IR given 2–3 × daily; extended-release [ER] given 1 × daily)					
Timolol • Only available generically • 20–60 mg/day					

Combination products:

Atenolol/chlorthalidone (Tenoretic)
Bisoprolol/hydrochlorothiazide (Ziac)

Metoprolol tartrate/hydrochlorothiazide (Lopressor HCT)
Metoprolol succinate/hydrochlorothiazide (Dutoprol)

Nadolol/bendroflumethiazide (Corzide)
Nebivolol/valsartan (Byvalson)
Propranolol/hydrochlorothiazide (only available generically)

Angiotensin-Converting Enzyme Inhibitors

Generic • Brand • Dose	Contra-indications	Primary Side Effects	Key Monitoring	Pertinent Drug Interactions	Med Pearl
Mechanism of action – inhibit angiotensin-converting enzyme and prevent the conversion of angiotensin I to angiotensin II → vasodilation, ↓ aldosterone production; also inhibit degradation of bradykinin					
Benazepril☆ • Lotensin • 5–40 mg/day Captopril • Only available generically • 12.5–450 mg/day Enalapril☆ • Epaned, Vasotec • 2.5–40 mg/day Fosinopril☆ • Only available generically • 5–80 mg/day Lisinopril☆ • Prinivil, Qbrelis, Zestril • 2.5–40 mg/day Moexipril • Univasc • 3.75–30 mg/day Perindopril • Aceon • 4–16 mg/day Quinapril☆ • Accupril • 10–80 mg/day Ramipril☆ • Altace • 1.25–20 mg/day Trandolapril☆ • Mavik • 0.5–4 mg/day	• Pregnancy • History of angioedema or renal failure with prior use • Hyperkalemia • Bilateral renal artery stenosis • Concurrent use with aliskiren in DM	• Hyperkalemia • Renal impairment • Cough (dry) • Angioedema	• BP • BUN/SCr • K+	• Use with K+ supplements, K+-sparing diuretics, ARAs, or NSAIDs may ↑ risk of hyperkalemia • Use with ARBs or aliskiren may ↑ risk of hyperkalemia and renal impairment (avoid concurrent use with aliskiren in DM and CrCl <60 mL/min) • May ↑ risk of lithium toxicity • Use with sirolimus, temsirolimus, or everolimus may ↑ risk of angioedema	• Captopril has shortest duration of action • Enalapril also available as oral solution (Epaned) and injection (enalaprilat) • If patient has intolerable dry cough, may switch to ARB • Hyperkalemia and renal impairment also likely to occur with ARBs (risk of angioedema cross-sensitivity with ARBs controversial)

Combination products:

Benazepril/amlodipine (Lotrel)
Benazepril/hydrochlorothiazide (Lotensin HCT)
Captopril/hydrochlorothiazide (only available generically)

Enalapril/hydrochlorothiazide (Vaseretic)
Fosinopril/hydrochlorothiazide (only available generically)
Lisinopril/hydrochlorothiazide (Zestoretic)

Moexipril/hydrochlorothiazide (Uniretic)
Perindopril/amlodipine (Prestalia)
Quinapril/hydrochlorothiazide (Accuretic)
Trandolapril/verapamil (Tarka)

Angiotensin II Receptor Blockers

Generic • Brand • Dose	Contra-indications	Primary Side Effects	Key Monitoring	Pertinent Drug Interactions	Med Pearl
Mechanism of action – inhibit the binding of angiotensin II to the angiotensin type 1 (AT_1) receptor $\rightarrow$ vasodilation, ↓ aldosterone production; no effect on bradykinin					
Azilsartan • Edarbi • 40–80 mg/day	Same as for ACEIs	• Same as for ACEIs (except no cough) • Sprue-like enteropathy (olmesartan)	Same as for ACEIs	• Use with K⁺ supplements, K⁺-sparing diuretics, ARAs, or NSAIDs may ↑ risk of hyperkalemia • Use with ACEIs or aliskiren may ↑ risk of hyperkalemia or renal impairment (avoid concurrent use with aliskiren in DM and CrCl <60 mL/min) • May ↑ risk of lithium toxicity	Hyperkalemia and renal impairment also likely to occur with ACEIs (risk of angioedema cross-sensitivity with ACEIs is controversial)
Candesartan • Atacand • 4–32 mg/day					
Eprosartan • Teveten • 400–800 mg/day					
Irbesartan☆ • Avapro • 75–300 mg/day					
Losartan☆ • Cozaar • 25–100 mg/day					
Olmesartan☆ • Benicar • 20–40 mg/day					
Telmisartan☆ • Micardis • 20–80 mg/day					
Valsartan☆ • Diovan • 80–320 mg/day					

Combination products:

Azilsartan/chlorthalidone (Edarbyclor)
Candesartan/hydrochlorothiazide (Atacand HCT)
Eprosartan/hydrochlorothiazide (Teveten HCT)
Irbesartan/hydrochlorothiazide (Avalide)
Losartan/hydrochlorothiazide (Hyzaar)

Olmesartan/amlodipine (Azor)
Olmesartan/amlodipine/hydrochlorothiazide (Tribenzor)
Olmesartan/hydrochlorothiazide (Benicar HCT)
Telmisartan/amlodipine (Twynsta)

Telmisartan/hydrochlorothiazide (Micardis HCT)
Valsartan/amlodipine (Exforge)
Valsartan/hydrochlorothiazide (Diovan HCT)
Valsartan/amlodipine/hydrochlorothiazide (Exforge HCT)

Renin Inhibitor

Generic • Brand • Dose	Contra-indications	Primary Side Effects	Key Monitoring	Pertinent Drug Interactions	Med Pearl
Mechanism of action — inhibits renin and prevents the conversion of angiotensinogen to angiotensin I, which then ↓ production of angiotensin II					
Aliskiren ☆ • Tekturna • 150–300 mg/day	• Pregnancy • History of ACEI- or ARB-induced angioedema • Hyperkalemia • Bilateral renal artery stenosis • Use with ACEIs or ARBs in DM	• Headache • Dizziness • Diarrhea • Hyperkalemia • Renal impairment	• BP • BUN/SCr • K+	• Use with K+ supplements, K+-sparing diuretics, ARAs, or NSAIDs may ↑ risk of hyperkalemia • Use with ACEIs or ARBs may ↑ risk of hyperkalemia or renal impairment (avoid concurrent use in DM and CrCl <60 ml/min) • Itraconazole or cyclosporine may ↑ effects; avoid concurrent use • May ↓ effects of furosemide	• Use with caution in patients with CrCl <30 mL/min • Avoid taking with high-fat meals
Combination products: Aliskiren/hydrochlorothiazide (Tekturna HCT)					

Calcium Channel Blockers

Generic • Brand • Dose	Contra-indications	Primary Side Effects	Key Monitoring	Pertinent Drug Interactions	Med Pearl
Mechanism of action – bind to L-type channels in heart and coronary/peripheral arteries to block inward movement of calcium (Ca^{2+}) $\longrightarrow$ vascular smooth-muscle relaxation (vasodilation); all (except for amlodipine and felodipine) have negative inotropic effects ($\downarrow$ contractility) • Dihydropyridines (DHPs) – more selective to vasculature; more potent vasodilators; have no effect on cardiac conduction • Non-DHPs – cause less peripheral vasodilation than DHPs; have negative chronotropic properties ($\downarrow$ HR)					
DHPs:					
Amlodipine ☆ • Norvasc • 2.5–10 mg/day Felodipine ☆ • Only available generically • 2.5–20 mg/day Isradipine • Only available generically • 5–10 mg/day Nicardipine • Cardene • 60–120 mg/day Nifedipine ☆ • Adalat CC, Afeditab CR, Procardia XL • 30–180 mg/day Nisoldipine • Sular • ER: 10–40 mg/day • Geomatrix: 17–34 mg/day	None	• Reflex tachycardia • Headache • Flushing • Peripheral edema • Gingival hyper-plasia • HF exacerbation (except amlodipine and felodipine)	• BP • HR • S/S of HF	• Cytochrome P450 (CYP) 3A4 substrates • CYP3A4 inhibitors may $\uparrow$ effects • CYP3A4 inducers may $\downarrow$ effects	• Sublingual nifedipine should not be used $\rightarrow$ may $\uparrow$ risk of MI, death • Do not use grapefruit juice • Nicardipine also available as injection
Non-DHPs:					
Diltiazem ☆ • Cardizem, Cardizem CD, Cardizem LA, Cartia XT, Taztia XT, Tiazac • 120–540 mg/day Verapamil ☆ • Calan, Calan SR, Isoptin SR, Verelan, Verelan PM • 120–360 mg/day (IR given 2–3 × daily, sustained-release [SR] given 1–2 × daily)	• ≥2nd degree heart block (in absence of pace-maker) • HFrEF	• Bradycardia/heart block • Constipation • Peripheral edema • Gingival hyper-plasia • HF exacerbation	Same as for DHPs	• CYP3A4 substrates and inhibitors • CYP3A4 inhibitors may $\uparrow$ effects • CYP3A4 inducers may $\downarrow$ effects • May $\uparrow$ effect/toxicity of CYP3A4 substrates • Use with other negative chronotropes (e.g., digoxin, β-blockers, clonidine, or ivabradine) may $\uparrow$ risk of bradycardia • May $\uparrow$ risk of digoxin toxicity	• Do not use grapefruit juice • Verapamil and diltia-zem also available as injection

α_1-Receptor Antagonists

Generic • Brand • Dose	Contra-indications	Primary Side Effects	Key Monitoring	Pertinent Drug Interactions	Med Pearl
Mechanism of action – block the α_1 receptor on peripheral blood vessels $\rightarrow$ arterial and venous vasodilation					
Doxazosin ☆ • Cardura • 1–16 mg/day Prazosin • Minipress • 1–20 mg/day Terazosin ☆ • Only available generically • 1–20 mg/day	Should not be used with phosphodiesterase (PDE)-5 inhibitors (e.g., avanafil, sildenafil, tadalafil, vardenafil) $\rightarrow$ $\uparrow$ risk of hypotension	• Orthostatic hypotension • Reflex tachycardia • Peripheral edema • Headache • Drowsiness • Priapism	• BP • HR	$\uparrow$ risk of hypotension with PDE-5 inhibitors (avoid concurrent use)	• Take dose at bedtime to minimize risk of orthostatic hypotension • ALLHAT trial $\rightarrow$ 25% $\uparrow$ in cardiovascular events with doxazosin • $\uparrow$ risk of intraoperative floppy iris syndrome in patients undergoing cataract surgery • Also used for benign prostatic hyperplasia

Central α_2-Receptor Agonists

Generic • Brand • Dose	Contra-indications	Primary Side Effects	Key Monitoring	Pertinent Drug Interactions	Med Pearl
Mechanism of action – stimulate α_2 receptors in brain $\rightarrow$ $\downarrow$ sympathetic outflow (release of norepinephrine) $\rightarrow$ $\downarrow$ BP and HR					
Clonidine ☆ • Catapres, Catapres-TTS • Oral: 0.2–2.4 mg/day • Transdermal: 0.1–0.3 mg weekly Methyldopa • Only available generically • 250–1,000 mg/day	Methyldopa: Liver disease	• Sedation • Orthostatic hypotension • Depression • Peripheral edema • Dry mouth • Bradycardia • Hepatitis (methyldopa)	• BP • HR • Liver function tests (LFTs) (methyldopa)	Use with other negative chronotropes (e.g., digoxin, verapamil, diltiazem, β-blockers, or ivabradine) may $\uparrow$ risk of bradycardia	• Clonidine patch should be applied once weekly • Abrupt discontinuation (especially in presence of β-blockers) may cause angina, MI, or hypertensive emergency; need to taper over 2 wks • When starting clonidine patch, overlap with oral for 2–3 days, then discontinue oral • Should not be used as first-line therapy • Clonidine also available as epidural injection (for pain) • Clonidine also used to treat attention-deficit/hyperactivity disorder • Methyldopa also available as injection • Methyldopa safe to use in pregnant women with HTN

Direct Vasodilators

Generic • Brand • Dose	Contra-indications	Primary Side Effects	Key Monitoring	Pertinent Drug Interactions	Med Pearl
Mechanism of action – ↑ cyclic GMP → arterial vasodilation					
Hydralazine • Only available generically • 25–300 mg/day	• Acute MI • Aortic dissection	• Reflex tachycardia • Orthostatic hypotension • Peripheral edema • Lupus-like syndrome (hydralazine) • Hirsutism (minoxidil)	• BP • HR • S/S of lupus (e.g., stabbing chest pain, joint pain, fever, rash)	None	• Should not be used as first-line therapy • Minoxidil is usually absolutely last-line therapy (because of side effects) • Hydralazine also available as injection • Minoxidil also available as topical solution/foam to stimulate hair growth
Minoxidil • Only available generically • 2.5–100 mg/day					

Storage and Administration Pearls

- When initiating antihypertensive drug therapy in older adults, initiate at a low dose and slowly titrate to achieve goal BP ("start low and go slow").

Patient Education Pearls

- Diuretics should be taken in the morning to avoid nocturia. Patients receiving diuretics should wear sunscreen and protective clothing. Also, they should report any episodes of muscle cramps, as this may be a symptom of hypokalemia or hypomagnesemia.

- Patients receiving K^+-sparing diuretics, ARAs, ACEIs, ARBs, or aliskiren should avoid excessive intake of foods high in K^+ (e.g., green leafy vegetables, potatoes, apricots, bananas, dates, oranges, avocados) and K^+-containing salt substitutes.

- α_1-receptor antagonists should be taken at bedtime to minimize the risk of developing orthostatic hypotension.

- Patients receiving α_1-receptor antagonists, α_2-receptor agonists, or direct vasodilators should rise slowly from a sitting position.

- Patients receiving ACEIs or ARBs should call 911 immediately if he/she experiences lip, tongue, or facial swelling or has difficulty breathing.

- ACEIs, ARBs, and aliskiren should be avoided in pregnant patients. Antihypertensive drugs that can be safely used in pregnancy include methyldopa, labetalol, or CCBs.

DYSLIPIDEMIA

Definitions

Dyslipidemia can refer to any lipid disorder including ↑ total cholesterol (TC), low-density lipoprotein cholesterol (LDL-C), and triglycerides (TGs), and ↓ high-density lipoprotein cholesterol (HDL-C). Dyslipidemia can predispose patients to the development of cardiovascular disease, cerebrovascular disease, or PAD. While most forms of dyslipidemia are due to genetic factors, certain drugs may also cause elevated lipid concentrations, including β-blockers, diuretics, corticosteroids, isotretinoin, protease inhibitors, cyclosporine, and estrogens.

Diagnosis

- Fasting lipid profile should be obtained in adults ≥20 years every 5 years.
- The Friedewald LDL equation (applies if TG <400 mg/dL) is LDL = TC − (HDL-C + TG/5).
- Factors that need to be considered when evaluating whether or not a patient is a candidate for statin therapy:
  - Presence of clinical atherosclerotic cardiovascular disease (ASCVD)
    - » Acute coronary syndromes (ACS), history of MI, stable/unstable angina, coronary or other arterial revascularization, stroke/TIA, or PAD
  - Age
  - LDL-C level
  - Presence of DM
  - 10-year ASCVD risk
    - » Do NOT need to estimate risk in patients with ASCVD or LDL-C ≥190 mg/dL
    - » Do NOT need to calculate on exam; however, should know implications of various risk categories

Signs and Symptoms

- Most patients with dyslipidemias are asymptomatic until a significant degree of atherosclerosis occurs.
- Complications of dyslipidemias may include MI, stroke, PAD, erectile dysfuction, and sudden cardiac death.

Guidelines

Stone NJ, Robinson JG, Lichtenstein AH, et al. 2013 ACC/AHA guideline on the treatment of blood cholesterol to reduce atherosclerotic cardiovascular risk in adults: a report of the American College of Cardiology/American Heart Association Task Force on Practice Guidelines. *Circulation* 2014;129(25 suppl 2):S1–45.

Guidelines Summary

- Achievement of specific LDL-C goals is *no longer* recommended in the most recent dyslipidemia guidelines.
- Four groups most likely to benefit from statin therapy are:
  - Clinical ASCVD (secondary prevention)
  - LDL-C ≥190 mg/dL (primary prevention)
  - Age 40–75 yr with DM **AND** LDL-C 70–189 mg/dL (primary prevention)
  - Age 40–75 yr without clinical ASCVD or DM, and with LDL-C 70–189 mg/dL and 10-yr ASCVD risk ≥7.5%
- Heart-healthy lifestyle habits should be encouraged for all patients.
- Pharmacologic therapy:
  - Statin therapy recommendations for four major benefit groups:

Major Benefit Groups	Statin Therapy Recommendations
Clinical ASCVD	• Age ≤75 yr → High-intensity statin therapy • Age >75 yr **OR** if not a candidate for high-intensity statin therapy → Moderate-intensity statin therapy
LDL-C ≥190 mg/dL	High-intensity statin therapy (moderate-intensity if not candidate for high-intensity therapy)
Age 40–75 yr with DM **AND** LDL-C 70–189 mg/dL	• 10-yr ASCVD risk <7.5% → Moderate-intensity statin therapy • 10-yr ASCVD risk ≥7.5% → High-intensity statin therapy
Age 40–75 yr without clinical ASCVD or DM, and with LDL-C 70–189 mg/dL and 10-yr ASCVD risk ≥7.5%	Moderate–high intensity statin therapy

- High- versus moderate-intensity statin therapy
  - » High-intensity: ↓ LDL-C by ≥50%
    - Atorvastatin 40–80 mg daily
    - Rosuvastatin 20–40 mg daily
  - » Moderate-intensity: ↓ LDL-C by 30–<50%
    - Atorvastatin 10–20 mg daily
    - Rosuvastatin 5–10 mg daily
    - Simvastatin 20–40 mg daily
    - Pravastatin 40–80 mg daily
    - Lovastatin 40 mg daily
    - Fluvastatin XL 80 mg daily
    - Fluvastatin 40 mg twice daily
    - Pitavastatin 2–4 mg daily

- Nonstatin therapy can be considered in selected high-risk patients (clinical ASCVD, LDL-C ≥190 mg/dL, or age 40–75 yr with DM and LDL-C 70–189 mg/dL) who are/have:
  » Less than anticipated response to statin therapy
  » Unable to tolerate a less than recommended intensity of statin therapy
  » Completely intolerant to statin therapy

Lipid-Lowering Effects of Various Drug Classes

Drug Class	Effect on LDL-C	Effect on HDL-C	Effect on TGs
Bile acid resins	↓ 15–30%	↑ 3–5%	↑ 1–10%
Niacin	↓ 5–25%	↑ 15–35%	↓ 20–50%
Fibric acid derivatives	↓/↑ 5–20%	↑ 10–20%	↓ 20–50%
Statins	↓ 18–55%	↑ 5–15%	↓ 7–30%
Cholesterol absorption inhibitors	↓ 15–20%	↑ 1%	↓ 8%
PCSK9 inhibitors	↓ 40–75%	↑ 4–9%	↓ 2–16%

Bile Acid Resins

Generic • Brand • Dose	Contra-indications	Primary Side Effects	Key Monitoring	Pertinent Drug Interactions	Med Pearl
Mechanism of action – bind bile acids in intestines, forming insoluble complex that is excreted in feces → ↓ in bile acids causes liver to convert cholesterol into bile acids, which then ↓ cholesterol stores → ↑ demand for cholesterol in liver → upregulation of LDL receptors → ↑ LDL-C clearance from bloodstream					
Cholestyramine • Prevalite • 4–24 g/day Colesevelam ☆ • Welchol • 3.75 g/day Colestipol • Colestid • Granules: 5–30 g/day • Tablets: 2–16 g/day	Complete biliary obstruction	• Constipation • Bloating • Abdominal pain • Nausea/vomiting (N/V) • Flatulence • ↑ TGs	Lipid panel	Bind to and ↓ absorption of many drugs (e.g., warfarin, digoxin, thiazides, levothyroxine, mycophenolate)	• Used to ↓ LDL-C • Can be used in patients with liver disease • Do not use in patients with ↑ TGs • Colesevelam has fewer gastrointestinal (GI) side effects and drug interactions

Niacin

Generic • Brand • Dose	Contra-indications	Primary Side Effects	Key Monitoring	Pertinent Drug Interactions	Med Pearl
Mechanism of action – ↓ production of very low density lipoproteins (VLDL) in liver → ↓ synthesis of LDL-C					
Niacin☆ • Niaspan; also available as over-the-counter (OTC) product • 500–3,000 mg/day	• Hepatic impairment • Active gout • Active peptic ulcer disease	• Flushing/itching • Nausea • Orthostatic hypotension • ↑ LFTs • Myopathy • Hyperuricemia • Hyperglycemia	• Lipid panel • LFTs • Creatine kinase (CK) (if muscle aches) • Uric acid • Blood glucose (if patient has DM)	None significant	• Used to ↓ LDL-C, ↓ TGs, and ↑ HDL-C • Most effective drug for ↑ HDL-C • Do not ↑ dose by >500 mg in 4-week period • Avoid use of OTC SR products (↑ risk of hepatotoxicity)

Fibric Acid Derivatives

Generic • Brand • Dose	Contra-indications	Primary Side Effects	Key Monitoring	Pertinent Drug Interactions	Med Pearl
Mechanism of action – ↑ activity of lipoprotein lipase → ↑ catabolism of VLDL → ↓ TGs					
Fenofibrate/fenofibric acid☆ • Antara, Fenoglide, Fibricor, Lipofen, Tricor, Triglide, Trilipix • 30–200 mg/day (depending on brand) Gemfibrozil☆ • Lopid • 1,200 mg/day	• Hepatic impairment • Severe renal impairment • Gallbladder disease • Concurrent use with statins, repaglinide, or dasabuvir (gemfibrozil)	• Nausea/vomiting/diarrhea (N/V/D) • Abdominal pain • ↑ LFTs • Myopathy	• Lipid panel • LFTs • CK (if muscle aches)	• Gemfibrozil is CYP2C8 inhibitor • Avoid using gemfibrozil with statins (↑ risk of myopathy), repaglinide (↑ risk of hypoglycemia), and dasabuvir (↑ risk of QT interval prolongation) • ↑ effects of warfarin and sulfonylureas • ↓ cyclosporine levels	• Used to ↓ TGs and/or ↑ HDL-C • Fenofibrate preferred with statins • Adjust dose in renal impairment

Omega-3 Fatty Acids (Fish Oil)

Generic • Brand • Dose	Contra-indications	Primary Side Effects	Key Monitoring	Pertinent Drug Interactions	Med Pearl
Mechanism of action – ↓ production of TGs in the liver					
Icosapent ethyl • Vascepa • 4 g/day	Fish allergy	Arthralgia	Lipid panel	May ↑ risk of bleeding with antithrombotic agents	• Used to ↓ TGs • Minimal effect on LDL-C • Take with meals
Omega-3-Acid Ethyl Esters☆ • Epanova, Lovaza, Omtryg; also available as OTC product • 2–4 g/day • Omtryg: 4.8 g/day	Fish allergy	• Belching ("fishy taste") • Dyspepsia	Lipid panel	May ↑ risk of bleeding with antithrombotic agents	• Used to ↓ TGs • May ↑ LDL-C • Take Omtryg with meals

HMG-CoA Reductase Inhibitors (Statins)

Generic • Brand • Dose	Contra-indications	Primary Side Effects	Key Monitoring	Pertinent Drug Interactions	Med Pearl
Mechanism of action – inhibit HMG-CoA reductase → prevent the conversion of HMG-CoA to mevalonate (rate-limiting step in cholesterol synthesis)					
Atorvastatin☆ • Lipitor • 10–80 mg/day Fluvastatin • Lescol, Lescol XL • 20–80 mg/day Lovastatin☆ • Altoprev • 20–80 mg/day Pitavastatin • Livalo • 1–4 mg/day Pravastatin☆ • Pravachol • 10–80 mg/day Rosuvastatin☆ • Crestor • 5–40 mg/day Simvastatin☆ • Zocor • 10–40 mg/day	• Hepatic impairment • Pregnancy • Concomitant use with cyclosporine (pitavastatin and atorvastatin) • Concomitant use with strong CYP3A4 inhibitors (lovastatin) • Concomitant use with strong CYP3A4 inhibitors, cyclosporine, or danazol (simvastatin)	• ↑ LFTs • Myopathy • N/V • Constipation	• Lipid panel • LFTs • CK (if muscle aches)	• Atorvastatin, lovastatin, and simvastatin are CYP3A4 substrates; CYP3A4 inhibitors may ↑ risk of side effects; may ↑ effects of warfarin • Fluvastatin, rosurastatin, and pitavastatin are CYP2C9 substrates; may ↑ effects of warfarin • Pravastatin not metabolized by CYP enzymes	• Most effective drugs for ↓ LDL-C • Lower maximum dosage of atorvastatin when used with clarithromycin, darunavir/ritonavir, fosamprenavir, fosamprenavir/ritonavir, itraconazole, nelfinavir, or saquinavir/ritonavir • Lower maximum dosage of fluvastatin when used with cyclosporine or fluconazole • Lower maximum dosage of lovastatin when used with amiodarone, dronedarone, verapamil, diltiazem, danazol, or lomitapide • Lower maximum dosage of pitavastatin when used with erythromycin or rifampin • Lower maximum dosage of pravastatin when used with clarithromycin • Lower maximum dosage of rosuvastatin when used with cyclosporine, gemfibrozil, lopinavir/ritonavir, atazanavir/ritonavir, or simeprevir • Lower maximum dosage of simvastatin when used with amiodarone, amlodipine, diltiazem, dronedarone, niacin, ranolazine, verapamil, or lomitapide • Adjust dose of pitavastatin and rosuvastatin in renal impairment
Combination products:		Atorvastatin/amlodipine (Caduet)		Simvastatin/ezetimibe (Vytorin)	

Cholesterol Absorption Inhibitor

Generic • Brand • Dose	Contra-indications	Primary Side Effects	Key Monitoring	Pertinent Drug Interactions	Med Pearl
Mechanism of action – prevents absorption of cholesterol from small intestine					
Ezetimibe ☆ • Zetia • 10 mg/day	None	• Headache • Diarrhea	Lipid panel	• Cyclosporine and fibrates may ↑ effects • ↑ cyclosporine levels • ↑ effects of warfarin	• Used to ↓ LDL-C • Can add to statin to further ↓ LDL-C or if dose-limiting side effects occur with statin

Microsomal Triglyceride Transfer Protein (MTP) Inhibitor

Generic • Brand • Dose	Contra-indications	Primary Side Effects	Key Monitoring	Pertinent Drug Interactions	Med Pearl
Mechanism of action – inhibits MTP and prevents the assembly of apo-B containing lipoproteins, which results in ↓ LDL-C					
Lomitapide • Juxtapid • 5–60 mg/day	• Pregnancy • Concomitant use with moderate or strong CYP3A4 inhibitors • Hepatic impairment	• ↑ LFTs • N/V/D	• Lipid panel • LFTs (monitor before every dose ↑)	• CYP3A4 substrate • CYP3A4 inhibitors may ↑ risk of side effects • May ↑ effects of warfarin • May ↑ risk of side effects with simvastatin and lovastatin (limit statin dose) • May ↑ effect/toxicity of P-glycoprotein (P-gp) substrates	• Used to ↓ LDL-C in patients with homozygous familial hypercholesterolemia • Has REMS program • Lower maximum dosage when used with weak CYP3A4 inhibitor (alprazolam, amiodarone, amlodipine, atorvastatin, bicalutamide, cilostazol, cimetidine, cyclosporine, fluoxetine, fluvoxamine, isoniazid, lapatinib, nilotinib, oral contraceptives, pazopanib, ranitidine, ranolazine, ticagrelor, or zileuton) • Take ≥2 hr after evening meal with glass of water (food ↑ GI side effects) • Take daily vitamin supplement (containing 400 IU vitamin E and ≥200 mg linoleic acid, 210 mg alpha-linoleic acid, 110 mg eicosapentaenoic acid, and 80 mg docosahexaenoic acid)

PCSK9 Inhibitors

Generic • Brand • Dose	Contra-indications	Primary Side Effects	Key Monitoring	Pertinent Drug Interactions	Med Pearl
Mechanism of action – inhibit binding of proprotein convertase subtilisin kexin type 9 (PCSK9) to LDL receptors on the surface of the hepatocyte, which ↑ number of LDL receptors available to clear circulating LDL and lowers LDL-C					
Alirocumab • Praluent • 75–150 mg subcut q2wk	None	• Hypersensitivity reactions • ↑ LFTs • Diarrhea	Lipid panel	None	Used to ↓ LDL-C (by up to 60%)
Evolocumab • Repatha • 140 mg subcut q2wk or 420 mg subcut monthly	None	Hypersensitivity reactions	Lipid panel	None	• Used to ↓ LDL-C (by up to 60%) • To administer 420 mg dose, give 3 consecutive injections within 30 min

Storage and Administration Pearls

- Bile acid resins:
  - Cholestyramine available as powder; colestipol available as granules and tablets; colesevelam available as tablets.
  - Should be administered with meals.
  - Powder can be mixed in applesauce, pudding, oatmeal, Jell-O, etc. to improve its palatability (do not mix in carbonated beverages).
  - Give other medications 1 hour *before* or 4 hours *after* cholestyramine or colestipol.
- Niacin: Give at bedtime (so flushing reaction can occur while patient is sleeping)
- Fibric acid derivatives: Can be administered with meals to ↓ GI effects
- Statins: IR lovastatin administered with meals; ER lovastatin administered at bedtime
- Most statins administered in the evening (at bedtime)—most hepatic cholesterol production occurs during the night (~2 A.M.); atorvastatin, rosuvastatin, and pitavastatin administered in the morning or evening
- Lomitapide: Administer ≥2 hours after evening meal (giving with food may ↑ GI effects)
- PCSK9 inhibitors: Store alirocumab and evolocumab in refrigerator; administer subcutaneous injection into thigh, abdomen, or upper arm
- After initiating lipid-lowering therapy, lipid profile reassessed in 6 weeks to determine if any changes in therapy are needed.

Patient Education Pearls

- Fiber/fiber supplements may help minimize GI side effects associated with bile acid resins.

- Any episodes of muscle pain/aches or dark urine should be reported.

- Flushing reaction associated with niacin may be minimized by taking aspirin (325 mg) or an NSAID at least 30 minutes before dose, taking with food, slowly titrating the dose, and avoiding alcohol or hot beverages. Tolerance usually develops.

- Statins and lomitapide should be avoided if the patient is pregnant.

HEART FAILURE

Definition

HF is a condition in which the heart is unable to pump out enough blood (CO) to meet the metabolic demands of the body. The decrease in CO leads to the activation of numerous compensatory mechanisms, which attempt to improve CO. There are two types of HF: HFrEF (previously known as systolic HF) (pumping function/contractility impaired; left ventricular ejection fraction [LVEF] ≤40%) or HF with preserved ejection fraction (HFpEF) (previously known as diastolic HF) (impaired ability to relax, which leads to underfilling; normal LVEF [>40%]). The majority of HF cases are due to either CAD or HTN. A number of drugs can also precipitate or worsen HF by causing negative inotropic effects (e.g., β-blockers, CCBs [except amlodipine and felodipine], antiarrhythmics [except amiodarone and dofetilide], itraconazole, terbinafine), causing Na^+ and water retention (e.g., corticosteroids, NSAIDs, thiazolidinediones), causing vasoconstriction (e.g., sympathomimetics), or acting as a direct cardiotoxin (e.g., anthracyclines, cyclophosphamide, trastuzumab).

Diagnosis

- Diagnosis is primarily based on the patient's physical exam findings in conjunction with the past medical history and results from laboratory and diagnostic tests.

- Echocardiogram provides information regarding LV function and can reflect whether the patient has HFrEF or HFpEF.

- B-type natriuretic peptide (BNP) concentration can also be obtained to help differentiate between acute HF and other causes of dyspnea (e.g., pneumonia, bronchitis, COPD, pulmonary embolus) (>500 pg/mL in patients with acute decompensated HF [ADHF]).

Signs and Symptoms

- Signs and symptoms of left-sided HF (reflect pulmonary congestion)
  - Symptoms: Dyspnea, orthopnea, paroxysmal nocturnal dyspnea, cough
  - Signs: Rales (usually bibasilar), pulmonary edema, pleural effusion, S_3 gallop
- Signs and symptoms of right-sided HF (reflect systemic congestion)
  - Symptoms: Anorexia, N/V, constipation, abdominal pain, bloating
  - Signs: Jugular venous distention, (+) hepatojugular reflux, ascites, peripheral edema, hepatomegaly, splenomegaly

Classification of HF

New York Heart Association (NYHA) Functional Classification	American College of Cardiology/ American Heart Association Staging System
• Functional class I = Patients have LV dysfunction but no physical limitations; lack symptoms with ordinary physical activity ("well compensated")	• Stage A = At high risk for development of HF but have no structural heart disease or symptoms of HF; includes patients with HTN, DM, and CAD
• Functional class II = Slight limitation of physical activity; symptoms with ordinary physical activity (e.g., walking two blocks)	• Stage B = Structural heart disease (e.g., LVH, previous MI, LV systolic dysfunction, or valvular heart disease) but no symptoms of HF (NYHA class I)
• Functional class III = Marked limitation of physical activity; minimal activity (e.g., activities of daily living) causes symptoms	• Stage C = Structural heart disease with current or previous symptoms of HF (NYHA class I, II, III, or IV)
• Functional class IV = Unable to carry on physical activity without discomfort; symptoms at rest	• Stage D = Refractory symptoms of HF at rest despite maximal medical therapy (often hospitalized) (end-stage HF) (NYHA class IV)

Guidelines

Yancy CW, Jessup M, Bozkurt B, et al. 2016 ACC/AHA/HFSA focused update on new pharmacological therapy for heart failure: an update of the 2013 ACCF/AHA guideline for the management of heart failure: a report of the American College of Cardiology/ American Heart Association Task Force on Clinical Practice Guidelines and the Heart Failure Society of America. *Circulation* 2016 May 17. Available at: http://circ.ahajournals.org/content/early/2016/05/18/CIR.0000000000000435. Accessed July 20, 2016.

Yancy CW, Jessup M, Bozkurt B, et al. 2013 ACCF/AHA guideline for the management of heart failure: a report of the American College of Cardiology Foundation/American Heart Association Task Force on Practice Guidelines. *Circulation* 2013;128:e240–327.

Guidelines Summary

The goals of therapy are to relieve symptoms, improve quality of life, improve survival, reduce hospitalizations, and slow the progression of disease.

- Nonpharmacologic therapy: Regular low-intensity physical activity, ↓ Na^+ (≤3 g/day), ↓ fluid intake (<2 L/day), weight loss (if obese), alcohol restriction, and smoking cessation

- Pharmacologic therapy:
  - Stage A: Modify risk factors and control HTN, DM, CAD, and dyslipidemia; ACEI or ARB in patients with risk factors for vascular disease
  - Stage B: ACEI + β-blocker
  - Stage C: ACEI (or ARB or sacubitril/valsartan) + β-blocker + diuretic
    - » Other drugs to be considered:
      - – Sacubitril/valsartan: NYHA class II-III patients who tolerate an ACEI or ARB (to be used in place of ACEI or ARB)
      - – ARA: NYHA class II-IV patients who are already receiving ACEI (or ARB) and β-blocker; NYHA class II patients should have history of prior cardiovascular hospitalization or ↑ BNP level to be considered for ARA therapy
      - – ARBs: Patients who cannot tolerate an ACEI due to intractable cough or angioedema
      - – Digoxin: Patients who remain symptomatic despite optimal therapy with ACEI (or ARB), β-blocker, and diuretic
      - – Hydralazine/isosorbide dinitrate (HDZ/ISDN): Patients with intolerance or contraindications (renal insufficiency, hyperkalemia) to ACEI or ARB; African-American patients with NYHA class III or IV symptoms who remain symptomatic despite optimal therapy with ACEI (or ARB) and β-blocker
      - – Ivabradine: NYHA class II-III patients with stable HFrEF (LVEF ≤35%) and in sinus rhythm who are receiving a β-blocker at a maximally tolerated dose and having a resting heart rate ≥70 bpm
  - Stage D: Chronic positive inotrope therapy (e.g., dobutamine, milrinone), mechanical circulatory support (e.g., LV assist device), heart transplant, end-of-life care/hospice

Chronic HFrEF Treatment Summary

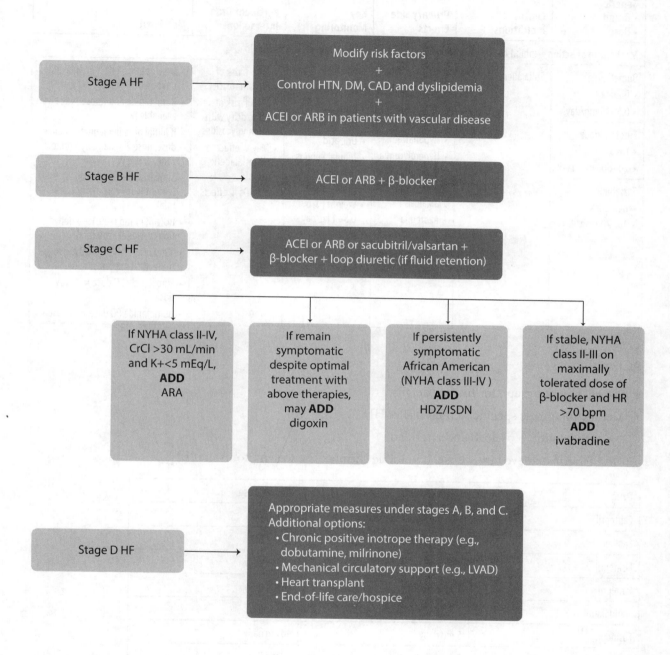

Stage A HF → Modify risk factors
+
Control HTN, DM, CAD, and dyslipidemia
+
ACEI or ARB in patients with vascular disease

Stage B HF → ACEI or ARB + β-blocker

Stage C HF → ACEI or ARB or sacubitril/valsartan +
β-blocker + loop diuretic (if fluid retention)

If NYHA class II-IV, CrCl >30 mL/min and K+<5 mEq/L, **ADD** ARA

If remain symptomatic despite optimal treatment with above therapies, may **ADD** digoxin

If persistently symptomatic African American (NYHA class III-IV) **ADD** HDZ/ISDN

If stable, NYHA class II-III on maximally tolerated dose of β-blocker and HR >70 bpm **ADD** ivabradine

Stage D HF → Appropriate measures under stages A, B, and C.
Additional options:
• Chronic positive inotrope therapy (e.g., dobutamine, milrinone)
• Mechanical circulatory support (e.g., LVAD)
• Heart transplant
• End-of-life care/hospice

Loop Diuretics

Generic • Brand • Dose	Contra-indications	Primary Side Effects	Key Monitoring	Pertinent Drug Interactions	Med Pearl
Mechanism of action – inhibit Na$^+$ reabsorption in the ascending limb of loop of Henle; ↓ preload					
Bumetanide • Bumex • 0.5–10 mg/day Furosemide ☆ • Lasix • 20–600 mg/day Torsemide • Demadex • 10–200 mg/day	Sulfa allergy	• Hypocalcemia • Hypokalemia • Hypomagne-semia • Hyponatremia • Hyperglycemia • Hyperuricemia • Metabolic alkalosis • Azotemia	• BP • Electrolytes • BUN/SCr • Blood glucose • Uric acid • Jugular venous pressure • Urine output • Weight (↓ by 0.5–1 kg/day initially)	• May ↑ risk of lithium toxicity • May ↑ risk of ototoxicity with aminoglycosides • May ↓ effect of antidiabetic agents • NSAIDs ↓ effects	• ↓ symptoms; effect on mortality unknown • Bumetanide and furosemide also available IV • If initial dose inadequate, double dose, dose 2 × daily, add metola-zone, or use IV • Similar side effects as thiazides (except loops cause hypocalce-mia) • BUN/SCr ratio >20:1 → dehydra-tion (prerenal azotemia) • 1 mg bumetanide = 20 mg torse-mide = 40 mg furosemide • Furosemide PO dose = 2 × IV dose • Bumetanide PO dose = IV dose

ACE Inhibitors

- See HTN monograph for further details
- Medication pearls specific to their use in HF:
    - ↓ mortality; ↓ preload and afterload
    - Strive to achieve target dose, if possible (titrate dose to symptoms, not BP)

Drug	Initial Dose	Target Dose
Captopril	6.25 mg TID	50 mg TID
Enalapril	2.5 mg BID	10 mg BID
Lisinopril	2.5 mg daily	40 mg daily
Ramipril	1.25 mg daily	10 mg daily
Trandolapril	1 mg daily	4 mg daily
Fosinopril	5 mg daily	40 mg daily
Quinapril	5 mg BID	20 mg BID
Perindopril	2 mg daily	16 mg daily

β-Blockers

Generic • Brand • Dose	Contra-indications	Primary Side Effects	Key Monitoring	Pertinent Drug Interactions	Med Pearl
Mechanism of action – ↓ activation of the sympathetic nervous system; slow and potentially reverse detrimental effects (e.g., ventricular remodeling) of catecholamines					
Bisoprolol • Zebeta • 1.25–10 mg/day • Target dose: 10 mg daily Carvedilol☆ • Coreg, Coreg CR • IR: 6.25–100 mg/day (in two divided doses) • Target dose: <85 kg = 25 mg BID; >85 kg = 50 mg BID • CR: 10–80 mg/day (1 × daily) • Target dose: 80 mg daily Metoprolol succinate☆ • Toprol XL • 12.5–200 mg/day • Target dose: 200 mg daily	• Symptomatic bradycardia • ≥2nd-degree heart block (in absence of pacemaker) • SBP <85 mmHg • Severe asthma • Decompensated HF	See HTN section	• BP • HR • S/S of HF • Weight	Carvedilol may ↑ digoxin levels	• ↓ mortality • Metoprolol succinate (not tartrate) approved for HF • Patient should be fairly euvolemic before starting • Strive to achieve target dose, if possible • Dose can be doubled every 2–4 wk to achieve target dose (unless side effects) • Manage worsening HF by ↑ diuretic dose • If hypotension occurs, may ↓ dose of ACEI, ARB, or other vasodilator (more common with carvedilol) • If bradycardia occurs, ↓ dose • Abrupt discontinuation may cause worsening HF

Angiotensin II Receptor Blockers

- See HTN monograph for further details
- Medication pearls specific to their use in HF:
  - Only candesartan, losartan, or valsartan recommended for the management of HF (only candesartan and valsartan approved for HF)
  - Should not be considered equivalent or superior to ACEIs

Drug	Initial Dose	Target Dose
Candesartan	4–8 mg daily	32 mg daily
Losartan	25–50 mg daily	150 mg daily
Valsartan	20–40 mg BID	160 mg BID

Sacubitril/Valsartan

Generic • Brand • Dose	Contra- indications	Primary Side Effects	Key Monitoring	Pertinent Drug Interactions	Med Pearl
Mechanism of action – sacubitril: prodrug, inhibits neprilysin (neutral endopeptidase) → ↑ levels of peptides (including natriuretic peptides); valsartan: ARB					
Sacubitril/valsartan • Entresto • Sacubitril 49–97 mg/valsartan 51–103 mg BID • New or previously low-dose user of ACEI/ARB: Start with sacubitril 24 mg/valsartan 26 mg BID • Target dose: sacubitril 97 mg/valsartan 103 mg BID	• Pregnancy • History of angioedema with prior ACEI/ARB use • Concurrent use with ACEI • Concurrent use with aliskiren in DM	• Angioedema • Hypotension • Renal impairment • Hyperkalemia	• BP • BUN/SCr • K+	• Use with K+ supplements, K+-sparing diuretics, ARAs, or NSAIDs may ↑ risk of hyperkalemia • Use with ACEI ↑ risk of angioedema (contraindicated) • Use with aliskiren may ↑ risk of hyperkalemia and renal impairment (avoid concurrent use in DM and CrCl <60 mL/min) • May ↑ risk of lithium toxicity	• ↓ cardiovascular death and hospitalizations • Do not give within 36 hr of change from/to ACEI • Double dose every 2–4 wk to achieve target dose (unless side effects) • Adjust dose in renal or hepatic impairment

Digoxin

Generic • Brand • Dose	Contra- indications	Primary Side Effects	Key Monitoring	Pertinent Drug Interactions	Med Pearl
Mechanism of action – inhibits Na+/K+ ATPase pump → ↑ intracellular Ca2+→ ↑ myocardial contractility; also ↓ neurohormonal activation					
Digoxin ☆ • Lanoxin • 0.125–0.25 mg/day (loading doses not necessary in HF)	≥2nd-degree heart block (in absence of pacemaker)	• Bradycardia/heart block • S/S of digoxin toxicity (visual disturbances, N/V, confusion, anorexia, arrhythmias)	• HR • Electrolytes (predisposed to toxicity if hypokalemia, hypomagnesemia, or hypercalcemia) • BUN/SCr • Digoxin concentrations	• P-gp substrate • Amiodarone, dronedarone, quinidine, verapamil, clarithromycin, lapatinib, propafenone, and ritonavir may ↑ levels • Antacids may ↓ levels (separate by 1–2 hours) • Use with other negative chronotropes (e.g., β-blockers, verapamil, diltiazem, clonidine, or ivabradine) may ↑ risk of bradycardia	• Improves symptoms, ↓ hospitalizations; no effect on mortality • Used to ↑ contractility in HFrEF and to ↓ HR in atrial fibrillation (AF) • Abrupt discontinuation may cause worsening HF • ↓ dose by 50% when starting amiodarone or dronedarone • Adjust dose renal impairment • Target level: 0.5–0.9 ng/mL (↑ mortality if >0.9 ng/mL)

Aldosterone Receptor Antagonists

Generic • Brand • Dose	Contra- indications	Primary Side Effects	Key Monitoring	Pertinent Drug Interactions	Med Pearl
Mechanism of action – inhibit the effects of aldosterone → ↓ remodeling and Na⁺/water retention • Spironolactone is nonselective ARA (also blocks androgen and progesterone receptors → associated with endocrine side effects) • Eplerenone is selective ARA (not associated with endocrinologic side effects)					
Eplerenone • Inspra • 25–50 mg/day Spironolactone • Aldactone • 12.5–25 mg/day	• K^+ >5 mEq/L • SCr >2.5 mg/dL (men) or >2 mg/dL (women) (or CrCl ≤30 mL/min) • Concomitant ACEI **and** ARB use • Concurrent use of eplerenone with strong CYP3A4 inhibitors (e.g., ritonavir, ketoconazole, itraconazole, nefazodone, clarithromycin, nelfinavir)	• Hyperkalemia • Also for spironolactone: Gynecomastia, breast tenderness, menstrual changes, hirsutism	• BP • K^+ • BUN/SCr	• Eplerenone is CYP3A4 substrate • CYP3A4 inhibitors may ↑ effects • Use with ACEIs, ARBs, K^+ supplements, or NSAIDs may ↑ risk of hyperkalemia	• ↓ mortality • Should consider discontinuing or ↓ dose of K^+ supplements • Eplerenone tends to be used in patients who develop endocrine side effects (i.e., gynecomastia) with spironolactone • Lower maximum dosage of eplerenone when used with erythromycin, saquinavir, verapamil, or fluconazole

Hydralazine/Isosorbide Dinitrate

Generic • Brand • Dose	Contra- indications	Primary Side Effects	Key Monitoring	Pertinent Drug Interactions	Med Pearl
Mechanism of action: • Hydralazine – causes arterial vasodilation (↓ afterload) • Isosorbide dinitrate – causes venous vasodilation (↓ preload)					
Hydralazine • Only available generically • 40–300 mg/day	None	• Headache • Dizziness • Reflex tachycardia • Peripheral edema (hydralazine) • Lupus-like syndrome (hydralazine)	• BP • HR	None	• ↓ mortality (when used together) • Combination often used in patients who cannot tolerate ACEIs or ARBs due to renal impairment, hyperkalemia, or angioedema • Do not use hydralazine alone (↑ mortality)
Isosorbide dinitrate ☆ • Isordil • 30–120 mg/day	None				
Combination product: Hydralazine/isosorbide dinitrate (BiDil) – approved for African-American patients with NYHA class III or IV HF due to LV systolic dysfunction (LVEF ≤40%) who are receiving an ACEI (or ARB) and a β-blocker (can also use individual products together if there are financial concerns)					

I$_f$ Channel Inhibitor

Generic • Brand • Dose	Contra-indications	Primary Side Effects	Key Monitoring	Pertinent Drug Interactions	Med Pearl
Mechanism of action – blocks hyperpolarization-activated cyclic nucleotide-gated channel responsible for cardiac pacemaker I$_f$ current in sinoatrial node, resulting in ↓ in HR					
Ivabradine • Corlanor • 2.5–7.5 mg BID	• ADHF • BP <90/50 mmHg • Sick sinus syndrome or 3rd-degree heart block (in absence of pacemaker) • HR <60 bpm (at baseline) • Severe hepatic impairment • Pacemaker dependence • Concurrent use of strong CYP3A4 inhibitors	• Bradycardia • Heart block • AF • Phosphenes	• HR • Electrocardiogram (ECG)	• CYP3A4 substrate • CYP3A4 inhibitors may ↑ effects • CYP3A4 inducers may ↓ effects (avoid use) • Use with other negative chronotropes (e.g., β-blockers, verapamil, diltiazem, digoxin, or clonidine) may ↑ risk of bradycardia	• ↓ hospitalizations; no effect on mortality • Titrate dose by 2.5 mg BID to achieve target resting HR of 50–60 bpm

Intravenous Drugs for Treatment of ADHF

Drug	Mechanism of Action	Primary Side Effects	Med Pearl
Vasodilators			
Nitroglycerin (NTG)	• Venous vasodilation → ↓ preload • Can cause arterial vasodilation at higher doses	• Hypotension • Tachycardia • Headache • Tolerance	• Especially useful in patients with myocardial ischemia • Tolerance can develop (overcome by ↑ infusion rate)
Nitroprusside	Arterial and venous vasodilation → ↓ preload and afterload	• Hypotension • N/V • Cyanide/thiocyanate toxicity (risk ↑ if infusion >24 hours)	Avoid in patients with renal impairment
Nesiritide (Natrecor)	• BNP • Arterial and venous vasodilation → ↓ preload and afterload	• Hypotension • Headache	Infusion should not be titrated more frequently than every 3 hours

Intravenous Drugs for Treatment of ADHF *(cont'd)*

Drug	Mechanism of Action	Primary Side Effects	Med Pearl
Positive Inotropes			
Dopamine	• 0.5–3 mcg/kg/min → Stimulates dopamine receptors → ↑ urine output • 3–10 mcg/kg/min → Stimulates β_1 receptors → ↑ CO, ↑ HR • >10 mcg/kg/min → Stimulates α_1 receptors → ↑ BP	• Arrhythmias • Tachycardia • Myocardial ischemia • N/V	Avoid in patients with myocardial ischemia
Dobutamine	β_1 and β_2 receptor agonist and weak α_1 receptor agonist → ↑ CO and vasodilation	• Arrhythmias • Tachycardia • Myocardial ischemia • Hypokalemia • Tremor	• Avoid in patients with myocardial ischemia • Should not be used in patients receiving chronic β-blocker therapy • Tolerance can develop
Milrinone	PDE III inhibitor → ↑ CO and vasodilation	• Hypotension • Arrhythmias	• Can be used in patients receiving chronic β-blocker therapy, or in those not responding to or tolerating dobutamine • Tolerance does not develop • Use lower initial dose in patients with renal impairment

Storage and Administration Pearls

- Administer captopril at least 1 hour *before* or 2 hours *after* meals.
- Administer carvedilol with food to minimize the risk of orthostatic hypotension.
- Administer ivabradine with meals.
- Nitroprusside infusions should be protected from light.

Patient Education Pearls

- If a patient is taking >1 dose of diuretic each day, the last dose should be taken before 5 P.M. to minimize nocturia.
- Patients should weigh themselves daily (first thing in the morning after urinating) and should contact their healthcare provider if they gain more than 3–5 pounds in a week.
- Patients receiving diuretics should wear sunscreen and protective clothing. Also, they should report any episodes of muscle cramps, as this may be a symptom of hypokalemia or hypomagnesemia.
- A patient who is receiving an ARA, ACEI, ARB, or sacubitril/valsartan should avoid excessive intake of foods high in K^+ (e.g., green leafy vegetables, potatoes, apricots, bananas, dates, oranges, avocados) and K^+-containing salt substitutes.
- A patient who is receiving an ACEI, ARB, or sacubitril/valsartan should call 911 immediately if he/she experiences lip, tongue, or facial swelling or is having difficulty breathing.

- ACEIs, ARBs, and sacubitril/valsartan should be avoided in patients who are pregnant.
- Patients should not stop their β-blocker or digoxin therapy abruptly, as this may cause a sudden worsening of HF symptoms.
- Patients should not be taking an ACEI while taking sacubitril/valsartan.

ANTIARRHYTHMIC DRUGS

Class IA

Generic • Brand • Dose	Contra-indications	Primary Side Effects	Key Monitoring	Pertinent Drug Interactions	Med Pearl
Mechanism of action – Na+ channel blockers; slow conduction velocity, prolong refractoriness, ↓ automaticity					
Disopyramide • Norpace, Norpace CR • 400–1,600 mg/day	• HF • ≥2nd-degree heart block (in absence of pacemaker) • Long QT syndrome	• Dry mouth • Urinary retention • Blurred vision • Constipation • HF exacerbation • Hypotension • Torsade de pointes (TdP)	• ECG (QTc interval, QRS duration) • BP • S/S of HF • Electrolytes • Disopyramide concentrations	• CYP3A4 substrate • CYP3A4 inhibitors and anticholinergics may ↑ risk of side effects • CYP3A4 inducers may ↓ effects • ↑ risk of TdP with other drugs that prolong QT interval	• Used for atrial and ventricular arrhythmias • Therapeutic range: 2–5 mcg/mL • Adjust dose in renal impairment
Procainamide • Only available generically • IV: • *Loading dose:* 15–17 mg/kg over 25–60 min • *Maintenance dose:* 1–4 mg/min continuous infusion	• ≥2nd-degree heart block (in absence of pacemaker) • Long QT syndrome	• Lupus-like syndrome • TdP • Hypotension • Agranulocytosis	• ECG (QTc interval, QRS duration) • BP • S/S of lupus (e.g., stabbing chest pain, joint pain, rash) • Procainamide/N-acetylprocainamide (NAPA) concentrations • Complete blood count (CBC) with differential • Electrolytes	↑ risk of TdP with other drugs that prolong QT interval	• Used for atrial and ventricular arrhythmias • Therapeutic range: 4–10 mcg/mL (procainamide); 15–25 mcg/mL (NAPA); 10–30 mcg/mL (total) • Use with caution, if at all, in renal impairment
Quinidine • Only available generically • Sulfate: 800–2,400 mg/day • Gluconate: 648–2,916 mg/day	• ≥2nd-degree heart block (in absence of pacemaker) • Long QT syndrome • Concurrent use of ritonavir	• Diarrhea • Stomach cramps • TdP • Hypotension • Cinchonism (tinnitus, blurred vision, headache) • Thrombocytopenia	• ECG (QTc interval, QRS duration) • BP • Quinidine concentrations • CBC with differential • LFTs • Electrolytes	• CYP3A4 substrate and CYP2D6 inhibitor • CYP3A4 inhibitors may ↑ risk of side effects • CYP3A4 inducers may ↓ effects • ↑ risk of digoxin toxicity • May ↑ toxicity of CYP2D6 substrates • ↑ risk of TdP with other drugs that prolong QT interval	• Used for atrial and ventricular arrhythmias • Therapeutic range: 2–5 mcg/mL • Administer with food to minimize GI effects

- Avoid all Class IA antiarrhythmics in patients with structural heart diseas (i.e., HF, CAD, left ventricular hypertrophy, valvular disease)

Class IB

Generic • Brand • Dose	Contra-indications	Primary Side Effects	Key Monitoring	Pertinent Drug Interactions	Med Pearl
Mechanism of action – Na⁺ channel blockers; little effect on conduction velocity, shorten refractoriness, ↓ automaticity					

Lidocaine
• Xylocaine
• IV:
  • *Loading dose:* 1–1.5 mg/kg, up to 3 mg/kg (total)
  • *Maintenance dose:* 1–4 mg/min
	≥2nd-degree heart block (in absence of pacemaker)	CNS toxicity (dizziness, blurred vision, slurred speech, confusion, paresthesias, seizures)	• ECG (QRS duration)
			• BP
			• Neurologic exam
			• Lidocaine concentrations (if duration of therapy >24 hours)
				Amiodarone may ↑ risk of toxicity	• Used only for ventricular arrhythmias
					• Therapeutic range: 1.5–5 mcg/mL
					• Use lower infusion rate in elderly, HF or hepatic impairment

Mexiletine • Only available generically • 600–1,200 mg/day	Same as for lidocaine	• CNS toxicity (same as lidocaine) • N/V	• ECG (QRS duration) • BP • LFTs • Neurologic exam	• CYP1A2 and CYP2D6 substrate • ↑ risk of theophylline toxicity • CYP1A2 and CYP2D6 inhibitors may ↑ risk of toxicity	• Used only for ventricular arrhythmias • Take with food to minimize GI effects • ↓ dose in HF or hepatic impairment

- Class IB antiarrhythmics do not cause TdP

Class IC

Generic • Brand • Dose	Contra-indications	Primary Side Effects	Key Monitoring	Pertinent Drug Interactions	Med Pearl
Mechanism of action – Na$^+$ channel blockers (most potent); markedly slow conduction velocity, no effect on refractoriness, ↓ automaticity; propafenone also has nonselective β-blocking properties					
Flecainide • Only available generically • *Loading dose (for AF conversion): 200–300 mg × 1 dose* • *Maintenance dose: 100–400 mg/day*	• ≥2nd-degree heart block (in absence of pacemaker) • History of MI • HF	• Dizziness • Tremor • HF exacerbation • Ventricular tachycardia (VT)	• ECG (QRS duration) • Echocardiogram (at baseline to evaluate LV function) • Electrolytes	↑ risk of digoxin toxicity	• Used for atrial and ventricular arrhythmias • Adjust dose in renal impairment

Propafenone
• Rythmol, Rythmol SR
• IR:
  • *Loading dose (for AF conversion): 450–600 mg × 1*
  • *Maintenance dose: 450–900 mg/day (in 3 divided doses)*
• SR:
  • *Maintenance dose: 450–950 mg/day (in 2 divided doses)*
	• ≥2nd-degree heart block (in absence of pacemaker)
	• Bradycardia
	• Bronchospastic disorders
	• HF
	• History of MI
		• Bradycardia/heart block
		• HF exacerbation
		• Bronchospasm
		• Taste disturbances
		• VT
			• ECG (QRS duration, PR interval)
			• BP
			• HR
			• Echocardiogram (at baseline to evaluate LV function)
			• Electrolytes
				• ↑ risk of digoxin toxicity
				• ↑ effects of warfarin
				• Use with other negative chronotropes (e.g., β-blockers, digoxin, verapamil, diltiazem, clonidine, or ivabradine) may ↑ risk of bradycardia
					• Used for atrial and ventricular arrhythmias

- Avoid Class IC antiarrhythmics in patients with structural heart disease
- Class IC antiarrhythmics do not cause TdP

Class II

(See medication chart in HTN section for discussion on β-blockers)

Class III

Generic • Brand • Dose	Contra-indications	Primary Side Effects	Key Monitoring	Pertinent Drug Interactions	Med Pearl
Mechanism of action – K+ channel blockers; no effect on conduction velocity or automaticity; amiodarone and dronedarone also have Na+-channel blocking, β-blocking, and CCB properties; sotalol also has nonselective β-blocking properties					

Amiodarone ☆
• Cordarone, Nexterone, Pacerone
• Loading dose (IV):
  • *Stable VT:* 150 mg over 10 min
  • *Pulseless VT / ventricular fibrillation:* 300 mg IV push
  • *AF:* 5 mg/kg over 30–60 min
• Loading dose (PO):
  • *Ventricular arrhythmias:* 1,200–1,600 mg/day (in 2–3 divided doses)
  • *Atrial arrhythmias:* 800–1,200 mg/day (in 2–3 divided doses) until 10 g total
• Maintenance dose:
  • IV: 1 mg/min × 6 hr, then 0.5 mg/min
  • PO: 100–400 mg/day
	≥2nd-degree heart block (in absence of pacemaker)	IV:
		• Hypotension
		• Bradycardia/ heart block
		• Phlebitis
		PO:
		• Hypo-/ hyperthyroidism
		• Pulmonary fibrosis
		• Bradycardia/ heart block
		• Corneal microdeposits
		• Optic neuritis
		• N/V
		• ↑ LFTs
		• Ataxia
		• Paresthesias
		• Photosensitivity
		• Blue-gray skin discoloration
			• ECG (QTc interval, QRS duration, PR interval)
			• BP
			• HR
			• Chest x-ray (baseline; then every 12 months)
			• Pulmonary function tests (baseline; then if symptoms develop)
			• High-resolution chest CT scan (if symptoms develop)
			• Thyroid function tests (TFTs) (baseline; then every 6 months)
			• LFTs (baseline; then every 6 months)
			• Ophthalmologic exam (baseline if visual impairment present; then if symptoms develop)
				• CYP2C8 and CYP3A4 substrate
				• CYP1A2, CYP2C9, CYP2D6, and CYP3A4 inhibitor
				• CYP3A4 inhibitors may ↑ risk of side effects
				• CYP3A4 inducers may ↓ effects
				• ↑ risk of digoxin toxicity (↓ digoxin dose by 50%)
				• ↑ effects of warfarin (↓ warfarin dose by 30%)
				• Use with other negative chronotropes (e.g. β-blockers, digoxin, verapamil, diltiazem, clonidine, or ivabradine) or sofosbuvir-containing regimens may ↑ risk of bradycardia
				• May ↑ cyclosporine or phenytoin levels
				• May ↑ risk of side effects of simvastatin and lovastatin
					• Used for atrial and ventricular arrhythmias
					• Safe to use in HF
					• Half-life = 40–60 days
					• If pulmonary fibrosis or blurred vision occur, discontinue therapy
					• If TFTs abnormal, treat thyroid disorder
					• If ↑ LFTs occur, ↓ amiodarone dose or discontinue therapy if LFTs >2x upper limit of normal
					• Take with food to minimize GI effects
					• Advise patients to wear sunscreen

Class III (cont'd)

Generic • Brand • Dose	Contra-indications	Primary Side Effects	Key Monitoring	Pertinent Drug Interactions	Med Pearl
Dronedarone • Multaq • 400 mg BID with meals	• Permanent AF • NYHA class IV HF or NYHA class II–III HF with recent decompensation requiring hospitalization or referral to specialized HF clinic • ≥2nd-degree heart block (in absence of pacemaker) • Bradycardia • Concurrent use of strong CYP3A4 inhibitors or strong CYP3A4 inducers • Concurrent use of other drugs that prolong QT interval • QTc interval ≥500 msec • PR interval >280 msec • Severe hepatic impairment • Liver or lung toxicity related to previous amiodarone use • Pregnancy	• N/V/D • ↑ SCr/acute renal failure • Bradycardia • ↑ LFTs • New-onset or worsening HF	• ECG (QTc interval, PR interval) • HR • BUN/SCr • S/S of HF • LFTs	• CYP3A4 substrate • CYP2D6 and CYP3A4 inhibitor • May ↑ toxicity of CYP2D6 and CYP3A4 substrates • CYP3A4 inhibitors may ↑ risk of side effects • CYP3A4 inducers may ↓ effects • ↑ risk of digoxin toxicity (↓ digoxin dose by 50% or consider discontinuing) • Use with other negative chronotropes (e.g., β-blockers, digoxin, verapamil, diltiazem, clonidine, or ivabradine) may ↑ risk of bradycardia • ↑ effects of dabigatran (↓ dose of dabigatran to 75 mg BID if CrCl 30–50 mL/min) • May ↑ risk of side effects of simvastatin and lovastatin	• Used only for atrial arrhythmias • Structurally related to amiodarone (does not have iodine component); less likely to cause thyroid toxicity; also has shorter half-life
Dofetilide • Tikosyn • 500 mcg BID	• CrCl <20 mL/min • QTc interval >440 msec • Hypokalemia/hypomagnesemia • Concurrent use of verapamil, ketoconazole, cimetidine, trimethoprim, prochlorperazine, hydrochlorothiazide, dolutegravir, megestrol, or other drugs that prolong QT interval	TdP	• ECG (QTc interval) • SCr • Electrolytes	↑ risk of TdP with other drugs that prolong QT interval	• Used only for atrial arrhythmias • Adjust dose based on renal function and QT interval • Must be initiated in hospital • Safe to use in HF

Class III *(cont'd)*

Generic • Brand • Dose	Contra-indications	Primary Side Effects	Key Monitoring	Pertinent Drug Interactions	Med Pearl
Ibutilide • Corvert • IV: 1 mg over 10 min; repeat × 1, if needed	• QTc interval >440 msec • Hypokalemia/hypo-magnesemia • Concurrent use of other drugs that prolong QT interval	TdP	• ECG (QTc interval) • Electrolytes	↑ risk of TdP with other drugs that prolong QT interval	Used only for atrial arrhythmias
Sotalol • Betapace, Betapace AF, Sorine, Sotylize • PO: 160–640 mg/day (in 2 divided doses)	• ≥2nd-degree heart block (in absence of pacemaker) • Concurrent use of other drugs that prolong QT interval • CrCl <40 mL/min (for AF) • Long QT syndrome • HF	• TdP • Bradycardia/heart block • Bronchospasm • HF exacerbation	• ECG (QTc interval, PR interval) • HR • SCr • Electrolytes	• ↑ risk of TdP with other drugs that prolong QT interval • Use with other negative chronotropes (e.g., β-blockers, digoxin, verapamil, diltiazem, clonidine, or iv-abradine) may ↑ risk of bradycardia	• Used for atrial and ventricular arrhythmias • Adjust dosing interval in renal impairment • Also available as oral solution and injection

Class IV Antiarrhythmics

(See medication chart in HTN section for discussion on non-DHP CCBs)

ANTITHROMBOTIC DRUGS

Vitamin K Antagonist

Generic • Brand • Dose	Contra-indications	Primary Side Effects	Key Monitoring	Pertinent Drug Interactions	Med Pearl
Mechanism of action – interferes with synthesis of vitamin-K dependent clotting factors of the liver (II, VII, IX, and X) as well as protein C and S					
Warfarin • Coumadin, Jantoven • Usual initial dose: 5–10 mg daily (2.5–10 mg daily in older adults)	• Pregnancy • Recent surgery	• Bleeding • Skin necrosis (especially in patients with protein C deficiency) • Purple toe syndrome	• Prothrombin time (PT)/international normalized ratio (INR) • Hemoglobin (Hgb)/hematocrit (Hct) • Bleeding	• CYP2C9 and CYP3A4 substrate • CYP2C9 and CYP3A4 inhibitors may ↑ effects and risk of bleeding • CYP3A4 inducers may ↓ effects and ↑ risk of clotting	• Vitamin K is antidote (PO preferred) • Full effect of a particular dose not seen for 3–4 days

Direct Thrombin Inhibitor

Generic • Brand • Dose	Contra-indications	Primary Side Effects	Key Monitoring	Pertinent Drug Interactions	Med Pearl
Mechanism of action – oral direct thrombin inhibitor					

Dabigatran
• Pradaxa
• AF:
  • CrCl >30 mL/min: 150 mg BID
  • CrCl 15–30 mL/min: 75 mg BID
  • CrCl <15 mL/min: Not recommended
• Treatment of deep venous thrombosis (DVT)/pulmonary embolism (PE):
  • CrCl >30 mL/min: 150 mg BID (after 5–10 days of parenteral anticoagulation)
  • CrCl ≤30 mL/min: No dosing recommendations
• Prevention of recurrent DVT/PE:
  • CrCl >30 mL/min: 150 mg BID
  • CrCl ≤30 mL/min: No dosing recommendations
• Prevention of DVT/PE after hip replacement surgery:
  • CrCl >30 mL/min: 110 mg 1–4 hr after surgery, then 220 mg daily × 28–35 days
  • CrCl ≤30 mL/min: No dosing recommendations
	• Active bleeding
	• Mechanical prosthetic heart valve
		• Bleeding
		• Dyspepsia
			• Hgb/Hct
			• Bleeding
				• P-gp substrate
				• P-gp inhibitors may ↑ effects and risk of bleeding
				• Rifampin ↓ effects and ↑ risk of clotting (avoid concurrent use)
				AF:
				• ↓ dabigatran dose to 75 mg BID when used with dronedarone or ketoconazole if CrCl 30–50 mL/min (avoid concurrent use with P-gp inhibitors if CrCl <30 mL/min)
				DVT/PE treatment/prevention (including after hip replacement surgery):
				• Avoid concurrent use with P-gp inhibitors if CrCl <50 mL/min
					• When converting from warfarin, discontinue warfarin and start dabigatran when INR <2
					• When converting to warfarin, adjust starting time of warfarin based on CrCl
					• When converting from parenteral anticoagulant, start dabigatran 0–2 hr before time of next dose of or at time of discontinuation of parenteral anticoagulant
					• When converting to parenteral anticoagulant, wait 12–24 hr (based on CrCl) after last dose of dabigatran before starting therapy with parenteral anticoagulant
					• Antidote = idarucizumab (Praxbind); 2.5 g IV; repeat dose in 15 min

Factor Xa Inhibitors

Generic • Brand • Dose	Contra-indications	Primary Side Effects	Key Monitoring	Pertinent Drug Interactions	Med Pearl
Mechanism of action – oral factor Xa inhibitor					

Apixaban
• Eliquis
• AF:
  • 5 mg BID
  • If patient has ≥2 of the following (age ≥80 yr, weight ≤60 kg, SCr ≥1.5 mg/dL): 2.5 mg BID
• Postoperative DVT/PE prophylaxis:
  • 2.5 mg BID (× 35 days for hip replacement; × 12 days for knee replacement)
• Treatment of DVT/PE:
  • 10 mg BID × 7 days, then 5 mg BID
• Prevention of recurrent DVT/PE:
  • 2.5 mg BID after ≥6 mo of treatment for DVT/PE
	Active bleeding	Bleeding	• Hgb/Hct
			• Bleeding
				• CYP3A4 and P-gp substrate
				• CYP3A4 and P-gp inhibitors may ↑ effects and risk of bleeding (if receiving 5 mg BID or 10 mg BID dose, ↓ apixaban dose by 50% when used with strong dual inhibitors of CYP3A4 and P-gp; if receiving 2.5 mg BID dose, avoid concurrent use with strong dual inhibitors of CYP3A4 and P-gp)
				• CYP3A4 and P-gp inducers ↓ effects and ↑ risk of clotting (avoid concurrent use)
					• When converting from warfarin, discontinue warfarin and start apixaban when INR <2
					• When converting to warfarin, discontinue apixaban and start parenteral anticoagulant and warfarin at the time the next dose of apixaban would have been taken; discontinue parenteral anticoagulant when desired INR achieved
					• When converting from parenteral anticoagulant, discontinue parenteral anticoagulant and start apixaban at the usual time of the next dose of parenteral anticoagulant
					• When converting to parenteral anticoagulant, discontinue apixaban and initiate parenteral anticoagulant at time the next dose of apixaban would have been taken
					• No antidote currently available

Factor Xa Inhibitors *(cont'd)*

Generic • Brand • Dose	Contra-indications	Primary Side Effects	Key Monitoring	Pertinent Drug Interactions	Med Pearl
Edoxaban • Savaysa • AF: • CrCl >95 mL/min: Avoid use • CrCl 51–95 mL/min: 60 mg daily • CrCl 15–50 mL/min: 30 mg daily • Treatment of DVT/PE: • CrCl ≥51 mL/min: 60 mg daily (after 5–10 days of parenteral anticoagulation) • CrCl 15-50 mL/min or weight ≤60 kg: 30 mg daily (after 5–10 days of parenteral anticoagulation)	Active bleeding	Bleeding	• Hgb/Hct • Bleeding	• P-gp substrate • P-gp inhibitors may ↑ effects and risk of bleeding • Rifampin may ↓ effects and ↑ risk of clotting (avoid concurrent use) Treatment of DVT/PE: • ↓ edoxaban dose to 30 mg daily when used with verapamil, quinidine, azithromycin, clarithromycin, erythromycin, itraconazole, or ketoconazole	• When converting from warfarin, discontinue warfarin and start edoxaban when INR ≤2.5 • When converting to warfarin, ↓ dose of edoxaban (60 mg to 30 mg daily; 30 mg to 15 mg daily) and begin warfarin concurrently; discontinue edoxaban when desired INR achieved; may also discontinue edoxaban and start parenteral anticoagulant and warfarin at the time the next dose of edoxaban would have been taken; discontinue parenteral anticoagulant when desired INR achieved • When converting from low molecular weight heparin (LMWH), start edoxaban at the time of the next dose of LMWH (and discontinue LMWH); for unfractionated heparin (UFH), discontinue infusion and start edoxaban 4 hr later • When converting to parenteral anticoagulant, discontinue edoxaban and initiate parenteral anticoagulant at time the next dose of edoxaban would have been taken • No antidote currently available

Factor Xa Inhibitors *(cont'd)*

Generic • Brand • Dose	Contra-indications	Primary Side Effects	Key Monitoring	Pertinent Drug Interactions	Med Pearl

Rivaroxaban
• Xarelto
• AF:
  • CrCl >50 mL/min: 20 mg daily with evening meal
  • CrCl 15–50 mL/min: 15 mg daily with evening meal
• Postoperative DVT/PE prophylaxis:
  • 10 mg daily (× 35 days for hip replacement; × 12 days for knee replacement)
• Treatment of DVT/PE:
  • 15 mg BID with food × 21 days, then 20 mg daily with food
• Prevention of recurrent DVT/PE:
  • 20 mg daily with food
	Active bleeding	Bleeding	• Hgb/Hct
			• Bleeding
				• CYP3A4 and P-gp substrate
				• CYP3A4 and P-gp inhibitors may ↑ effects and risk of bleeding (avoid concurrent use with combined P-gp and strong CYP3A4 inhibitors)
				• CYP3A4 and P-gp inducers ↓ effects and ↑ risk of clotting (avoid concurrent use with combined P-gp and strong CYP3A4 inducers)
					• When converting from warfarin, discontinue warfarin and start rivaroxaban when INR <3
					• When converting to warfarin, discontinue rivaroxaban and start parenteral anticoagulant and warfarin at the time the next dose of rivaroxaban would have been taken; discontinue parenteral anticoagulant when desired INR achieved
					• When converting from parenteral anticoagulant, start rivaroxaban 0–2 hr before time of next dose of parenteral anticoagulant (and discontinue parenteral anticoagulant); for UFH, discontinue infusion and start rivaroxaban
					• When converting to parenteral anticoagulant, discontinue rivaroxaban and initiate parenteral anticoagulant at time the next dose of rivaroxaban would have been taken
					• No antidote currently available

ISCHEMIC HEART DISEASE

Definitions

Ischemic heart disease (IHD) is characterized by a lack of oxygen resulting from inadequate perfusion of the myocardium, which is often due to narrowing or blockage in a coronary artery. Patients with IHD may present with chronic stable angina, vasospastic angina (variant or Prinzmetal's angina), or an ACS. ACS can include UA, non–ST-segment-elevation MI (NSTEMI), or ST-segment–elevation MI (STEMI). An ACS is precipitated by rupture of an atherosclerotic plaque, followed by formation of a thrombus at the site of plaque rupture. In NSTEMI, the thrombus tends to contain more platelets than fibrin ("white clot") and does not completely occlude the vessel. In STEMI, the thrombus contains more fibrin and red blood cells than platelets ("red clot") and completely occludes the vessel.

This section reviews the management of NSTEMI and STEMI.

Diagnosis

- If ischemic-like chest pain persists for at least 20 minutes, ACS should be suspected.
  - An ECG should be performed and serial cardiac enzymes (troponin, CK-MB) should be obtained.

Findings	UA	NSTEMI	STEMI
Cardiac enzymes (troponin, CK-MB)	Negative	Positive	Positive
ECG changes	ST-segment depression, T-wave inversion, or no ECG changes (any changes are usually transient)	ST-segment depression, T-wave inversion, or no ECG changes	ST-segment elevation

Signs and Symptoms

- Chest pain/pressure (substernal, crushing) that may radiate to the left arm, jaw, shoulders, and back are common symptoms.
- Other symptoms include dyspnea, diaphoresis, N/V.
- When compared to chronic stable angina, pain in ACS may be more severe, occur at rest, occur more frequently, be precipitated by less exertion, and be refractory to sublingual NTG.
- Patients may also present with signs/symptoms of HF or with arrhythmias.

Guidelines

Amsterdam EA, Wenger NK, Brindis RG, et al. 2014 ACC/AHA guidelines for the management of patients with non-ST-elevation acute coronary syndrome: a report of the American College of Cardiology/American Heart Association Task Force on Practice Guidelines. *Circulation* 2014;130:e334–e426.

American College of Emergency Physicians; Society for Cardiovascular Angiography and Interventions, O'Gara PT, Kushner FG, Ascheim DD, et al. 2013 ACCF/AHA guideline for the management of ST-elevation myocardial infarction: a report of the American College of Cardiology Foundation/American Heart Association Task Force on Practice Guidelines. *J Am Coll Cardiol* 2013;61(4):e78–140.

ACUTE PHARMACOLOGIC MANAGEMENT OF UA/NSTEMI

Anti-Ischemic and Analgesic Therapy

Morphine

- May be reasonable for patients who continue to have chest discomfort despite maximally tolerated anti-ischemic medications
- Dose: 1–5 mg IV every 5–30 minutes as needed for pain

NTG

- Can be given to patients with ongoing chest discomfort (0.4 mg sublingually every 5 min × 3 doses); following these doses, give IV NTG within the initial 48 hours if patients continue to have ischemia, or if they present with HF or are hypertensive
- Dose: 5–10 mcg/min continuous infusion; can be titrated up to 100 mcg/min for relief of symptoms
- Adverse effects: Reflex tachycardia, hypotension, headache

β-Blockers

- Oral β-blockers: Given within the first 24 hours to patients who **do not** have signs/symptoms of HF, risk factors for developing cardiogenic shock (age >70 years, SBP <120 mmHg, HR >110 bpm, or prolonged duration since presenting with UA/NSTE-MI), PR interval >0.24 sec, ≥2nd-degree heart block, or severe reactive airway disease
- IV β-blockers no longer recommended

CCBs

- A non-DHP CCB (verapamil or diltiazem) can be used alternatively if the patient has a contraindication to β-blocker therapy and does not have evidence of LV dysfunction
- A long-acting non-DHP CCB can be used in patients who have recurrent ischemia despite being on a β-blocker and nitrate therapy

ACEIs

- Should be given to all patients with LVEF ≤40% and in those with HTN, DM, or stable CKD, provided they have no contraindications
- May be reasonable in all other patients with cardiac or other vascular disease
- An ARB can be used alternatively in patients who cannot tolerate ACEIs

Antiplatelet Therapy

Aspirin

- All patients should receive 162–325 mg (non–enteric-coated) at the onset of chest pain (should be chewed and swallowed).
- Patients should continue to receive 81–325 mg daily indefinitely (regardless of whether the patient undergoes PCI)

Clopidogrel (Plavix)

- Prodrug; must be converted via CYP2C19 to active drug
- Avoid concurrent use of omeprazole or esomeprazole (use pantoprazole if PPI needed)
- The following loading and maintenance doses should be given (**with** aspirin):
  - Early invasive strategy (PCI ± stent)
    - » Loading dose = 600 mg × 1
    - » Maintenance dose = 75 mg daily
    - » Continue for ≥12 months
  - Ischemia-guided strategy
    - » Loading dose = 300 mg × 1
    - » Maintenance dose = 75 mg daily
    - » Continue for up to 12 months
- Can also be used as an alternative to aspirin in patients who are allergic or have a major GI intolerance to aspirin
- Discontinue ≥5 days before CABG

Prasugrel (Effient)

- Prodrug
- Alternative to clopidogrel in patients with ACS managed with early invasive strategy
- Initiate only in patients with known coronary artery anatomy (after angiography, but before PCI)
- Achieves faster inhibition of platelet aggregation than clopidogrel
- Administered as a loading dose of 60 mg prior to PCI, followed by maintenance dose of 10 mg daily (↓ dose to 5 mg daily in patients <60 kg)
- Not recommended for patients ≥75 years unless they have DM or history of MI (↑ risk of bleeding), in patients with prior history of stroke or TIA, or in patients requiring triple antithrombotic therapy
- Continue for ≥12 months
- Discontinue ≥7 days before CABG

Ticagrelor (Brilinta)

- NOT a thienopyridine
  - Reversibly binds to the P2Y12 receptor
  - Does not require conversion to an active metabolite (NOT a prodrug)
- Alternative to clopidogrel in patients with ACS managed with early invasive or ischemia-guided strategy
- Contraindicated in severe hepatic impairment
- Drug interactions
  - CYP3A4 substrate; CYP3A4 and P-gp inhibitor
  - Avoid concurrent use with strong CYP3A4 inhibitors or inducers
  - Avoid simvastatin or lovastatin doses >40 mg/day
  - May ↑ digoxin levels
- Administered as a loading dose of 180 mg prior to PCI, followed by maintenance dose of 90 mg BID (dose of aspirin during maintenance therapy should not exceed 100 mg/day); if continued >12 months, ↓ dose to 60 mg BID
- Continue for
  - ≥12 months (early invasive strategy) or up to 12 months (ischemia-guided strategy)
- Discontinue ≥5 days before CABG

Glycoprotein IIb/IIIa Receptor Blockers (GPBs)

- PCI planned: Clopidogrel (or ticagrelor) and/or GPB (eptifibatide or tirofiban) can be initiated prior to angiography. Do not need GPB if bivalirudin + 300 mg loading dose of clopidogrel (given ≥6 hours before angiography) are used.
- Conservative strategy: Adding eptifibatide or tirofiban to clopidogrel or ticagrelor can be considered (especially if patient has recurrent ischemia and requires angiography).

Anticoagulant Therapy

- Early invasive strategy: UFH, enoxaparin, fondaparinux, or bivalirudin should be added to antiplatelet therapy.
- Ischemia-guided strategy: UFH, enoxaparin, or fondaparinux should be added to antiplatelet therapy.

ACUTE PHARMACOLOGIC MANAGEMENT OF STEMI

Anti-Ischemic and Analgesic Therapy

Morphine, NTG, β-Blockers, ACEIs

- Same recommendations as for UA/NSTEMI

Antiplatelet Therapy

Aspirin

- Same recommendations as for UA/NSTEMI

Clopidogrel

- The following loading and maintenance doses should be given:
  - Patients undergoing primary PCI:
    - » Loading dose = 600 mg × 1
    - » Maintenance dose = 75 mg daily
  - Patients receiving fibrinolytic therapy and patients who do not receive reperfusion therapy:
    - » Loading dose = 300 mg × 1 (no loading dose in patients age ≥75 years)
    - » Maintenance dose = 75 mg daily
- Can also be used as an alternative to aspirin in patients who are allergic or have a major GI intolerance to aspirin.
- Clopidogrel should be continued (**with** aspirin) for the following durations of time:
  - Bare metal stent (BMS) or drug-eluting stent (DES): 12 months
  - No stent: At least 14 days (can be considered for up to 1 year)
- Discontinue ≥ 5 days before CABG

Prasugrel

- Same recommendations as for UA/NSTEMI

Ticagrelor

- Same recommendations as for UA/NSTEMI

GPBs

- Can be used if patient undergoing primary PCI

Fibrinolytic Therapy

- Should be used in patients presenting to a hospital without the capability to perform PCI or cannot perform PCI within 120 minutes of first medical contact ("door-to-balloon" time)
- Should be initiated within 30 minutes of presenting to the hospital ("door-to-needle" time)

Anticoagulant Therapy

- Fibrinolytic administered: UFH, enoxaparin, or fondaparinux can be used; should be continued for up to 8 days; UFH should only be used if the treatment duration is <48 hours because of risk for heparin-induced thrombocytopenia (HIT) with prolonged therapy.
- Primary PCI: UFH or bivalirudin can be used.

SECONDARY PREVENTION OF MI

- **Aspirin:** See recommendation above regarding dosing and duration of therapy.
- **Clopidogrel, prasugrel, or ticagrelor:** See recommendations in respective NSTEMI and STEMI sections regarding dosing and duration of therapy.
- **β-blockers:** Continue indefinitely.
- **ACEIs:** Should be given and continued indefinitely in all patients; ARB can be used in patients intolerant of ACEIs.
- **ARAs:** Should be given to patients with LVEF ≤40% receiving optimal ACEI and β-blocker therapy who have DM or HF.
- **Statins:** Should be given and continued indefinitely in all patients.

Glycoprotein IIb/IIIa Receptor Blockers

Generic • Brand • Dose	Contra-indications	Primary Side Effects	Key Monitoring	Pertinent Drug Interactions	Med Pearl
Mechanism of action – block the glycoprotein IIb/IIIa receptor on platelets to prevent the binding of fibrinogen → Inhibit platelet aggregation					
Abciximab • ReoPro • *Loading dose:* 0.25 mg/kg IV bolus • *Maintenance dose:* 0.125 mcg/kg/min (max of 10 mcg/min); continue for 12 hr after PCI	• Active bleeding • Prior stroke within past 30 days or any hemorrhagic stroke • History of intracranial neoplasms or aneurysm • Thrombocytopenia • BP >180/110 mmHg • Dialysis-dependent (for eptifibatide)	• Bleeding • Thrombocytopenia	• CBC • PT/activated partial thromboplastin time (aPTT) • Activated clotting time (ACT) (with PCI) • S/S bleeding • SCr (baseline)	Anticoagulants and other anti-platelets may ↑ risk of bleeding	Adjust dose of maintenance infusion of tirofiban and eptifibatide in renal impairment
Eptifibatide • Integrilin • *Loading dose:* 180 mcg/kg (max of 22.6 mg) IV bolus × 2 (given 10 min apart) • *Maintenance dose:* 2 mcg/kg/min (max of 15 mg/hr); continue for 18–24 hr after PCI					

Tirofiban
• Aggrastat
• NSTEMI:
  • *Loading dose:* 25 mcg/kg IV over ≤5 min
  • *Maintenance dose:* 0.15 mcg/kg/min; continue for up to 18 hr after PCI
• STEMI (with PCI):
  • *Loading dose:* 25 mcg/kg IV bolus
  • *Maintenance dose:* 0.15 mcg/kg/min; continue for 18–24 hr after PCI					

Anticoagulants

Generic • Brand • Dose	Contra-indications	Primary Side Effects	Key Monitoring	Pertinent Drug Interactions	Med Pearl
Mechanism of action: • UFH: Potentiates the action of antithrombin III, which inactivates the clotting factors, IIa (thrombin), IXa, Xa, XIa, and XIIa, and ultimately prevents the conversion of fibrinogen to fibrin • Enoxaparin: LMWH; similar mechanism as UFH, but primarily inhibits factor Xa • Fondparinux: Selective inhibitor of factor Xa • Bivalirudin: Direct thrombin inhibitor					
UFH • Only available generically • *Loading dose:* 60 units/kg IV bolus (max = 4,000 units) • *Maintenance dose:* 12 units/kg/hr (max = 1,000 units/hr)	• Active bleeding • History of HIT • Recent stroke	• Bleeding • Thrombocytopenia (UFH and LMWH)	• PT/aPTT (only for UFH) • CBC • Anti-Xa levels (for enoxaparin) (consider in obese or renal impairment) • S/S bleeding	Antiplatelets and other anticoagulants may ↑ risk of bleeding	• If platelets <100,000 or ↓ by >50% from baseline, test for HIT; discontinue UFH and start direct thrombin inhibitor (e.g., argatroban, bivalirudin) • Protamine can be used to reverse effects
Enoxaparin • Lovenox • *Loading dose:* 30 mg IV × 1 (for STEMI only) • *Maintenance dose:* 1 mg/kg subcut every 12 hr					• ↓ enoxaparin dose to 1 mg/kg every 24 hr if CrCl <30 mL/min • Should not use in patients with suspected HIT • Protamine only partially reverses effects
Fondaparinux • Arixtra • 2.5 mg subcut daily	• Active bleeding • CrCl <30 mL/min				For STEMI, can give initial dose IV
Bivalirudin • Angiomax • *Loading dose:* 0.75 mg/kg IV bolus • *Maintenance dose:* 1.75 mg/kg/hr	Active bleeding		• PT/aPTT • ACT		Can also be used during PCI in patients with HIT

Fibrinolytic Agents

Generic • Brand • Dose	Contra-indications	Primary Side Effects	Key Monitoring	Pertinent Drug Interactions	Med Pearl
Mechanism of action – activate and convert plasminogen into plasmin, which then degrades fibrin (lyses the clot) to form fibrin degradation products					
Alteplase • Activase • 15 mg IV bolus, then 0.75 mg/kg (max = 50 mg) over 30 min, then 0.5 mg/kg (max = 35 mg) over 60 min	• Active bleeding • Any history of intracranial hemorrhage • Known intracranial neoplasm or arteriovenous malformation • Suspected aortic dissection • Significant closed head or facial trauma within 3 months	Bleeding	• CBC • ECG (for signs of reperfusion) • S/S bleeding	Antiplatelets and other anticoagulants may ↑ risk of bleeding	Alteplase also approved for treatment of acute ischemic stroke and pulmonary embolism
Reteplase (rPA) • Retavase • 10 units IV × 2 doses (separated by 30 min)					
Tenecteplase (TNK) • TNKase • All doses given as IV bolus: • <60 kg: 30 mg • 60–69.9 kg: 35 mg • 70–79.9 kg: 40 mg • 80–89.9 kg: 45 mg • ≥90 kg: 50 mg					

LEARNING POINTS

- **HTN**
  - For nonblack patients (in presence or absence of DM), a thiazide diuretic, ACEI, ARB, and/or CCB should be considered first-line therapy. For black patients (in presence or absence of DM), a thiazide diuretic and/or CCB should be considered first-line therapy. If patients have certain comorbidities, antihypertensive agent(s) that can also be used to treat this disease state should be initiated.

- **Dyslipidemia**
  - Statins are the most effective drugs for ↓ LDL-C.
  - Niacin is the most effective drug for ↑ HDL-C.
  - Myopathy and ↑ LFTs are potential side effects of niacin, fibric acid derivatives, and statins.

- **Heart Failure**
  - ACEIs, β-blockers, ARAs, and hydralazine/isosorbide dinitrate have been shown to ↓ mortality in patients with HFrEF.
  - β-blockers should not be initiated in patients who have evidence of fluid overload (peripheral or pulmonary); patients should be relatively euvolemic before starting β-blocker therapy.
  - Sacubitril/valsartan can be used in Stage C, class II-III HFrEF in place of an ACEI or ARB.
  - ARBs can be used in patients who develop intolerable cough from ACEI therapy.
  - Hyperkalemia and renal impairment can be associated with both ACEIs and ARBs. If patients are unable to tolerate ACEIs or ARBs because of hyperkalemia or renal insufficiency, hydralazine/isosorbide dinitrate can be used as an alternative.

- **Antiarrhythmic Drugs**
  - Know which antiarrhythmic drugs belong in which class and their basic mechanism of action (e.g., Na^+-channel blocker)
  - Dosages of disopyramide, procainamide, flecainide, sotalol, and dofetilide must be adjusted in patients with renal impairment.
  - Amiodarone and dofetilide are the antiarrhythmics of choice in patients with AF who have HF.
  - Dronedarone should not be used in patients with severe HF.
  - Class IA and IC antiarrythmics should be avoided in patients with structural heart disease.
  - Lidocaine and mexiletine are only effective for ventricular arrhythmias.

- Amiodarone has a large volume of distribution and a very long half-life. It can be associated with toxicities that affect just about every organ system in the body. Chest x-ray should be performed annually while TFTs and LFTs should be evaluated every 6 months. Pulmonary function tests can be performed if patient complains of symptoms, such as shortness of breath or cough. An ophthalmologic exam can be performed if patient complains of visual changes.

- **Ischemic Heart Disease**

  - Fibrinolytic drugs should only be used for STEMI.

  - For patients undergoing PCI and receiving a DES, clopidogrel, prasugrel, or ticagrelor should be administered for at least 12 months.

  - Know examples of GPBs, LMWHs, factor Xa inhibitors, direct-thrombin inhibitors, and fibrinolytic drugs.

  - Drugs used for the secondary prevention of MI include aspirin, statins, β-blockers, ACEIs, clopidogrel/prasugrel/ticagrelor, and ARAs.

PRACTICE QUESTIONS

1. Which of the following drugs may be associated with bradycardia? (Select ALL that apply.)

    (A) Amlodipine
    (B) Bisoprolol
    (C) Clonidine
    (D) Enalapril
    (E) Ivabradine

2. A patient has been taking simvastatin 80 mg PO at bedtime for 3 weeks and is now complaining of muscle pain. Which of the following laboratory tests should be obtained?

    (A) Blood glucose
    (B) Creatine kinase
    (C) Complete blood count
    (D) Simvastatin blood concentration
    (E) Thyroid function tests

3. Which of the following is a common side effect of nitroglycerin?

    (A) Arrhythmias
    (B) Bleeding
    (C) Headache
    (D) Hyperkalemia
    (E) Stevens-Johnson syndrome

4. Which of the following drugs is considered a positive inotrope?

    (A) Dobutamine
    (B) Hydralazine
    (C) Nesiritide
    (D) Nitroglycerin
    (E) Verapamil

5. Which of the following drugs antagonize both β_1 and β_2 receptors at low doses?

    (A) Atenolol
    (B) Bisoprolol
    (C) Carvedilol
    (D) Metoprolol
    (E) Nebivolol

6. Which of the following statements regarding niacin is TRUE?

   (A) It is also available over-the-counter.
   (B) Patients should be advised to take acetaminophen 30 minutes before each dose.
   (C) It can increase a patient's risk for developing hypoglycemia.
   (D) It is contraindicated in patients with hypertriglyceridemia.
   (E) The dose should be titrated up on a weekly basis until a daily dose of 3,000 mg is achieved.

7. Which of the following drugs has been shown to improve survival in patients with heart failure with reduced ejection fraction (HFrEF)? (Select ALL that apply.)

   (A) Carvedilol
   (B) Digoxin
   (C) Enalapril
   (D) Ivabradine
   (E) Spironolactone

8. Which of the following oral antithrombotic agents is/are approved for the treatment of deep venous thrombosis (DVT) and pulmonary embolism (PE)? (Select ALL that apply.)

   (A) Apixaban
   (B) Aspirin
   (C) Dabigatran
   (D) Rivaroxaban
   (E) Ticagrelor

9. Nitroglycerin is available in which of the following formulations? (Select ALL that apply.)

   (A) Injection
   (B) Nasal spray
   (C) Sublingual tablets
   (D) Topical ointment
   (E) Transdermal patch

10. Which of the following drugs is considered a class IV antiarrhythmic?

   (A) Dofetilide
   (B) Diltiazem
   (C) Flecainide
   (D) Metoprolol
   (E) Procainamide

ANSWERS AND EXPLANATIONS

1. **B, C, E**

Bisoprolol (B), clonidine (C), and ivabradine (E) may cause bradycardia and/or heart block. The nondihydropyridine (non-DHP) calcium channel blockers (CCBs) (i.e., verapamil, diltiazem) also decrease atrioventricular (AV) nodal conduction and can cause bradycardia. However, the DHP CCBs, including amlodipine (A), have no effect on AV nodal conduction. Instead, these drugs can actually cause reflex tachycardia. Angiotensin-converting enzyme inhibitors (ACEIs), such as enalapril (D), have no effect on cardiac conduction.

2. **B**

For a patient on a statin who complains of muscle pain, a creatine kinase should be obtained. Therefore, choice (B) is correct.

3. **C**

Nitroglycerin could potentially cause headaches, so choice (C) is correct. Nitroglycerin does not cause cardiac arrhythmias (A), bleeding (B), hyperkalemia (D), or Stevens-Johnson syndrome (E).

4. **A**

Dobutamine (A) stimulates β_1 receptors in the heart and increases myocardial contractility and is therefore considered a positive inotrope. Hydralazine (B) is a direct arterial vasodilator. Nesiritide (C) is an arterial and venous vasodilator. While both of these drugs may increase cardiac output (CO), they do so by decreasing afterload and not by increasing myocardial contractility. Nitroglycerin (D) is a venous vasodilator and is used to reduce preload; it has no effect on CO. Verapamil (E) is a negative inotrope.

5. **C**

Carvedilol (C) is a nonselective β-blocker, antagonizing both the β_1 and β_2 receptors. Atenolol (A), bisoprolol (B), metoprolol (D), and nebivolol (E) are all considered cardioselective β-blockers (i.e., selectively block β_1 receptors), especially at low doses.

6. **A**

Niacin is available as a prescription product as well as an over-the-counter product (A). To prevent niacin-induced flushing, patients should be counseled to take either an aspirin or a nonsteroidal anti-inflammatory drug 30 minutes before each dose because this adverse reaction is mediated by prostaglandins. Acetaminophen (B) does not antagonize the effects of prostaglandins and would not reduce the incidence of niacin-induced flushing. Niacin has been associated with hyperglycemia, not hypoglycemia (C). Niacin is effective in lowering triglycerides and can be used in patients with hypertriglyceridemia (D). To minimize the flushing reactions, the dose of niacin should not be increased by more than 500 mg every 4 weeks (E).

7. **A, C, E**

ACEIs (C), certain β-blockers (carvedilol, metoprolol succinate, and bisoprolol) (A), aldosterone receptor antagonists (E), and isosorbide/dinitrate have all been associated with a reduction in mortality in patients with HFrEF. Although the use of digoxin (B) has been shown to reduce symptoms in patients with HFrEF, it has not been associated with a reduction in mortality. Although the use of ivabradine (D) has been associated with a reduction in hospitalizations in patients with HFrEF, it also has not been associated with a reduction in mortality.

8. **A, C, D**

All three of the novel oral anticoagulants—apixaban, dabigatran, and rivaroxaban—are currently approved by the FDA for the treatment of DVT and PE. Antiplatelet medications such as aspirin (B) or ticagrelor (E) would not be useful for the treatment of DVT or PE.

9. **A, C, D, E**

Nitroglycerin is currently available as an intravenous injection (A), sublingual tablet (C), topical ointment (D), and a transdermal patch (E). This drug is also available as a sublingual spray and rectal ointment (for chronic anal fissures). It is not available as a nasal spray (B).

10. **B**

The non-DHP CCBs—verapamil and diltiazem (B)—are considered class IV antiarrhythmics. Dofetilide (A) is primarily a K^+ channel blocker and is considered a class III antiarrhythmic. Flecainide (C) and procainamide (E) are Na^+ channel blockers and are considered class I antiarrhythmics, with flecainide designated a class Ic antiarrhythmic and procainamide a class Ia antiarrhythmic. β-blockers such as metoprolol (D) are considered class II antiarrhythmics.

Infectious Diseases

2

This chapter reviews various antibiotic agents, including antibacterial, antifungal, and antiviral agents. A brief overview of the recommended pharmacologic treatments of the following infections is also provided:

- **Urinary tract infections**
- **Pneumonia**
- **Meningitis**
- **Infective endocarditis**
- **Infectious diarrhea**
- **Otitis media**
- **Sexually transmitted diseases**
- **Skin and soft tissue infections**
- **Invasive fungal infections**
- **Human immunodeficiency virus**
- **Tuberculosis**

 Suggested Study Time: **5 hours**

PRINCIPLES OF ANTIBIOTIC THERAPY

Factors to Consider When Selecting Antibiotic Therapy

- Identity/susceptibility of bacteria
  - Important to know which bacteria may be causing the infection
    - » Can begin empiric antibiotic therapy without knowing the actual identity (or sensitivities) of the organism; select antibiotic(s) (usually broad-spectrum) based on the organism(s) *most* likely to cause a particular infection
    - » Once organism (and sensitivities) identified, adjust/narrow antibiotic therapy, as needed, to cover this organism

- Site of infection
  - Especially important for meningitis, urinary tract infections (UTIs), prostatitis, and osteomyelitis
    - » Only certain antibiotics can penetrate into these areas to target the infection; these drugs may need to be used at higher doses, especially for meningitis, prostatitis, and osteomyelitis
- Patient allergies
- Concomitant medications
  - May need to be concerned with potential drug interactions when selecting an antibiotic
- Hepatic and renal function
  - May need to adjust antibiotic dosages if hepatic or renal dysfunction present
- Past medical history
  - Certain antibiotics may need to be avoided in particular disease states (e.g., seizure disorders)
- Patient age
  - Some antibiotics are contraindicated in pediatric patients
- Pregnancy/breastfeeding
  - Some antibiotics are contraindicated in these patients

URINARY TRACT INFECTIONS

Common Organisms

Community-Acquired	Nosocomial (Hospital-Acquired)
• *E. coli* • *Staphylococcus saprophyticus* • *Klebsiella pneumoniae* • *Proteus mirabilis*	• *E. coli* • *Pseudomonas aeruginosa* • *Klebsiella pneumoniae* • *Proteus mirabilis* • *Enterobacter* spp. • *Staphylococcus aureus* • Fungus (e.g., *Candida*)

Diagnosis

- Confirmed by urinalysis
  - Bacteruria: $>10^2$ cfu/mL
  - Pyuria: $>5–10$ white blood cells (WBCs)/mm^3
  - Nitrite-positive
  - Leukocyte esterase–positive
  - Casts (may be present in pyelonephritis)

Signs and Symptoms

- Lower UTI (cystitis)
  - Dysuria
  - Urgency
  - Frequency
  - Nocturia
  - Suprapubic pressure/pain
- Upper UTI (pyelonephritis)
  - All lower UTI symptoms, *plus*
  - Flank pain
  - Fever
  - Nausea/vomiting (N/V)
- Complicated UTI factors
  - Male
  - Elderly
  - Pregnancy
  - Children
  - Nosocomial
  - Recent use of antibiotics
  - Diabetes
  - Immunosuppressed
  - Catheterized

Guidelines

Gupta K, Hooton TM, Naber KG, et al; Infectious Diseases Society of America; European Society for Microbiology and Infectious Diseases. International clinical practice guidelines for the treatment of acute uncomplicated cystitis and pyelonephritis in women: a 2010 update by the Infectious Diseases Society of America and the European Society for Microbiology and Infectious Diseases. *Clin Infect Dis* 2011;52:e103–20.

Guidelines Summary

Acute Uncomplicated Cystitis

First-line therapy	Nitrofurantoin 100 mg PO BID × 5 days
Second-line therapy	Trimethoprim/sulfamethoxazole (TMP/SMX) 160/800 mg (double-strength [DS]) PO BID × 3 days
Third-line therapy	Fosfomycin 3 g PO × 1 dose

- *Alternative agents:*
  - Fluoroquinolone (FQ) × 3 days
    - » Only use when other agents cannot be used
  - β-lactams (i.e., amoxicillin-clavulanate, cefdinir, cefaclor, cefpodoxime) × 3–7 days
    - » Avoid unless other agents are not appropriate

Acute Pyelonephritis (Outpatient Therapy)
- First-line therapy:
  - Ciprofloxacin 500 mg PO BID × 7 days
  - Cipro XR 1 g PO daily × 7 days
  - Levofloxacin 750 mg PO daily × 5 days
  - May be combined with either of the following:
    - Ceftriaxone 1 g IV × 1 day **OR**
    - Gentamicin 5–7 mg/kg IV × 1 day
- Second-line therapy: TMP/SMX DS PO BID × 14 days
  - May be combined with either of the following:
    - Ceftriaxone 1 g IV × 1 day **OR**
    - Gentamicin 5–7 mg/kg IV × 1 day
- Third-line therapy: Oral β-lactam (i.e., amoxicillin-clavulanate) × 10–14 days **AND** one-time dose of ceftriaxone 1 g IV or gentamicin 5–7 mg/kg IV

Acute Pyelonephritis (Inpatient Therapy)
- IV FQ
- Aminoglycoside +/– IV ampicillin
- IV extended-spectrum cephalosporin or penicillin +/– aminoglycoside
- IV carbapenem (e.g., imipenem/cilastatin)

Complicated UTIs
- Duration of therapy: 10–14 days

PNEUMONIA

Common Organisms

Community-Acquired	Hospital-Acquired (occurs ≥48 hours after admission)
• *Mycoplasma pneumoniae* • *Streptococcus pneumoniae* • *Haemophilus influenzae* • *Chlamydia pneumoniae* • *Legionella pneumophila* • *Moraxella catarrhalis* • Viruses	• *Staphylococcus aureus* • *Pseudomonas aeruginosa* • *Klebsiella pneumoniae* • *Enterobacter* • *E. coli* • *Acinetobacter* spp. • *Serratia* spp. • Anaerobes

Diagnosis

- Symptoms and auscultatory findings consistent with pneumonia, plus an infiltrate on chest x-ray

- Diagnosis can often be made on history and physical exam findings

Signs and Symptoms

- Fever, chills, dyspnea, cough (may or may not be productive), rigors, pleuritic pain
- Physical examination:
  - Tachypnea
  - Tachycardia
  - Dullness to percussion
  - Inspiratory crackles
  - ↓ breath sounds over affected area
- Laboratory findings
  - ↑ WBCs
- Infiltrate on chest x-ray

Guidelines

Mandell LA, Wunderink RG, Anzueto A; Infectious Diseases Society of America; American Thoracic Society. Infectious Diseases Society of America/American Thoracic Society consensus guidelines on the management of community-acquired pneumonia in adults. *Clin Infect Dis* 2007;44(suppl 2):S27–72.

Kalil AC, Metersky ML, Klompas M, et al. Management of adults with hospital-acquired and ventilator-associated pneumonia: 2016 clinical practice guidelines by the Infectious Diseases Society of America and the American Thoracic Society. *Clin Infect Dis* 2016;63;1–51.

Guidelines Summary

Diagnosis	Treatment	Duration
Community-acquired (ambulatory)	*Previously healthy and no antibiotic therapy in past 3 months:* Macrolide (clarithromycin or azithromycin) **OR** Doxycycline	≥5 days
	With comorbidities (see table notes)[1] that place patient at risk for drug-resistant Streptococcus pneumoniae or antibiotic use in past 3 months: FQ (moxifloxacin, gemifloxacin, or levofloxacin) **OR** Macrolide (or doxycycline) *plus* one of the following: • High-dose amoxicillin • Amoxicillin/clavulanate • Cephalosporin (ceftriaxone, cefuroxime, or cefpodoxime)	
Community-acquired (hospitalized)	*Not in Intensive Care Unit (ICU):* FQ (moxifloxacin, gemifloxacin, or levofloxacin) **OR** Macrolide (or doxycycline) *plus* one of the following: • Ampicillin • Ceftriaxone • Cefotaxime	
	In ICU: FQ (moxifloxacin, gemifloxacin, or levofloxacin) *plus* one of the following: • Ampicillin/sulbactam • Ceftriaxone • Cefotaxime **OR** Azithromycin *plus* one of the following: • Ampicillin/sulbactam • Ceftriaxone • Cefotaxime	

Guidelines Summary *(cont'd)*

Diagnosis	Treatment	Duration
Hospital-acquired	*Not at high risk for mortality (see below)[2] **AND** no factors increasing likelihood of methicillin-resistant S. aureus (MRSA) (see below)[3] (select one of the following drugs):* • Piperacillin/tazobactam • Cefepime • Levofloxacin • Imipenem/cilastatin or meropenem	7 days
	*Not at high risk for mortality (see below)[2] but **WITH** factors increasing the likelihood of MRSA (see below)[3]:* Vancomycin **OR** Linezolid **PLUS** one of the following: • Piperacillin/tazobactam • Ceftazidime • Cefepime • Levofloxacin or ciprofloxacin • Imipenem/cilastatin or meropenem • Aztreonam	
	High risk for mortality (see below)[2] or receipt of IV antibiotics in the past 90 days: Vancomycin **OR** Linezolid **PLUS** 2 of the following (avoid 2 β-lactams): • Piperacillin/tazobactam • Ceftazidime • Cefepime • Levofloxacin or ciprofloxacin • Imipenem/cilastatin or meropenem • Aztreonam • Amikacin, or gentamicin, or tobramycin	

[1] *Comorbidities: Chronic obstructive pulmonary disease (COPD), diabetes, chronic renal failure, chronic liver failure, heart failure (HF), cancer, asplenia, immunosuppressed*

[2] *Risk factors for mortality: Need for ventilatory support due to pneumonia and septic shock.*

[3] *Risk factors for MRSA infection: Prior IV antibiotic use in past 90 days, hospitalization in a unit where >20% of S. aureus isolates are methicillin-resistant or the prevalence of MRSA is unknown.*

MENINGITIS

Common Organisms

Age Group	Most Common Organisms
<1 mo	• *Streptococcus agalactiae* (Group B Strep) • *E. coli* • *Listeria monocytogenes* • *Klebsiella* spp.
1–23 mo	• *Streptococcus pneumoniae* • *Neisseria meningitidis* • Group B Strep • *Haemophilus influenzae* • *E. coli*
2–50 yr	• *Neisseria meningitidis* • *Streptococcus pneumoniae*
>50 yr	• *Streptococcus pneumoniae* • *Neisseria meningitidis* • *Listeria monocytogenes*

Diagnosis

- Confirmed by analysis of cerebrospinal fluid (CSF)
  - Bacterial meningitis: ↓ glucose, ↑ protein, ↑ WBCs
  - Gram stain can help identify organism

Signs and Symptoms

- Symptoms
  - Fever, chills
  - Headache, photophobia
  - Nuchal rigidity
  - N/V
  - Altered mental status
  - Petechiae/purpura (*Neisseria meningitidis*)
- Signs
  - Brudzinski's sign (flexion of hips and knees upon flexing the neck)
  - Kernig's sign (pain develops when the knee is extended after flexing the hip to 90 degrees)
  - Bulging fontanelle (children)

Guidelines

Tunkel AR, Hartman BJ, Kaplan SL, et al. Practice guidelines for the management of bacterial meningitis. *Clin Infect Dis* 2004;39:1267–84.

Guidelines Summary

Empiric Treatment

Age Group	Treatment
<1 mo	Ampicillin + aminoglycoside **OR** Ampicillin + cefotaxime
1–23 mo	Third-generation cephalosporin (cefotaxime or ceftriaxone) + vancomycin
2–50 yr	Third-generation cephalosporin (cefotaxime or ceftriaxone) + vancomycin
>50 yr	Third-generation cephalosporin (cefotaxime or ceftriaxone) + vancomycin + ampicillin

- Dexamethasone may be considered as adjunctive therapy for the following:
  - Infants and children: *H. influenzae* meningitis
  - Adults: *Streptococcus pneumoniae* meningitis

INFECTIVE ENDOCARDITIS

Common Organisms

- *Staphylococcus aureus*
- Viridans group streptococci (*Streptococcus sanguis, Streptococcus mutans, Streptococcus oralis, Streptococcus salivaris, Gemella morbillorium*)
- *Enterococcus* sp.
- Coagulase-negative staphylococci
- *Streptococcus bovis* (group D strep)
- HACEK group

Diagnosis

- Based on modified Duke criteria
  - Classified as definite infective endocarditis (IE), possible IE, or IE rejected

- Definite IE
  - 2 major criteria, **OR**
  - 1 major + 3 minor criteria, **OR**
  - 5 minor criteria
- Complicated IE
  - Large vegetations (>10 mm)
  - Severe valvular insufficiency
  - Abscess cavities or pseudoaneurysms
  - Valvular perforation or dehiscence
  - Decompensated HF

Modified Duke Criteria

Major Criteria	Minor Criteria
Blood culture positive for IE (one of the following): • Typical microorganisms consistent with IE from 2 separate blood cultures • Persistently positive cultures defined as: ≥2 positive cultures of blood samples drawn >12 hr apart or all 3 or a majority of ≥4 separate blood cultures (with 1st and last sample drawn ≥1 hr apart	Predisposition, predisposing heart condition, or injection drug use
Evidence of endocardial involvement	Fever (temperature >38°C)
Echocardiogram positive for IE (vegetation, abscess, or new partial dehiscence of prosthetic valve or new valvular regurgitation)	Vascular phenomena, major arterial emboli, septic pulmonary infarcts, mycotic aneurysm, intracranial hemorrhage, conjunctival hemorrhages, and Janeway lesions
	Immunological phenomena (e.g., glomerulonephritis, Osler nodes, Roth spots, rheumatoid factor)
	Microbiological evidence (positive blood culture but does not meet a major criterion) or serological evidence of active infection with organism consistent with IE

Signs and Symptoms

- Symptoms
  - Chills
  - Weakness
  - Dyspnea
  - Night sweats
- Signs
  - Heart murmur (new or change) (tricuspid, mitral, or aortic regurgitation)
  - Splenomegaly

- Embolic phenomenon (lungs, kidneys, brain)
- Peripheral manifestations
    - » Osler nodes: Purplish or erythematous subcutaneous papules or nodules on pads of fingers or toes that are painful or tender
    - » Janeway lesions: Flat, hemorrhagic plaques on palms of hands or soles of feet that are painless
    - » Splinter hemorrhages: Thin, linear hemorrhages under nail beds of fingers and/or toes
    - » Petechiae: Small, erythematous painless lesions usually on anterior trunk, buccal mucosa, palate, or conjunctiva
    - » Roth spots: Retinal infarct with central pallor and surrounding hemorrhage
    - » Finger clubbing

Guidelines

Baddour LM, Wilson WR, Bayer AS, et al. Infective endocarditis in adults: diagnosis, antimicrobial therapy, and management of complications: a scientific statement for healthcare professionals from the American Heart Association. *Circulation* 2015;132:1435–86.

Guidelines Summary, Empiric Treatment

Viridans Group Streptococci and *Streptococcus bovis* Highly Susceptible to Penicillin (MIC ≤0.12 mcg/mL): Native Valve IE

Treatment Regimen	Duration	Clinical Pearls
Penicillin G 12–18 million units/day IV in 4–6 divided doses **OR** Ceftriaxone 2 g IV/IM q24h	4 wk 4 wk	If patient has NO β-lactam allergy
Penicillin G 12–18 million units/day IV in 6 divided doses **OR** ceftriaxone 2 g IV/IM q24h **PLUS** Gentamicin 3 mg/kg IV q24h or 1 mg/kg IV q8h	2 wk 2 wk	Should not be used if patients have: • Cardiac or extracardiac abscess • CrCl <20 mL/min For gentamicin q8h dosing: • Target peak concentration = 3–4 mcg/mL • Target trough concentration <1 mcg/mL
Vancomycin 15 mg/kg IV q12h	4 wk	• For patients with β-lactam allergy • Target trough concentration = 10–15 mcg/mL

Viridans Group Streptococci and *Streptococcus bovis* Relatively Resistant to Penicillin (MIC >0.12 and <0.5 mcg/mL): Native Valve IE

Treatment Regimen	Duration	Clinical Pearls
Penicillin G 24 million units/day IV in 4–6 divided doses **PLUS** Gentamicin 3 mg/kg IV q24h or 1 mg/kg IV q8h	4 wk 2 wk	If organism susceptible to ceftriaxone, may use ceftriaxone monotherapy For gentamicin q8h dosing: • Target peak concentration = 3–4 mcg/mL • Target trough concentration <1 mcg/mL
Vancomycin 15 mg/kg IV q12h	4 wk	• For patients with β-lactam allergy • Target trough concentration = 10–15 mcg/mL

Viridans Group Streptococci and *Streptococcus bovis* Resistant to Penicillin (MIC ≥0.5 mcg/mL): Native Valve IE

- Treat as enterococcal IE

Viridans Group Streptococci and *Streptococcus bovis* Susceptible to Penicillin (MIC ≤0.12 mcg/mL): Prosthetic Valve IE

Treatment Regimen	Duration	Clinical Pearls
Penicillin G 24 million units/day IV in 4–6 divided doses **OR** ceftriaxone 2 g IV/IM q24h **WITH OR WITHOUT** Gentamicin 3 mg/kg IV q24h or 1 mg/kg IV q8h	6 wk 2 wk	Do NOT give gentamicin if patient's CrCl <30 mL/min For gentamicin q8h dosing: • Target peak concentration = 3–4 mcg/mL • Target trough concentration <1 mcg/mL
Vancomycin 15 mg/kg IV q12h	6 wk	• For patients with β-lactam allergy • Target trough concentration = 10–15 mcg/mL

Viridans Group Streptococci and *Streptococcus bovis* Relatively or Fully Resistant to Penicillin (MIC >0.12 mcg/mL): Prosthetic Valve IE

Treatment Regimen	Duration	Clinical Pearls
Penicillin G 24 million units/day IV in 4–6 divided doses **OR** Ceftriaxone 2 g IV/IM q24h **PLUS** Gentamicin 3 mg/kg IV q24h or 1 mg/kg IV q8h	6 wk 6 wk	For gentamicin q8h dosing: • Target peak concentration = 3–4 mcg/mL • Target trough concentration <1 mcg/mL
Vancomycin 15 mg/kg IV q12h	6 wk	• For patients with β-lactam allergy • Target trough concentration = 10–15 mcg/mL

Staphylococci: Native Valve IE

Treatment Regimen	Duration	Clinical Pearls
Oxacillin-susceptible strains:		
Nafcillin or oxacillin 12 g/day IV in 4–6 divided doses	6 wk (complicated, right-sided IE and uncomplicated, left-sided IE); ≥6 wk (complicated, left-sided IE); 2 wk (uncomplicated, right-sided IE)	
Cefazolin 2 g IV q8h	6 wk	For patients with non-anaphylactoidtype β-lactam allergy
Vancomycin 15 mg/kg IV q12h	6 wk	• For patients with anaphylactoid-type β-lactam allergy • Target trough concentration = 10–20 mcg/mL
Oxacillin-resistant strains:		
Vancomycin 15 mg/kg IV q12h	6 wk	Target trough concentration = 10–20 mcg/mL
Daptomycin ≥8 mg/kg/dose	6 wk	

Staphylococci: Prosthetic Valve IE

Treatment Regimen	Duration	Clinical Pearls
Oxacillin-susceptible strains:		
Nafcillin or oxacillin 2 g IV q4h **PLUS**	≥6 wk	Cefazolin may be substituted for nafcillin/ oxacillin in patients with non-anaphylactoid-type β-lactam allergy
Rifampin 300 mg IV/PO q8h **PLUS**	≥6 wk	Vancomycin may be substituted for nafcillin/oxacillin in patients with anaphylactoid-type β-lactam allergy
Gentamicin 3 mg/kg/day IV in 2–3 divided doses	2 wk	For gentamicin: • Target peak concentration = 3–4 mcg/mL • Target trough concentration <1 mcg/mL
Oxacillin-resistant strains:		
Vancomycin 15 mg/kg IV q12h **PLUS**	≥6 wk	Target vancomycin trough concentration = 10–20 mcg/mL
Rifampin 300 mg IV/PO q8h **PLUS**	≥6 wk	For gentamicin: • Target peak concentration = 3–4 mcg/mL
Gentamicin 3 mg/kg/day IV in 2–3 divided doses	2 wk	• Target trough concentration <1 mcg/mL

Enterococcus Species Susceptible to Penicillin and Gentamicin in Patients Who Can Tolerate β-Lactam Therapy: Native or Prosthetic Valve IE

Treatment Regimen	Duration	Clinical Pearls
Ampicillin 2 g IV q4h **OR** Penicillin G 18–30 million units IV in 6 divided doses **PLUS**	4–6 wk	Recommended for patients with CrCl >50 mL/min 4 wk of therapy recommended for patients with native valve IE with symptoms <3 mo
Gentamicin 3 mg/kg/day IV in 2–3 divided doses	4–6 wk	6 wk of therapy recommended for patients with native valve IE with symptoms >3 mo **OR** prosthetic valve IE For gentamicin: • Target peak concentration = 3–4 mcg/mL • Target trough concentration <1 mcg/mL
Ampicillin 2 g IV q4h **PLUS**	6 wk	Recommended for patients with CrCl <50 mL/min
Ceftriaxone 2 g IV q12h	6 wk	

Enterococcus Species Susceptible to Vancomycin and Gentamicin and Resistant to Penicillin in Patients Who Cannot Tolerate β-Lactam Therapy: Native or Prosthetic Valve IE

Treatment Regimen	Duration	Clinical Pearls
Vancomycin 15 mg/kg IV q12h **PLUS** Gentamicin 1 mg/kg IV q8h	6 wk	Target vancomycin trough concentration = 10–20 mcg/mL For gentamicin: • Target peak concentration = 3–4 mcg/mL • Target trough concentration <1 mcg/mL

Enterococcus Species Resistant to Penicillin, Aminoglycosides, and Vancomycin: Native or Prosthetic Valve IE

Treatment Regimen	Duration
Linezolid 600 mg IV/PO q12h **OR**	>6 wk
Daptomycin 10–12 mg/kg per dose	>6 wk

INFECTIOUS DIARRHEA

Common Organisms

- *Clostridium difficile*
- *E. coli*
- *Salmonella*
- *Shigella*
- *Giardia*
- *Campylobacter jejuni*
- Viruses

Diagnosis

- Infectious diarrhea = Diarrhea due to an infectious etiology that is often accompanied by N/V or abdominal cramps
- Categories of infectious diarrhea:
  - Community-acquired or traveler's diarrhea: Often accompanied by fever or blood in stool; perform fecal testing for:
    - » *Salmonella*
    - » *Shigella*

» *Campylobacter*

» *E. coli* O157:H7 (also known as Shiga toxin-producing *E. coli* [STEC])

» *C. difficile* toxins A and B (especially if history of treatment with antibiotics or chemotherapy within past 8 weeks)

- Nosocomial diarrhea: Onset after >3 days in hospital; perform fecal testing for:

  » *C. difficile* toxins A and B

  » If bloody stools, also include other organisms listed under Community-acquired or traveler's diarrhea

- Persistent diarrhea: >7 days (often occurs in immunosuppressed patients); perform fecal tests for:

  » *Giardia*

  » *Cryptosporidium*

  » *Cyclospora*

  » *Isospora belli*

  » *Microsporidia* (if HIV-positive)

  » *M. avium complex* (if HIV-positive)

Signs and Symptoms

- Symptoms
  - N/V/D
  - Abdominal pain
  - Cramps
  - Headache
  - Dehydration (lethargy, mental status changes, $\uparrow$ thirst)
- Signs
  - Blood or pus in stool
  - Dehydration ($\downarrow$ BP, tachycardia, $\downarrow$ urination, $\downarrow$ skin turgor)

Guidelines

Cohen SH, Gerding DN, Johnson S, et al. Clinical practice guidelines for *Clostridium difficile* infection in adults: 2010 update by the Society for Healthcare Epidemiology of America (SHEA) and the Infectious Diseases Society of America. *Infect Control Hosp Epidemiol* 2010;31:431–55.

Guerrant RL, Van Gilder T, Steiner TS, et al. Practice guidelines for the management of infectious diarrhea. *Clin Infect Dis* 2001;31:331–50.

Guidelines Summary

Organism	First-Line Treatment
Shigella	TMP/SMX or FQ
Salmonella	TMP/SMX or FQ
Campylobacter	Erythromycin
E. coli, enterotoxigenic	TMP/SMX or FQ
E.coli, enterohemorrhagic (STEC)	Avoid antimotility drugs and antibiotics
C. difficile	• Discontinue antibiotics and avoid antimotility agents • Mild-to-moderate: Metronidazole 500 mg PO TID × 10–14 days • Severe: Vancomycin 125 mg PO 4 times daily × 10–14 days
Giardia	Metronidazole
Cryptosporidium	Paromomycin (if severe)
Isospora	TMP/SMX
Cyclospora	TMP/SMX

OTITIS MEDIA

Definitions

- Acute otitis media (AOM): Rapid onset of signs/symptoms of inflammation and effusion (fluid) in the middle ear

- Otitis media with effusion (OME): Fluid and inflammation in the middle ear *without* evidence of signs/symptoms of acute infection

- Recurrent AOM: ≥3 episodes of AOM within previous 6 months **OR** 4 episodes of AOM within previous 12 months (with ≥1 episode within previous 6 months)

Common Organisms

- *Streptococcus pneumoniae*
- *Haemophilus influenzae*
- *Moraxella catarrhalis*

Diagnosis

- Key elements in diagnosis of AOM:
  - Acute (<48 hr) onset of signs/symptoms
  - Middle ear inflammation and erythema of tympanic membrane
  - Presence of middle ear effusion
    - » Leads to bulging of tympanic membrane → May lead to perforation and drainage (otorrhea)

Signs and Symptoms

- Otalgia
  - May be demonstrated by:
    - » Holding/tugging/rubbing of ear
    - » Excessive crying
    - » Fever
    - » Changes in sleep or behavior pattern
- Otoscopic findings:
  - Middle ear effusion
  - Tympanic membrane → Bulging and erythematous

Guidelines

Lieberthal AS, Carroll AE, Chonmaitree T, et al. The diagnosis and management of acute otitis media. *Pediatrics* 2013;131(3):e964–99.

Guidelines Summary

Initial Management of Uncomplicated AOM

Age	Otorrhea with AOM	Unilateral or Bilateral AOM with Severe Symptoms	Bilateral AOM without Otorrhea	Unilateral AOM without Otorrhea
6 months–2 years	Antibiotic therapy	Antibiotic therapy	Antibiotic therapy	Antibiotic therapy **OR** additional observation
≥2 years	Antibiotic therapy	Antibiotic therapy	Antibiotic therapy **OR** additional observation	Antibiotic therapy **OR** additional observation

Recommended Antibiotic Therapy for Management of Uncomplicated AOM

	First-Line Therapy	Alternative Therapy
Initial Immediate or Delayed Treatment	Amoxicillin (high-dose) 80–90 mg/kg/day PO in 2 divided doses **OR** *If history of amoxicillin use in past 90 days, concurrent purulent conjunctivitis, or history of recurrent AOM unresponsive to amoxicillin:* Amoxicillin-clavulanate (high-dose) 90 mg/kg/day of amoxicillin + 6.4 mg/kg/day PO of clavulanate in 2 divided doses	*If penicillin allergy:* Cefdinir **OR** Cefuroxime **OR** Cefpodoxime **OR** Ceftriaxone × 1 or 3 days
Treatment After 48–72 Hours of Failure of Initial Antibiotic Treatment	Amoxicillin-clavulanate (high-dose) 90 mg/kg/day + 6.4 mg/kg/day of clavulanate PO in 2 divided doses **OR** Ceftriaxone 50 mg IM or IV for 3 days	Clindamycin

Duration of Therapy

Age/Characteristic of Symptoms	Duration
<2 yr or severe symptoms	10 days
2–5 yr with mild–moderate symptoms	7 days
≥6 yr with mild–moderate symptoms	5–7 days

SEXUALLY TRANSMITTED DISEASES

Causative Organisms

Disease	Organisms
Chlamydia	*Chlamydia trachomatis*
Gonorrhea	*Neisseria gonorrhoeae*
Syphilis	*Treponema pallidum*

Diagnosis

- Chlamydia: Test performed on urine swab or endocervical/vaginal/male urethral swab

- Gonorrhea: Gram-stained smears or culture (endocervical/vaginal/male urethral/urine specimen)

- Syphilis: Dark field examination and direct fluorescent antibody stains of exudates
  - Serologic testing (diagnosis requires use of 2 tests, nontreponemal and treponemal)
    - » Nontreponemal: Venereal Disease Research Laboratory (VDRL) slide test, rapid plasma regain (RPR) test; used for screening
    - » Treponemal: Fluorescent treponemal antibody absorbed (FTA-ABS), *T. pallidum* particle agglutination (TP-PA); used to confirm diagnosis

Signs and Symptoms

- Chlamydia
  - Penile/vaginal discharge, dysuria
  - May also be asymptomatic
- Gonorrhea
  - Penile/vaginal discharge, dysuria, urinary frequency
  - May also be asymptomatic
- Syphilis
  - Primary (10–90 days after exposure): Presence of chancre
  - Secondary (2–8 weeks after development of primary stage): Variety of rashes/lesions, flu-like symptoms, and lymphadenopathy
  - Latent (positive serologic test but no clinical manifestations)
  - Tertiary: Cardiovascular (e.g., aortic insufficiency) and neurologic abnormalities (e.g., deafness, blindness, dementia, paresis)

Guidelines

Workowski KA, Bolan GA; Centers for Disease Control and Prevention (CDC). Sexually transmitted diseases treatment guidelines, 2015. *MMWR Recomm Rep* 2015;64 (RR-03):1–137.

Guidelines Summary

Disease	Treatment
Chlamydia	Azithromycin 1 g PO × 1 dose **OR** Doxycycline 100 mg PO q12h × 7 days
Gonorrhea	Ceftriaxone 250 mg IM × 1 dose **PLUS** Azithromycin 1 g PO × 1 dose
Syphilis	*Primary, secondary, or early latent syphilis (<1 yr in duration):* • Benzathine penicillin G 2.4 million units IM × 1 dose *Late latent syphilis (>1 yr in duration), latent syphilis of unknown duration, or tertiary syphilis (not neurosyphilis):* • Benzathine penicillin G 2.4 million units IM once weekly × 3 weeks *Neurosyphilis:* • Aqueous penicillin G 3–4 million units IV q4h or as continuous infusion × 10–14 days

SKIN AND SOFT TISSUE INFECTIONS

Common Organisms

- Community-acquired skin and soft tissue infections (SSTIs)
  - *Staphylococcus aureus* (especially methicillin-resistant *Staphylococcus aureus* [MRSA])
  - Group A streptococci (*Streptococcus pyogenes*)
- Nosocomial SSTIs
  - Gram-negative organisms (e.g., *Pseudomonas aeruginosa, E. coli*)
  - Anaerobes

Diagnosis

- Purulent SSTIs
  - Abscess: Collection of pus within the dermis and deeper skin tissues
    - » Painful, tender, fluctuant red nodules accompanied by a pustule and surrounded by rim of erythematous swelling

- Furuncle: Infection of the hair follicle ("boil"); pus extends into subcutaneous tissue
    - » Inflammatory nodules with overlying pustules through which hair emerges
- Carbuncle: Adjacent furuncles coalesce to form a single pus-filled mass
- Nonpurulent SSTIs
    - Cellulitis: Affects epidermis and dermis; may spread within superficial fascia
    - Erysipelas: Form of cellulitis that tends to be limited to upper dermis
    - Necrotizing fasciitis: Severe, life-threatening infection of subcutaneous tissue that results in progressive destruction of superficial fascia and subcutaneous fat

Signs and Symptoms

- Purulent (SSTIs)
    - Pus-filled, erythematous lesion(s)
    - Systemic signs/symptoms of infection uncommon
- Nonpurulent SSTIs
    - Rapidly spreading areas of erythema, swelling, tenderness, and warmth
    - Lymph nodes may become swollen
    - Systemic signs/symptoms of infection more common

Guidelines

Stevens DL, Bisno AL, Chambers HF, et al. Practice guidelines for the diagnosis and management of skin and soft tissue infections: 2014 update by the Infectious Diseases Society of America. *Clin Infect Dis* 2014;59(2):e10–52.

Guidelines Summary

Infection	Empiric Treatment
Purulent SSTIs	
Mild	Incision and drainage; no antibiotics
Moderate (with systemic signs of infection*)	Incision and drainage **PLUS** antibiotics: TMP/SMX **OR** Doxycycline
Severe (failed incision and drainage plus PO antibiotics **OR** have systemic signs of infection*, **OR** are immunocompromised)	Incision and drainage **PLUS** antibiotics: Vancomycin **OR** **OR** Daptomycin Dalbavancin **OR** **OR** Linezolid Oritavancin **OR** **OR** Telavancin Tedizolid **OR** Ceftaroline
Nonpurulent SSTIs	
Mild	Penicillin VK **OR** Cephalosporin (PO) **OR** Dicloxacillin **OR** Clindamycin (PO)
Moderate (with systemic signs of infection*)	Penicillin (IV) **OR** Ceftriaxone **OR** Cefazolin **OR** Clindamycin (IV)
Severe (failed PO antibiotics **OR** signs of systemic infection*, **OR** immunocompromised **OR** signs of deeper infection [e.g., bullae, skin sloughing, hypotension, evidence of organ dysfunction])	Emergent surgical inspection/debridement **PLUS** antibiotics: Vancomycin **AND** Piperacillin/tazobactam

* Signs of systemic infection: Temperature >38°C, heart rate >90 beats/minute, respiratory rate >24 breaths/minute, WBCs >12,000 cells/μL or <400 cells/μL

INVASIVE FUNGAL INFECTIONS

Drugs of Choice for Selected Invasive Fungal Infections

Organism	Disease	First-Line Therapy	Duration
Candida albicans, C. glabrata, C. krusei, C. tropicalis	Candidemia	*Nonneutropenic:* Echinocandin **OR** Fluconazole (if not critically ill) *Neutropenic:* Echinocandin **OR** Lipid amphotericin B **OR** Fluconazole (if not critically ill and no prior azole exposure) If *C. krusei*: Echinocandin, lipid amphotericin B, or voriconazole	14 days after first negative blood culture
	Urinary candidiasis	*Asymptomatic:* Eliminate predisposing factor (i.e., remove urinary catheter) Treat only if high-risk for dissemination: • Neutropenic: Treat as for candidemia (see above) • Undergoing urologic manipulation: Fluconazole (PO) **OR** amphotericin B *Symptomatic:* • Fluconazole-susceptible organism: Fluconazole (PO) • Fluconazole-resistant *C. glabrata*: Amphotericin B **OR** flucytosine • *C. krusei*: Amphotericin B	*Asymptomatic:* Treatment for urologic manipulation: Several days before and after procedure *Symptomatic:* • Fluconazole-susceptible organisms: 14 days • Fluconazole-resistant *C. glabrata*: 7–10 days • *C. krusei*: 1–7 days

Drugs of Choice for Selected Invasive Fungal Infections *(cont'd)*

Organism	Disease	First-Line Therapy	Duration
Blastomyces dermatitidis	Pulmonary blastomycosis	*Mild to moderate:* Itraconazole *Moderately severe to severe:* Amphotericin B × 1–2 wk, then itraconazole × 6–12 mo	6–12 mo
	Disseminated blastomycosis	*Mild to moderate:* Itraconazole *Moderately severe to severe:* Amphotericin B × 1–2 wk, then itraconazole × 12 mo	*Mild to moderate:* 6–12 mo *Moderately severe to severe:* 12 mo
	Immunosuppressed	Amphotericin B × 1–2 wk, then itraconazole × 12 mo	12 mo
Aspergillus fumigatus, A. flavus, A. niger	Pulmonary aspergillosis	Voriconazole	6–12 wk
Coccidioides immitis	Pulmonary coccidioidomycosis	Amphotericin B or high-dose fluconazole	1 yr
	Disseminated (nonmeningeal) coccidioidomycosis	Fluconazole or itraconazole	Prolonged (may be lifelong)
	Disseminated (meningeal) coccidioidomycosis	Fluconazole	Prolonged (may be lifelong)
Histoplasma capsulatum	Pulmonary histoplasmosis	*Mild to moderate:* Symptoms <4 wk: No treatment Symptoms >4 wk: Itraconazole *Moderately severe to severe:* Amphotericin B × 1–2 wk, then itraconazole × total of 12 wk	*Mild to moderate:* 6–12 wk *Moderately severe to severe:* 12 wk
Cryptococcus neoformans	Cryptococcal meningoencephalitis (in HIV-infected patients)	*Induction:* Amphotericin B + flucytosine *Consolidation:* Fluconazole	*Induction:* ≥2 wk *Consolidation:* ≥8 wk

Antibacterial Agents

Penicillins (β-Lactams)

Generic • Brand • Dose/Dosage Forms	Spectrum of Activity	Contraindications	Primary Side Effects	Pertinent Drug Interactions	Med Pearl
Mechanism of action – inhibit bacterial cell wall synthesis; bactericidal					
Natural Penicillins					
Penicillin G • Only available generically • 2–4 million units IV q4–6h • Injection Penicillin G benzathine • Bicillin LA • 1.2–2.4 million units IM at specified intervals • Injection Penicillin G procaine • Only available generically • 1.2–4.8 million units IM/day at specified intervals • Injection Penicillin VK☆ • Only available generically • 250–500 mg PO q6h • Solution, tabs	• *Strep. viridans* • *Strep. pyogenes* • *Strep. pneumoniae* (↑ resistance) • Mouth anaerobes	Allergy to penicillins, cephalosporins, or carbapenems	• Hypersensitivity reaction (rash, hives, dyspnea, throat swelling) • Nausea/vomiting/diarrhea (N/V/D) • Interstitial nephritis • Hemolytic anemia (with prolonged administration)	• Probenecid may ↑ effects (may be used for this purpose) • May ↓ effects of oral contraceptives	• Adjust dose in renal impairment • Penicillin G benzathine or procaine used for syphilis; benzathine also used for Strep throat • Take penicillin VK 1 hour before or 2 hours after meals
Penicillinase-Resistant Penicillins					
Dicloxacillin • Only available generically • 125–500 mg PO q6h • Caps Nafcillin • Only available generically • 500 mg–2 g IV q4–6h • Injection Oxacillin • Bactocill • 250 mg–2 g IV q4–6h • Injection	• *Staph aureus* (methicillin-sensitive, MSSA) • *Streptococcus*	Same as natural penicillins	Same as natural penicillins	Same as natural penicillins	• No need to adjust dose in renal impairment (cleared by biliary excretion) • Take dicloxacillin 1 hour before or 2 hours after meals • Patients on nafcillin (IV) or oxacillin (IV) can be switched to dicloxacillin (PO)

Penicillins (β-Lactams) *(cont'd)*

Generic • Brand • Dose/Dosage Forms	Spectrum of Activity	Contraindications	Primary Side Effects	Pertinent Drug Interactions	Med Pearl
Aminopenicillins					
Amoxicillin ☆ • Moxatag • Immediate-release (IR): 250–500 mg PO q8h or 500–875 mg PO q12h • Extended release (ER): 775 mg PO daily • Caps, chewable tabs, suspension, tabs (ER and IR)	• *Strep pneumoniae* • *H. influenzae* • *E. coli* • *Proteus mirabilis* • *Salmonella* • *Shigella*	Same as natural penicillins	Same as natural penicillins	Same as natural penicillins	• Amoxicillin can be used in 3-drug regimen for *H. pylori* • Adjust dose in renal impairment • Take ampicillin 1 hour before or 2 hours after meals
Ampicillin • Only available generically • 250–500 mg PO q6h • 250 mg–2 g IV q4–6h • Caps, injection, suspension					
Aminopenicillins + β-Lactamase Inhibitors					
Amoxicillin-clavulanate ☆ • Augmentin • IR: 250–500 mg PO q8h or 500–875 mg PO q12h • ER: 2,000 mg PO q12h • Chewable tabs, suspension, tabs (ER and IR)	• β-lactamase producing *Staph. aureus* (MSSA), *H. influenzae*, *M. catarrhalis*, *E. coli*, and *K. pneumoniae* • Anaerobes	Same as natural penicillins	Same as natural penicillins	Same as natural penicillins	• Adjust dose in renal impairment • Patients on ampicillin sulbactam (IV) can be switched to amoxicillin-clavulanate (PO) • Good anaerobic coverage
Ampicillin-sulbactam • Unasyn • 1.5–3 g IV q6h • Injection					
Antipseudomonal Penicillin + β-Lactamase Inhibitor					
Piperacillin-tazobactam • Zosyn • 3.375 IV q6h or 4.5 g IV q6–8h • Injection	• Same as amoxicillin-clavulanate and ampicillin-sulbactam • *Pseudomonas aeruginosa*	Same as natural penicillins	Same as natural penicillins	Same as natural penicillins	• Adjust dose in renal impairment • Primarily used for *Pseudomonas* infections • Good anaerobic coverage • Contains Na$^+$ (use with caution in volume-overloaded patients)

Cephalosporins (β-Lactams)

Generic • Brand • Dose/Dosage Forms	Spectrum of Activity	Contraindications	Primary Side Effects	Pertinent Drug Interactions	Med Pearl
Mechanism of action – inhibit bacterial cell wall synthesis; bactericidal • As drugs move from 1st through 4th generation, ↑ activity against Gram (−) organisms and ↓ activity against Gram (+) organisms					
First-Generation					
Cefadroxil • Only available generically • 500 mg–1 g PO q12h • Caps, suspension, tabs Cefazolin • Ancef • 250 mg–1 g IV q8h • Injection Cephalexin ☆ • Keflex • 250–500 mg PO q6h • Caps, suspension, tabs	• *Staph. aureus* (MSSA) • *Staph. epidermidis* • *Strep. pyogenes* • *Strep. pneumoniae* • *E. coli* • *P. mirabilis* • *K. pneumoniae*	Allergy to penicillins, cephalosporins, or carbapenems (up to 10% risk of cross-sensitivity)	Same as natural penicillins	Same as natural penicillins	• Adjust dose in renal impairment • Patients on cefazolin (IV) can be switched to cephalexin (PO) • Cefazolin often used for surgical prophylaxis
Second-Generation					
Cefaclor • Only available generically • 250–500 mg PO q8h • Caps, ER tabs, suspension Cefotetan • Cefotan • 1–2 g IV q12h • Injection Cefoxitin • Mefoxin • 1–2 g IV q6–8h • Injection Cefprozil • Only available generically • 250–500 mg q12–24h • Suspension, tabs Cefuroxime • Ceftin, Zinacef • 250–500 mg PO q12h • 500 mg–1.5 g IV q8h • Injection, suspension, tabs	• Gram (+) activity similar to 1st-generation agents • Same Gram (−) activity as 1st-generation agents, but with added activity against *Acinetobacter, Citrobacter, Enterobacter, Neisseria, Serratia,* and *H. influenzae* • Anaerobes (cefotetan and cefoxitin only)	Same as 1st-generation agents	• Same as natural penicillins • Bleeding/bruising (with cefotetan and cefoxitin)	• Same as natural penicillins • Disulfiram-like reaction may occur if alcohol is used during treatment with cefotetan • Cefotetan and cefoxitin may ↑ risk of bleeding with warfarin	• Adjust dose in renal impairment • Take cefaclor ER tabs and cefuroxime suspension with food to ↑ absorption

Cephalosporins (β-Lactams) *(cont'd)*

Generic • Brand • Dose/Dosage Forms	Spectrum of Activity	Contraindications	Primary Side Effects	Pertinent Drug Interactions	Med Pearl
Third-Generation					
Cefdinir☆ • Only available generically • 300 mg PO q12h or 600 mg PO daily • Caps, suspension	• Limited Gram (+) activity • More extensive Gram (−) activity vs. 2nd-generation agents • *Pseudomonas aeruginosa* (ceftazidime and ceftazidime-avibactam only)	• Same as 1st-generation agents • Ceftriaxone should be avoided in neonates (↑ risk of hyperbilirubine-mia, kernicterus)	Same as natural penicillins	• Same as natural penicillins • Antacids and iron may ↓ absorption of cefdinir • Antacids and H_2 antagonists may ↓ absorption of cefpodoxime • Ceftriaxone may cause precipitation if given with Ca^{2+}- containing solutions	• Adjust dose for all, except cefoperazone and ceftriaxone, in renal impairment • Take cefpo-doxime and cefditoren tabs with food to ↑ absorption • Take ceftibuten suspension 2 hours before or 1 hour after meals • Ceftriaxone often used for meningitis and sexually trans-mitted diseases (STDs) • Ceftazidime-avi-bactam indicated for complicated intra-abdominal infections (with metronidazole) and complicated UTIs • ↓ efficacy of ceftazidime-avibactam in patients with creatinine clearance (CrCl) 30–50 mL/min
Cefditoren • Spectracef • 200–400 mg PO q12h • Tabs					
Cefixime • Suprax • 400 mg PO daily • Caps, chewable tabs, suspension, tabs					
Cefotaxime • Claforan • 1–2 g IV q8h • Injection					
Cefpodoxime • Only available generically • 100-400 mg PO q12h • Suspension, tabs					
Ceftazidime • Fortaz, Tazicef • 1–2 g IV q8–12h • Injection					
Ceftazidime-avibactam • Avycaz • 2.5 g IV q8h • Injection					
Ceftibuten • Cedax • 400 mg PO daily • Caps, suspension					
Ceftriaxone • Only available generically • 1–2 g IV daily • Injection					

Cephalosporins (β-Lactams) *(cont'd)*

Generic • Brand • Dose/Dosage Forms	Spectrum of Activity	Contraindications	Primary Side Effects	Pertinent Drug Interactions	Med Pearl
Fourth-Generation					
Cefepime • Maxipime • 1–2 g IV q8–12h • Injection	• Gram (+) activity better than 3rd-generation agents • More extensive Gram (−) activity vs. 3rd-generation agents • *Pseudomonas aeruginosa*	Same as 1st-generation agents	Same as natural penicillins	Same as natural penicillins	Adjust dose in renal impairment
Fifth-Generation					
Ceftaroline • Teflaro • 600 mg IV q12h • Injection	• *Staph. aureus* (MSSA and MRSA [for skin infections only]) • *Strep. pyogenes* • *Strep. pneumoniae* • *Klebsiella* • *E. coli* • *H. influenzae*	Same as 1st-generation agents	Same as natural penicillins	Same as natural penicillins	• Indicated for SSTIs and community-acquired pneumonia • Adjust dose in renal impairment
Ceftolozane-tazobactam • Zerbaxa • 1.5 g IV q8h • Injection	• Active against Gram (+) and Gram (−) organisms, including drug-resistant organisms • *Pseudomonas aeruginosa* • Some activity against anaerobes (*Bacteroides fragilis*) • No activity against *Staph. aureus*				• Indicated for complicated intra-abdominal infections (with metronidazole) and complicated UTIs • Adjust dose in renal impairment • ↓ efficacy in patients with CrCl 30–50 mL/min

Carbapenems (β-Lactams)

Generic • Brand • Dose/Dosage Forms	Spectrum of Activity	Contraindications	Primary Side Effects	Pertinent Drug Interactions	Med Pearl
Mechanism of action – inhibit bacterial cell wall synthesis; bactericidal					
Doripenem • Doribax • 500 mg IV q8h • Injection Ertapenem • Invanz • 1 g IV daily • Injection Imipenem-cilastatin • Primaxin • 250 mg–1 g IV q6–12h • Injection Meropenem • Merrem • 500 mg–1 g IV q8h • Injection	• Broad-spectrum (active against Gram [+], Gram [−], and anaerobic organisms) • All, except ertapenem, are active against *Pseudomonas aeruginosa*	Allergy to penicillins, cephalosporins, or carbapenems	• Same as natural penicillins • Seizures (esp. in patients with renal impairment or history of seizure disorder)	• Same as natural penicillins • May ↓ valproic acid levels	• Adjust dose in renal impairment • Risk of seizures is highest with imipenem/cilastatin

Monobactam (β-Lactam)

Generic • Brand • Dose/Dosage Forms	Spectrum of Activity	Contraindications	Primary Side Effects	Pertinent Drug Interactions	Med Pearl
Mechanism of action – inhibits bacterial cell wall synthesis; bactericidal					
Aztreonam • Azactam, Cayston • IV: 500 mg–2 g IV q6–12h • Nebs: 75 mg via nebulization 3× daily (at least 4 hr apart) × 28 days • Injection, nebulizer solution	Only effective against Gram (−) organisms, including *Pseudomonas aeruginosa*	None	Same as natural penicillins	None	• Can be used in patients allergic to penicillins, cephalosporins, or carbapenems • Adjust dose for IV in renal impairment • Cayston used for patients with cystic fibrosis (*Pseudomonas*); do not repeat for 28 days after completion

Aminoglycosides

Generic • Brand • Dose/Dosage Forms	Spectrum of Activity	Contra indications	Primary Side Effects	Pertinent Drug Interactions	Med Pearl
Mechanism of action – inhibit bacterial protein synthesis by binding to the 30S subunit of the bacterial ribosome; bactericidal					
Amikacin • Only available generically • 15 mg/kg IV q24h or 5–7.5 mg/kg IV q8h • Injection Gentamicin • Gentak • 5–7 mg/kg IV q24h or 1–2.5 mg/kg IV q8–12h • Injection, ophthalmic ointment/solution, topical cream/ointment Neomycin • Only available generically • 500 mg–2 g PO q6–8h • Tabs, oral solution Streptomycin • Only available generically • 15 mg/kg/day IM • Injection Tobramycin • Bethkis, Kitabis Pak, TOBI, Tobrex • 5–7 mg/kg IV q24h or 1–2.5 mg/kg IV q8–12h • Caps for inhalation, injection, nebulizer solution, ophthalmic ointment/solution	• Primarily used for Gram (−) organisms (*E.coli, Klebsiella, P. mirabilis, Enterobacter, Acinetobacter, Serratia, Pseudomonas aeruginosa*) • Provide synergistic activity against *Staph., Strep.,* or *Enterococcus* when used with penicillins or vancomycin • Streptomycin and amikacin active against *Mycobacteria* • Neomycin used as prep for bowel surgery or for hepatic encephalopathy	None	• Nephrotoxicity • Ototoxicity (both related to dose and duration of therapy; may be reversible)	• May ↑ effects of neuromuscular blocking agents • ↑ risk of nephrotoxicity when used with amphotericin B, loop diuretics, tacrolimus, cyclosporine, or cisplatin	• Bactericidal effect is concentration-dependent • Target serum concentrations (for traditional dosing): *Amikacin:* Peak = Life-threatening infections: 25–40 mcg/mL; serious infections: 20–25 mcg/mL, UTIs: 15–20 mcg/mL; Trough <8 mcg/mL (The American Thoracic Society [ATS] recommends trough levels of <4–5 mcg/mL for patients with hospital-acquired pneumonia) *Tobramycin and gentamicin:* Peak = 4–10 mcg/mL, depending on the infection; Trough = 0.5–2 mcg/mL for serious infections; <1 mcg/mL for hospital-acquired pneumonia • Target serum concentrations (for extended-interval dosing) (peaks not routinely monitored): *Amikacin:* Trough <8 mcg/mL (The ATS recommends trough levels of <4–5 mcg/mL for patients with hospital-acquired pneumonia) *Tobramycin and gentamicin:* Trough = 0.5–2 mcg/mL for serious infections, <1 mcg/mL for hospital-acquired pneumonia • Bethkis, Kitabis Pak, and TOBI used for patients with cystic fibrosis (*Pseudomonas*)

Macrolides

Generic • Brand • Dose/Dosage Forms	Spectrum of Activity	Contraindications	Primary Side Effects	Pertinent Drug Interactions	Med Pearl
Mechanism of action – inhibit bacterial protein synthesis by binding to the 50S subunit of the bacterial ribosome; bacteriostatic					
Macrolides					
Azithromycin ☆ • AzaSite, Zithromax, Zmax • 250–500 mg PO/IV q24h • Zmax: 2 g PO × 1 • Injection, ophthalmic solution, suspension (IR and ER), tabs Clarithromycin ☆ • Biaxin • IR: 250–500 mg PO q12h • ER: 1,000 mg PO q24h • Suspension, tabs (IR and ER) Erythromycin • E.E.S, Erygel, EryPed, Ery-Tab, Erythrocin, PCE • 250–500 mg PO q6h • 500 mg–1 g IV q6h • Caps, injection, ophthalmic ointment, suspension, tabs, topical gel/ointment/solution Fidaxomicin • Dificid • 200 mg PO q12h • Tabs	• Gram (+) organisms (esp. *Streptococcus*); azithromycin and clarithromycin have better activity against *Streptococcus* than erythromycin • Gram (−) organisms • Atypical organisms (e.g., *Chlamydia pneumoniae*, *Legionella*, *Mycoplasma pneumoniae*) • Azithromycin and clarithromycin active against *Mycobacteria* • Fidaxomicin active against *Clostridium difficile*	QT interval prolongation or concurrent use with other drugs that prolong QT interval (azithromycin, clarithromycin, and erythromycin)	• Prolonged QT interval (azithromycin, clarithromycin, and erythromycin) • N/V/D • Phlebitis (erythromycin IV)	• Clarithromycin and erythromycin are major substrates and inhibitors of CYP3A4 (azithromycin less affected by CYP interactions) • CYP3A4 inhibitors may ↑ risk of side effects of clarithromycin and erythromycin • CYP3A4 inducers may ↓ effects of clarithromycin and erythromycin • Clarithromycin and erythromycin may ↑ effect/toxicity of CYP3A4 substrates • ↑ risk of torsade de pointes (TdP) with other drugs that prolong QT interval (azithromycin, clarithromycin, and erythromycin) • Azithromycin, clarithromycin, and erythromycin may ↑ risk of bleeding with warfarin • Azithromycin, clarithromycin, and erythromycin may ↑ risk of digoxin toxicity	• Azithromycin ER suspension is not interchangeable with IR formulations • 400 mg erythromycin ethylsuccinate (EES) = 250 mg erythromycin base or stearate • Azithromycin, clarithromycin, and erythromycin are good alternatives for patients allergic to penicillin • Take with food to ↓ gastrointestinal (GI) effect • Clarithromycin can be used in three-drug regimen for *H. pylori* • Erythromycin can be used for diabetic gastroparesis and acne • Take ER azithromycin suspension 1 hour before or 2 hours after meals • Take ER clarithromycin tabs with food to ↑ absorption • Azithromycin or erythromycin preferred in pregnancy • Fidaxomicin used to treat *Clostridium difficile*

Tetracyclines

Generic • Brand • Dose/Dosage Forms	Spectrum of Activity	Contraindications	Primary Side Effects	Pertinent Drug Interactions	Med Pearl
Mechanism of action – inhibit bacterial protein synthesis by binding to the 30S subunit of the bacterial ribosome; bacteriostatic					
Demeclocycline • Only available generically • 150 mg PO q6h or 300 mg PO q12h • Tabs Doxycycline ☆ • Acticlate, Doryx, Monodox, Oracea, Vibramycin • 100 mg IV/PO q12h • Caps, delayed-release caps/tabs, injection, suspension, syrup, tabs Minocycline ☆ • Minocin, Solodyn • 100 mg PO q12h • Caps, injection, tabs (IR and ER) Tetracycline • Only available generically • 250–500 mg PO q6–12h • Caps	• Gram (+) organisms • Gram (−) organisms • Atypical organisms	Children ≤8 yr and pregnant/breast-feeding women (may cause permanent teeth discoloration and impaired teeth/bone growth)	• N/V/D • Photosensitivity • Phlebitis (IV) • Vertigo (minocycline) • Intracranial hypertension (pseudotumor cerebri)	• Absorption ↓ with antacids, dairy products, and products containing iron, magnesium, aluminum, calcium, or zinc (separate by 2 hr) • Tetracycline is a CYP3A4 substrate • CYP3A4 inhibitors may ↑ risk of side effects of tetracycline • CYP3A4 inducers may ↓ effects • May ↑ risk of bleeding with warfarin • May ↓ effects of oral contraceptives • Use with isotretinoin may ↑ risk of intracranial hypertension	• Good alternative for patients allergic to penicillin • Demeclocycline also used to treat syndrome of inappropriate antidiuretic hormone secretion (SIADH) • Tetracycline can be used in four-drug regimen for *H. pylori* • All except demeclocycline can be used for acne • Doxycycline is drug of choice for Lyme disease • Take demeclocycline and tetracycline 1 hour before or 2 hours after meals • Do not use after expiration date (can cause Fanconi syndrome) • Adjust dose for all, except doxycycline, in renal impairment

Glycylcyclines

Generic • Brand • Dose/Dosage Forms	Spectrum of Activity	Contraindications	Primary Side Effects	Pertinent Drug Interactions	Med Pearl
Mechanism of action – inhibits bacterial protein synthesis by binding to the 30S subunit of the bacterial ribosome (mechanism similar to tetracyclines); bacteriostatic					
Tigecycline • Tygacil • 100 mg IV × 1, then 50 mg IV q12h • Injection	• Gram (+) organisms (MSSA, MRSA, vancomycin-sensitive *Enterococcus faecalis*) • Gram (−) organisms (*E. coli, Enterobacter, H. influenzae, Klebsiella, Legionella*)	Children ≤8 yr and pregnant/breast-feeding women (may cause permanent teeth discoloration and impaired teeth/bone growth)	• N/V/D • Infusion site reaction • Photosensitivity • Hepatotoxicity • Pancreatitis	May ↑ risk of bleeding with warfarin	• Indicated for complicated SSTIs, complicated intra-abdominal infections, and community-acquired pneumonia • Structurally similar to tetracyclines

Oxazolidinones

Generic • Brand • Dose/Dosage Forms	Spectrum of Activity	Contraindications	Primary Side Effects	Pertinent Drug Interactions	Med Pearl
Mechanism of action – inhibit bacterial protein synthesis by binding to the 50S subunit of the bacterial ribosome; bacteriostatic					
Linezolid ☆ • Zyvox • 400–600 mg IV/PO q12h • Injection, suspension, tabs	Gram (+) organisms (vancomycin-resistant *Enterococcus faecium* [VRE], MRSA, resistant *Strep. pneumoniae*)	• Concurrent or recent (within 2 wk) use of MAO inhibitors (MAOI) • Patients with uncontrolled hypertension, pheochromocytoma, thyrotoxicosis, and/or taking sympathomimetic agents (e.g., pseudoephedrine), vasopressor agents (e.g., epinephrine), or dopaminergic agents (e.g., dopamine) • Concurrent use of selective serotonin reuptake inhibitors, tricyclic antidepressants, 5-HT$_1$ receptor agonists (triptans), meperidine or buspirone	• N/V/D • Headache • Myelosuppression (more common if therapy >2 wk) • Peripheral/optic neuropathy (more common if therapy >4 wk) • Seizures	• Avoid taking with foods or beverages with high tyramine content (may ↑ risk of hypertensive crises) • Use with serotonergic agents may ↑ risk of serotonin syndrome; avoid concurrent use • Use with adrenergic agents (e.g., dopamine, epinephrine) may ↑ risk of hypertensive crises • Use with tramadol may ↑ risk of seizures • Use with insulin or oral hypoglycemic agents may ↑ risk of hypoglycemia	• Indicated for nosocomial/community-acquired pneumonia, SSTIs, and VRE • Weak MAOI • Monitor complete blood count (CBC) weekly if therapy >2 wk
Tedizolid • Sivextro • 200 mg IV/PO q24h × 6 days • Injection, tabs	Gram (+) organisms (MSSA, MRSA, *Enterococcus faecalis, Streptococcus*)	None	• N/V/D • Headache • Dizziness	None	• Indicated for SSTIs • Weak MAOI

Streptogramin

Generic • Brand • Dose/Dosage Forms	Spectrum of Activity	Contraindications	Primary Side Effects	Pertinent Drug Interactions	Med Pearl
Mechanism of action – inhibits bacterial protein synthesis by binding to the 50S subunit of the bacterial ribosome; bactericidal					
Quinupristin-dalfopristin • Synercid • 7.5 mg/kg IV q8–12h • Injection	Gram (+) organisms (MSSA and *Strep. pyogenes*)	None	• N/V/D • Infusion site reactions (pain, phlebitis) • Muscle/joint pain • ↑ bilirubin	• CYP3A4 inhibitor • May ↑ effect/toxicity of CYP3A4 substrates	• Indicated for complicated SSTIs • Flush line with D5W before and after infusion • If infusion reaction occurs, can ↑ volume of diluent or administer via central line

Fluoroquinolones

Generic • Brand • Dose/Dosage Forms	Spectrum of Activity	Contraindications	Primary Side Effects	Pertinent Drug Interactions	Med Pearl
Mechanism of action – inhibit bacterial DNA topoisomerase and gyrase → inhibit bacterial DNA replication; bactericidal					
Besifloxacin • Besivance • 1 drop TID • Ophthalmic solution Ciprofloxacin ☆ • Cetraxal, Ciloxan, Cipro, Cipro XR • IR: 250–750 mg PO q12h • ER: 500 mg–1 g PO q24h • IV: 200–400 mg IV q8–12h • Injection, ophthalmic ointment/solution, suspension, otic solution, tabs (ER and IR) Gatifloxacin • Zymaxid • 1 drop q2h while awake on day 1, then 1 drop 2–4 times/day while awake • Ophthalmic solution Gemifloxacin • Factive • 320 mg PO q24h • Tabs Levofloxacin ☆ • Levaquin • 250–750 mg IV/PO q24h • Injection, ophthalmic solution, solution, tabs Moxifloxacin ☆ • Avelox, Moxeza, Vigamox • 400 mg IV/PO q24h • Injection, ophthalmic solution, tabs Ofloxacin • Ocuflox • 200–400 mg PO q12h • Ophthalmic solution, otic solution, tabs	• Gram (+) organisms (levofloxacin, gemifloxacin, and moxifloxacin have greatest activity against *Streptococcus*) • Gram (−) organisms • Ciprofloxacin active against *Pseudomonas aeruginosa* • Atypical organisms	• Children <18 yr and pregnant/breastfeeding women (may cause impaired bone growth) • Concurrent use with other drugs that prolong QT interval • Myasthenia gravis	• N/D • Photosensitivity • Tendinitis/tendon rupture • Hyper-/hypoglycemia • Peripheral neuropathy • Seizures • Prolonged QT interval	• Absorption ↓ with antacids, dairy products, and products containing iron, magnesium, aluminum, calcium, or zinc (separate by 2 hours) • Use with corticosteroids may ↑ risk of tendon rupture • Use with nonsteroidal anti-inflammatory drugs (NSAIDs) may ↑ risk of seizures • Ciprofloxacin and ofloxacin are strong CYP1A2 inhibitors • Ciprofloxacin and ofloxacin may ↑ effects of CYP1A2 substrates • Ciprofloxacin may ↓ phenytoin levels • May ↑ risk of bleeding with warfarin • Use with antidiabetic agents may ↑ risk of hypoglycemia • ↑ risk of TdP with other drugs that prolong QT interval	• Ciprofloxacin ER and IR tabs are not interchangeable • Adjust dose for all, except moxifloxacin, in renal impairment • Take levofloxacin oral solution 1 hour before or 2 hours after meals • Patients with diabetes should monitor their blood glucose more frequently • Ciprofloxacin, levofloxacin, and moxifloxacin can be used to treat plague (*Yersinia pestis*) • Ophthalmic preparations used to treat bacterial conjunctivitis

Sulfonamide

Generic • Brand • Dose/Dosage Forms	Spectrum of Activity	Contraindications	Primary Side Effects	Pertinent Drug Interactions	Med Pearl
Mechanism of action – inhibits incorporation of para-aminobenzoic acid (PABA) into DNA → inhibits folic acid production and bacterial growth; bacteriostatic					
Trimethoprim/sulfamethoxazole ☆ • Bactrim, Septra, Sulfatrim • 1 double-strength tab PO q12h • 10–20 mg/kg/day of TMP IV in divided doses • Injection, suspension, tabs	• Gram (+) organisms (including MSSA, MRSA) • Gram (−) organisms • TMP/SMX is 1st-line drug to treat/prevent *Pneumocystis jiroveci* pneumonia (PJP)	• Sulfa allergy • Porphyria • Megaloblastic anemia • Infants and pregnant/breast-feeding women (↑ risk of kernicterus) • Glucose-6-phosphate dehydrogenase (G6PD) deficiency	• N/V/D • Rash • Stevens-Johnson syndrome • Photosensitivity • Folate deficiency • Hypoglycemia (in patients with diabetes)	• May ↑ effects/toxicity of methotrexate • May ↑ risk of bleeding with warfarin • Use with antidiabetic agents may ↑ risk of hypoglycemia	• Instruct patients to take with a full glass of water (to prevent crystalluria) • Adjust dose in renal impairment

Cyclic Lipopeptide

Generic • Brand • Dose/Dosage Forms	Spectrum of Activity	Contraindications	Primary Side Effects	Pertinent Drug Interactions	Med Pearl
Mechanism of action – binds to bacterial cell membranes and causes rapid depolarization → inhibits protein, DNA, and RNA synthesis; bactericidal					
Daptomycin • Cubicin • 4–6 mg/kg IV q24h • Injection	Gram (+) organisms (MSSA, MRSA, vancomycin-sensitive *Enterococcus faecalis*)	Children <1 yr (↑ risk of muscular, neuromuscular, and/or central nervous system [CNS] toxicity)	• N/D • Infusion site reactions • Myopathy/rhabdomyolysis • Peripheral neuropathy	Use with statins may ↑ risk of myopathy; consider discontinuing statin therapy throughout treatment	• Monitor creatine kinase levels weekly • Adjust dose in renal impairment • Indicated for complicated SSTIs and *Staph. aureus* bloodstream infections

Glycopeptides

Generic • Brand • Dose/Dosage Forms	Spectrum of Activity	Contraindications	Primary Side Effects	Pertinent Drug Interactions	Med Pearl
Mechanism of action – inhibit bacterial cell wall synthesis; bactericidal					
Dalbavancin • Dalvance • 1,000 mg IV × 1, then 500 mg IV 1 wk later **OR** 1,500 mg IV × 1 • Injection	Gram (+) organisms (MSSA, MRSA, *Streptococcus*, vancomycin-sensitive Enterococcus faecalis)	None	• Hypersensitivity reactions • Headache • N/D • Red-man syndrome (flushing, hypotension, erythema, pruritus)	None	• Indicated for SSTIs • Adjust dose in renal impairment • If red-man syndrome occurs, ↓ infusion rate
Oritavancin • Orbactiv • 1,200 mg IV × 1 • Injection	Gram (+) organisms (MSSA, MRSA, *Streptococcus*, vancomycin-sensitive *Enterococcus faecalis*)	Use of IV unfractionated heparin × 5 days after administration	• Hypersensitivity reactions • Headache • N/V/D • Red-man syndrome	May ↑ risk of bleeding with warfarin	• Indicated for SSTIs • If red-man syndrome occurs, ↓ infusion rate • May falsely ↑ prothrombin time (PT), international normalized ratio (INR), activated partial thromboplastin time (aPTT), and activated clotting time (ACT) (PT/INR effects can last up to 12 hr after discontinuation; aPTT effects can last up to 5 days after discontinuation; ACT effects can last up to 24 hr after discontinuation)

Glycopeptides *(cont'd)*

Generic • Brand • Dose/Dosage Forms	Spectrum of Activity	Contraindications	Primary Side Effects	Pertinent Drug Interactions	Med Pearl
Telavancin • Vibativ • 10 mg/kg IV q24h • Injection	Gram (+) organisms (MSSA, MRSA, *Streptococcus*, vancomycin-sensitive *Enterococcus faecalis*)	• Pregnancy • Concurrent use of IV unfractionated heparin	• Hypersensitivity reactions • Insomnia • Headache • Nephrotoxicity • Red-man syndrome • Metallic taste • N/V/D • QT interval prolongation	• ↑ risk of nephrotoxicity when used with amphotericin B, loop diuretics, tacrolimus, cyclosporine, or cisplatin • ↑ risk of TdP with other drugs that prolong QT interval	• Indicated for complicated SSTIs and hospital-acquired and ventilator-associated pneumonia • ↑ risk of mortality in hospital-acquired and ventilator-associated pneumonia in patients with CrCl ≤50 mL/min • Adjust dose in renal impairment • Monitor renal function • If red-man syndrome occurs, ↓ infusion rate • May falsely ↑ PT, INR, aPTT, and ACT (can last up to 18 hr after discontinuation) • Has REMS program
Vancomycin • Vancocin • 125–250 mg PO q6h • 500 mg–1 g IV q12h • Caps, injection	• Gram (+) organisms (MSSA, MRSA) • *Clostridium difficile*	None	• Red-man syndrome • Nephrotoxicity • Ototoxicity	↑ risk of nephrotoxicity when used with amphotericin B, loop diuretics, tacrolimus, cyclosporine, or cisplatin	• Bactericidal effect is time-dependent • Adjust dose in renal impairment • Often used in patients with penicillin allergy • Use PO (NOT IV) to treat *Clostridium difficile* (PO not effective for any other type of infection) • If red-man syndrome occurs, ↓ infusion rate • Target serum concentrations (peaks not routinely monitored); trough ≥10 mcg/mL (15–20 mcg/mL for complicated infections)

Miscellaneous Antibacterial Agents

Generic • Brand • Dose/Dosage Forms	Spectrum of Activity	Contraindications	Primary Side Effects	Pertinent Drug Interactions	Med Pearl
Mechanism of action – inhibits bacterial protein synthesis by binding to the 50S subunit of the bacterial ribosome; bacteriostatic					
Chloramphenicol • Only available generically • 12.5–25 mg/kg IV q6h • Injection	• Gram (+) organisms (VRE) • Gram (−) organisms	Neonates (↑ risk of gray-baby syndrome)	• N/V/D • Myelosuppression (anemia, leukopenia, thrombocytopenia, aplastic anemia) • Gray-baby syndrome (vomiting, lethargy, respiratory depression, death) • Optic neuritis	• Phenobarbital and rifampin may ↓ effects • May ↑ effects of warfarin and phenytoin	• Only used for life-threatening infections • Monitor CBC frequently • Target serum concentrations: Peak = 15–25 mcg/mL; Trough = 5–10 mcg/mL
Mechanism of action – inhibits bacterial protein synthesis by binding to the 50S subunit of the bacterial ribosome; bacteriostatic					
Clindamycin ☆ • Cleocin, Clindagel, Clindesse, Evoclin • 150–450 mg PO q6h • 300–900 mg IV q8h • Caps, injection, solution, topical foam/gel/lotion/pledgets/solution, vaginal cream/suppository	• Gram (+) organisms • Anaerobes	History of pseudomembranous colitis or ulcerative colitis	• N/V/D • Pseudomembranous colitis (*Clostridium difficile*) (highest incidence) • Metallic taste	None	• Also used for acne (topical) • Patients using intravaginally should avoid intercourse (↓ efficacy of condoms and diaphragms)
Mechanism of action – interferes with bacterial DNA synthesis; bactericidal					
Metronidazole ☆ • Flagyl, Metro, Metrocream, Metrogel, Metrolotion, Noritate, Nuvessa, Vandazole • 250–500 mg PO q8–12h • 500 mg IV q8–12h • Caps, injection, tabs (ER and IR), topical cream/gel/lotion, vaginal gel	• Anaerobes • *Clostridium difficile*	Pregnancy (1st trimester)	• N/D • Confusion • Dizziness • Peripheral neuropathy • Metallic taste	• Disulfiram-like reaction may occur if alcohol is used during treatment • May ↑ effects of warfarin and lithium • Phenobarbital and phenytoin may ↓ effects • Cimetidine may ↑ effects	• Can be used in four-drug regimen for *H. pylori* • Drug of choice for *Clostridium difficile* • Take ER tabs 1 hour before or 2 hours after meals

Antifungal Agents

Azole Antifungals

Generic • Brand • Dose/Dosage Forms	Spectrum of Activity	Contraindications	Primary Side Effects	Pertinent Drug Interactions	Med Pearl
Mechanism of action – inhibit synthesis of ergosterol (essential component of fungal cell membrane) • Imidazoles: butoconazole, clotrimazole, econazole, efinaconazole, ketoconazole, luliconazole, miconazole, oxiconazole, sulconazole, tioconazole • Triazoles: fluconazole, itraconazole, isavuconazonium terconazole, posaconazole, voriconazole					
Fluconazole ☆ • Diflucan • 100–800 mg IV/PO q24h • Injection, suspension, tabs	• *Candida* spp. • *Coccidioides* spp. • *Histoplasma* spp. • *Cryptococcus* spp.	None	• Headache • N/V/D • Abdominal pain • Rash • ↑ liver function tests (LFTs) • Prolonged QT interval	• CYP2C9, CYP2C19, and CYP3A4 inhibitor • May ↑ effect/toxicity of CYP2C9, CYP2C19, and CYP3A4 substrates • Rifampin may ↓ effects • ↑ risk of TdP with other drugs that prolong QT interval	• Adjust dose in renal impairment • Conversion from IV to PO is 1:1 • Monitor LFTs
Isavuconazonium • Cresemba • 372 mg IV/PO q8h × 6 doses (48 hr), then 372 mg IV/PO q24h • Caps, injection	• *Aspergillus* spp. • *Mucormycetes* spp.	• Concurrent use of strong CYP3A4 inhibitors or inducers • Familial short QT syndrome	• ↑ LFTs • Infusion reactions • Rash • N/V/D • Headache • Shortened QT interval	• CYP3A4 substrate and inhibitor • CYP3A4 inhibitors may ↑ risk of side effects • CYP3A4 inducers may ↓ effects • May ↑ effect/toxicity of CYP3A4 substrates • ↑ risk of digoxin toxicity	Monitor LFTs
Itraconazole • Sporanox, Onmel • 100–400 mg/day PO • Caps, solution, tabs	• *Candida* spp. • *Coccidioides* spp. • *Histoplasma* spp. • *Cryptococcus* spp. • *Aspergillus* spp.	• Concurrent use of dofetilide, ergot alkaloids, lovastatin, midazolam, pimozide, quinidine, simvastatin, or triazolam • HF	• Nausea • Abdominal pain • Rash • ↑ LFTs • Prolonged QT interval	• CYP3A4 substrate and inhibitor • CYP3A4 inhibitors may ↑ risk of side effects • CYP3A4 inducers may ↓ effects • May ↑ effect/toxicity of CYP3A4 substrates • ↑ risk of digoxin toxicity • Absorption ↓ with antacids, H$_2$ antagonists, and proton pump inhibitors (PPIs) (acidic environment required for absorption) (separate by 2 hr) • ↑ risk of TdP with other drugs that prolong QT interval	• Caps and solution cannot be used interchangeably (bioavailability of solution > caps) • Potent negative inotrope • Monitor LFTs
Ketoconazole ☆ • Extina, Nizoral, Xolegel • 200–400 mg PO q24h • Rx: Tabs, topical cream/foam/gel/shampoo • OTC: Shampoo	• *Candida* spp. • *Coccidioides* spp. • *Histoplasma* spp. • *Cryptococcus* spp.	• Concurrent use of ergot alkaloids • Hepatic impairment	• N/V • Gynecomastia • Sexual dysfunction • ↑ LFTs • Prolonged QT interval	Same as itraconazole	• May ↓ testosterone levels • Monitor LFTs

Azole Antifungals *(cont'd)*

Generic • Brand • Dose/Dosage Forms	Spectrum of Activity	Contraindications	Primary Side Effects	Pertinent Drug Interactions	Med Pearl
Posaconazole • Noxafil • 300 mg IV/PO (tabs) q12h × 1 day, then 300 mg IV/PO (tabs) q24h • 200 mg PO TID (suspension) (for prophylaxis); 100 mg PO BID × 1 day, then 100 mg PO q24h × 13 days (suspension) (for treatment) • Injection, suspension, tabs	• *Candida* spp. • *Aspergillus* spp.	Concurrent use of ergot alkaloids, quinidine, pimozide, sirolimus, atorvastatin, lovastatin, or simvastatin	• Headache • N/V • Rash • ↑ LFTs • Prolonged QT interval	• CYP3A4 inhibitor • May ↑ effect/toxicity of CYP3A4 substrates • Absorption of suspension ↓ with cimetidine and esomeprazole (avoid concurrent use) • Metoclopramide may ↓ effects of suspension • Efavirenz, fosamprenavir, rifabutin, and phenytoin may ↓ effects • ↑ risk of TdP with other drugs that prolong QT interval	• Tabs and suspension cannot be used interchangeably • Take tabs with food to ↑ absorption • Suspension must be taken with full meal (or liquid nutritional supplement or acidic carbonated beverage) to ↑ absorption • IV and tabs ONLY used for prophylaxis of invasive *Aspergillus* or *Candida* infections • Use PO when CrCl <50 mL/min (diluent in IV can accumulate) • Monitor LFTs
Voriconazole • Vfend • 6 mg/kg IV q12h × 24 hr, then 3–4 mg/kg IV q12h or 100–300 mg PO q12h • Injection, suspension, tabs	• *Candida* spp. • *Aspergillus* spp.	Concurrent use of pimozide, quinidine, long-acting barbiturates, carbamazepine, ergot alkaloids, rifampin, rifabutin, ritonavir (≥ 800 mg/day), efavirenz (≥ 800 mg/day), St. John's wort, or sirolimus	• Visual disturbances (transient) (blurred vision, photophobia, altered perception of color) • Rash • Photosensitivity • ↑ LFTs • Hallucinations • N/V • Prolonged QT interval	• CYP2C9 and CYP2C19 substrate • CYP2C9, CYP2C19, and CYP3A4 inhibitor • May ↑ effect/toxicity of CYP2C9, CYP2C19, and CYP3A4 substrates • CYP2C9 and CYP2C19 inhibitors may ↑ risks of side effects • CYP2C9 and CYP2C19 inducers may ↓ effects • May ↑ efavirenz levels • Efavirenz may ↓ effects • ↑ risk of TdP with other drugs that prolong QT interval	• ↓ dose of cyclosporine by 50% • When using with efavirenz, ↑ voriconazole dose and ↓ efavirenz dose • ↑ dose of voriconazole when using with phenytoin • Use PO when CrCl <50 mL/min (diluent in IV can accumulate) • Take PO 1 hour before or after meals • Monitor LFTs and vision

Echinocandins

Generic • Brand • Dose/Dosage Forms	Spectrum of Activity	Contraindications	Primary Side Effects	Pertinent Drug Interactions	Med Pearl
Mechanism of action – inhibit synthesis of 1,3-β-d-glucan (essential component of fungal cell wall)					
Anidulafungin • Eraxis • 100–200 mg IV on day 1, then 50–100 mg IV q24h • Injection	• *Candida* spp. • *Aspergillus* spp. (caspofungin only)	None	• N/V • Headache • Hypokalemia • Rash • Fever • ↑ LFTs • Phlebitis	None	Monitor LFTs
Caspofungin • Cancidas • 70 mg IV on day 1, then 50 mg IV q24h • Injection				• Rifampin, carbamazepine, dexamethasone, efavirenz, nevirapine, and phenytoin may ↓ effects • May ↓ tacrolimus levels • Cyclosporine may ↑ risk of side effects	• ↑ dose of caspofungin to 70 mg/day when used with rifampin, carbamazepine, dexamethasone, efavirenz, nevirapine, or phenytoin • Adjust dose in moderate hepatic impairment • Monitor LFTs
Micafungin • Mycamine • 50–150 mg IV q24h • Injection				None	Monitor LFTs

Amphotericin B

Generic • Brand • Dose/Dosage Forms	Spectrum of Activity	Contraindications	Primary Side Effects	Pertinent Drug Interactions	Med Pearl
Mechanism of action – bind to ergosterol in cell membrane → produce a channel in cell membrane ($\uparrow$ permeability) → allow K^+ and Mg^{2+} to leak out of cell ("leaky membrane") → cell death					
Amphotericin B desoxycholate • Only available generically • Test dose of 1 mg IV should be given over 20–30 min (monitor patient for 2–4 hr before starting infusion) • 0.5–1.5 mg/kg/day IV • Injection Amphotericin B lipid complex (ABLC) • Abelcet • 5 mg/kg IV q24h • Injection Liposomal amphotericin B (L-AmB) • AmBisome • 3–6 mg/kg IV q24h • Injection	• *Candida* spp. • *Coccidioides* spp. • *Blastomyces* spp. • *Histoplasma* spp. • *Cryptococcus* spp. • *Aspergillus* spp.	None	• Nephrotoxicity (less common with lipid-based formulations) • Infusion reactions (fever, chills, hypotension, nausea, tachypnea) • Phlebitis • Electrolyte disturbances (i.e., hypokalemia, hypomagnesemia)	$\uparrow$ risk of nephrotoxicity when used with aminoglycosides, loop diuretics, tacrolimus, cyclosporine, or cisplatin	• May premedicate with acetaminophen, NSAIDs, diphenhydramine, and/or corticosteroid to prevent infusion reactions (give 30–60 min before infusion); meperidine may be used for rigors • Infusion reactions less common with lipid-based formulations (amphotericin B deoxycholate > ABLC > L-Amb) • Infusion reactions $\downarrow$ after first few doses • Sodium loading (500 mL of 0.9% NaCl IV before and after infusion) may $\downarrow$ risk of nephrotoxicity with amphotericin B desoxycholate • Monitor blood urea nitrogen (BUN)/serum creatinine (SCr), potassium, and magnesium

Other Antifungals

Generic • Brand • Dose/Dosage Forms	Spectrum of Activity	Contraindications	Primary Side Effects	Pertinent Drug Interactions	Med Pearl
Mechanism of action – similar to amphotericin B					
Nystatin ☆ • Nystop • Suspension: 400,000–600,000 units 4 times/day • Topical: Apply 2–3 times daily • Suspension, tabs, topical cream/ointment/powder	*Candida* spp.	None	• N/V/D • Abdominal pain	None	Suspension should be swished and swallowed
Mechanism of action – inhibits squalene epoxidase → inhibits synthesis of ergosterol					
Terbinafine ☆ • Lamisil • PO: 250 mg q24h • Topical: Apply 1–2 times daily • Rx: Granules, tabs, topical solution • OTC: Topical cream/gel/solution	*Trichophyton* spp.	• Hepatic impairment • CrCl <50 mL/min	• Headache • N/V/D • ↑ LFTs	• CYP2D6 inhibitor • May ↑ effect/toxicity of CYP2D6 substrates • May ↓ cyclosporine levels	• Oral used for onychomycosis or tinea capitis (scalp ringworm); topical used for tinea pedis (athlete's foot), tinea corporis (ringworm), or tinea cruris (jock itch) • Give for 6 wk for fingernail infection; 12 wk for toenail infection • Monitor LFTs
Mechanism of action – inhibits fungal protein synthesis					
Tavaborole • Kerydin • Apply once daily × 48 wk • Topical solution	*Trichophyton* spp.	None	Application reactions	None	Indicated for onychomycosis

Other Antifungals *(cont'd)*

Generic • Brand • Dose/Dosage Forms	Spectrum of Activity	Contraindications	Primary Side Effects	Pertinent Drug Interactions	Med Pearl
Mechanism of action – enters fungal cell wall → converted into 5-fluorouracil, which interferes with fungal RNA and protein synthesis					
Flucytosine • Ancobon • 25–37.5 mg/kg PO q6h (administered with amphotericin B) • Caps	• *Candida* spp. • *Cryptococcus* spp.	None	• Confusion • Hallucinations • Ataxia • Headache • N/V/D • ↑ LFTs • Renal impairment • Bone marrow depression	None	• Should not be used as monotherapy • Adjust dose in renal impairment • Monitor LFTs, BUN/SCr, and CBC • Flucytosine concentrations: Peak: 50–100 mcg/mL; Trough: 25–50 mcg/mL
Mechanism of action – inhibits fungal cell mitosis					
Griseofulvin • Gris-PEG • Microsize: 500–1,000 mg/day PO • Ultramicrosize: 375 mg/day PO • Microsize: Suspension, tabs • Ultramicrosize: Tabs	*Trichophyton* spp.	• Hepatic impairment • Porphyria	• Rash/hives • N/V/D • Headache • Confusion • Photosensitivity	• Barbiturates may ↓ effects • May ↓ effects of cyclosporine and warfarin • Disulfiram-like reaction may occur if alcohol is used during treatment	• Monitor LFTs • Administer with high-fat meal to ↑ absorption

Antiviral Agents

Drugs for Treatment of Herpes Simplex Virus and Varicella-Zoster Virus

Generic • Brand • Dose/Dosage Forms	Spectrum of Activity	Contraindications	Primary Side Effects	Pertinent Drug Interactions	Med Pearl
Mechanism of action – inhibit viral DNA polymerase → inhibit replication of viral DNA					
Acyclovir☆ • Sitavig, Zovirax • *Genital herpes (initial episode):* 200 mg PO 5 times/day × 7–10 days **OR** 5 mg/kg IV q8h × 5–7 days • *Herpes labialis (cold sores):* 400 mg PO 5 times/day × 5 days • *Varicella (chickenpox):* 800 mg PO q6h × 5 days **OR** 10 mg/kg IV q8h × 7 days • *Herpes zoster (shingles):* 800 mg PO 5 times/day × 7–10 days **OR** 10 mg/kg IV q8h × 7 days • Buccal tabs, caps, injection, suspension, tabs, topical cream/ointment	• Herpes simplex virus (HSV)-1 (herpes labialis) and HSV-2 (genital herpes) • Varicella zoster virus (causes chickenpox and shingles)	None	• N/V/D • Headache • Phlebitis (IV acyclovir) • Renal impairment (IV acyclovir) • Seizures (esp. in patients with renal impairment)	None	• Adjust dose for all, except penciclovir, in renal impairment • To avoid renal damage with IV acyclovir (can crystallize), infuse slowly and keep patient hydrated • Sitavig is a buccal tab for treatment of recurrent cold sores
Famciclovir☆ (prodrug of penciclovir) • Famvir • *Genital herpes (initial episode):* 250 mg PO q8h × 7–10 days • *Cold sores:* 1,500 mg PO × 1 • *Herpes zoster:* 500 mg PO q8h × 7 days • Tabs					
Penciclovir • Denavir • *Cold sores:* Apply q2h while awake × 4 days • Topical cream					
Valacyclovir☆ (prodrug of acyclovir) • Valtrex • *Genital herpes (initial episode):* 1 g PO q12h × 10 days • *Genital herpes (recurrence):* 500 mg PO q12h × 3 days • *Cold sores:* 2 g PO q12h × 1 day • *Herpes zoster:* 1 g PO q8h × 7 days • Tabs					

Drugs for Treatment of Cytomegalovirus

Generic • Brand • Dose/Dosage Forms	Spectrum of Activity	Contraindications	Primary Side Effects	Pertinent Drug Interactions	Med Pearl
Mechanism of action – inhibit replication of viral DNA					
Cidofovir • Only available generically • 5 mg/kg IV once weekly × 2 wk, then q2 wk • Injection	• Cytomegalovirus • HSV (foscarnet) • Acute herpetic keratitis (ophthalmic gangiclovir)	• SCr >1.5 mg/dL, CrCl ≤55 mL/min, or proteinuria • Use of other nephrotoxic drugs within 7 days	• Nephrotoxicity • Neutropenia • Metabolic acidosis • ↓ intraocular pressure • Uveitis/iritis	Use of antiretroviral drugs may ↑ risk of side effects	• Monitor BUN/SCr • To minimize renal damage, administer 1 L of 0.9% NaCl before and after each infusion; also give 2 g of probenecid 3 hr before each infusion and then 1 g at 2 hr and 8 hr after each infusion • If SCr ↑ by 0.3–0.4 mg/dL above baseline, ↓ dose to 3 mg/kg; if SCr ↑ by ≥0.5 mg/dL, discontinue • Advise patients to use effective contraception
Foscarnet • Foscavir • 60 mg/kg IV q8h **OR** 90 mg/kg IV q12h × 14–21 days, then 90–120 mg/kg IV q24h • Injection		None	• Nephrotoxicity • N/V • Anemia • Electrolyte disturbances • Genital sores • Seizures	• ↑ risk of nephrotoxicity when used with amphotericin B, aminoglycosides, loop diuretics, tacrolimus, cyclosporine, or cisplatin • Zidovudine may ↑ risk of anemia	• Adjust dose in renal impairment • Monitor BUN/SCr • To minimize renal damage, administer 1 L of 0.9% NaCl IV with each infusion • Rapid infusion associated with seizures and arrhythmias
Ganciclovir • Cytovene, Zirgan • IV: 5 mg/kg q12h × 14–21 days, then either 5 mg/kg/day 7 times/wk or 6 mg/kg/day 5 times/wk • Ophth: 1 drop 5 times/day until ulcer heals, then 1 drop 3 times/day × 7 days • Injection, ophthalmic gel		• Neutropenia • Thrombocytopenia • Anemia	• Myelosuppression • Fever • Rash • Phlebitis (IV ganciclovir) • ↑ LFTs • Nephrotoxicity • Seizures • N/V/D	• ↑ risk of myelosuppression when used with other immunosuppressive drugs • ↑ risk of nephrotoxicity when used with amphotericin B, aminoglycosides, loop diuretics, tacrolimus, cyclosporine, or cisplatin • May ↑ effects/toxicity of zidovudine	• Adjust dose in renal impairment • Advise patients to use effective contraception during treatment and for at least 90 days after treatment • Take valganciclovir with food
Valganciclovir (prodrug of ganciclovir) • Valcyte • 900 mg PO q12h × 21 days, then 900 mg PO q24h • Solution, tabs					

Drugs for Treatment of Influenza

Generic • Brand • Dose/Dosage Forms	Spectrum of Activity	Contraindications	Primary Side Effects	Pertinent Drug Interactions	Med Pearl
Mechanism of action – inhibit the enzyme (neuraminidase) responsible for releasing the newly formed mature virus from the host cell					
Oseltamivir • Tamiflu • *Prophylaxis:* 75 mg PO q24h × ≥10 days (6 wk for community outbreak) • *Treatment:* 75 mg PO q12h × 5 days • Caps, suspension	• Influenza A and B • H1N1 influenza	None	• N/V/D • Headache • Rash • Neuropsychiatric events (e.g., confusion, delirium, hallucinations, self-injury)	None	• For prophylaxis, initiate therapy within 2 days of contact with infected person • For treatment, initiate therapy within 2 days of onset of symptoms • Adjust dose in renal impairment • ↓ flu severity and duration by ~ 1 day • Can be used in children ≥1 yr (prophylaxis) or ≥2 wk (treatment)
Peramivir • Rapivab • *Treatment:* 600 mg IV × 1 • Injection			• Rash • Neuropsychiatric events (e.g., confusion, delirium, hallucinations, self-injury)		• Initiate therapy within 2 days of onset of symptoms • For adults only • Adjust dose in renal impairment
Zanamivir • Relenza • *Prophylaxis:* 2 inhalations q24h × 10 days (28 days for community outbreak) • *Treatment:* 2 inhalations q12h × 5 days • Powder for oral inhalation		Asthma/COPD	• Bronchospasm • Cough • Headache • N/D • Rash • Neuropsychiatric events (e.g., confusion, delirium, hallucinations, self-injury)		• For prophylaxis, initiate therapy within 1.5 days (5 days in community setting) of contact with infected person • For treatment, initiate therapy within 2 days of onset of symptoms • ↓ flu severity and duration by ~ 1 day • Can be used in children ≥5 yr (prophylaxis) or ≥7 yr (treatment)

HUMAN IMMUNODEFICIENCY VIRUS

Definitions

HIV is a human retrovirus that infects lymphocytes and other cells that bear the CD4 surface protein. Infection leads to CD4 T-cell depletion, impaired cell-mediated immunity, and polyclonal B-cell activation. Over time, this immune system dysfunction leads to acquired immune deficiency syndrome (AIDS) and illnesses such as opportunistic infections and malignancies.

Diagnosis

- The CDC recommends routine HIV screening for adults, adolescents and pregnant women in healthcare settings in the United States.
- Persons at a high risk for HIV infection should be screened for HIV at least annually:
  - Healthcare workers, intravenous drug users, men who have sex with men, hemophiliacs, sexual partners of persons living with HIV, commercial sex workers and their partners, persons with a history of sexually transmitted infections, and persons with multiple sex partners or those with a history of unprotected sexual encounters
- Pregnant women should receive HIV testing during the routine panel of prenatal screening tests.
- Laws requiring informed consent for HIV testing vary depending upon the state. Most states have adopted the "opt-out" testing strategy recommended by the CDC. This strategy notifies a patient that HIV screening will be taking place unless the patient declines.
- Screening for HIV is performed with an enzyme-linked immunosorbent assay (ELISA) test. Positive results must always be confirmed with a Western blot.

Signs and Symptoms

Acute HIV infection most commonly presents with a "flu-like" illness that resolves within 2–4 weeks. After acute infection, patients may remain symptom-free for ≥8–9 years. As the virus continues to multiply and destroy immune cells, the patient may develop chronic symptoms such as:

- Swollen lymph nodes, diarrhea, weight loss, rash, fever, cough, and shortness of breath

When a patient's CD4 cell count declines to <200 cells/mm^3, the immune system is significantly compromised and the patient is at an increased risk for opportunistic infections such as:

- Oropharyngeal candidiasis, *PJP* pneumonia, *Toxoplasma gondii*, *Cryptococcus neoformans*, and *Mycobacterium avium intracellulare*

Guidelines

Panel on Antiretroviral Guidelines for Adults and Adolescents. Guidelines for the use of antiretroviral agents in HIV-1-infected adults and adolescents. Department of Health and Human Services. Available at www.aidsinfo.nih.gov/ContentFiles/AdultandAdolescentGL.pdf. Accessed July 20, 2016.

Panel on Opportunistic Infections in HIV-Infected Adults and Adolescents. Guidelines for the prevention and treatment of opportunistic infections in HIV-infected adults and adolescents: recommendations from the Centers for Disease Control and Prevention, the National Institutes of Health, and the HIV Medicine Association of the Infectious Diseases Society of America. Available at http://aidsinfo.nih.gov/contentfiles/lvguidelines/adult_oi.pdf. Accessed July 20, 2016.

Guidelines Summary

For the NAPLEX®, make learning the names of the medications and their respective classes a priority.

- Memorize the non-nucleoside reverse transcriptase inhibitors (NNRTIs)
  - Efavirenz, nevirapine, etravirine, rilpivirine
- All protease inhibitors (PIs) end in "-navir"
  - Examples: Darunavir, atazanavir, ritonavir
- There are only three integrase inhibitors: Dolutegravir, raltegravir, elvitegravir
- There is only one fusion inhibitor: Enfuvirtide
- There is only one CCR5 inhibitor: Maraviroc
- The remaining agents are nucleoside reverse transcriptase inhibitors (NRTIs)
  - Tenofovir, emtricitabine, abacavir, lamivudine, zidovudine, didanosine, stavudine

For the exam, know that antiretroviral therapy is now recommended for ALL HIV-infected patients (regardless of CD4 count). Increased urgency to initiate antiretroviral therapy in following patient populations:

- AIDS-defining condition (including HIV-associated dementia and AIDS-associated malignancies)
- Acute opportunistic infection
- CD4 count <200 cells/mm^3
- HIV-associated nephropathy
- Hepatitis B or hepatitis C co-infection
- Pregnancy
- Acute HIV infection

For the exam, know the signature side effects for the major drug classes (NNRTIs, NRTIs, and PIs) and know the five antiviral regimens that are recommended for starting therapy in treatment-naïve patients:

- Darunavir + ritonavir + tenofovir (disoproxil fumarate or alafenamide) + emtricitabine

- Dolutegravir + abacavir + lamivudine (only for patients who are HLA-B*5701 negative)

- Dolutegravir + tenofovir (disoproxil fumarate or alafenamide) + emtricitabine

- Elvitegravir + cobicistat + tenofovir (disoproxil fumarate or alafenamide) + emtricitabine

- Raltegravir + tenofovir (disoproxil fumarate or alafenamide) + emtricitabine

A summary of acceptable initial combination regimens for antiretroviral naïve patients follows:

- PI-based regimen: PI (boosted with ritonavir or cobicistat) + 2 NRTIs
- Integrase inhibitor-based regimen: Integrase inhibitor + 2 NRTIs

Drugs of Choice

Prophylaxis of First-Episode Opportunistic Infections in Patients with HIV

Opportunistic Infection	Indication	First-Line Therapy
PJP	CD4 count <200 cells/mm^3 **OR** Oropharyngeal candidiasis **OR** History of AIDS-defining illness	TMP/SMX 1 DS tablet PO daily **OR** TMP/SMX 80/400 mg (single-strength [SS]) PO daily
Toxoplasma gondii encephalitis	Toxoplasma IgG (+) with CD4 count <100 cells/mm^3	TMP/SMX 1 DS tablet PO daily
Mycobacterium avium complex (MAC) disease	CD4 count <50 cells/mm^3	Azithromycin 1200 mg PO 1 × weekly **OR** Clarithromycin 500 mg PO BID **OR** Azithromycin 600 mg PO 2 × weekly

Treatment and Secondary Prophylaxis of AIDS-Associated Opportunistic Infections

Opportunistic Infection	First-Line Therapy/Duration
PJP	*Treatment:* TMP/SMX (IV/PO) ± corticosteroids* × 21 days *Secondary Prophylaxis:* TMP/SMX 1 DS tablet PO daily **OR** TMP/SMX 1 SS tablet PO daily
Toxoplasma gondii encephalitis	*Treatment:* Pyrimethamine (PO) + sulfadiazine (PO) + leucovorin† (PO) × ≥6 wk *Secondary Prophylaxis:* Pyrimethamine + sulfadiazine + leucovorin†
MAC disease	*Treatment:* Clarithromycin (or azithromycin) (PO) + ethambutol (PO) × ≥12 mo *Secondary Prophylaxis:* Clarithromycin (or azithromycin) + ethambutol
Mucocutaneous candidiasis	*Treatment:* Oropharyngeal: Fluconazole (PO) **OR** clotrimazole (troche) **OR** miconazole (buccal) × 7–14 days Esophageal: Fluconazole (IV/PO) **OR** itraconazole (PO) × 14–21 days *Secondary Prophylaxis:* Usually not recommended unless patients have frequent or severe recurrences
Cryptococcal meningitis	*Treatment:* Induction: Liposomal amphotericin B (IV) + Flucytosine (PO) × ≥2 wk Consolidation: Fluconazole (IV/PO) × ≥8 wk *Secondary Prophylaxis:* Fluconazole (PO)
Cytomegalovirus retinitis	*Treatment:* Ganciclovir (or foscarnet) (via intravitreal injection) × 1–4 doses over 7–10 days + valganciclovir (PO) x 14-21 days *Secondary Prophylaxis:* Valganciclovir (PO)

* Indications for adjunctive corticosteroid therapy for PJP include PaO_2 <70 mmHg (room air) **OR** alveolar-arterial O_2 gradient >35 mmHg.

†Leucovorin reduces the risk of bone marrow suppression associated with pyrimethamine.

Non-Nucleoside Reverse Transcriptase Inhibitors (NNRTIs)

Generic • Brand • Dose/Dosage Forms	Contraindications	Primary Side Effects	Key Monitoring	Pertinent Drug Interactions	Med Pearl
Mechanism of action – bind to an allosteric site on reverse transcriptase that results in a conformational change to the enzyme's active site					
Efavirenz • Sustiva • 600 mg PO QHS • Caps, tabs	None	• Rash • ↑ LFTs • Hyperlipidemia • Drowsiness • Dizziness • Insomnia • Abnormal vivid dreaming • Agitation • Depression • Suicidal thoughts • Hallucinations • Fat redistribution	LFTs	• CYP2B6 and CYP3A4 substrate • CYP2C9 and CYP2C19 inhibitor • CYP2B6 and CYP3A4 inducer	• Can cause a false positive cannabinoid or benzodiazepine screening test • Take on an empty stomach
Etravirine • Intelence • 200 mg PO BID • Tabs	None	• Rash • Nausea • Hypersensitivity reaction • ↑ LFTs • Fat redistribution		• CYP3A4, CYP2C9, and CYP2C19 substrate • CYP2C9 and CYP2C19 inhibitor • CYP3A4 inducer	• May disperse tabs in water • Take with food
Nevirapine • Viramune, Viramune XR • IR: 200 mg PO daily × 2 wk, then 200 mg PO BID • ER: 200 mg PO daily (of IR) × 2 wk, then 400 mg PO daily (of ER) • Suspension, tabs (IR and ER)	Moderate or severe hepatic impairment	• Rash • ↑ LFTs • Fat redistibution		CYP2B6 and CYP3A4 substrate and inducer	• Risk of hepatotoxicity in men and women with CD4 count >400 and >250 cells/mm³, respectively • Hepatotoxicity often associated with a rash • 2-wk lead-in period with IR helps to ↓ rash
Rilpivirine • Edurant • 25 mg PO daily • Tabs	Concurrent use with carbamazepine, oxcarbazepine, phenobarbital, phenytoin, rifampin, rifapentine, PPIs, dexamethasone, and St. John's wort	• Rash • ↑ LFTs • Depression • Insomnia • Headache • Fat redistribution		• CYP3A4 substrate • Does not inhibit or induce CYP450 enzymes • H₂-antagonists, PPIs, and antacids may ↓ absorption (avoid concomitant use of PPIs; may use H₂-antagonists or antacids [need to space administration])	• Requires ≥500-calorie meal • ↑ virologic failure with high baseline HIV RNA (>100,000 copies/mL)

Nucleoside Reverse Transcriptase Inhibitors (NRTIs)

Generic • Brand • Dose/Dosage Forms	Contraindications	Primary Side Effects	Key Monitoring	Pertinent Drug Interactions	Med Pearl
Mechanism of action – triphosphate moiety competes with natural substrates for incorporation into proviral DNA that is developed by reverse transcriptase					
Abacavir • Ziagen • 300 mg PO BID or 600 mg PO daily • Solution, tabs	• Discontinue drug promptly and do not rechallenge in patients with hypersensitivity • HLA-B*5701 positive • Moderate or severe hepatic impairment	• Hypersensitivity reaction • Lactic acidosis • Hepatomegaly with steatosis • Fat redistribution	Hypersensitivity symptoms (fever, rash, N/V/D, abdominal pain, malaise, fatigue, dyspnea, cough)	None	Perform HLA-B*5701 test prior to initiating therapy: only use if negative
Didanosine • Videx, Videx EC • ER: ≥60 kg: 400 mg PO daily (250 mg PO daily when used with tenofovir disoproxil fumarate); 25 to <60 kg: 250 mg PO daily (200 mg PO daily when used with tenofovir disoproxil fumarate) • Solution: ≥60 kg: 200 mg PO BID (250 mg PO daily when used with tenofovir disoproxil fumarate); <60 kg: 125 mg PO BID (200 mg PO daily when used with tenofovir disoproxil fumarate) • ER caps, solution	Concurrent use with allopurinol or ribavirin	• Peripheral neuropathy • Pancreatitis • Lactic acidosis • Hepatomegaly with steatosis • Hepatotoxicity • Fat redistribution • N/V/D • Optic neuritis	LFTs	• Tenofovir ↑ levels (↓ didanosine dose) • Ganciclovir ↑ levels • Methadone ↓ levels (use ER didanosine) • ↓ FQ, ketoconazole, and itraconazole levels (space administration)	• Do not crush or open ER caps • Reconstitute powder for oral solution with water or antacid • Adjust dose in renal impairment • Take on an empty stomach (0.5 hr before or 2 hr after meal)
Emtricitabine • Emtriva • Caps: 200 mg PO daily • Solution: 240 mg PO daily • Caps, solution	None	• N/V/D • Hyperpigmentation of palms/soles • Lactic acidosis • Hepatomegaly with steatosis • Fat redistribution	None	None	Adjust dose in renal impairment

Nucleoside Reverse Transcriptase Inhibitors (NRTIs) *(cont'd)*

Generic • Brand • Dose/Dosage Forms	Contraindications	Primary Side Effects	Key Monitoring	Pertinent Drug Interactions	Med Pearl
Lamivudine • Epivir • 150 mg PO BID or 300 mg PO daily • Solution, tabs	None	• N/V/D • Pancreatitis • Lactic acidosis • Hepatomegaly with steatosis • Fat redistribution	None	None	• Also active against hepatitis B (Epivir HBV) • Adjust dose in renal impairment
Stavudine • Zerit • ≥60 kg: 40 mg PO BID • <60 kg: 30 mg PO BID • Caps, solution	None	• Peripheral neuropathy • Pancreatitis • Lactic acidosis • Hepatomegaly with steatosis • Hepatotoxicity • Fat redistribution • Hyperlipidemia	LFTs	Additive risk of pancreatitis with concurrent didanosine	Adjust dose in renal impairment
Tenofovir • Viread (disoproxil fumarate) • 300 mg PO daily • Powder, tabs • NOTE: Tenofovir alafenamide only available in combo products	CrCl <30 mL/min (alafenamide)	• Renal impairment (> with disoproxil fumarate) • Fanconi syndrome • ↓ bone mineral density (> with disoproxil fumarate) • Lactic acidosis • Hepatomegaly with steatosis • Fat redistribution • Headache • N/V/D	• SCr • Bone mineral density	• ↓ atazanavir levels • ↑ didanosine levels (↓ didanosine dose) • Lopinavir/ritonavir, atazanavir/ritonavir, darunavir/ritonavir, acyclovir, valacyclovir, ganciclovir, valganciclovir, aminoglycosides, and NSAIDs ↑ levels	• Also active against hepatitis B • Oral powder can be used if patient unable to swallow tabs • Oral powder should be mixed in soft food (NOT liquids) • Adjust dose of disoproxil fumarate in renal impairment • Alafenamide associated with ↓ risk of renal impairment and reduced bone density
Zidovudine • Retrovir • 300 mg PO BID • 1 mg/kg IV q4h until PO can be taken • Caps, injection, solution, tabs	Concurrent ribavirin due to additive toxicity	• Anemia • Neutropenia • Headache • N/V • Myopathy • Lactic acidosis • Hepatomegaly with steatosis • Fat redistribution • Hyperlipidemia • Nail pigmentation	CBC with differential	None	• Can be used to prevent maternal-fetal HIV transmission • Adjust dose in renal impairment

Protease Inhibitors (PIs)

Generic • Brand • Dose/Dosage Forms	Contraindications	Primary Side Effects	Key Monitoring	Pertinent Drug Interactions	Med Pearl
Mechanism of action – inhibit HIV protease enzyme from processing the gag-pol polyprotein precursor, thereby preventing development and maturation of new HIV particles					
Atazanavir • Reyataz • Therapy naïve: 300 mg PO daily (400 mg PO daily when used with efavirenz) + ritonavir 100 mg PO daily (or cobicistat 150 mg PO daily) **OR** 400 mg PO daily (if unable to tolerate ritonavir) • Therapy experienced: 300 mg PO daily + ritonavir 100 mg PO daily (or cobicistat 150 mg PO daily) • Caps, powder	Concurrent use with alfuzosin, rifampin, irinotecan, triazolam, ergot derivatives, St. John's wort, lovastatin, simvastatin, pimozide, sildenafil (for pulmonary hypertension), indinavir, and nevirapine	• Indirect hyper-bilirubinemia • PR interval prolongation • Hyperlipidemia • Hepatotoxicity • N/V • Hyperglycemia • Fat redistribution • Cholelithiasis • Nephrolithiasis • Renal impairment • Rash	• LFTs • Bilirubin • Lipids • Blood glucose • Electrocardiogram (ECG)	• CYP3A4 inhibitor and substrate • H$_2$-antagonists, PPIs, and antacids may ↓ absorption (follow guidelines for using in combination)	• Oral powder used in children ≥3 mo old and 10 to <25 kg • Oral powder can be used in adults if patient unable to swallow tabs • Take with food • Adjust dose in hepatic impairment
Darunavir • Prezista • Therapy naïve or therapy experienced (with no darunavir mutations): 800 mg PO daily + ritonavir 100 mg PO daily (or cobicistat 150 mg PO daily) • Therapy experienced (with ≥1 darunavir resistance associated substitution): 600 mg PO BID + ritonavir 100 mg PO BID • Suspension, tabs	Concurrent use with alfuzosin, dronedarone, colchicine, ranolazine, rifampin, triazolam, ergot derivatives, St. John's wort, lovastatin, simvastatin, pimozide, and sildenafil (for pulmonary hypertension)	• Hyperlipidemia • Rash • Hepatotoxicity • N/V/D • Headache • Hyperglycemia • Fat redistribution	• LFTs • Lipids • Blood glucose	• CYP3A4 inhibitor and substrate • CYP2C9 inducer	• Perform genotypic and/or phenotypic testing prior to initiating therapy • Use with caution in patients with sulfa allergy • Take with food
Fosamprenavir • Lexiva • Therapy naïve: 1,400 mg PO BID **OR** 1,400 mg PO daily + ritonavir 100–200 mg PO daily **OR** 700 mg PO BID + ritonavir 100 mg PO BID • Therapy experienced: 700 mg PO BID + ritonavir 100 mg PO BID • Suspension, tabs	Concurrent use with alfuzosin, flecainide, propafenone, rifampin, triazolam, ergot derivatives, St. John's wort, lovastatin, simvastatin, pimozide, and sildenafil (for pulmonary hypertension)	• Hyperlipidemia • Rash • Headache • Hepatotoxicity • N/V/D • Hyperglycemia • Fat redistribution • Nephrolithiasis	• LFTs • Lipids • Blood glucose	• CYP3A4 inhibitor and substrate • H$_2$-antagonists ↓ levels	• Use with caution in patients with sulfa allergy • Adjust dose in hepatic impairment • Adults should take suspension without food; children should take suspension with food • Take tabs with meals if taking with ritonavir

Protease Inhibitors (PIs) *(cont'd)*

Generic • Brand • Dose/Dosage Forms	Contraindications	Primary Side Effects	Key Monitoring	Pertinent Drug Interactions	Med Pearl
Indinavir • Crixivan • 800 mg PO q8h **OR** 800 mg PO BID + ritonavir 100–200 mg PO BID • Caps	Concurrent use with alfuzosin, amiodarone, triazolam, alprazolam, ergot derivatives, lovastatin, simvastatin, pimozide, and sildenafil (for pulmonary hypertension)	• Hyperlipidemia • Hepatotoxicity • N/V/D • Nephrolithiasis • Indirect hyper-bilirubinemia • Hyperglycemia • Fat redistribution	• LFTs • Lipids • Bilirubin • Blood glucose	CYP3A4 inhibitor and substrate	• Patients are advised to drink six 8 oz glasses of water per day • Adjust dose in hepatic impairment • If taking *without* ritonavir, take with water 1 hr before or 2 hr after meals
Lopinavir/ritonavir • Kaletra • Lopinavir 400 mg/ritonavir 100 mg PO BID **OR** lopinavir 800 mg/ritonavir 200 mg PO daily • BID regimen must be used if patient has ≥3 lopinavir resistance associated substitutions • Solution, tabs	Concurrent use with alfuzosin, rifampin, triazolam, ergot derivatives, St. John's wort, lovastatin, simvastatin, pimozide, and sildenafil (for pulmonary hypertension)	• Hyperlipidemia • Pancreatitis • Hepatotoxicity • N/V/D • Hyperglycemia • Fat redistribution • PR interval prolongation • QT interval prolongation	• LFTs • Lipids • Blood glucose • ECG	CYP3A4 substrate and inhibitor	• Recommended PI for pregnant women (BID dosing only) • Oral solution contains alcohol and propylene glycol • Take oral solution with food
Nelfinavir • Viracept • 1,250 mg PO BID **OR** 750 mg PO TID • Tabs	Concurrent use with alfuzosin, amiodarone, quinidine, rifampin, triazolam, ergot derivatives, St. John's wort, lovastatin, simvastatin, pimozide, and sildenafil (for pulmonary hypertension)	• N/D • Hyperlipidemia • Hyperglycemia • Fat redistribution • Hepatotoxicity	• LFTs • Lipids • Blood glucose	• CYP3A4 and CYP2C19 substrate • CYP3A4 inhibitor	• May disperse tabs in water • Take with food
Ritonavir • Norvir • 100–400 mg/day in 1–2 divided doses to boost other PIs • Caps, solution, tabs	Concurrent use with alfuzosin, amiodarone, flecainide, propafenone, quinidine, voriconazole (with ritonavir doses ≥800 mg/day), triazolam, ergot derivatives, St. John's wort, lovastatin, simvastatin, pimozide, and sildenafil (for pulmonary hypertension)	• Hyperlipidemia • Hepatotoxicity • N/V/D • Hyperglycemia • Fat redistribution • Paresthesia • Taste disturbance	• LFTs • Lipids • Blood glucose • ECG	• CYP3A4 and CYP2D6 substrate and inhibitor • CYP1A2, CYP2C9, and CYP2C19 inducer	• Only used for boosting • Oral solution contains alcohol • Take with food • Do NOT refrigerate oral solution

Protease Inhibitors (PIs) *(cont'd)*

Generic • Brand • Dose/Dosage Forms	Contraindications	Primary Side Effects	Key Monitoring	Pertinent Drug Interactions	Med Pearl
Saquinavir • Invirase • 1,000 mg PO BID + ritonavir 100 mg PO BID • Caps, tabs	• QT interval prolongation or concurrent use with other drugs that prolong QT interval • Complete atrioventricular block (in absence of pacemaker) • Severe hepatic impairment • Concurrent use with alfuzosin, amiodarone, cobicistat, dofetilide, lidocaine, flecainide, propafenone, quinidine, trazodone, rifampin, triazolam, ergot derivatives, St. John's wort, lovastatin, simvastatin, pimozide, and sildenafil (for pulmonary hypertension)	• PR interval prolongation • QT interval prolongation • Hyperlipidemia • Hepatotoxicity • N/V/D • Headache • Hyperglycemia • Fat redistribution	• LFTs • Lipids • Blood glucose • ECG	CYP3A4 substrate and inhibitor	Take with food
Tipranavir • Aptivus • Therapy experienced: 500 mg PO BID + ritonavir 200 mg PO BID • Caps, solution	• Moderate or severe hepatic impairment • Concurrent use with alfuzosin, amiodarone, flecainide, propafenone, quinidine, rifampin, triazolam, ergot derivatives, St. John's wort, lovastatin, simvastatin, pimozide, and sildenafil (for pulmonary hypertension)	• Hepatotoxicity • Intracranial hemorrhage • Rash • N/V/D • Hyperlipidemia • Hyperglycemia • Fat redistribution	• LFTs • Lipids • Blood glucose	• CYP3A4 substrate • CYP2D6 inhibitor • CYP1A2, CYP2C19, and CYP3A4 inducer • Antiplatelets, anticoagulants, and vitamin E ↑ risk of bleeding	• Not for therapy naïve patients • Use with caution in patients with sulfa allergy • Take with food if used with ritonavir tabs • Oral solution contains propylene glycol • Do NOT refrigerate oral solution

Integrase Inhibitors

Generic • Brand • Dose/Dosage Forms	Contraindications	Primary Side Effects	Key Monitoring	Pertinent Drug Interactions	Med Pearl
Mechanism of action – inhibit integration of proviral DNA into host CD4 T-cell genome					
Dolutegravir • Tivicay • Therapy naïve or therapy experienced, integrase inhibitor naïve: 50 mg PO daily • Integrase inhibitor experienced with certain integrase inhibitor associated resistance substitutions: 50 mg PO BID • Tabs	Concurrent use with dofetilide	• Hypersensitivity reaction • Insomnia • Headache • Depression or suicidal thoughts (primarily in patients with pre-existing psychiatric conditions)	None	• ↑ dofetilide and metformin levels • Etravirine, efavirenz, nevirapine, fosamprenavir/ritonavir, and tipranavir/ritonavir ↓ levels • Carbamazepine, oxcarbazepine, phenytoin, phenobarbital, St. John's wort, and rifampin ↓ levels • Absorption ↓ with antacids and products containing iron, magnesium, aluminum, calcium, or zinc (give dolutegravir 2 hr before or 6 hr after these medications)	↑ dose to 50 mg PO BID when used with carbamazepine, efavirenz, fosamprenavir/ritonavir, tipranavir/ritonavir, or rifampin
Elvitegravir • Vitekta • Therapy experienced: 85 mg PO daily + atazanavir 300 mg PO daily + ritonavir 100 mg PO daily **OR** 85 mg PO daily + lopinavir 400 mg PO BID + ritonavir 100 mg PO BID **OR** 150 mg PO daily + darunavir 600 mg PO BID + ritonavir 100 mg PO BID **OR** 150 mg PO daily + fosamprenavir 600 mg PO BID + ritonavir 100 mg PO BID **OR** 150 mg PO daily + tipranavir 500 mg PO BID + ritonavir 200 mg PO BID • Tabs	None	• N/D • Depression or suicidal thoughts (primarily in patients with pre-existing psychiatric conditions)	None	• CYP3A4 substrate • Atazanavir, lopinavir/ritonavir, ketoconazole ↑ levels • Carbamazepine, efavirenz, didanosine, bosentan, oxcarbazepine, phenytoin, phenobarbital, rifampin, rifabutin, dexamethasone, and St. John's wort ↓ levels • Absorption ↓ with antacids and products containing iron, magnesium, aluminum, calcium, or zinc (space administration by ≥2 hr) • May ↑ ketoconazole, rifabutin, bosentan, and buprenorphine levels • May ↓ naloxone and methadone levels	Take with food

Integrase Inhibitors *(cont'd)*

Generic • Brand • Dose/Dosage Forms	Contraindications	Primary Side Effects	Key Monitoring	Pertinent Drug Interactions	Med Pearl
Raltegravir • Isentress • 400 mg PO BID • Chewable tabs, powder for suspension, tabs	None	• N/D • Headache • Rash • ↑ creatinine kinase • Muscle weakness • Insomnia • Depression or suicidal thoughts (primarily in patients with pre-existing psychiatric conditions)	None	• Rifampin ↓ levels • Absorption ↓ with antacids containing aluminum or magnesium (space administration)	• ↑ dose to 800 mg PO BID when used with rifampin • Chewable tabs and suspension for children

Cytochrome P450 Inhibitor

Generic • Brand • Dose/Dosage Forms	Contraindications	Primary Side Effects	Key Monitoring	Pertinent Drug Interactions	Med Pearl
Mechanism of action – CYP3A inhibitor used to ↑ systemic exposure to the CYP3A substrates, atazanavir and darunavir					
Cobicistat • Tybost • Therapy naïve or experienced: 150 mg PO daily + atazanavir 300 mg PO daily **OR** 150 mg PO daily + darunavir 800 mg PO daily • Tabs	Concurrent use with alfuzosin, drone-darone, irinotecan, rifampin, triazolam, ergot derivatives, St. John's wort, lovastatin, simvas-tatin, pimozide, lur-asidone, sildenafil (for pulmonary hypertension), ne-virapine, indinavir, carbamazepine, phenytoin, pheno-barbital, ranolazine, colchicine	• ↑ SCr/↓ CrCl (monitor closely if SCr ↑ by >0.4 mg/dL) • Jaundice • Nausea	SCr/CrCl	• CYP2D6 and CYP3A substrate and inhibitor • ↑ risk of renal impairment when used with tenofovir (do not use combi-nation if CrCl <70 mL/min)	• ↑ SCr by inhibiting renal tubular secretion • Take with food

CCR5 Inhibitor

Generic • Brand • Dose/Dosage Forms	Contraindications	Primary Side Effects	Key Monitoring	Pertinent Drug Interactions	Med Pearl
Mechanism of action – acts as an antagonist for the CCR5 receptor, a chemokine coreceptor that can facilitate HIV entry into CD4 T-cells					
Maraviroc • Selzentry • Use with strong CYP3A4 inhibitors (including PIs [except tipranavir/ritonavir] and elvitegravir/ritonavir): 150 mg PO BID • Use with strong CYP3A4 inducers (including efavirenz, etravirine, rifampin, phenytoin, phenobarbital, and carbamazepine): 600 mg PO BID • Use with other medications (including tipranavir/ritonavir, nevirapine, raltegravir, NRTIs and enfuvirtide): 300 mg PO BID • Tabs	• CrCl <30 mL/min • Concurrent use of strong CYP3A4 inhibitors or inducers	• Abdominal pain • Cough • Dizziness • Joint/muscle pain • Rash • Hepatotoxicity • Orthostatic hypotension	• Tropism testing • LFTs • Blood pressure	CYP3A4 substrate	• Only for patients with CCR5-tropic HIV • Hepatotoxicity may be preceded by systemic hypersensitivity reaction (rash, eosinophilia) • Adjust dose in renal impairment

Fusion Inhibitor

Generic • Brand • Dose	Contraindications	Primary Side Effects	Key Monitoring	Pertinent Drug Interactions	Med Pearl
Mechanism of action – blocks conformational changes in gp41 on the surface of HIV that are required for HIV fusion with CD4 cell membranes					
Enfuvirtide • Fuzeon • 90 mg subcut BID • Injection	None	• Local injection site reactions (pain, erythema, induration, nodules and cysts, pruritus, ecchymosis) • Pneumonia • Hypersensitivity reactions	Injection sites	None	Only HIV medication available as subcut injection

Combination Products: See individual drug components for important points		
Brand	Components	Dosing
Atripla	Efavirenz, tenofovir disoproxil fumarate, emtricitabine	1 tablet PO daily
Combivir	Lamivudine, zidovudine	1 tablet PO BID
Complera	Rilpivirine, tenofovir disoproxil fumarate, emtricitabine	1 tablet PO daily
Descovy	Emtricitabine, tenofovir alafenamide	1 table PO daily
Epzicom	Abacavir, lamivudine	1 tablet PO daily
Evotaz	Atazanavir, cobicistat	1 tablet PO daily
Genvoya	Elvitegravir, cobicistat, emtricitabine, tenofovir alafenamide	1 tablet PO daily
Odefsey	Emtricitabine, rilpivirine, tenofovir alafenamide	1 tablet PO daily
Prezcobix	Darunavir, cobicistat	1 tablet PO daily
Stribild	Elvitegravir, cobicistat, emtricitabine, tenofovir disproxil fumarate	1 tablet PO daily
Triumeq	Dolutegravir, abacavir, lamivudine	1 tablet PO daily
Trizivir	Abacavir, lamivudine, zidovudine	1 tablet PO BID
Truvada	Emtricitabine, tenofovir disoproxil fumarate	1 tablet PO daily

TUBERCULOSIS

Definitions

Tuberculosis (TB) is a communicable infection caused by *Mycobacterium tuberculosis*. It can produce a silent, latent infection, as well as an active disease state. Although TB is far less common today in the United States, it remains the most prevalent infection on the planet. Effective therapy for *Mycobacterium tuberculosis* infections require combination chemotherapy designed to prevent the emergence of resistant organisms. Increased resistance to the conventional antituberculous agents has led to the use of more complex regimens.

Diagnosis

- Diagnosis relies on skin testing with the tuberculin purified protein derivative (PPD).
- PPD should be performed on high-risk patients.
  - High-risk patients include HIV-infected, hospital employees, nursing home staff and residents, workers in prisons, immigrants, and healthcare students.
- The intracutaneous PPD injection should produce a small, raised, blanched wheal. This test should be read by an experienced professional in 48 to 72 hours.
  - Measured area >5 mm is considered positive for HIV-infected persons, recent contact of a person with TB disease, persons with fibrotic changes on chest radiograph consistent with prior TB, patients with organ transplants, and persons who are immunosuppressed for other reasons.
  - Measured area >10 mm is considered positive for recent immigrants from high-prevalence countries, injection drug users, residents and employees of high-risk congregate settings, mycobacteriology laboratory personnel, persons with clinical conditions that place them at high risk, children <4 years of age, and infants, children, and adolescents exposed to adults in high-risk categories.
  - Measured area >15 mm is considered positive for any person, including persons with no known risk factors for TB.
- After a positive PPD skin test, a diagnostic test must be performed to rule out active disease.
  - Confirmatory diagnosis is performed with chest radiographs and microbiologic examination or sputum.
  - A total of three sputum samples should be collected and sent for acid-fast bacillus testing.

Signs and Symptoms

TB can present with generalized symptoms of weight loss, malaise, fever, and night sweats. As the disease progresses, the patient may develop a persistent cough, which is often productive of sputum. Frequently, the onset of TB is insidious and the diagnosis may not be considered until a chest radiograph is performed.

Guidelines

Blumberg HM, Burman WJ, Chaisson RE, et al; American Thoracic Society, Centers for Disease Control and Prevention and the Infectious Diseases Society. American Thoracic Society/Centers for Disease Control and Prevention/Infectious Diseases Society of America: treatment of tuberculosis. *Am J Respir Crit Care Med* 2003;167:603–62.

Guidelines Summary

The overall goals for treatment of TB are: (1) To cure the individual patient, and (2) to minimize the transmission of *Mycobacterium tuberculosis* to other persons.

- Risk factors
  - Location of birth (New York, New Jersey, California, Florida, and Texas account for 92% of cases)
  - Close contact (>40 hours per week) with TB patients
  - Increase in age
  - Race and ethnicity: Hispanics, African Americans, and Asian Pacific Islanders
- Successful treatment of TB has benefits for both the individual patient and the community in which the patient resides.
- Prescribing physician responsibility for treatment completion is a fundamental principle in TB control.
- Treatment of patients with TB is most successful within a comprehensive framework that addresses both clinical and social issues of relevance to the patient.
- It is strongly recommended that patient-centered care be the initial management strategy, regardless of the source of supervision. This strategy should always include an adherence plan that emphasizes directly observed therapy (DOT).
- Patients with TB caused by drug-susceptible organisms usually are treated initially with a four-drug regimen (rifampin, isoniazid, pyrazinamide, and ethambutol [RIPE]) followed by a two-drug continuation phase (rifampin and isoniazid).

Antitubercular Drugs

Generic • Brand • Dose/Dosage Forms	Contraindications	Primary Side Effects	Key Monitoring	Pertinent Drug Interactions	Med Pearl
Mechanism of action – inhibits mycolic acid synthesis resulting in disruption of the bacterial cell wall					
Isoniazid • Only available generically • Latent: 5 mg/day (max = 300 mg) PO daily × 6–9 mo **OR** 15 mg/kg (max = 900 mg) PO weekly × 6–9 mo • Active: multiple scenarios • Injection, syrup, tabs	• Hepatic impairment • Previous severe reactions (drug fever, chills, arthritis)	• Depression • Flushing • Jaundice	• LFTs • Sputum cultures	CYP2C19 and CYP2D6 inhibitor	• Severe and sometimes fatal hepatitis may occur within 3 mo of treatment • Drinking alcohol not recommended during treatment • Pyridoxine should be administered to prevent peripheral neuropathy
Mechanism of action – inhibits bacterial RNA synthesis by binding to the beta subunit of DNA-dependent RNA polymerase, blocking RNA transcription					
Rifampin • Rifadin • 10 mg/kg/day PO/IV (max = 600 mg/day) • Caps, injection	Concurrent use with PIs	• Numbness • Flu-like syndrome • Rash • Red discoloration of bodily fluids • Neutropenia/leukopenia	• LFTs • CBC • Sputum cultures • Chest x-ray	CYP1A2, CYP2C9, CYP2C19 and CYP3A4 inducer	None
Mechanism of action – kills mycobacteria replicating in macrophages; exact mechanism is not known					
Pyrazinamide • Only available generically • 40–55 kg: 1,000 mg/day PO • 56–75 kg: 1,500 mg/day PO • 76–90 kg: 2,000 mg/day PO (max dose) • Tabs	• Acute gout • Hepatic impairment	• Malaise • Anorexia • Hepatotoxicity	• LFTs • Uric acid levels • Sputum cultures • Chest x-ray	None	Typically used for the first 2 months of therapy
Mechanism of action – suppresses mycobacteria multiplication by interfering with RNA synthesis					
Ethambutol • Myambutol • 15–25 mg/kg/day (max = 1,600 mg/day) • Tabs	Optic neuritis	• Myocarditis • Headache • Gout • Hepatotoxicity	• Baseline and periodic (monthly) visual testing • LFTs	Aluminum hydroxide ↓ absorption (separate by 4 hours)	Optic neuritis manifests as ↓ red-green color perception, ↓ visual field

LEARNING POINTS

- Compliance is a must with antiretroviral therapy. If a patient is going to stop the prescribed regimen, all the antiretrovirals must be stopped at the same time to prevent resistance.

- Patients receiving antibiotics should complete the entire course of therapy.

- Be aware of the patient's allergies when selecting antibiotic therapy (especially penicillin and sulfa allergies).

- Know agents to treat unique organisms:

  - MRSA: Vancomycin, linezolid, tedizolid, tigecycline, daptomycin, dalbavancin, oritavancin, telavancin, ceftaroline

  - *Pseudomonas aeruginosa*: Piperacillin/tazobactam, ticarcillin/clavulanic acid, aztreonam, aminoglycosides, ciprofloxacin, ceftazidime, cefepime, ceftazidime-avibactam, ceftolozane-tazobactam, carbapenems (except ertapenem)

  - Anaerobes: Metronidazole, clindamycin, piperacillin/tazobactam, ticarcillin/clavulanic acid, cefoxitin, cefotetan, ceftolozane-tazobactam, carbapenems

- Know important/notable side effects and drug interactions of antibiotics:

  - Which ones cause nephrotoxicity?

  - Which ones are associated with QT interval prolongation?

  - Which ones cause myelosuppression?

  - Which ones are associated with a disulfiram reaction?

  - Which ones should be avoided with antacids or products containing di-/trivalent cations?

  - Which ones cause photosensitivity?

- Isoniazid is currently the drug of choice for a positive PPD and in combination-treatments for TB.

PRACTICE QUESTIONS

1. Which of the following medications should NOT be given to a 1-year-old child?

    (A) Amoxicillin
    (B) Cefuroxime
    (C) Clindamycin
    (D) Penicillin
    (E) Tetracycline

2. Which of the following medications would be appropriate for the treatment of *Pseudomonas aeruginosa*?

    (A) Ampicillin
    (B) Cefepime
    (C) Ceftriaxone
    (D) Erythromycin
    (E) Clindamycin

3. A patient admitted to the hospital is diagnosed with aspergillosis. Which of the following antimicrobial agents would be MOST appropriate to initiate in this patient?

    (A) Acyclovir
    (B) Caspofungin
    (C) Chloramphenicol
    (D) Nystatin
    (E) Tigecycline

4. Patients taking which of the following antimicrobial agents should be counseled to wear sunscreen because of the risk of photosensitivity? (Select ALL that apply.)

    (A) Bactrim
    (B) Biaxin
    (C) Cleocin
    (D) Factive
    (E) Vibramycin

5. Which of the following drugs used in the treatment of tuberculosis can cause orange-red discoloration of a patient's urine?

    (A) Isoniazid
    (B) Ethambutol
    (C) Pyrazinamide
    (D) Rifampin
    (E) Streptomycin

6. A woman diagnosed with a sexually transmitted disease picks up her antibiotic prescription at her local pharmacy. The pharmacist counsels her that she should not drink alcoholic beverages while taking this medication because it may lead to an unpleasant reaction. Which of the following antibiotics has MOST likely been prescribed for this patient?

   (A) Azithromycin
   (B) Cefixime
   (C) Doxycycline
   (D) Metronidazole
   (E) Penicillin VK

7. An 85-year-old female patient has been hospitalized with an infection. She has a creatinine clearance of 25 mL/min. Which of the following antibiotics does NOT need to be dose-adjusted in this patient?

   (A) Ceftriaxone
   (B) Gentamicin
   (C) Meropenem
   (D) Piperacillin-tazobactam
   (E) Vancomycin

8. Which of the following antibiotics is the first-line treatment for *Pneumocystis jiroveci* pneumonia?

   (A) Acyclovir
   (B) Azithromycin
   (C) Ciprofloxacin
   (D) Fluconazole
   (E) Trimethoprim-sulfamethoxazole

9. Which of the following is an acceptable antiviral regimen for a treatment-naïve patient with HIV?

   (A) Abacavir + didanosine + zidovudine
   (B) Efavirenz + nevirapine + emtricitabine
   (C) Darunavir + ritonavir + atazanavir
   (D) Tenofovir + emtricitabine + raltegravir
   (E) Dolutegravir + tipranavir + stavudine

10. Acyclovir is available in which of the following formulations?
    (Select ALL that apply.)

    (A) Capsule
    (B) Injection
    (C) Sublingual film
    (D) Topical ointment
    (E) Transdermal patch

KAPLAN MEDICAL

ANSWERS AND EXPLANATIONS

1. E

Tetracycline should not be given to children younger than 9 years of age, as it can cause enamel hypoplasia or permanent tooth discoloration, therefore choice (E) is correct. The other medications can be administered safely to children.

2. B

Cefepime, a fourth-generation cephalosporin, is the only antibiotic listed that would treat an infection caused by *Pseudomonas aeruginosa*; therefore, choice (B) is correct.

3. B

Aspergillosis is a serious fungal infection. Both caspofungin (B) and nystatin (D) are considered antifungal agents; however, nystatin is used topically (as an oral suspension for thrush or as topical cream/ointment/powder) for local infections caused by *Candida* spp. Caspofungin is administered intravenously and can be used for the treatment of aspergillosis; thus, choice (B) is correct. Acyclovir (A) is an antiviral agent. Tigecycline (E) and chloramphenicol (C) are used for bacterial infections.

4. A, D, E

Fluoroquinolones, sulfonamides, and tetracyclines are associated with an increased risk of photosensitivity. Therefore, patients receiving Bactrim (trimethoprim/sulfamethoxazole) (A), Factive (gemifloxacin) (D), or Vibramycin (doxycycline) (E) should be counseled to wear sunscreen during the course of therapy. Neither Biaxin (clarithromycin) (B) nor Cleocin (clindamycin) (C) is associated with photosensitivity.

5. D

Rifampin (D) can cause an orange-red discoloration of all bodily fluids (e.g., tears, saliva, urine). Rifabutin can also cause this discoloration of bodily fluids. Isoniazid (A), ethambutol (B), pyrazinamide (C), and streptomycin (E) do not cause discoloration of the urine.

6. **D**

Metronidazole should not be taken with alcohol as this may lead to a disulfiram-like reaction, which can manifest as severe flushing, headache, nausea, vomiting, or chest and abdominal pain. Although patients generally should not take any of their medications with alcohol, the concomitant use with metronidazole can lead specifically to this very unpleasant reaction; therefore, answer (D) is correct.

7. **A**

Ceftriaxone (A) is eliminated via both biliary and renal excretion. Therefore, the dose of this antibiotic does not need to be adjusted in patients with renal impairment. The dose of gentamicin (B), meropenem (C), piperacillin-tazobactam (D), and vancomycin (E) would all need to be adjusted in this patient with a CrCl of 25 mL/min.

8. **E**

Trimethoprim/sulfamethoxazole (E) is the drug of choice for the treatment of *Pneumocystis jiroveci* pneumonia, provided that the patient does not have a sulfa allergy. Alternative medications, including dapsone, pentamidine, or atovaquone, can be used for the treatment of this opportunistic infection in patients with a sulfa allergy.

9. **D**

The regimen consisting of tenofovir + emtricitabine + raltegravir (D) is an acceptable approach for management of a treatment-naïve patient with HIV because it contains 2 nucleoside reverse transcriptase inhibitors (NRTIs) (tenofovir and emtricitabine) and an integrase inhibitor (raltegravir). Other acceptable antiviral regimens include those that contain a protease inhibitor (PI) (boosted with ritonavir or cobicistat) + 2 NRTIs. Choice (A) contains 3 NRTIs (abacavir + didanosine + zidovudine). Choice (B) contains 2 non-nucleoside reverse transcriptase inhibitors (NNRTIs) (efavirenz and nevirapine) + 1 NRTI (emtricitabine). Choice (C) contains 3 PIs (darunavir + ritonavir + atazanavir). Choice (E) contains an integrase inhibitor (dolutegravir), a PI (tipranavir), and a NRTI (stavudine). None of these four regimens is acceptable for the management of a treatment-naïve patient with HIV.

10. **A, B, D**

Acyclovir is available as a capsule (A), an intravenous injection (B), and a topical ointment (D). This drug is also available as a tablet, oral suspension, buccal tablet, and topical cream. Acyclovir is not available as a sublingual film (C) or a transdermal patch (E).

Pulmonary Disorders 3

This chapter covers the following diseases:

- **Asthma**
- **Chronic obstructive pulmonary disease**

 Suggested Study Time: **40 minutes**

ASTHMA

Definitions

Asthma is a disease of the airways characterized by airway inflammation and bronchoconstriction of the smooth muscles. This hyperactivity is due to a wide variety of stimuli or triggers. Common triggers include: pollen, dust, chemicals, changes in weather, perfumes, smoke, heartburn, mold, and exercise. The hallmark features of asthma include airflow obstruction that is reversible, bronchial hyperresponsiveness, and airway inflammation. The hyperactivity and inflammation lead to obstruction of the airways, cough, dyspnea, chest tightness, and wheezing. The inflammatory cell infiltration mainly consists of neutrophils (especially in sudden-onset, fatal asthma exacerbations, and in patients who smoke), eosinophils, lymphocytes, mast cell activation, and epithelial cell injury and is called remodeling.

Diagnosis

To diagnose asthma, a patient has to have episodes of airway obstruction or airway hyper-responsiveness and at least partially reversible airway obstruction, all alternative diagnoses excluded.

- Pulmonary function tests (PFTs) provide an objective means to diagnose asthma.
    - Measured using spirometry and demonstrate an obstructive pattern of a reduction in expiratory flow rates.
- Spirometry measures forced vital capacity (FVC) and forced expiratory volume (FEV1).
    - FVC is the volume of air forcibly exhaled from the point of maximal inspiration
    - FEV1 is the volume of aired exhaled during the first second.
- The guidelines recommend that spirometry measurements of FEV1, FVC, and FEV1/FEV are used before and after the patient inhales a short-acting bronchodilator to assess bronchodilation. Improvements are defined as an increase of FEV1 by >12%, which is diagnostic of asthma.

Signs and Symptoms

- Shortness of breath
- Wheezing
- Chest tightness
- Coughing
- Worsening of symptoms at night
- Nasal polyps

Guidelines

National Heart, Lung and Blood Institute, National Asthma Education and Prevention Program, Expert Panel Report 3: Guidelines for the Diagnosis and Management of Asthma—Full Report, 2007. www.nhlbi.nih.gov/files/docs/guidelines/asthgdln.pdf.

Global Initiative for Asthma. Global Strategy for Asthma Management and Prevention, 2016. www.ginasthma.org

Guidelines Summary

There are four components to asthma management:

- Measurement of assessment and monitoring
- Controlling environmental factors and comorbid conditions
- Education for asthma care
- Pharmacologic therapy

The goals of therapy are as follows:

- Patient education is a must.
- Daily usage of peak flow meter will provide an objective FEV1.
- Implementation of an action plan:
  - Green zone ("I feel good"), yellow zone ("I do not feel good"), red zone ("I feel awful")
  - Green zone = FEV1 >80% of personal best
  - Yellow zone = FEV1 >50–80% of personal best
  - Red zone = FEV1 <50% of personal best
- Attempt to identify triggers:
  - Consider subcutaneous allergen immunotherapy.
  - Management of gastrointestinal reflux disease (GERD) can greatly improve symptoms.
  - Avoid aspirin therapy due to prostaglandin inhibition; can cause bronchoconstriction.
  - Smoking cessation is recommended.
  - Consider clean home, dust, plastic case over mattress.
- Ensure adherence with medications.
- Identify frequency of symptoms and nighttime awakenings.
- Identify use of short-acting beta-2 agonists and lung function.
  - Ensure proper inhaler technique.
  - Use a stepwise approach to treatment.
  - Long-term medications should include anti-inflammatory mechanism.
- Consider addition of tiotropium to standard step therapy in severe persistent patients (step 4 or 5) with history of exacerbations.

Asthma Treatment Summary

Asthma Stepwise Therapy

Abbreviations: ICS = inhaled corticosteroid; LABA = long-acting β-2 agonist; prn = as needed; SABA = short-acting β-2 agonist

Medications for Asthma

Generic • Brand • Dose/Dosage Forms	Contraindications	Primary Side Effects	Key Monitoring	Pertinent Drug Interactions	Med Pearl
Mechanism of action – glucocorticoid receptor agonist with an affinity for the receptor resulting in anti-inflammatory and immunosuppressive properties, and antiproliferative actions					
Fluticasone • Flovent Diskus, Flovent HFA • 88–440 mcg BID	Primary treatment of acute broncho-spasm	• Throat irritation • Cough • Oral candidiasis • Upper respiratory tract infection • Sinusitis	• FEV1 • Peak flow • Other PFTs • Hypothalamic-pituitary-adrenal axis suppression	• CYP3A4 substrate • Cobicistat (component of Stribild) and ritonavir may ↑ levels	• HFA formulation for Flovent • Most potent corticosteroid
Fluticasone furoate☆ • Arnuity Ellipta • 100–200 mcg daily					
Budesonide☆ • Pulmicort Flex-haler, Pulmicort Respules • Flexhaler: 180–720 mcg BID • Respules: 0.25-1 mg/day					Respules are the only nebulized corticosteroid
Mometasone • Asmanex HFA, Asmanex Twisthaler • HFA: 100-200 mcg BID • 110–880 mcg/day					True once daily
Beclomethasone☆ • QVAR • 40–320 mcg BID					HFA formulation
Flunisolide • Aerospan • 160–320 mcg BID					HFA formulation
Ciclesonide • Alvesco • 80 mcg BID (max = 640 mcg/day)					Drug is a solution aerosol so no shaking is required

Medications for Asthma *(cont'd)*

Generic • Brand • Dose/Dosage Forms	Contraindications	Primary Side Effects	Key Monitoring	Pertinent Drug Interactions	Med Pearl
Mechanism of action – long-acting beta-2 agonists					
Salmeterol • Serevent Diskus • 50 mcg/inhalation • 1 inhalation BID (max = 2 puffs/day)	• Use as an acute bronchodilator • Presence of tachyarrhythmias	• Headache • Hypertension • Dizziness • Chest pain • Throat irritation	• FEV1 • Peak flow • Other PFTs	• Cobicistat (component of Stribild) • Ritonavir	Long-acting beta-2 agonists may increase the risk of asthma-related deaths; should be used only in adjunct therapy with inhaled corticosteroids
Mechanism of action – prevents the mass cells from releasing histamine and leukotrienes					
Cromolyn • Only available generically • 60–80 mg/day • Nebulization solution	Primary treatment for acute bronchospasms	• Cough and irritation • Unpleasant taste • ↑ sneezing	PFTs	None	• Safety is the primary advantage of this drug • May take 4–6 wk for full benefit • Approved for adults and children >2 yr
Mechanism of action – IgG monoclonal antibody which inhibits IgE receptor on mast cells and basophils					
Omalizumab • Xolair • 150–375 mg subcut every 2–4 wk, based on weight and serum IgE	Acute bronchospasms	• Pain and bruising of injection sites • Anaphylaxis • Neuromuscular pain	Be prepared for anaphylaxis	None	Do not administer more than 150 mg per injection site
Mechanism of action – interleukin-5 antagonist which ↓ production and survival of eosinophils; however, the mechanism of action in asthma has not been definitively established					
Mepolizumab • Nucala • 100 mg subcut every 4 wk	Hypersensitivity	• Anaphylaxis • Injection site reaction • Antibody development • Herpes zoster activation	• FEV1 • Peak flow • Other PFTs	None	• Add-on therapy for severe asthma with eosinophilic phenotype • Zoster vaccination recommended prior to use
Reslizumab • Cinqair • 3 mg/kg IV every 4 wk	Hypersensitivity	• Anaphylaxis • ↑ creatine kinase • Antibody development	• FEV1 • Peak flow • Other PFTs • S/S of infection	None	Add-on therapy for severe asthma with eosinophilic phenotype

Medications for Asthma *(cont'd)*

Generic • Brand • Dose/Dosage Forms	Contraindications	Primary Side Effects	Key Monitoring	Pertinent Drug Interactions	Med Pearl
Mechanism of action – selective leukotriene-receptor antagonist of leukotrienes D4 and E4					
Montelukast☆ • Singulair • 4–10 mg PO HS • Tabs, chewable tabs, and granules	Hypersensitivity	• Behavioral changes (agitation, hostility, anxiety, depression, hallucinations, insomnia, irritability, suicidal thoughts) • Headache • Churg-Strauss syndrome (rare)	Behavioral changes	None	Approved for adults and children ≥1 yr
Zafirlukast • Accolate • 10–20 mg PO BID		• ↑ liver function tests (LFTs) • Headache • Insomnia • Depression	LFTs	• CYP2C9 substrate • CYP2C9 and CYP3A4 inhibitor • May ↑ effects of warfarin • CYP2C9 inhibitors may ↑ effects • CYP2C9 inducers may ↓ effects	Must be taken on empty stomach
Mechanism of action – 5-lipoxygenase inhibitor limits neutrophil and monocyte aggregation					
Zileuton • Zyflo, Zyflo CR • IR: 600 mg PO 4x/ day • CR: 1,200 mg PO BID	Acute liver disease	• ↑ LFTs • Headache	• LFTs at baseline, then q4 wk × 3 mo, then q2–3 mo for the rest of the yr, then periodically • Peak flow	• CYP1A2, CYP2C9, and CYP3A4 substrate • CYP1A2 inhibitor • May ↑ effects/ toxicity of theophylline and warfarin	• 4 × /day dose is disadvantage for IR • CR should be taken with food
Mechanism of action – methylxanthine causes bronchodilation by ↑ tissue concentrations of cyclic adenine monophosphate					
Theophylline☆ • Theo-24, Theocron, Elixophyllin • 10 mg/kg/day PO up to 600 mg/day • Liquid, sustained-release tabs, and caps	Allergy to corn-derived dextrose	• Tachycardia • Nausea/vomiting • Central nervous system (CNS) stimulation • Theophylline toxicity (persistent, repetitive vomiting)	• Theophylline concentrations (10–20 mcg/mL) • Heart rate • CNS effects	• CYP1A2 substrate • CYP1A2 inhibitors may ↑ effects/ toxicity • CYP1A2 inducers may ↓ effects	Dosage adjustments should be in small increments (maximum: 25%); ↓ dose by 25% in older adult patients
Aminophylline • Only available generically • Dose is diagnosis- and age-dependent • Injection	Hypersensitivity to theophylline	• Tachycardia • Tremor • CNS stimulation	• Theophylline concentrations (10–20 mcg/mL) • Heart rate • CNS effects	• CYP1A2 substrate • CYP1A2 inhibitors may ↑ effects/ toxicity • CYP1A2 inducers may ↓ effects	Theophylline dose is 80% of aminophylline dose

Medications for Asthma *(cont'd)*

Generic • Brand • Dose/Dosage Forms	Contraindications	Primary Side Effects	Key Monitoring	Pertinent Drug Interactions	Med Pearl
Mechanism of action – relaxes bronchial smooth muscle by acting on beta-2 receptors					
Albuterol ☆ • Ventolin HFA, Proventil HFA, Pro Air HFA • MDI: 2 inhalations q4-6 hr prn (90 mcg/inhalation) • Neb: 2.5 mg 3-4x/ day prn	Hypersensitivity	• Dose-dependent • Angina • Arrhythmias • Chest discomfort • Cough • Tremor	• FEV1 • Peak flow • Blood pressure • HR	Nonselective beta-blockers ↓ effects	• Excessive use can ↑ risk of death • Nebulizer is compatible with budesonide, cromolyn, ipratropium
Levalbuterol ☆ • Xopenex, Xopenex HFA • MDI: 2 inhalations q4-6 hr prn (45 mcg/inhalation) • Neb: 0.63 mg TID	Hypersensitivity	• Tremor • Rhinitis • Tachycardia			Fewer cardiac side effects than albuterol

Combination Products: See individual drug components for important points		
Brand	**Components**	**Dosing**
Advair Diskus, Advair HFA	Fluticasone + Salmeterol	Diskus: 1 inhalation BID HFA: 2 inhalations BID
Breo Ellipta	Fluticasone + Vilanterol	1 inhalation daily
Dulera	Mometasone + Formoterol	2 inhalations BID
Symbicort	Formoterol + Budesonide	2 inhalations BID

Storage and Administration Pearls

- Metered-dose inhaler (MDI) requires hand coordination and proper technique.
- Dry powder inhaler (DPI) is breath-actuated and requires less coordination.
- Spacer with non–breath-actuated MDIs and mouth washing and spitting after inhalation reduces local side effects.
- Hydrofluoroalkane (HFA) is an earth-friendly alternative to CFCs.

Patient Education Pearls

- Using a spacer with inhaled corticosteroids allows for better deposition into the lungs and helps to prevent thrush.
- Proper inhaler/device technique should be reviewed with each patient.

- Patient should rinse and spit to avoid thrush from inhaled corticosteroids.
- Adherence is a must with all asthma medications; patients should be educated on the difference between rescue and controller medications.

CHRONIC OBSTRUCTIVE PULMONARY DISEASE

Definitions

Chronic obstructive pulmonary disease (COPD) is characterized by persistent and largely irreversible airflow obstruction causing dyspnea, which does not fluctuate like asthma. Airflow obstruction is generally progressive and associated with abnormal inflammatory responses of lungs to noxious particles and gases. It is a disease entity with a spectrum of manifestations depending on the lung region affected. Chronic bronchitis affects the larger airways; emphysema affects the smaller airways, called alveolar sacs.

Diagnosis

If COPD is suspected, perform spirometry because diagnosis has to be confirmed with spirometry. FEV1 is gathered from using spirometry and aids in determining the severity of COPD.

- History of cigarette smoking is a factor.
- α_1-antitrypsin deficiency in nonsmokers is a factor.
- Nocturnal symptoms are unusual.
- Chest x-ray often shows low and flattened diaphragms.
- FEV1 and all measurements of expiration airflow are reduced.
- FEV1 is the standard way to assess clinical course for response to therapy.
- FEV1/FVC < 0.70 confirms diagnosis of airflow limitation that is not reversible.

Signs and Symptoms

- Cough with mucus
- Dyspnea and dyspnea on exertion
- FEV1/FVC < 0.70
- Chest tightness
- Wheezing
- Tachypnea
- Pursed lip breathing
- Hyperinflation of the lungs
- Use of accessory muscles for breathing

Classification of Airflow Severity

- GOLD I: mild COPD: FEV1 ≥80% predicted
- GOLD II: moderate COPD: 50% ≤FEV1 <80% predicted
- GOLD III: severe COPD: 30% ≤FEV1 <50% predicted
- GOLD IV: very severe COPD: FEV1 <30% predicted

Classification of COPD Exacerbation Risk

- Group A: mild to moderate airflow limitation, low risk of exacerbation
- Group B: mild to moderate airflow limitation, low risk of exacerbation with more symptoms than group A
- Group C: severe to very severe airflow limitation, high risk of exacerbation
- Group D: severe to very severe airflow limitation, high risk of exacerbation with more symptoms than group C

Guidelines

Global Initiative for Chronic Obstructive Lung Disease. Global Strategy for the Diagnosis, Management, and Prevention of Chronic Obstructive Pulmonary Disease. 2016. www.goldcopd.org

Guidelines Summary

- **Global Initiative for Chronic Obstructive Lung Disease (GOLD)**
  - Spirometry should be used to diagnose airway obstruction in symptomatic patients >40 years old.
  - Smoking cessation should be encouraged for all patients who smoke.
  - Inhaled bronchodilator therapy, prescribed either as needed or scheduled, is the mainstay of treatment for COPD.
  - May combine bronchodilators from different classes to improve efficacy.
  - Inhaled corticosteroids may be used to prevent exacerbations.
  - Consider influenza and pneumococcal vaccines.
  - Oral corticosteroids may be used to prevent exacerbations.
  - Antibiotics may be given if the patient has ↑ dyspnea, sputum production, and sputum purulence.

COPD Treatment Summary

Medications for COPD

Generic • Brand • Dose	Contraindications	Primary Side Effects	Key Monitoring	Pertinent Drug Interactions	Med Pearl
Mechanism of action — long-acting beta2-adrenergic agonist; relaxes bronchial smooth muscle					
Indacaterol • Arcapta Neohaler • 75 mcg daily	Monotherapy in the treatment of asthma	• Cough • Chest pain • Headache • Nasopharyn-gitis	• PFTs • HR	Nonselective β-blockers	• Indcaterol, arformoterol, formoterol, and olodaterol not approved for the treatment of asthma • Arformoterol and formoterol available as nebulizer solution
Arformoterol • Brovana • 15 mcg BID					
Formoterol • Perforomist • 20 mcg BID					
Salmeterol • Serevent Diskus • 50 mcg/ inhalation • 1 inhalation BID					
Olodaterol • Striverdi Respimat • 2 inhalations daily					

Medications for COPD *(cont'd)*

Generic • Brand • Dose	Contraindications	Primary Side Effects	Key Monitoring	Pertinent Drug Interactions	Med Pearl
Mechanism of action – inhibits phosphodiesterase-4 leading to an accumulation of cyclic AMP					
Roflumilast • Daliresp • 500 mcg daily	Hepatic impairment (Child-Pugh class B or C)	• Diarrhea • Weight loss • Nausea • Gynecomastia	• Weight • LFTs	• CYP1A2 and CYP3A4 substrate • CYP1A2 and CYP3A4 inhibitors may ↑ effects • CYP1A2 and CYP3A4 inducers may ↓ effects	Not indicated for relieving acute bronchospasms or for use as monotherapy of COPD
Mechanism of action – blocks acetylcholine at the parasympathetic sites in bronchial smooth muscle, causing bronchodilation					
Ipratropium ☆ • Atrovent HFA • MDI: 2 inhalations 4×/day (max = 12 puffs/24 hrs) • Nebulizer: 500 mcg every 6–8 hr	• Hypersensitivity • Peanut allergy (due to soya lecithin) • Does not apply to Atrovent HFA	• Upper respiratory tract infection • Palpitation • Xerostomia • Pharyngeal irritation	• FEV1 • Peak flow • Other PFTs	Avoid use with other anticholinergic inhalers	• Not recommended for initial treatment of acute episode of bronchospasm • Anticholinergic side effects are possible. Be careful in BPH, narrow-angle glaucoma, and myasthenia gravis
Tiotropium ☆ • Spiriva Handihaler, Spiriva Respimat • Handihaler: 1 cap (18 mcg) via inhalation daily • Respimat: 2 inhalations daily	Contains lactose				
Aclidinium • Tudorza Pressair • 1 inhalation BID	Hypersensitivity to milk protein				
Umeclidinium • Incruse Ellipta • 1 inhalation daily	Hypersensitivity to milk protein				
Glycopyrrolate • Seebri Neohaler • 1 cap (15.6 mcg) by inhalation BID	Hypersensitivity	• Upper respiratory tract infection • Nasopharyngitis			

Combination Products: See individual drug components for important points		
Brand	Components	Dosing
Advair Diskus	Fluticasone + Salmeterol	1 inhalation BID
Anoro Ellipta	Umeclidinium + Vilanterol	1 inhalation daily
Breo Ellipta	Fluticasone + Vilanterol	1 inhalation daily
Combivent Respimat	Ipratropium + Albuterol	1 inhalation 4 × /day
Stiolto Respimat	Tiotropium + Olodaterol	2 inhalations daily
Symbicort	Budesonide + Formoterol	2 inhalations BID
Bevespi Aerosphere	Glycopyrrolate + Formoterol	2 inhalations BID
Utibron Neohaler	Glycopyrrolate + Indacaterol	1 cap inhaled BID

Storage and Administration Pearls

- Tiotropium: Do not store capsules in Handihaler device. Capsules should be used within 2 days of removal from blister pack.
- Umeclidinium/vilanterol and fluticasone/vilanterol: Discard inhaler 6 weeks after opening foil pack.
- Fluticasone/salmeterol: Discard inhaler 4 weeks after opening foil pack.
- Budesonide/fomoterol: Discard inhaler 3 months after opening foil pack.

Patient Education Pearls

- Using a spacer with inhaled corticosteroids allows for better deposition into the lungs and helps to prevent thrush.
- Proper inhaler/device technique should be reviewed with each patient.
- Patient should rinse and spit to avoid thrush from inhaled corticosteroids.

LEARNING POINTS

- Inhaled corticosteroids are the primary treatment for asthma. They prevent re-modeling, improve symptoms, and prevent exacerbations as compared to the other medications.

- Peak flow meters are crucial to the maintenance of asthma. They should be used to determine a patient's personal best, and used every morning to identify an early exacerbation.

- All patients with asthma should have a short-acting bronchodilator for rescue therapy.

- Smoking cessation will help slow the progression of COPD and is the most important intervention when dealing with patients who have COPD.

PRACTICE QUESTIONS

1. What is Zyflo's mechanism of action?

    (A) Selective leukotriene-receptor antagonist of leukotrienes D4 and E4
    (B) 5-lipoxygenase inhibitor limits neutrophil and monocyte aggregation
    (C) Methylxanthine causes bronchodilation by increasing tissue concentrations of cyclic adenine monophosphate
    (D) Relaxes bronchial smooth muscle by stimulating beta-2 receptors

2. The device used to measure forced vital capacity is called a

    (A) tonometer.
    (B) optomyometer.
    (C) sphygmomanometer.
    (D) spirometer.
    (E) gonioscope.

3. QVAR is indicated for which of the following scenarios? (Select ALL that apply.)

    (A) Asthma
    (B) Emphysema
    (C) Chronic brochitis
    (D) Smoking cessation

4. Which of the following include fluticasone as an active ingredient? (Select ALL that apply.)

    (A) Flonase
    (B) Flovent
    (C) Foradil
    (D) Pulmicort

5. Patient counseling that includes the need for the patient to rinse his or her mouth and spit after use is applicable to which medication?

    (A) Breo Ellipta
    (B) Arcapta Neohaler
    (C) Xopenex HFA
    (D) Servent Diskus

6. Which of the following should be used in combination with an inhaled corticosteroid in the treatment of asthma?

    (A) Budesonide
    (B) Cromolyn
    (C) Formoterol
    (D) Levalbuterol

ANSWERS AND EXPLANATIONS

1. B

The challenging aspect of this question is that Zyflo is classified as a leukotriene modifier (A), like Accolate or Singulair, but the two have different mechanisms of action. Zyflo's mechanism is an inhibitor of 5-lipoxygenase versus an antagonist at the receptor. Choice (C) is the mechanism of theophylline and choice (D) is the mechanism of albuterol.

2. D

A spirometer is a gasometer used for measuring respiratory gases, so (D) is correct. A tonometer (A) determines pressure or tension within the eye. An optomyometer (B) is an instrument for determining the relative power of the extrinsic muscles of the eye. A sphygmomanometer (C) measures arterial blood pressure. A gonioscope (E) measures the lens angle in relationship to the eye.

3. A

QVAR is an inhaled corticosteroid that is indicated only for the maintenance and prophylactic treatment of asthma, so (A) is the only correct answer.

4. A, B

Flonase and Flovent contain fluticasone. Foradil (C) contains formoterol. Pulmicort (D) contains budesonide.

5. A

Breo Ellipta contains fluticasone, which is an inhaled corticosteroid. Counseling for inhaled corticosteroids should include having the patient rinse his or her mouth with water and spit it out to reduce the risk of thrush or hoarseness. The other medications listed do not contain an inhaled corticosteroid and therefore do not require the patient to rinse his or her mouth after use.

6. C

Formoterol is a long-acting beta-2 agonist that needs to be administered in conjunction with an inhaled corticosteroid. Use of long-acting beta-2 agonists without the use of an inhaled corticosteroid has been associated with increased risk of asthma-related deaths. Budesonide is an inhaled corticosteroid and should not be used with another inhaled corticosteroid. Cromolyn and levalbuterol do not need to be administered with an inhaled corticosteroid, although they often are.

Endocrine Disorders

4

This chapter covers the following diseases:

- **Diabetes mellitus**
- **Hypothyroidism**
- **Hyperthyroidism**
- **Polycystic ovarian syndrome**

 Suggested Study Time: **40 minutes**

DIABETES MELLITUS

Definition—Type 1

Diabetes mellitus (DM) type 1 accounts for fewer than 10% of all cases of diabetes, occurs in younger persons, and is caused by insulin deficiency that results from an immune-mediated destruction of the pancreatic-islet beta cells. Exogenous insulin is required to control blood glucose, prevent diabetic ketoacidosis (DKA), and preserve life. A transient period of insulin independence ("honeymoon phase") or reduced insulin requirement may occur early in the course of type 1 DM.

Definition—Type 2

DM type 2 accounts for >90% of all cases of DM. While it is most commonly diagnosed in adults, it is increasing in prevalence in younger age groups. Obesity, insulin resistance, and relative insulin deficiency are characteristic findings.

Diagnosis

- Impaired fasting glucose (IFG) is defined by a fasting plasma glucose between 100 and 125 mg/dL and is indicative of prediabetes.

- Impaired glucose tolerance (IGT) is defined by a 2-hour oral glucose tolerance test plasma glucose between 140 and 199 mg/dL and is indicative of prediabetes.
- A1c 5.7% to 6.4% is considered "increased risk for diabetes."
- Diagnostic test results:
  - A1c ≥ 6.5%; **OR**
  - Plasma glucose ≥126 mg/dL after fasting for ≥8 hr; **OR**
  - Symptoms of diabetes and random plasma glucose ≥200 mg/dL; **OR**
  - Oral glucose tolerance test indicating a plasma glucose ≥200 mg/dL 2 hours after a 75-g glucose load.
- Confirmation requires a second positive test on a subsequent day (any of the above).

Signs and Symptoms

- Polyuria is a symptom, which is characterized by excessive excretion of urine.
- Polyphagia is a symptom, which is characterized by excessive eating.
- Polydipsia is a symptom, which is characterized by excessive thirst that is relatively prolonged.
- Weight loss is due to excretion of glucose in the urine when blood sugars >180 mg/dL. The excretion of glucose results in loss of calorie retention. In addition, the excessive polyuria leads to polyphagia and polydipsia.

Diabetes Complications

- Retinopathy—Diabetic retinopathy is caused by damage to blood vessels in the eye over a long period of the disease. There are two stages of retinopathy: nonproliferative: blood vessel leakage in the eye leads to macular edema; and proliferative: abnormal blood vessels form in the eye. The growth of these vessels can lead to vitreous hemorrhage and retinal detachment, both of which can cause blindness.
- Neuropathy—Neuropathies are common in patients with diabetes and can lead to pain and other complications. There are two main types of neuropathies: distal polyneuropathy: demyelination in sensory nerves causes numbness, tingling, and paresthesias as these nerves lose function; and autonomic neuropathy: Functions of the sympathetic and parasympathetic nervous systems are lost. Examples of autonomic neuropathies include gastroparesis, orthostatic hypotension, and erectile dysfunction.
- Nephropathy—Nephropathy occurs in patients with diabetes as a result of dysfunction in the glomeruli of the kidney. The symptoms of this disease are preceded by a period of hyperfiltration, followed by glomerular changes that cause proteinuria. As the damage progresses, proteinuria worsens until end-stage renal failure is reached, accompanied by massive proteinuria.

- Atherosclerosis—Diabetes is a major risk factor for atherosclerosis and subsequent cardiovascular diseases, including myocardial infarction, stroke, and peripheral arterial disease.

Guidelines

American Diabetes Association. *Diabetes Care*, no. 39 (Suppl 1) (2016): http://care.diabetesjournals.org.

American Association of Clinical Endocrinologists. *Endocrine Practice*, no. 17 (Suppl 2) (March/April 2011): www.aace.com/publications/guidelines.

Guidelines Summary

- American Diabetes Association (ADA) Guideline Goals
  - Preprandial glucose 80–130 mg/dL
  - Postprandial glucose <180 mg/dL
  - A1c <7%
  - Blood pressure <140/90 mmHg
  - Goals should be individualized
- American Association of Clinical Endocrinologists (AACE) Guideline Goals
  - Preprandial glucose <110 mg/dL
  - Postprandial glucose <140 mg/dL
  - A1c <6.5%

Patient education is integral to successful management of diabetes. Diabetes education should be conducted through an interdisciplinary approach.

Dietary education should focus on medical nutrition therapy provided by a registered dietitian.

Exercise should include 150 min/week of moderate intensity aerobic activity or 75 min/week of vigorous aerobic activity.

- Insulin replacement is necessary in type 1 DM and is generally initiated at 0.5–1 units/kg/day.
  - Analog-based basal bolus regimen (50% basal, 50% bolus [divided into 3 meals]); OR
  - Human insulin–based split-mixed regimen (70% A.M.; 30% P.M. [each dose ⅔ NPH to ⅓ Regular])
- Insulin regimens are adjusted based upon patient response (self-monitored blood glucose [SMBG]).

- Metformin is first-line therapy for patients with type 2 DM unless contraindicated.

- Second-line options include insulin, sulfonylureas, DPPIV inhibitors, GLP1 agonists, SGLT-2 inhibitors, and thiazolidinediones.

- Second-line selection is made based upon patient-specific considerations of efficacy needed, risk of hypoglycemia/weight gain, other side effects, and cost.

- New data is emerging indicating potential cardiovascular risk reduction with the use of empagliflozin and liraglutide.

Treatment Algorithm

Medications for Diabetes (Insulin)

Generic • Brand	Onset	Peak	Duration	Comments
Rapid-acting				• Hypoglycemia is the most common side effect. It is defined as blood sugar <70 mg/dL and must be treated as soon as recognized.
Aspart ☆ • NovoLog	5–15 min	30–90 min	<5 hr	
Lispro U-100 ☆ Lispro U-200 • Humalog	5–15 min	30–90 min	<5 hr	• Insulin dosage is individually based due to sensitivity; 0.5–1.0 units/kg/day for the average nonobese patient.
Glulisine • Apidra	5–15 min	30–90 min	<5 hr	
Short-acting				• Duration of action is prolonged in renal failure.
Regular ☆ • Humulin R (OTC)	30–60 min	2–3 hr	5–8 hr	
Inhaled, regular • Afrezza	30–60 min	2–3 hr	5–8 hr	
Intermediate, basal				
NPH (Neutral Protamine Hagedorn) ☆ • Humulin N (OTC)	2–4 hr	4–10 hr	10–16 hr	
Long-acting, basal				
Glargine U-100 ☆ • Basaglar, Lantus	2–4 hr	No peak	20–24 hr	
Detemir ☆ • Levemir	3–8 hr	No peak	6–24 hr	
Glargine U-300 • Toujeo	2–4 hr	No peak	22–24 hr	
Degludec • Tresiba	1–3 hr	No peak	42 hr	

Medications for Diabetes (Insulin) (cont'd)

Generic • Brand	Onset	Peak	Duration	Comments
Premixed				[same as above]
75% Lispro protamine /25% lispro • Humalog Mix 75/25	5–15 min	Dual	10–16 hr	
50% Lispro protamine / 50% lispro • Humalog Mix 50/50	5–15 min	Dual	10–16 hr	
50% Aspart protamine / 50% aspart • NovoLog Mix 50/50	5–15 min	Dual	10–16 hr	
70% Aspart protamine / 30% aspart • NovoLog Mix 70/30	5–15 min	Dual	10–16 hr	
70% Degludec/30% aspart • Ryzodeg	5–15 min	Dual	<5 hr (aspart); 42 hr (degludec)	
70% NPH / 30% regular • 70/30 (OTC)	30–60 min	Dual	10–16 hr	
• OTC insulin is available without a prescription. • Rapid-acting insulin should be given at time of meal ingestion, no more than 15 minutes from eating. • Regular insulin should be given 30 minutes prior to meal due to delayed onset of action.				

Medications for Diabetes (Non-Insulin)

Generic • Brand • Dose & Max	Contraindications	Primary Side Effects	Key Monitoring	Pertinent Drug Interactions	Med Pearl
Sulfonylureas, first generation – stimulate insulin release from the pancreatic beta cells					
Tolbutamide • Only available generically • 250 mg–3 g daily Tolazamide • Only available generically • 100 mg–1 g daily Chlorpropamide • Diabinese • 100–500 mg daily	• Type 1 DM • Sulfa allergy • Creatinine clearance (CrCl) <50 mL/min (chlorpropamide)	• Hypoglycemia • Weight gain	• Fasting plasma glucose (FPG) • A1c every 3 mo • S/S hypoglycemia	• Tolbutamide = CYP2C9 substrate and inhibitor • Chlorpropamide = CYP2C9 substrate • Chronic ethanol ingestion may ↓ hypoglycemic effect	Response plateaus after half maximum dose

Medications for Diabetes (Non-Insulin) *(cont'd)*

Generic • Brand • Dose & Max	Contraindications	Primary Side Effects	Key Monitoring	Pertinent Drug Interactions	Med Pearl
Sulfonylureas, second generation – stimulate insulin release from the pancreatic beta cells					
Glyburide☆ • DiaBeta, Glynase • 1.25–20 mg/day (given daily BID) • Micronized: 0.75–12 mg/day (given daily BID) Glipizide☆ • Glucotrol, Glucotrol XL • 2.5–40 mg/day Glimepiride☆ • Amaryl • 1–8 mg daily	• Type 1 DM • Sulfa allergy	• Hypoglycemia • Weight gain	• FPG • A1c every 3 mo • S/S hypoglycemia	• CYP2C9 substrates • CYP2C9 inhibitors may ↑ effects • CYP2C9 inducers may ↓ effects • Chronic ethanol ingestion may ↓ hypoglycemic effect	• Response plateaus after half maximum dose • Administer with meals
Meglitinides – stimulates insulin release from the pancreatic beta cells					
Repaglinide • Prandin • 0.5–16 mg/day (taken BID–4 × /day)	• Type 1 DM • Concurrent use of gemfibrozil	• Hypoglycemia • Weight gain	• Postprandial plasma glucose • A1c every 3 mo • S/S hypoglycemia	• CYP2C8 and CYP3A4 substrate • CYP2C8 and CYP3A4 inhibitors may ↑ effects • CYP2C8 and CYP3A4 inducers may ↓ effects	• Faster acting and shorter duration than sulfonylureas • Recommended for postprandial hyperglycemia • Administer each dose 15–30 min before meals
Nateglinide • Starlix • 60–120 mg TID	Type 1 DM			• CYP2C9 and CYP3A4 substrate • CYP2C9 and CYP3A4 inhibitors may ↑ effects • CYP2C9 and CYP3A4 inducers may ↓ effects	
Biguanide – ↓ hepatic glucose production, ↓ intestinal absorption of glucose, and improves insulin sensitivity					
Metformin☆ • Glucophage, Glucophage XR • IR: 500–2,550 mg/day (in 2–3 divided doses) • XR: 500–2,000 mg daily	• CrCl < 30 mL/min • Lactic acidosis • Severe heart failure • Radiocontrast dyes (discontinue 48 hr before and after procedure)	• Diarrhea • Flatulence • Lactic acidosis • Vitamin B_{12} deficiency	• Serum creatinine (SCr) • Hgb/Hct • Vitamin B_{12} concentrations • FPG • A1c every 3 months	Cimetidine may ↑ effects	• Black box warning: lactic acidosis • Maximum daily dose for immediate release is 2,550 mg

Medications for Diabetes (Non-Insulin) *(cont'd)*

Generic • Brand • Dose & Max	Contraindications	Primary Side Effects	Key Monitoring	Pertinent Drug Interactions	Med Pearl
Alpha-glucosidase inhibitors – inhibit pancreatic alpha-amylase and alpha-glucosidases, block carbohydrate hydrolysis to glucose; ↓ postprandial blood glucose					
Acarbose • Precose • 25–100 mg TID	• Cirrhosis • Inflammatory bowel disease • Intestinal obstruction	• Abdominal pain • Diarrhea • Flatulence	• Liver function tests (LFTs) every 3 mo × 1 yr • Postprandial plasma glucose • A1c every 3 mo	Sulfonylureas and insulin ↑ risk of hypoglycemia	• Must treat hypoglycemia with simple carbohydrate such as glucose • Administer with food
Miglitol • Glyset • 25–100 mg TID			• Postprandial plasma glucose • A1c every 3 mo		
Thiazolidinediones – PPAR-gamma activator, which improves insulin sensitivity					
Rosiglitazone • Avandia • 2–8 mg daily	• Liver disease • Unstable heart failure • Previous myocardial infarction • Osteopenia or osteoporosis • History of bladder cancer	• Edema • Hepatotoxicity	• LFTs at baseline and periodically • FPG • A1c every 3 months	• CYP2C8 substrates • CYP2C8 inhibitors may ↑ effects • CYP2C8 inducers may ↓ effects	Potential link to ↑ risk of cardiovascular events; controversial
Pioglitazone☆ • Actos • 15–45 mg daily					Thought to have better lipid profile than rosiglitazone
Amylinomimetic – amylin cosecreted with insulin ↓ postprandial blood sugars, prolonging gastric emptying, ↓ postprandial glucagon secretion, and caloric intake through centrally mediated appetite suppression					
Pramlintide • Symlin • 15–120 mcg subcut daily	• Gastroparesis • Hypoglycemia unawareness	• Nausea • Severe hypoglycemia	• Blood sugars (before and after meals and HS) • A1c every 3 mo • S/S hypoglycemia	• May delay absorption of other drugs due to ↑ gastric emptying time (administer other medications 1 hr prior to pramlintide) • Sulfonylureas and insulin ↑ risk of hypoglycemia (↓ dose of mealtime insulin by 50% when starting pramlintide)	Adjunctive treatment *with* mealtime insulin

Medications for Diabetes (Non-Insulin) *(cont'd)*

Generic • Brand • Dose & Max	Contraindications	Primary Side Effects	Key Monitoring	Pertinent Drug Interactions	Med Pearl
GLP-1 agonist – glucagon-like peptide (GLP) which ↑ insulin secretion, ↑ B-cell growth/replication, slows gastric emptying, and ↓ food intake					
Exenatide ☆ • Byetta (IR) • 5–10 mcg subcut BID • Bydureon (ER) • 2 mg subcut once weekly	• CrCl <30 mL/min • Family history of medullary thyroid carcinoma (ER) • Multiple endocrine neoplasia syndrome type 2 (ER)	• Nausea • Hypoglycemia • ↓ appetite • Weight loss • Pancreatitis • Thyroid tumors	• FPG • A1c every 3 mo • S/S pancreatitis • S/S hypoglycemia • Thyroid tumors	• May delay absorption of other drugs due to ↑ gastric emptying time (administer other medications 1 hour prior) • Sulfonylureas and insulin ↑ risk of hypoglycemia	• IR: Administer within 60 min before main meals of day • ER: Reconstitute prior to injection, must be injected immediately after reconstitution; administer without regard to meals; administer missed dose within 3 days
Liraglutide • Victoza • 0.6–1.8 mg subcut daily	• Family history of medullary thyroid carcinoma • Multiple endocrine neoplasia syndrome type 2				• Administer without regard to meals • Saxenda used for chronic weight management
Albiglutide • Tanzeum • 30–50 mg subcut once weekly					• Reconstitute prior to injection, must be injected within 8 hours of reconstitution • Administer without regard to meals • Administer missed dose within 3 days
Lixisenatide • Adlyxin • 10 mcg subcut daily × 14 days then 20 mcg subcut daily					Administer within 1 hr of 1st meal of day
Dulaglutide • Trulicity • 0.75–1.5 mg subcut once weekly		• Nausea • Hypoglycemia • ↓ appetite • Weight loss • Pancreatitis • Thyroid tumors • Tachycardia • PR interval prolongation • AV block	• FPG • A1c every 3 mo • S/S pancreatitis • S/S hypoglycemia • Thyroid tumors • Heart rate • Electrocardiogram		• Administer without regard to meals • Administer missed dose within 3 days

Medications for Diabetes (Non-Insulin) *(cont'd)*

Generic • Brand • Dose & Max	Contraindications	Primary Side Effects	Key Monitoring	Pertinent Drug Interactions	Med Pearl
Dipeptidyl-peptidase 4 inhibitors – prolong the active incretin levels of GLP and glucose-dependent insulinotropic polypeptide (GIP)					
Sitagliptin ☆ • Januvia • 25–100 mg daily	None	• Hypoglycemia • Arthralgias • Pancreatitis	• Renal function • FPG • A1c every 3 mo • S/S pancreatitis • S/S hypoglycemia	• Sulfonylureas and insulin ↑ risk of hypoglycemia • May ↑ digoxin concentrations	• 100-mg dose is preferred unless patient has renal impairment • Adjust dose in renal impairment
Saxagliptin • Onglyza • 2.5–5 mg daily		• Hypoglycemia • Arthralgias • Pancreatitis • Heart failure	• Renal function • FPG • A1c every 3 mo • S/S pancreatitis • S/S hypoglycemia • S/S heart failure	• CYP3A4 substrate • CYP3A4 inhibitors may ↑ effects; ↓ dose to 2.5 mg daily when used with strong CYP3A4 inhibitors • CYP3A4 inducers may ↓ effects • Sulfonylureas and insulin ↑ risk of hypoglycemia	Adjust dose in renal impairment
Linagliptin • Tradjenta • 5 mg daily		• Hypoglycemia • Arthralgias • Pancreatitis	• FPG • A1c every 3 mo • S/S pancreatitis • S/S hypoglyce-mia	• CYP3A4 and P-glycoprotein (P-gp) substrate • CYP3A4 or P-gp inhibitors may ↑ effects • CYP3A4 or P-gp inducers may ↓ effects • Sulfonylureas and insulin ↑ risk of hypoglycemia	No renal dose adjustment
Alogliptin • Nesina • 25 mg daily		• Hypoglycemia • Arthralgias • Pancreatitis • Heart failure	• Renal function • FPG • A1c every 3 mo • S/S pancreatitis • S/S hypoglyce-mia • S/S heart failure • LFTs (at baseline)	• Sulfonylureas and insulin ↑ risk of hypoglycemia	Adjust dose in renal and hepatic impairment

Medications for Diabetes (Non-Insulin) *(cont'd)*

Generic • Brand • Dose & Max	Contraindications	Primary Side Effects	Key Monitoring	Pertinent Drug Interactions	Med Pearl
Sodium-glucose cotransporter 2 (SGLT2) inhibitors – ↓ reabsorption of filtered glucose from tubular lumen, ↑ glucosuria					
Canagliflozin • Invokana • 100–300 mg daily	CrCl <30 mL/min	• Genitourinary infections (especially in females) • Dehydration • Hyperkalemia • Hypotension • DKA • Fractures • Acute kidney injury • Hypoglycemia • ↑ low-density lipoprotein cholesterol (LDL-C)	• Renal function • FPG • A1c every 3 mo • S/S hypoglycemia • Blood pressure • Serum K+ • LDL-C • S/S heart failure • LFTs (at baseline) • S/S genital fungal infections or UTIs	• Rifampin, phenytoin, phenobarbital, and ritonavir may ↓ effects • May ↑ digoxin concentrations • Diuretics may ↑ risk of volume depletion and hypotension • Sulfonylureas and insulin ↑ risk of hypoglycemia	Administer before first meal of the day
Dapagliflozin • Farxiga • 5–10 mg daily				• Diuretics may ↑ risk of volume depletion and hypotension • Sulfonylureas and insulin ↑ risk of hypoglycemia	
Empagliflozin • Jardiance • 10–25 mg daily	• CrCl < 45 mL/min				• Administer in AM • Administer without regard to meals

Medications for Diabetes (Non-Insulin): Combination Products

See individual drug components for important points		
Brand	**Components**	**Maximum Daily Dose**
Actoplus Met, Actoplus Met XR	Actoplus Met = Pioglitazone + Metformin Actoplus Met XR = Pioglitazone + Metformin ER	Actoplus Met: Pioglitazone 45 mg/metformin 2,550 mg Actoplus Met XR: Pioglitazone 45 mg/metformin ER 2,000 mg
Avandamet	Rosiglitazone + Metformin	Rosiglitazone 8 mg/metformin 2,000 mg
Avandaryl (only available generically)	Rosiglitazone + Glimepiride	Rosiglitazone 8 mg/glimepiride 4 mg
Duetact	Pioglitazone + Glimepiride	Pioglitazone 45 mg/glimepiride 8 mg
Glucovance	Glyburide + Metformin	Glyburide 20 mg/metformin 2,000 mg
Glyxambi	Empagliflozin + Linagliptin	Empagliflozin 25 mg/linagliptin 5 mg
Invokamet	Canagliflozin + Metformin	Cangliflozin 300 mg/metformin 2,000 mg
Janumet, Janumet XR	Janumet = Sitagliptin + Metformin Janumet XR = Sitagliptin + Metformin ER	Janumet: Sitagliptin 100 mg/metformin 2,000 mg Janumet XR: Sitagliptin 100 mg/metformin ER 2,000 mg

Medications for Diabetes (Non-Insulin): Combination Products *(cont'd)*

Brand	Components	Maximum Daily Dose
Jentadueto, Jentadueto XR	Jentadueto = Linagliptin + Metformin Jentadueto = Linagliptin + Metformin ER	Jentadueto: Linagliptin 5 mg/metformin 2,000 mg Jentadueto XR: Linagliptin 5 mg/metformin ER 2,000 mg
Kazano	Alogliptin + Metformin	Alogliptin 25 mg/metformin 2,000 mg
Kombiglyze XR	Saxagliptin + Metformin ER	Saxagliptin 5 mg/metformin ER 2,000 mg
Metaglip (only available generically)	Glipizide + Metformin	Glipizide 20 mg/metformin 2,000 mg
Oseni	Alogliptin + Pioglitazone	Alogliptin 25 mg/pioglitazone 45 mg
Prandimet	Repaglinide + Metformin	Repaglinide 10 mg/metformin 2,500 mg
Synjardy	Empagliflozin + Metformin	Empagliflozin 25 mg/metformin 2,000 mg
Xigduo XR	Dapagliflozin + Metformin ER	Dapagliflozin 10 mg/metformin ER 2,000 mg

Storage and Administration Pearls

- Unopened containers of insulin should be stored in the refrigerator.
- If not refrigerated, use insulin within 28 days and protect from heat and light.
- Do not freeze insulin or other injectable products.
- Once opened or in use, vials or pens may be stored in refrigerator or at room temperature for up to 28 days (42 days for detemir).
- IV insulin infusion: May be kept stable for 24 hours at room temperature.
- Weekly exenatide and albiglutide must be reconstituted prior to injection.

Patient Education Pearls

- A patient who is on alpha-glucosidase inhibitors must use a simple sugar to treat hypoglycemia anytime.
- Rotate insulin injection sites.
- Mixing rule: "Clear, then cloudy" is the rule. It still applies to NPH (cloudy), regular (clear), fast-acting (clear).
- The exceptions: Never mix detemir, glargine, or degludec (clear) with any other insulin or injectable product.
- May take several weeks to see the full effect of thiazolidinediones.

HYPOTHYROIDISM

Definitions

Primary hypothyroidism accounts for more than 90% of cases. It is due to actual disease of the thyroid itself and not from a feedback or hypothalamus issue. Hashimoto's disease is the most common cause and may be associated with Addison's disease (chronic adrenocortical insufficiency) and other endocrine deficits.

Diagnosis

Plasma thyroid-stimulating hormone (TSH) is the best initial diagnostic test. A TSH that is markedly elevated (>20 mcgU/mL) confirms the diagnosis.

Signs and Symptoms

- Most symptoms are nonspecific and develop gradually.
- Typical symptoms are cold intolerance, fatigue, weight gain, dry skin, somnolence, poor memory, and depression.
- Atypical symptoms are constipation, menorrhagia, myalgias, and hoarseness.
- Physical exam will often show slow tendon reflexes, bradycardia, and facial and periorbital edema.
- Myxedema coma (acute, severe hypothyroidism) presents with mental status, non pitting edema, and hypothermia.

Guidelines

American Association of Clinical Endocrinologists/American Thyroid Association. *Endocrine Practice* vol. 18 no. 6 (Nov/Dec 2012): www.aace.com/publications/guidelines.

Guidelines Summary

The treatment and management of chronic thyroiditis and clinical hypothyroidism must be tailored to the individual patient. Many clinical endocrinologists treat the goiter of chronic thyroiditis with levothyroxine, even in patients with normal levels of TSH, and all physicians will treat clinical hypothyroidism with levothyroxine replacement therapy.

- TSH is the primary marker for medication monitoring. Because thyroid hormone functions on a negative feedback loop, elevated levels indicate hypothyroid state and low levels indicate hyperthyroid state.
- Initial dose of levothyroxine is 1.7 mcg/kg/day. Adjust doses in 10–25 mcg/day increments based upon clinical response. Half-life of levothyroxine is approximately 1 week. TSH monitoring and dose adjustments occur at 4–8 week intervals.

Medications for Hypothyroidism

Generic • Brand • Dose	Contraindications	Primary Side Effects	Key Monitoring	Pertinent Drug Interactions	Med Pearl
Mechanism of action – T4 is c onverted to T3 and exerts many metabolic effects through control of DNA transcription and protein synthesis					
Levothyroxine ☆ (T4) • Synthroid, Levoxyl, Unithroid • Tab: 25–300 mcg daily • Also available as injection	• Recent myocardial infarction or thyrotoxicosis • Uncorrected adrenal insufficiency	• Angina • Anxiety • Alopecia • ↑ LFTs • Tachycardia	• TSH • T3 • T4 • Free T4 • Heart rate • Blood pressure • Weight	Absorption may be ↓ by: cholestyramine, aluminum-containing medications, sucralfate, sodium polystyrene sulfonate, phenytoin, carbamazepine, rifampin	• T4: not the active compound; must be converted to T3 to become active • Thyroid treatment may also be used to augment depression treatment • Narrow therapeutic index drug • Often involved in medication errors
Liothyronine (T3) • Cytomel, Triostat • Tab: 5–100 mcg daily • Also available as injection					
Desiccated thyroid ☆ T4 (80%) T3 (20%) • Armour, Thyroid • Tab: 15–120 mg daily	• Hypersensitivity to beef or pork • Recent myocardial infarction or thyrotoxicosis • Uncorrected adrenal insufficiency				• Same as above • Origin: hog, cow, sheep • 80% T4 and 20% T3 is to mimic natural physiologic production
Liotrix • Thyrolar • Levothyroxine 12.5–100 mcg/liothyronine 3.1–25 mcg daily	• Uncorrected adrenal cortical insufficiency • Untreated thyrotoxicosis				Liotrix is LT4/LT3 which is T4:T3 ratio; this ratio is 4:1

Storage and Administration Pearls

- Levothyroxine: Administer on an empty stomach
- Levothyroxine injection at room temperature (59–86°F)
  - Do not mix IV solution with other IV infusion solutions
  - Dilute vial with 5 mL of normal saline and inject immediately

Patient Education Pearls

- Thyroid supplementation is ineffective and potentially toxic for weight reduction (in euthyroid patients).
- Recheck TSH 4–8 weeks following initiation of therapy or dose change.

HYPERTHYROIDISM

Definitions

Hyperthyroidism includes Graves' disease, which causes most cases of hyperthyroidism, especially in young patients. This autoimmune disorder may cause exophthalmos (protrusion of the eyes) and pretibial myxedema (nodules and plaques on skin). Toxic multinodular goiter is a common cause. Other causes can be drug-induced (e.g., amiodarone) or radiographic contrast media and thyroid adenomas.

Diagnosis

- Plasma TSH is the best initial diagnostic test. The TSH will be markedly suppressed (<0.1 mcg/mL).

Signs and Symptoms

- Typical symptoms: Heat intolerance, insomnia, weight loss, weakness, palpitations, oligomenorrhea, and anxiety
- Sinus tachycardia, atrial fibrillation, and exacerbation of coronary artery disease
- Brisk tendon reflexes, fine tremor, proximal weakness, stare, and eyelid lag
- Thyroid storm: Presents as an acute life-threatening exaggeration of usual hyperthyroid symptoms

Guidelines

American Association of Clinical Endocrinologists/American Thyroid Association. *Endocrine Practice* vol. 17 no. 3 (May/June 2011): www.aace.com/publications/guidelines.

Guidelines Summary

Three types of therapy are available for Graves' disease: surgical intervention, antithyroid drugs, and radioactive iodine.

- In the United States, radioactive iodine is currently the treatment of choice for Graves' disease. Many clinical endocrinologists prefer an ablative dose of radioactive iodine, but some prefer use of a smaller dose in an attempt to render the patient euthyroid. Ablative therapy with radioactive iodine yields quicker resolution of the hyperthyroidism than does small-dose therapy, and thereby minimizes potential hyperthyroid-related morbidity.
- Although thyroidectomy for Graves' disease was frequently used in the past, it is now uncommonly performed in the United States unless coexistent thyroid cancer is suspected.

- Antithyroid medications methimazole and propylthiouracil have been used since the 1940s and are prescribed in an attempt to achieve a remission. The remission rates are variable, and relapses are frequent. Patients in whom remission is most likely to be achieved are those with mild hyperthyroidism and small goiters. Antithyroid drug treatment is not without the risk of adverse reactions, including minor rashes, and, in rare instances, agranulocytosis and hepatitis.

Medications for Hyperthyroidism

Generic • Brand • Dose	Contraindications	Primary Side Effects	Key Monitoring	Pertinent Drug Interactions	Med Pearl
Mechanism of action – inhibits synthesis of thyroid hormones by blocking the oxidation of iodine in the thyroid gland					
Propylthiouracil • Only available generically • Initial: 300–600 mg/day in 3–4 divided doses • Maintenance: 50–300 mg/day in 2–3 divided doses	Hypersensitivity	• Benign transient leukopenia (white blood cell [WBC] count <4,000/mm^3) • Pruritic maculo-papular rash • Arthralgias • Fever • Hepatotoxicity • Lupus-like syndrome	• WBC with differential • LFTs • TSH • T3 • T4	May $\uparrow$ effects of warfarin	• Clinical improvement approx. 4–8 weeks • Side effects with propylthio-uracil more common with higher doses and in children • Rash may be treated with antihistamine • Severe side effects may require discontinuation of therapy • "PTU" is an error-prone abbreviation; avoid use • Tapering doses may start once clinical improvement seen • Correction of hyperthyroid-ism may alter disposition of beta-blockers, digoxin, and theophylline • Propylthiouracil preferred in pregnancy
Methimazole • Tapazole • Initial: 15–60 mg/day in 3 divided doses • Maintenance: 5–30 mg/day	Hypersensitivity				

Storage and Administration Pearls

- On the NAPLEX and in the work force, PTU is an error-prone abbreviation and is not recommended for use on prescription pads, verbally, or within your computer system.

Patient Education Pearls

- Both propylthiouracil and methimazole cross the placenta. Methimazole has been associated with teratogenic effects; propylthiouracil has been associated with hepatotoxicity in pregnancy. Propylthiouracil preferred during 1st trimester of pregnancy; methimazole preferred during second and third trimesters of pregnancy.

POLYCYSTIC OVARY SYNDROME

Definitions

Polycystic ovary syndrome (PCOS) is a metabolic disorder involving infertility, hirsutism, obesity, and amenorrhea. The fundamental defect of PCOS is unknown but is thought to be from adrenal androgen excess of obesity, which results in enhanced extraglandular formation of estrogen. The dysfunctional uterine bleeding is usually due to estrogen excess.

Diagnosis

- History and physical examination, including the onset and duration of various signs of androgen excess; menstrual history; family history of DM and cardiovascular disease; lifestyle factors; evaluation of blood pressure, body mass index (BMI), and waist-hip ratio; and presence of acne, hirsutism, androgenic alopecia, and acanthosis nigricans

- Laboratory tests, including documentation of biochemical hyperandrogenemia (total testosterone and/or bioavailable or free testosterone); exclusion of other causes of hyperandrogenism, such as thyroid dysfunction, hyperprolactinemia, nonclassical congenital adrenal hyperplasia, and Cushing's syndrome; evaluation for metabolic abnormalities; and fasting lipid and lipoprotein level

- Optional tests to consider:
  - Ultrasound evaluation of ovaries
  - Gonadotropin determinations
  - Fasting insulin levels
  - 24-hour urine test

Signs and Symptoms

- Infertility: Inability to become pregnant
- Hirsutism: Caused by excess androgen levels
- Obesity: BMI > 29 kg/m^2
- Anovulation: Lack of ovulation; however, the woman may experience withdrawal bleeding after progestogen administration

Guidelines

Legro RS, Arslanian SA, Ehrmann DA, et al. Diagnosis and treatment of polycystic ovary syndrome: an Endocrine Society clinical practice guideline. *J Clin Endocrinol Metab.* 2013;98:4565–92.

Guidelines Summary

Treatment is based on a symptoms approach for anovulation, amenorrhea, ovulation induction, and hirsutism.

Anovulation and Amenorrhea

- Hormonal contraceptives (oral, patch, or vaginal ring) are first-line therapy to regulate or restore irregular or absent menses. The agents also improve symptoms of hirsutism and acne.
- Weight-reduction through a combination of calorie restriction and exercise are important; they affect and improve insulin resistance.
- Progestin, including medroxyprogesterone acetate, is often used to induce menses.
- Insulin-sensitizing agents, including metformin, pioglitazone, and rosiglitazone, are used to ↓ insulin resistance primarily in patients with type 2 diabetes or in those with impaired fasting glucose.

Ovulation Induction

- Lifestyle modifications, especially weight loss, will assist with ovulation induction.
- Clomiphene citrate is used to induce ovulation for up to 6 months.
- Ovarian drilling with laser or diathermy can be considered but is not recommended.
- Insulin-sensitizing agents, such as metformin and thiazolidinediones, can induce ovulation.

Hirsutism

- Oral contraceptives can reduce hair growth.
- Antiandrogens, including spironolactone, flutamide, insulin-sensitizing agents, and eflornithine can be used to ↓ hair growth.
- Mechanical hair removal, such as shaving, plucking, waxing, depilatory creams, electrolysis, and laser vaporization, can also be used.

Medications for Polycystic Ovary Syndrome

Generic • Brand • Dose	Contraindications	Primary Side Effects	Key Monitoring	Pertinent Drug Interactions	Med Pearl
Mechanism of action – inhibits secretion of pituitary gonadotropins, which prevents follicular maturation and ovulation; causes endometrial thinning					
Medroxyprogester-one☆ • Provera • Amenorrhea: 5–10 mg daily × 10 days	• History of deep venous thrombosis or pulmonary embolism • Pregnancy	• Headache • Weight changes • Edema • Menstrual irregularities	• Pregnancy should be ruled out • Symptoms of migraine	CYP3A4 substrate	Long-term use can lead to ↓ bone mineral density
Mechanism of action – Enclomiphene is less potent in inducing ovulation; however, it is rapidly absorbed and metabolized, allowing for the more potent zuclomiphene to act. Zuclomiphene inhibits normal estrogen negative feedback, which results in release of luteinizing hormone and follicle stimulating hormone; more potent than enclomiphene					
Clomiphene citrate (38% zuclomi-phene; 62% enclomiphene) • Clomid • 50–100 mg daily × 5 days	• Liver disease • Abnormal uterine bleeding • Ovarian cysts • Uncontrolled thyroid or adrenal dysfunction • Pregnancy	• Ovarian enlarge-ment • Hot flashes • Breast discom-fort • Nausea • Bloating	• Pregnancy test • Menstrual cycle	May ↑ effects of ospemifene	Dosages ≥150 mg do not im-prove symptoms for PCOS
Mechanism of action – competes with aldosterone receptor sites in the distal tubules					
Spironolactone☆ • Aldactone • 50–200 mg daily	• Acute renal failure • Hyperkalemia • Pregnancy	• Gynecomastia • Hyperkalemia • Nausea • Cramping	• Blood pressure • Renal function • K^+	Use with angioten-sin-converting enzyme inhibi-tors, angiotensin receptor blockers, K^+ supplements, or nonsteroidal anti-inflammato-ry drugs may ↑ risk of hyperka-lemia	Adjust dose in renal impair-ment
Mechanism of action – nonsteroidal antiandrogen that inhibits androgen uptake or inhibits binding to androgen in target tissue					
Flutamide • Only available generically • 125–250 mg BID-TID	• Severe hepatic impairment • Pregnancy	• Gynecomastia • Hot flashes • Breast tender-ness • Galactorrhea • ↓ libido	LFTs monthly for 4 mo, then periodi-cally	1A2 substrate	Most cases of liver failure occur within first 3 months of therapy

Medications for Polycystic Ovary Syndrome *(cont'd)*

Generic • Brand • Dose	Contraindications	Primary Side Effects	Key Monitoring	Pertinent Drug Interactions	Med Pearl
Mechanism of action – inhibitor of 5-alpha reductase which results in the inhibition of conversion of testosterone to dihydrotestosterone					
Finasteride ☆ • Proscar, Propecia • 2.5–5 mg daily	• Pregnancy	• Impotence • Ejaculation disturbances • ↓ libido • Orthostatic hypotension	Absolute need for dual forms of birth control	None	Women should avoid contact with crushed or broken tablets and the semen from a male partner exposed to finasteride (teratogen)
Mechanism of action – inhibits ornithine decarboxylase, the rate-limiting enzyme in biosynthesis of putrescine, spermin, and spermidine (rapid dividing cell most susceptible)					
Eflornithine • Vaniqa • Apply BID	Hypersensitivity	• Acne • Pruritus • Alopecia • Stinging	None	None	• Used to ↓ unwanted facial hair • Do not wash affected area for 8 hours following application • Onset of action 4–8 wk

Storage and Administration Pearls

- Women should avoid contact with crushed or broken tablets and the semen from a male partner exposed to finasteride

Patient Education Pearls

- Prolonged use of medroxyprogesterone may result in a loss of bone mineral density.

LEARNING POINTS

- The basic diagnoses for type 1 and type 2 DM are identical. However, patients with type 2 will go undiagnosed for as long as 10 years, whereas type 1 is usually diagnosed within 6 months. As a result, it is important to consider and assess risk factors for type 2 DM.

- For the NAPLEX, it is important that you understand the different mechanisms of action of the diabetes medications to ensure you can catch duplication of actions within the patient's drug profile.

- Hypothyroidism and hyperthyroidism have opposite side effects (i.e., somnolence with hypothyroid; insomnia with hyperthyroidism).

- PCOS has become more common as obesity rates have risen and as more women want to become pregnant.

- Remember, many women with diabetes may have PCOS and may be placed on an insulin sensitizer such as a glitazone. As a result, it is important to counsel the patient on an increased risk for ovulation if her uterus is still intact.

PRACTICE QUESTIONS

1. Patients with overactive thyroid may present with which of the following symptoms?

    (A) Weight loss
    (B) Heat intolerance
    (C) Heart palpitations
    (D) Goiter
    (E) All of the above

2. A patient comes to the pharmacy and tells you that her blood sugars were 126 and 127 mg/dL fasting on two occasions. She wants some advice because her doctor didn't have time to talk with her. What is the main point you will be addressing with this woman?

    (A) This patient does not have diabetes because the doctor did the same test.
    (B) This patient has diabetes but it's not bad and will not need medication.
    (C) This patient has diabetes but does not need education; she should just watch what she eats and exercise more.
    (D) This patient doesn't have diabetes but might develop it soon.
    (E) This patient has diabetes, needs a formal diabetes education class, and is likely a candidate for a medication called metformin.

3. How many days can Humalog stay out of the refrigerator and be considered safe to administer?

    (A) 1 day
    (B) 28 days
    (C) 56 days
    (D) 90 days
    (E) 180 days

4. A 62-year-old woman (5′2″, 180 lb) with type 2 diabetes, history of medullary thyroid carcinoma, osteopenia, and stage 3 chronic kidney disease (CrCl = 45 mL/min) presents for routine follow-up. Current medications include metformin 1 g BID, lisinopril 10 mg PO daily, calcium carbonate/vitamin D 600/400 BID, and aspirin 81 mg PO daily. Labs today include A1c 7.6%, AST 20 IU/L, ALT 22 IU/L and K 4.2 mEq/L. Which of the following is the most appropriate recommendation?

    (A) Initiate Bydureon 2 mg SC once each week.
    (B) Initiate pioglitazone 30 mg PO once daily.
    (C) Initiate insulin glargine 40 units once daily.
    (D) Initiate sitagliptin 50 mg PO daily.

5. Which of the following medications is contraindicated in a patient with heart failure?

   (A) Exenatide
   (B) Sitagliptin
   (C) Glimepiride
   (D) Pioglitazone

6. Which of the following medications is most likely to cause hypoglycemia?

   (A) Metformin
   (B) Glipizide
   (C) Sitagliptin
   (D) Exenatide

7. Which of the following mechanisms most accurately describes the action of exenatide?

   (A) Mimics glucagon-like peptide-1
   (B) Inhibits gluconeogenesis in the liver
   (C) Inhibits the dipeptidyl peptidase IV enzyme
   (D) Increases insulin sensitivity in the periphery

8. A 65-year-old woman (5'2", 182 lb) with hypertension, heart failure (NHYA Class I), and history of pancreatitis is newly diagnosed with type 2 diabetes. Medications include lisinopril 20 mg PO daily, carvedilol 6.25 mg PO BID, and aspirin 81 mg PO daily. Serum laboratory results today include A1c 8.3%, creatinine 1.6 mg/dL, ALT 35 IU/L, and BNP 20 pg/mL. A prescription is written for metformin. Which of the following statements is the best evaluation of this therapy?

   (A) Appropriate drug; no contraindications present
   (B) Inappropriate drug; contraindicated due to pancreatitis
   (C) Inappropriate drug; contraindicated due to heart failure
   (D) Inappropriate drug; contraindicated due to renal function

9. A 72-year-old man with hypothyroidism is treated with levothyroxine 88 mcg
    PO daily for 6 weeks. His TSH returns at 18 mIU/L (normal range 0.4–4 mIU/L).
    Which of the following is the most appropriate recommendation?

    (A) Increase levothyroxine dose to 100 mcg PO daily, recheck TSH in 2 weeks.
    (B) Increase levothyroxine dose to 100 mcg PO daily, recheck TSH in 6 weeks.
    (C) Decrease levothyroxine dose to 75 mcg PO daily, recheck TSH in 2 weeks.
    (D) Decrease levothyroxine dose to 75 mcg PO daily, recheck TSH in 6 weeks.

10. Which of the following is an appropriate patient education to provide for a patient
    on oral levothyroxine?

    (A) Take medication after a high-fat meal.
    (B) Take medication on an empty stomach.
    (C) Take medication without regard to meals.
    (D) Take medication with a glass of milk.

ANSWERS AND EXPLANATIONS

1. E

Weight loss, heat intolerance, heart palpitations, and goiter are all commonly seen symptoms with hyperthyroid disorders. Other common symptoms include nervousness, emotional lability, bowel frequency, irregular menses, and increased appetite.

2. E

This patient has diabetes and needs a formal diabetes education class. The newest guidelines suggest starting all eligible patients on metformin at the time of diagnosis. Choice (A) is not correct because this woman does have diabetes—her fasting blood sugar was verified and was ≥126 mg/dL. Although the doctor caught the disease early, the patient still needs to seek formal education as this will lead to the best management.

3. B

Most unopened insulin preparations are stable at normal temperatures for 28 days. They should not be used if frozen or exposed to temperature greater than 98.6°F. Once opened (in use), vials may be stored in the refrigerator or for up to 28 days at room temperature.

4. D

Sitagliptin 50 mg PO daily is an appropriate agent to lower the A1c as needed and at an appropriate dose for renal function (30–50 mL/min = 50 mg daily). Bydureon (A) would be inappropriate for this patient due to the history of medullary thyroid carcinoma. Pioglitazone (B) would not be a good choice due to its potential to decrease bone mineral density; this patient has osteopenia. Although insulin glargine (C) would be an appropriate option, the dose of 40 units daily is too high for a starting dose.

5. D

Pioglitazone is contraindicated in a patient with heart failure. Thiazolidinediones have a side effect profile that includes fluid retention/edema and have demonstrated increases in heart failure exacerbations. The class should be avoided in patients with heart failure, especially NYHA classes III and IV.

6. B

Sulfonylureas such as glipizide have the greatest risk of hypoglycemia among the listed agents. Metformin (A) does not cause hypoglycemia as monotherapy. Although sitagliptin (C) and exenatide (D) can cause hypoglycemia, the risk is significantly lower than with secretagogues.

7. **A**

Exenatide is a glucagon-like peptide agonist that, by mimicking this incretin hormone, results in glucose-dependent insulin secretion, slowed gastric emptying, and diminished glucagon secretion postprandially.

8. **D**

Metformin is contraindicated in female patients with serum creatinine ≥1.4 mg/dL and males with serum creatinine ≥1.5 mg/dL. Pancreatitis (B) is not a contraindication to the use of metformin. Decompensated heart failure (C) is a contraindication to the medication, but this patient's heart failure is currently compensated (NYHA class I).

9. **B**

The TSH elevation indicates that the patient remains hypothyroid and requires a higher dose of levothyroxine. The half-life of levothyroxine is ~1 week; therefore, TSH levels are checked at 4–8 weeks to allow medication to reach steady state.

10. **B**

Levothyroxine is best and most consistently absorbed when taken on an empty stomach. Taking it with a high-fat meal (A), other food (C), or milk (D) would decrease absorption.

Neurological Disorders

5

This chapter covers the following disease states:

- **Multiple sclerosis**
- **Epilepsy**
- **Parkinson's disease**
- **Migraine headache**
- **Alzheimer's disease**

 Suggested Study Time: **55 minutes**

MULTIPLE SCLEROSIS

Definitions

Multiple sclerosis (MS) is a disease of the central nervous system (CNS) characterized by inflammation within the brain and spinal cord that results in areas of plaque formation and sclerosis and leads to neurological symptoms. The basic pathophysiological defect in MS is the demyelinization of the sheath surrounding the neurons in the CNS.

Diagnosis

The diagnosis of MS is based primarily on clinical presentation and requires ≥2 episodes of neurologic symptoms that cannot be attributed to another cause; represent distinct areas of CNS involvement; and occur at least 3 months apart. The McDonald criteria are often used to diagnose MS. These criteria require 2 lesions separated by 3 months but allow for the use of MRI and cerebrospinal fluid analysis to be used as identification of a second attack. MRI is useful for confirming diagnosis of MS because it is highly selective for MS lesions.

Signs and Symptoms

- The most common symptoms of early MS include weakness/numbness of limbs and visual disturbances.
- The clinical presentation of MS varies among patients and is classified as relapsing-remitting, primary progressive, or secondary progressive.
  - Relapsing-remitting MS: Most common (85%) and characterized by frequent symptomatic episodes of ≥24 hours' duration followed by periods of remission of at least 30 days. During remission, residual symptoms and increasing clinical deficit are common.
  - Primary progressive MS: Occurs in ~10% of patients and consists of persistently progressive disease from the time of disease onset that does not include remissions or relapses. This classification is associated with a poor prognosis.
  - Secondary progressive MS: Occurs in ~5% of patients. Many patients originally classified as relapsing-remitting may be reclassified as secondary progressive during the course of illness.

Guidelines

The Use of Disease Modifying Therapies in Multiple Sclerosis: Principles and Current Evidence. Multiple Sclerosis Coalition Consensus Paper. 2015. www.nationalmssociety.org.

Medical Advisory Board of the National Multiple Sclerosis Society. Recommendations Regarding Corticosteroids in the Management of Multiple Sclerosis Expert Opinion Paper. 2008. www.nationalmssociety.org.

Guidelines Summary

The clinical management of MS should include consideration of treatment for acute exacerbations, altering the disease process, and alleviating ongoing symptoms related to the disease.

Disease-modifying drugs (DMDs) are used to alter the disease process. Treatment with interferon beta or glatiramer should be initiated as soon as possible after diagnosis in patients with relapsing disease. Therapies should be continued indefinitely except in the case of intolerable side effects, clear lack of benefit, or new therapy considerations.

Acute exacerbations—The cornerstone of therapy for acute exacerbations is IV corticosteroids. Methylprednisolone is most commonly used at 50–100 mg/day for 3 to 10 days. Oral prednisone may also be considered, but there is not strong evidence for using oral corticosteroids. Although corticosteroids have been shown to be very effective in the treatment of acute exacerbations, they do not alter the disease process.

Altering disease process—DMDs are the therapy of choice in altering the MS disease process. The 13 currently approved DMDs include: interferon-β1a (Avonex and Rebif), interferon-β1b

(Betaseron and Extavia), peginterferon β1a (Plegridy), glatiramer acetate (Copaxone), natalizumab (Tysabri), mitoxantrone (Novantrone), dimethyl fumarate (Tecfidera), teriflunomide (Aubagio), fingolimod (Gilenya), alemtuzumab (Lemtrada), and daclizumab (Zinbryta).

- The interferon agents and glatiramer acetate are considered first-line DMDs, whereas natalizumab is reserved for patients who do not respond to those therapies.
- Natalizumab may be considered if a patient cannot tolerate or has a poor response to another MS medication.
- Dimethyl fumarate, teriflunomide, fingolimod, alemtuzumab, and daclizumab are approved for relapsing MS.
- Mitoxantrone is approved to treat worsening relapsing-remitting MS and secondary progressive MS.
- Patients are generally treated with one DMD at a time, but worsening disease can be treated with combination DMD + mitoxantrone pulse therapy.

Symptom management—Dalfampridine (Ampyra) is used to improve walking in patients with MS.

Disease-Modifying Drugs

Generic • Brand • Dose & Max	Contraindications	Primary Side Effects	Key Monitoring Parameters	Pertinent Drug Interactions	Med Pearls
Disease-Modifying Drugs					
Mechanism of action – anti-inflammatory and immunomodulatory effects are exerted through binding of interferon to human cell-surface receptors and subsequent ↓ T-cell production of pro-inflammatory cytokines, ↓ production of pro-inflammatory lymphocytes, and ↑ production of anti-inflammatory lymphocytes					
Interferon-β1a • Avonex, Rebif • Avonex: 30 mcg IM weekly • Rebif: 4.4–8.8 mcg subcut 3 times weekly × 2 wk, then 11–22 mcg subcut 3 times weekly × 2 wk, then 22–44 mcg 3 times weekly Interferon-β1b • Betaseron, Extavia • 0.0625 mg subcut every other day; ↑ dose by 0.0625 mg every 2 wk to target dose of 0.25 mg subcut every other day Peginterferon-β1a • Plegridy • 63 mcg subcut on day 1, then 94 mcg subcut on day 15, then 125 mcg subcut every 2 wk starting on day 29	• Hypersensitivity to interferon–β or human albumin • Allergy to other interferons	• Flu-like symptoms (fever, chills, fatigue, muscle aches) • Injection site reactions • Anemia • Thrombocytopenia • Hepatotoxicity • Depression	• Liver function tests (LFTs) • Complete blood count (CBC)	None	• Acetaminophen or nonsteroidal anti-inflammatory drugs (NSAIDs) can ↓ flu-like symptoms • Neutralizing antibodies may develop, rendering the drug less efficacious

Disease-Modifying Drugs (cont'd)

Generic • Brand • Dose & Max	Contraindications	Primary Side Effects	Key Monitoring Parameters	Pertinent Drug Interactions	Med Pearls
Mechanism of action – influences immature CD4 cells to become less inflammatory, thereby suppressing demyelination and preventing nerve fiber damage					
Glatiramer acetate • Copaxone, Glatopa • 20 mg subcut daily or 40 mg subcut 3 times/week	Hypersensitivity to the drug or to mannitol	• Injection site reactions • Postinjection reactions (chest pain, palpitations)	Injection reactions	• Natalizumab • Live vaccines • Tofacitinib • Tacrolimus • Pimecrolimus	Does not produce neutralizing antibodies
Mechanism of action – ↓ central inflammation by binding to sphingosine 1-phosphate receptors					
Fingolimod • Gilenya • 0.5 mg PO daily	• Myocardial infarction • Unstable angina • Transient ischemic attack/cerebrovascular accident • New York Heart Association class III/IV or decompensated heart failure (HF) • Atrioventricular (AV) block/sick sinus syndrome • QTc interval ≥500 msec • Concurrent use with class Ia or III antiarrhythmic	• Bradycardia • AV block • Hypertension • Infection • Macular edema • Dyspnea • ↑ LFTs • Diarrhea • Headache • Flu-like syndrome • HF • QT interval prolongation • Hypersensitivity reactions • Posterior reversible encephalopathy syndrome (PRES) • Progressive multifocal leukoencephalopathy (PML)	• Heart rate (HR) • Blood pressure (BP) • CBC • Electrocardiogram (ECG) • Ophthalmologic exam • LFTs • S/S of HF • S/S of PRES or PML • S/S of infection	• Class Ia and class III antiarrhythmics may ↑ risk of bradycardia and AV block • Avoid use of live vaccines • Use with QT-interval prolonging agents may ↑ risk of torsades de pointes (TdP)	Give zoster vaccination prior to administration, if needed
Mechanism of action – monoclonal antibody inhibits pro-inflammatory interactions within vascular endothelial cells and parenchymal brain cells					
Natalizumab • Tysabri • 300 mg IV infusion every 4 wk	• Hypersensitivity • Current or history of PML	• Infusion reactions (rash, drowsiness, fever, chills, hypotension, nausea, shortness of breath) • ↑ LFTs • Infection • Headache • Fatigue • Arthralgia • PML	• Magnetic resonance imaging (MRI) (baseline and then in PML suspected) • LFTs • Infusion reactions • S/S of infection	Other DMDs ↑ risk of PML	• Reserved for patients who have not responded to other DMDs • Should be used as monotherapy only; combining with other DMDs ↑ risk of PML • Available only through a restrictive prescribing program (MS-TOUCH) • Also indicated for Crohn's disease

Disease-Modifying Drugs (cont'd)

Generic • Brand • Dose & Max	Contraindications	Primary Side Effects	Key Monitoring Parameters	Pertinent Drug Interactions	Med Pearls
Mechanism of action – ↓ migration of T cells into the CNS by arresting the cell cycle and interfering with DNA repair and RNA synthesis					
Mitoxantrone • Only available generically • 12 mg/m² IV infusion every 3 mo; max cumulative dose = 140 mg/m²	Hypersensitivity	• HF • Nausea • Neutropenia • Alopecia • Menstrual irregularities • Infection	• Echocardiogram (left ventricular ejection fraction [LVEF] at baseline and prior to each IV infusion) • CBC with differential • LFTs • S/S of infection	Avoid use of live vaccines	Discontinue therapy if LVEF <50% or clinically significant decline in LVEF
Mechanism of action – activates nuclear factor–like 2 (Nrf 2) pathway, ↓ inflammatory response to oxidative stress					
Dimethyl fumarate • Tecfidera • 120 mg PO BID × 7 days, then 240 mg PO BID	Hypersensitivity	• Dermatitis • Flushing • ↑ LFTs • Lymphopenia • Nausea/vomiting/diarrhea (N/V/D) • Hypersensitivity reaction • PML • Infection	• CBC with differential (baseline, 6 mo, then every 6-12 mo) • S/S of PML • S/S of infection • LFTs	May ↓ effectivness and ↑ toxicity of live vaccines	May give with food or give aspirin 325 mg 30 min before to ↓ flushing
Mechanism of action – inhibits pyrimidine synthesis, ↓ proliferation and inflammation					
Teriflunomide • Aubagio • 7–14 mg PO daily	• Hypersensitivity • Severe hepatic impairment • Pregnancy • Women of childbearing age without adequate contraception	• Hepatotoxicity • Rash • Hypersensitivity reaction • Hypertension • Infection • Interstitial lung disease • Peripheral neuropathy • Neutropenia • Headache • Alopecia • N/D	• CBC with differential • LFTs (monthly for first 6 months) • BP • Renal function • PPD (prior to initiation) • Pregnancy test (prior to initiation) • S/S of infection	• CYP2C8 inhibitor • CYP1A2 inducer • May ↓ effects of warfarin • Avoid use of live vaccines	Counsel males and females on appropriate use of contraception during therapy (teratogenic)

Disease-Modifying Drugs *(cont'd)*

Generic • Brand • Dose & Max	Contraindications	Primary Side Effects	Key Monitoring Parameters	Pertinent Drug Interactions	Med Pearls
Mechanism of action – monocolonal antibody to CD52 receptors which causes the depletion of lymphocytes to CD52 receptors which causes the depletion of lymphocytes					
Alemtuzumab • Lemtrada • 12 mg IV daily × 5 days, then 12 mg daily × 3 days 12 months later	HIV infection	• Autoimmune conditions • Bone marrow suppression • Infection • Infusion reactions • Pulmonary fibrosis • PML • Thyroid disease • Malignancy (melanoma)	• CBC with differential • S/S of infection • Thyroid stimulating hormone • S/S of infusion reactions • S/S of PML • Malignancy • S/S of pulmonary fibrosis • Renal function • Urinalysis • Skin exam	Avoid use of live vaccines	• REMS program • Premedicate with corticosteroids for first 3 days of each treatment course • Initiate antiviral therapy on 1st day of therapy and continue for 2 mo or until CD4+ cell count >200/m³
Mechanism of action – monoclonal antibody inhibitor of IL-2					
Daclizumab • Zinbryta • 150 mg subcut monthly	• Hypersensitivity • impairment • Autoimmune hepatitis	• Hepatotoxicity • Autoimmune disorders • Photosensitivity • N/D • Hypersensitivity reaction • Infection • Depression • Suicidal thoughts	• LFTs • S/S of infection	Avoid use of live vaccines	• REMS program • Screen for TB and hepatitis B/C prior to initiating therapy
Symptom Management					
Mechanism of action – potassium channel blocker; ↑ action potential in demyelinated axon					
Dalfampridine • Ampyra • 10 mg PO every 12 hr	• History of seizures • Moderate–severe renal impairment (creatinine clearance ≤50 mL/min) • Hypersensitivity	• Seizures • Anaphylaxis • Urinary tract infection • Dizziness • Insomnia • Headache • Nausea • Balance disturbance	• Renal function • Walking ability	None	• Indicated to improve walking in patients with MS • Seizure risk is dose-dependent

Storage and Administration Pearls

- Interferon β1a, interferon β1b, glatiramer acetate, natalizumab, and mitoxantrone should be refrigerated to 2–8°C (36–46°F). These products should not be frozen and should be protected from light.

- Interferon β1 products and glatiramer acetate are available in prefilled syringes.

- Interferon β1 products and glatiramer acetate can be self-administered. Natalizumab, mitoxantrone, and alemtuzumab are administered via IV infusion by qualified health-care professionals.

- Alemtuzumab should be refrigerated prior to dilution. This product should not be frozen and should be protected from light. Diluted product can be stored at room temperature or frozen and should be used within 8 hours.

- Daclizumab, a single-dose, prefilled syringe, should be refrigerated to 2–8°C (36–46°F). The medication should not be frozen and if it is has, it should then be discarded. Daclizumab may be stored up to 30°C (86°F) if protected from light for up to 30 days. Once the medication has reached room temperature, it should not be placed back into the refrigerator, but instead be discarded.

Patient Education Pearls

- For self-injectable therapies:
  - Use the auto-injector supplied by the manufacturer (when available).
  - Apply ice to the injection site prior to injection.
  - Allow the medication to reach room temperature prior to injection.
  - Rotate injection sites.

- For those newly initiated on therapy, a natalizumab medication guide should be provided. Both patient and provider must be enrolled in TOUCH prescribing program.

- Dimethyl fumarate should not be crushed or chewed. It may irritate mucous membranes on contact.

- Teriflunomide requires a reliable form of contraception.

EPILEPSY

Definitions

Epilepsy is a symptom of disturbed electrical activity within the brain. Epilepsy is a general term that encompasses a wide variety of symptomatic presentations that include periodic and recurrent seizures with or without convulsions. Seizures are classified as partial, generalized, or status epilepticus.

Partial seizures begin in one hemisphere of the brain and result in symptoms that are asymmetrical. Partial seizures can be classified as simple (no impairment of consciousness), complex (with impaired consciousness), or secondarily generalized (partial onset which becomes generalized).

Generalized seizures are bilateral/symmetrical in symptoms and can be classified as absence, myoclonic, clonic, tonic, tonic-clonic, atonic, or infantile spasms. The most common types are absence and tonic-clonic.

Diagnosis

The diagnosis of epilepsy is based on comprehensive history and physical, electroencephalography (EEG), and brain imaging by computed tomography (CT) scan or MRI. Differential diagnosis is important with exclusion of potential underlying causes of seizure including metabolic abnormalities (ruled out with evaluation of routine laboratory chemistries), traumatic head injury (determined by history), and presence of underlying structural abnormalities such as tumor (ruled out through brain imaging studies).

Signs and Symptoms

The clinical presentation of epilepsy is dependent on the classification of seizure type.

- Partial seizures result in asymmetrical alterations in motor function and in sensory or somatosensory symptoms, and may or may not involve a loss of consciousness. Nervous ticks, aberrations of normal behavior, and memory loss are also possible.
- Generalized seizures have symptoms that indicate involvement of both hemispheres of the brain. Motor symptoms are bilateral and there may be a loss of consciousness.
  - Absence seizures manifest as sudden interruption of ongoing activities, a blank stare, or an upward rotation of the eyes.
  - Tonic-clonic seizures consist of sharp tonic muscle contractions, rigidity, and clonic movement that are accompanied by a loss of consciousness and may be preceded by an aura.

Guidelines

Efficacy and tolerability of the new antiepileptic drugs I: treatment of new onset epilepsy: report of the Therapeutics and Technology Assessment Subcommittee and Quality Standards Subcommittee of the American Academy of Neurology and the American Epilepsy Society. *Neurology* 2004;62: 1252–60. http://www.guideline.gov/summary/summary.aspx?ss=15&doc_id=5183&nbr=3565.

Evidence-based guideline: treatment of convulsive status epilepticus in children and adults: report of the Guideline Committee of the American Epilepsy Society. *Epilepsy Currents.* 2016;16: 48–61.

Guidelines Summary

- Goals of treatment include a lack of seizure activity, minimal medication side effects of treatment, and improved quality of life.

- Treatment with antiepileptic drugs (AEDs) is warranted for patients that experience multiple seizures or have significantly affected quality of life. AED choice is based on the specific seizure type, the patient's age, comorbidities, ability to adhere to the regimen, and insurance coverage.

- AED monotherapy is preferred, but some patients may require combination therapy.

- First-line AEDs for partial seizures include carbamazepine, phenytoin, lamotrigine, valproic acid, and oxcarbazepine.

- First-line AEDs for generalized absence seizures include valproic acid and ethosuximide.

- First-line AEDs for tonic-clonic seizures include phenytoin, carbamazepine, and valproic acid.

- Alternative AEDs include gabapentin, topiramate, levetiracetam, zonisamide, tiagabine, primidone, felbamate, lamotrigine, phenobarbital, lacosamide, vigabatrin, and perampanel.

- The Food and Drug Administration (FDA) issued an alert regarding the relationship between the use of AEDs and suicidality (including suicidal behavior or ideation). Pooled analyses completed by the FDA indicated a significant ↑ of suicidality for patients treated with AEDs when compared to those given placebo. All AEDs appear to ↑ the risk similarly. Manufacturers of all AEDs are now required to include a boxed warning in their prescribing information and to include a medication guide for patients in their product labeling regarding the risk of suicide.

Antiepileptic Drugs

Generic • Brand • Dose/Dosage Forms	Contraindications	Primary Side Effects	Key Monitoring Parameters	Med Pearls
Mechanism of action – inhibits voltage-gated sodium channels, thereby depressing electrical transmission in the nucleus ventralis anterior of the thalamus				
Carbamazepine☆ • Carbatrol, Epitol, Equetro, Tegretol, Tegretol XR • 200–1,600 mg/day in 2 divided doses • ER cap, ER tabs, suspension, tabs	• Bone marrow suppression • Concomitant use with monoamine oxidase inhibitors (MAOIs) or non-nucleoside transcriptase inhibitors	• Dizziness • Drowsiness • Unsteadiness • N/V • Blurred vision • Aplastic anemia • Agranulocytosis • Rash (Stevens-Johnson syndrome possible) • Hyponatremia	• CBC with differential • Suicidality • Serum drug concentrations (4–12 mcg/mL) • Serum Na+ concentrations	• First-line for partial seizures and generalized tonic-clonic seizures • ↑ risk of Stevens-Johnson syndrome in patients with HLA-B*1502 allele (Asian descent)
Mechanism of action – thought to ↑ gamma amino butyric acid (GABA) concentrations in the brain				
Valproic acid (divalproex sodium)☆ • Depakote, Depakote ER, Depakene, Depacon • 10–60 mg/kg/day • Caps, delayed-release caps/tabs, ER tabs, injection, solution, sprinkle caps	• Hepatic impairment • Urea cycle disorders	• Hepatotoxicity • Thrombocytopenia • Hyperammonemia • Weight gain • Pancreatitis • Headache • Somnolence • Dizziness • Alopecia	• Serum drug concentrations (50–100 mcg/mL) • LFTs • CBC • Serum ammonia concentrations • Suicidality	• First-line for partial, generalized, tonic-clonic, and absence seizures • Highly teratogenic
Mechanism of action – promotes neuronal sodium efflux, thereby stabilizing the threshold against hyperexcitability				
Phenytoin☆ • Dilantin • 100–200 mg TID • Caps, chewable tabs, injection, suspension	Hypersensitivity	• Nystagmus • Ataxia • Slurred speech • Dizziness • Insomnia • Headache • Tremor • Gingival hyperplasia • Rash (Stevens-Johnson syndrome possible)	• Serum drug concentrations (10–20 mcg/mL) • Suicidality	• First-line option for partial and generalized tonic-clonic seizures • Abrupt discontinuation should be avoided (may precipitate status epilepticus) • Takes 7–10 days to reach steady state • Therapeutic concentration must be corrected for hypoalbuminemia (serum albumin <4 g/dL): corrected phenytoin concentration = measured total concentration/([0.2*albumin] + 0.1) • ↑ risk of Stevens-Johnson syndrome in patients with HLA-B*1502 allele (Asian descent)

Antiepileptic Drugs (cont'd)

Generic • Brand • Dose/Dosage Forms	Contraindications	Primary Side Effects	Key Monitoring Parameters	Med Pearls
Mechanism of action – depresses motor cortex and elevates the threshold of the CNS to convulsive stimuli				
Ethosuximide • Zarontin • 250–1,500 mg/day in divided doses • Caps, solution	Hypersensitivity	• Ataxia • Drowsiness • N/V/D • Blood dyscrasias • Rash (Stevens-Johnson syndrome possible)	• CBC • Suicidality • Serum drug concentration (40–100 mcg/mL)	Used ONLY for absence seizures
Mechanism of action – blocks voltage-sensitive sodium channels, resulting in stabilization of hyperexcitable neuronal membranes				
Oxcarbazepine ☆ • Oxtellar XR, Trileptal • IR: 300–600 mg BID • ER: 600–1,200 mg daily • ER tabs, suspension, tabs	Hypersensitivity	• Sedation • Dizziness • Ataxia • Nausea • Rash (Stevens-Johnson syndrome possible) • Hyponatremia • Angioedema	• Suicidality • Serum Na+ concentrations	• Adjust dose in renal impairment • 25-30% risk of cross-sensitivity in patients allergic to carbamazepine • ↑ risk of Stevens-Johnson syndrome in patients with HLA-B*1502 allele (Asian descent)
Felbamate • Felbatol • 1,200–3,600 mg/day in 3-4 divided doses • Suspension, tabs	• Hypersensitivity • Blood dyscrasias • Hepatic impairment	• Aplastic anemia • Acute liver failure • Anorexia • N/V • Insomnia • Headache	• CBC • LFTs • Suicidality	• AST or ALT ≥2 × upper limit of normal requires discontinuation • Not a first-line agent; reserved for refractory cases
Lamotrigine ☆ • Lamictal, Lamictal XR • IR: 25–700 mg/day in 1-2 divided doses • ER: 25-600 mg daily • Chewable tabs, ER tabs, ODTs, tabs	Hypersensitivity	• Rash (Stevens-Johnson syndrome possible) • Blood dyscrasias • Aseptic meningitis • Diplopia • Dizziness • Headache	• Rash • Suicidality • S/S of aseptic meningitis • CBC	• Risk of rash ↑ when combined with valproate • First-line option for partial seizures • Slow dose titration necessary (to minimize risk for rash) • May cause false-positive for phencyclidine (PCP) • Adjust dose in hepatic impairment
Lacosamide • Vimpat • 50-200 mg BID • Injection, solution, tabs	None	• N/V • Ataxia • Dizziness • PR interval prolongation • AV block • Headache • Fatigue • Diplopia • Tremor	• Suicidality • ECG (in patients with conduction abnormalities, on negative chronotropic drugs or with cardiovascular disease) at baseline and at steady state or when receiving IV	• Schedule V controlled substance • Adjust dose in renal or hepatic impairment

Antiepileptic Drugs *(cont'd)*

Generic • Brand • Dose/Dosage Forms	Contraindications	Primary Side Effects	Key Monitoring Parameters	Med Pearls
Mechanism of action – although structurally similar to GABA, pharmacological effects in epilepsy are not fully understood				
Gabapentin ☆ • Neurontin • 300–1,200 mg TID • Caps, solution, tabs	Hypersensitivity	• Dizziness • Fatigue • Somnolence • Ataxia • Weight gain • Angioedema • Behavioral disturbances (aggression, agitation, anger, anxiety, depression, hostility, nervousness) • Difficulty concentrating • Restlessness	• Suicidality	• No significant drug interactions • Adjust dose in renal impairment • Also used for various neuropathies
Mechanism of action – blocks voltage-dependent sodium channels, augments GABA activity, antagonizes glutamate receptors				
Topiramate ☆ • Qudexy XR, Topamax, Trokendi XR • IR: 25–200 mg BID • ER: 50–400 mg daily • ER caps, sprinkle caps, tabs	Hypersensitivity	• Difficulty concentrating • Confusion • Memory issues • Speech problems • Depression • Somnolence • Fatigue • Dizziness • Headache • Weight loss • Kidney stones • Angle closure glaucoma • Visual field defects • ↓ sweating • Hyperthermia • Metabolic acidosis • Hyperammonemia • Encephalopathy • Paresthesia	• Suicidality • Serum bicarbonate concentrations • Serum ammonia concentration (if unexplained lethargy, vomiting, or mental status changes) • Intraocular pressure	• Adjust dose in renal impairment • Slow titration necessary to minimize side effects • Teratogenic • Also indicated for migraines

Antiepileptic Drugs *(cont'd)*

Generic • Brand • Dose/Dosage Forms	Contraindications	Primary Side Effects	Key Monitoring Parameters	Med Pearls
Mechanism of action – not well understood, thought to inhibit calcium channels and facilitate GABA transmission				
Levetiracetam ☆ • Keppra, Spritam • IR: 500–1500 mg BID • ER: 1,000–3,000 mg daily • ER tabs, injection, ODTs, solution, tabs	None	• Dizziness • Behavioral disturbances (aggression, agitation, anger, anxiety, depression, hostility, nervousness) • Psychotic symptoms • Somnolence • Fatigue • Rash (Stevens-Johnson syndrome possible) • Ataxia • Anemia • Neutropenia • Hypertension	• Renal function • Suicidality • CNS disturbances • BP (in children) • CBC with differential	• Adjust dose in renal impairment • No significant drug interactions • Do not chew or crush IR tabs
Mechanism of action – elevates seizure threshold by ↓ postsynaptic excitability through stimulation of postsynaptic GABA inhibitory responses				
Phenobarbital ☆ • Only available generically • 60–200 mg/day in 2–3 divided doses • Elixir, injection, solution, tabs	• Severe liver impairment • Hypersensitivity • Porphyria • Dyspnea or airway obstruction	• Sedation • Nystagmus • Ataxia • Agitation • Hyperactivity • Headache • Nausea • Agranulocytosis • Rash (Stevens-Johnson syndrome possible) • Behavior changes • Intellectual blunting • Mood change • Respiratory depression (IV)	• Serum concentrations 20–40 mcg/mL • CBC with differential • LFTs • Suicidality	• Schedule IV controlled substance • Drug of choice for neonatal seizures • Frequency of side effects limits use • Titrate dose slowly to minimize side effects • Takes 3–4 wk to reach steady-state
Primidone • Mysoline • 750–2,000 mg/day in 3–4 divided doses • Tabs			• Serum concentrations 5–12 mcg/mL • CBC with differential • LFTs • Suicidality	Metabolized to phenobarbital
Mechanism of action – potent and specific inhibitor of GABA uptake into neuronal elements, thereby enhances GABA activity by ↓ its removal from the neuronal space				
Tiagabine • Gabitril • 32–56 mg/day in 2–4 divided doses • Tabs	Hypersensitivity	• Dizziness • Fatigue • Difficulty concentrating • Speech problems • Confusion • Somnolence • Rash (Stevens-Johnson syndrome possible) • Nervousness • Tremor • Blurred vision • Depression • Weakness	Suicidality	Take with food

Antiepileptic Drugs (cont'd)

Generic • Brand • Dose/Dosage Forms	Contraindications	Primary Side Effects	Key Monitoring Parameters	Med Pearls
Mechanism of action – irreversible inhibition of gamma-aminobutyric acid transaminase (GABA-T), thereby ↑ the levels of GABA within the brain				
Vigabatrin • Sabril • 500 mg BID, then ↑ daily dose by 500 mg at weekly intervals (max dose = 1,500 mg BID) • Packet for oral solution, tabs	None	• Permanent vision loss • Anemia • Fatigue • Somnolence • Peripheral neuropathy • Edema • Tremor • Memory impairment • Weight gain • Confusion	• Ophthalmologic exam (every 3 mo) • Suicidality • CBC	• Adjust dose in renal impairment • Black box warning due to ophthalmologic effects • Available only through special REMS program
Mechanism of action – blocks voltage-dependent sodium and calcium channels, thereby ↓ repetitive neuronal firing				
Zonisamide ☆ • Zonegran • 100–600 mg/day in 1–2 divided doses • Caps	Hypersensitivity to zonisamide or sulfonamides	• Depression • Psychotic symptoms • Difficulty concentrating • Speech problems • Somnolence • Fatigue • Dizziness • Nausea • Rash (Stevens-Johnson syndrome possible) • Aplastic anemia • Agranulocytosis • ↓ sweating • Hyperthermia • Metabolic acidosis • Kidney stones • ↑ blood urea nitrogen/ serum creatinine	• Suicidality • Renal function • Serum bicarbonate concentrations	• Takes up to 2 wk to achieve steady-state • Teratogenic
Mechanism of action – modulates calcium influx at the nerve terminals, thereby inhibiting excitatory neurotransmitter release				
Pregabalin ☆ • Lyrica • 150–600 mg/day in 2–3 divided doses • Caps, solution	Hypersensitivity	• Angioedema • Somnolence • Dizziness • Peripheral edema	• Suicidality • Presence of edema	• Schedule V controlled substance • Adjust dose in renal impairment

Antiepileptic Drugs *(cont'd)*

Generic • **Brand** • **Dose/Dosage Forms**	Contraindications	Primary Side Effects	Key Monitoring Parameters	Med Pearls
Mechanism of action – antagonistic effects of ionotropic alpha-amino-3-hydroxy-5-methyl-4-isoxazolepropionic acid (AMPA) glutamate receptor				
Perampanel • Fycompa • 2–12 mg at bedtime • Suspension, tabs	None	• Dizziness • Gait disturbance • Headache • Somnolence • Fatigue • Behavioral disturbances (aggression, agitation, anger, anxiety, depression, hostility, nervousness) • Depression • Weight gain	• Suicidality • Weight	• Adjust dose in renal impairment • Schedule III controlled substance
Mechanism of action – Mechanism is not well understood, but may be attributed to selective affinity for synaptic vesicle protein 2A (SV2A)				
Brivaracetam • Briviact • 25–100 mg BID • Injection, solution, tabs	Hypersensitivity	• Somnolence • Dizziness • Fatigue • Gait disturbance • Behavioral disturbances (aggression, agitation, anger, anxiety, depression, hostility, nervousness) • Psychotic symptoms • Angioedema • N/V	Suicidality	• Schedule V controlled substance • Adjust dose in hepatic impairment

Selected AED Drug Interactions

AED	Interacting Medication	Effect
Carbamazepine • 3A4 substrate • Strong CYP1A2, CYP2C19, CYP2C8, CYP2C9, and CYP3A4 inducer	Abiraterone Apixaban Bortezomib Cimetidine Clozapine Dabigatran Dolutegravir Doxycycline Dronedarone Erythromycin Everolimus Fluoxetine Ibrutinib Isoniazid Itraconazole Oral contraceptives Perampanel Phenobarbital Phenytoin Rivaroxaban Theophylline Warfarin	↓ Abiraterone ↓ Apixaban ↓ Bortezomib ↑ Carbamazepine ↓ Clozapine ↓ Dabigatran ↓ Dolutegravir ↓ Doxycycline ↓ Dronedarone ↑ Carbamazepine ↓ Everolimus ↑ Carbamazepine ↓ Ibrutinib ↑ Carbamazepine ↓ Itraconazole ↓ Contraceptives ↓ Perampanel ↓ Carbamazepine, ↓ phenobarbital ↓ Carbamazepine, ↓ phenytoin ↓ Rivaroxaban ↓ Theophylline ↓ Warfarin
Valproic acid	Carbamazepine Lamotrigine Phenobarbital Phenytoin Primidone	↓ Valproic acid, ↑ carbamazepine ↑ Toxicity of lamotrigine ↓ Valproic acid, ↑ phenobarbital ↓ Valproic acid, ↓ phenytoin ↓ Valproic acid, ↑ phenobarbital
Phenytoin • CYP2C19 and CYP2C9 substrate • Strong CYP2C19, CYP2C8, CYP2C9, and CYP3A4 inducer	Abiraterone Antacids Apixaban Carbamazepine Cimetidine Clozapine Dabigatran Dolutegravir Dronederone Fluconazole Isoniazid Oral contraceptives Perampanel Phenobarbital RivaroxabanTicagrelor Warfarin	↓ Abiraterone ↓ Phenytoin ↓ Apixaban ↓ Phenytoin ↑ Phenytoin ↓ Clozapine ↓ Dabigatran ↓ Dolutegravir ↓ Dronederone ↑ Phenytoin ↑ Phenytoin ↓ Contraceptives ↓ Perampanel ↑ or ↓ Phenytoin ↓ Rivaroxaban ↓ Ticagrelor ↑ Phenytoin, ↑ anticoagulant effect

Selected AED Drug Interactions *(cont'd)*

AED	Interacting Medication	Effect
Ethosuximide • CYP3A4 substrate	Phenytoin Valproic acid	↑ Phenytoin ↑ or ↓ Ethosuximide
Oxcarbazepine • CYP3A4 inducer	Cobicistat Dolutegravir Elvitegravir Ledipasvir Oral contraceptives Perampanel Phenobarbital Phenytoin Sofosbuvir	↓ Cobicistat ↓ Dolutegravir ↓ Elvitegravir ↓ Ledipasvir ↓ Contraceptives ↓ Perampanel, ↑ oxcarbazepine ↓ Oxcarbazepine ↓ Oxcarbazepine ↓ Sofosbuvir
Felbamate • CYP3A4 substrate	Carbamazepine Phenobarbital Phenytoin Valproic acid	↓ Carbamazepine, ↓ felbamate ↑ Phenobarbital, ↓ felbamate ↑ Phenytoin, ↓ felbamate ↑ Valproic acid
Perampanel • CYP3A4 substrate	Buprenorphine Carbamazepine Oxcarbazepine Phenytoin Progestins	↑ CNS depressant effect ↓ Perampanel ↓ Perampanel ↓ Perampanel ↓ Progestins
Lacosamide • CYP2C19, CYP2C9, and CYP3A4 substrate	Carbamazepine Phenobarbital Phenytoin	↓ Lacosamide ↓ Lacosamide ↓ Lacosamide
Lamotrigine	Carbamazepine Phenobarbital Phenytoin Primidone Valproic acid	↓ Lamotrigine ↓ Lamotrigine ↓ Lamotrigine ↓ Lamotrigine ↑ Lamotrigine
Topiramate	Carbamazepine Oral contraceptives Phenytoin Simeprevir Valproic acid	↓ Topiramate ↓ Contraceptives ↓ Topiramate ↓ Simeprevir ↓ Valproic acid
Phenobarbital • CYP2C19 substrate • Strong CYP1A2, CYP2C8, CYP2C9, and CYP3A4 inducer	Apixaban Dronederone Felbamate Oral contraceptives Phenytoin Rivaroxaban Simeprevir Valproic acid	↓ Apixaban ↓ Dronederone ↑ Phenobarbital ↓ Contraceptives ↑ Phenobarbital ↓ Rivaroxaban ↓ Simeprevir ↑ Phenobarbital

Selected AED Drug Interactions *(cont'd)*

AED	Interacting Medication	Effect
Primidone • Strong CYP1A2, CYP2C8, CYP2C9, and CYP3A4 inducer	Carbamazepine Corticosteroids Phenytoin Valproic acid	↓ Primidone, ↑ phenobarbital ↓ Corticosteroids ↓ Primidone, ↑ phenobarbital ↑ Primidone, ↓ phenobarbital
Tiagabine • CYP3A4 substrate	Carbamazepine Phenytoin	↓ Tiagabine ↓ Tiagabine
Vigabatrin	Clonazepam Phenytoin	↑ Clonazepam ↓ Phenytoin
Zonisamide • CYP3A4 substrate	Carbamazepine Phenobarbital Phenytoin	↓ Zonisamide ↓ Zonisamide ↓ Zonisamide
Brivaracetam • CYP2C19 substrate	Phenytoin	↓ Brivaracetam

Storage and Administration Pearls

- Valproic acid: Extended-release divalproex sodium should be swallowed whole and should not be chewed, crushed, or split. Divalproex sodium sprinkle caps may be swallowed whole or may be opened and sprinkled on a small amount (around a teaspoon) of soft food, such as pudding or applesauce.

- Oxcarbazepine oral suspension should be shaken well before administration and should be used within 7 weeks of opening the bottle.

- Topiramate: Topiramate XR should be swallowed whole and should not be chewed, crushed, or split.

- Levetiracetam: Levetiracetam XR should be swallowed whole and should not be chewed, crushed, or split.

Patient Education Pearls

- AEDs should not be abruptly discontinued, as this may result in increasing and emergent seizure activity; need to taper therapy.

- Any skin rash that develops should be reported to a health care provider immediately.

- When taking any new medications, patients should consult with their pharmacist, as multiple drug interactions are possible.

- AEDs have been associated with an ↑ risk of suicidal thoughts and behaviors. Patients should consult with their health care provider immediately if they experience any thoughts of harming themselves.

PARKINSON'S DISEASE

Definitions

Parkinson's disease (PD) is a syndrome characterized by tremor, rigidity, bradykinesia, and/or postural instability caused by a progressive depletion of dopamine neurons in the substantia nigra of the basal ganglia. Symptoms are a result of the dopamine deficiency and subsequent relative acetylcholine excess.

Diagnosis

Diagnosis of PD is based on careful clinical history and physical exam. There are no agreed-upon objective or definitive lab or imaging criteria for diagnosis. Generally, patients need 2 of the 4 main symptoms (tremor, bradykinesia, rigidity, postural instability) to be diagnosed with PD.

Signs and Symptoms

PD has an insidious onset and begins with nonspecific symptoms such as malaise and fatigue. Tremor is generally the first of the cardinal signs and is generally unilateral and occurring at rest rather than upon intention. Rigidity of the limbs manifests as resistance to passive movement of the joints, and bradykinesia as slow movements or difficulty moving. Symptoms generally begin unilaterally and progress asymmetrically.

Summary of Treatment Recommendations

- Initial therapy generally consists of either a dopamine agonist or carbidopa/levodopa.
  - Patients ≥65 years of age or those with significant disability due to their PD should receive carbidopa/levodopa as initial therapy.
  - Patients <65 years of age should receive a dopamine agonist as initial therapy.
  - Inadequate response to maximum tolerable doses of initial therapy with a dopamine agonist or carbidopa/levodopa should result in the addition of the alternate medication.
  - Subsequently, COMT inhibitors may be added to ongoing carbidopa/levodopa therapy, and adjunctive therapies such as amantadine or anticholinergics may also be utilized.
  - Anticholinergic agents are primarily useful for the treatment of tremor-predominant PD but should be used with caution in elderly patients and avoided in patients with pre-existing cognitive impairment.
  - Because dopamine agonists and carbidopa/levodopa are aimed at increasing the available dopamine in the CNS, side effects such as hallucinations and delusions are possible. Psychiatric side effects which occur at the lowest effective doses of these drugs may be treated with the antipsychotic medication, quetiapine.

Medications for Parkinson's Disease

Generic • Brand • Dose/Dosage Forms	Contraindications	Primary Side Effects	Key Monitoring Parameters	Pertinent Drug Interactions	Med Pearls
Mechanism of action – unknown, thought to enhance dopamine release and inhibit dopamine reuptake, also acts as an NMDA receptor antagonist					
Amantadine • Only available generically • 100–200 mg BID • Caps, solution, tabs	Hypersensitivity	• Confusion • Nightmares • Hallucinations • Insomnia • Nervousness • Irritability	• Response to therapy • Presence of side effects	Triamterene ↑ effects	Adjust dose in renal impairment
Mechanism of action – monoamine-oxidase (MAO) B inhibitors: inhibit the catabolism of dopamine by selectively inhibiting the monoamine oxidase B enzyme					
Selegiline • Eldepryl, Zelapar • Cap/tab: 5 mg BID • ODT: 1.25–2.5 mg daily • Caps, ODTs, tabs	• Hypersensitivity • Concurrent use with meperidine, methadone, dextromethorphan, tramadol, or MAOIs	• Nausea • Hallucinations • Insomnia • Depression • Orthostasis • Impulse control disorders • Hypertensive crisis (if high-tyramine foods are ingested)	• BP • Response to therapy • Presence of side effects	Use with meperidine, other opioid analgesics, dextromethorphan, tramadol, selective serotonin reuptake inhibitors (SSRIs), or serotonin-norepinephrine reuptake inhibitors (SNRIs), tricyclic antidepressants (TCAs), cyclobenzaprine, triptans, or St. John's wort may ↑ risk of serotonin syndrome	• Avoid tyramine-containing foods • Should not be abruptly discontinued • Discontinue 14 days prior to surgery if possible; should not be taken with general anesthesia • Transdermal patch (Emsam) used for depression
Rasagiline • Azilect • 0.5–1 mg daily • Tabs	• Hypersensitivity • Concurrent use with meperidine, methadone, tramadol, MAOIs, cyclobenzaprine, dextromethorphan, or St. John's wort	• Hypertension • Nausea • Orthostasis • Somnolence • Hallucinations • Impulse control disorders • Hypertensive crisis (if high-tyramine foods are ingested)	• Response to therapy • Presence of side effects • BP	• CYP1A2 substrate • CYP1A2 inhibitors may ↑ effects • CYP1A2 inducers may ↓ effects • Use with meperidine, other opioid analgesics, dextromethorphan, tramadol, SSRIs, SNRIs, TCAs, cyclobenzaprine, triptans, or St. John's wort may ↑ risk of serotonin syndrome	• Avoid tyramine-containing foods • Should not be abruptly discontinued • Adjust dose in hepatic impairment

Medications for Parkinson's Disease (cont'd)

Generic • Brand • Dose/Dosage Forms	Contraindications	Primary Side Effects	Key Monitoring Parameters	Pertinent Drug Interactions	Med Pearls
Mechanism of action – levodopa is a direct precursor to dopamine and is converted to dopamine once it crosses the blood-brain barrier; carbidopa is a dopa decarboxylase inhibitor; it is necessary to combine carbidopa with levodopa in order to prevent the peripheral degradation of levodopa prior to entry into the blood-brain barrier.					
Carbidopa/levodopa ☆ • Duopa, Rytary, Sinemet, Sinemet CR • Carbidopa 75–300 mg/ day in 3–4 divided doses (75 mg required, side effects if >300 mg/ day) • Levodopa 100–2,000 mg/day in 3–4 divided doses • Enteral suspension, CR caps, ER tabs, ODTs, tabs	• Hypersensitivity • Narrow-angle glaucoma • Concurrent use with MAOIs	• N/V • Orthostasis • Confusion • Hallucinations • Wearing-off fluctuations • Dyskinesias • Somnolence • Impulse control disorders	• Response to therapy • Presence of side effects • BP	• Nonselective MAOIs may cause hypertensive crisis • Pyridoxine (vitamin B6) ↓ effectiveness of levodopa	• IR tabs and CR caps/tabs often used simultaneously; IR tabs can treat wearing-off symptoms of CR caps/tabs • CR is less bioavailable (~30% less) than IR • Duopa is indicated for PEG-J tube administration
Mechanism of action – dopamine agonists: directly stimulate striatal dopamine receptors					
Bromocriptine (ergot derivative) • Parlodel • 1.25–50 mg BID • Caps, tabs	• Uncontrolled hypertension • Sensitivity to ergot alkaloids • Pregnancy • Postpartum with history of coronary artery disease	• Valvular fibrosis • Nausea • Hallucinations • Dizziness • Drowsiness • Orthostasis • Impulse control disorders	• Response to therapy • Presence of side effects • BP	• ↓ levodopa dose by 20–30% when initiating • Metoclopramide and antipsychotics ↓ effects	Cardiac side effects ↓ clinical use; nonergot derivatives used much more commonly
Pramipexole ☆ (nonergot derivative) • Mirapex, Mirapex ER • IR: 0.125–1.5 mg TID • ER: 0.375–4.5 mg daily • ER tabs, tabs	None	• N/V • Constipation • Orthostasis • Hallucinations • Somnolence • Syncope • Impulse control disorders	• Response to therapy • Presence of side effects • BP	• ↓ levodopa dose by 20–30% when initiating • Metoclopramide and antipsychotics ↓ effects	• Adjust dose in renal impairment • Titrate dose slowly and taper upon discontinuation • Also indicated for restless leg syndrome
Ropinirole ☆ (nonergot derivative) • Requip, Requip XL • IR: 0.25–8 mg TID • ER: 2–24 mg daily • ER tabs, tabs	Hypersensitivity				• Titrate dose slowly and taper upon discontinuation • Also indicated for restless leg syndrome

Medications for Parkinson's Disease *(cont'd)*

Generic • Brand • Dose/Dosage Forms	Contraindications	Primary Side Effects	Key Monitoring Parameters	Pertinent Drug Interactions	Med Pearls
Rotigotine • Neupro • 2–8 mg daily • Transdermal patch	Hypersensitivity	• Application site reactions • N/V • Orthostasis • Hallucinations • Somnolence • Syncope • Impulse control disorders • Hypertension • Tachycardia • Edema	• Response to therapy • Presence of side effects • BP • HR		• Apply patch daily • Titrate dose slowly and taper upon discontinuation • Also indicated for restless leg syndrome

Mechanism of action – COMT inhibitors: inhibit the degradation of dopamine through inhibition of the catechol-O-methyltransferase enzyme

Tolcapone • Tasmar • 100–200 mg TID • Tabs	• Hypersensitivity • Hepatic impairment • History of nontraumatic rhabdomyolysis or hyperpyrexia and confusion due to medication	• Liver failure • Dyskinesias • N/V/D • Orthostasis • Hallucinations • Somnolence • Syncope • Impulse control disorders • Rhabdomyolysis	• LFTs • Response to therapy • Presence of side effects • BP	• May ↑ effects of MAOIs (avoid concurrent use of nonselective MAOIs) • ↑ activity of drugs known to be metabolized by COMT (dopamine, dobutamine, isoproterenol, methyldopa)	• Reserved for third-line therapy in patients that do not respond adequately to carbidopa/levodopa and dopamine agonists • Should be used with carbidopa/levodopa
Entacapone • Comtan • 200–1,600 mg daily (divided up to 8 × daily; administered with each dose of carbidopa/levodopa) • Tabs	Hypersensitivity	• Dyskinesias • N/V/D • Hallucinations • Urine discoloration (brown-orange) • Orthostasis • Hallucinations • Somnolence • Syncope • Impulse control disorder	• Response to therapy • Presence of side effects • BP	• May ↑ effects of MAOIs (avoid concurrent use of nonselective MAOIs) • ↑ activity of drugs known to be metabolized by COMT (dopamine, dobutamine, isoproterenol, methyldopa)	• Reserved for third-line therapy in patients that do not respond adequately to carbidopa/levodopa and dopamine agonists • Preferred over tolcapone, as no fatal liver injury has been reported with this agent

Combination product: Levodopa/carbidopa/entacapone (Stalevo)

Medications for Parkinson's Disease *(cont'd)*

Generic • **Brand** • **Dose/Dosage Forms**	Contraindications	Primary Side Effects	Key Monitoring Parameters	Pertinent Drug Interactions	Med Pearls
Mechanism of action – anticholinergics: through diminished activity of acetylcholine, help to ↓ the relative ↑ in activity compared to dopamine, thereby ↓ tremor					
Benztropine ☆ • Cogentin • 0.5–6 mg/day in 2–4 divided doses • Injection, tabs	Hypersensitivity	• Dry mouth • Blurred vision • Constipation • Urinary retention • Confusion • Memory impairment • Hallucinations	• Response to therapy • Presence of side effects	Additive anticholinergic side effects when co-administered with other anticholinergic medications	• Use with caution in elderly patients who are at risk for mental status changes with anticholinergic medications • Primarily used for tremor and/or drooling
Trihexyphenidyl ☆ • Only available generically • 1–15 mg/day in 3–4 divided doses • Solution, tabs	None				
Mechanism of action – 2nd generation atypical antipsychotic; inverse agonist and antagonist activity at 5-HT2A and 5-HT2C receptors					
Pimavanserin • Nuplazid • 34 mg daily • Tabs	None	• Edema • Confusion • Hallucination • Gait disturbance • QT interval prolongation	• ECG • Response to therapy	• CYP3A4 substrate • CYP3A4 inhibitors may ↑ toxicity/effect (↓ pimavanserin dose) • CYP3A4 inducers may ↓ effect • Use with QT-interval prolonging agents may ↑ risk of torsades de pointes (TdP)	Indicated to treat hallucinations and delusions associated with PD psychosis

Storage and Administration Pearls

- Selegiline ODTs should be taken in the morning before any food or water. Tablets dissolve on the tongue, and food/drink should be avoided for 5 minutes after dose.

- Carbidopa/levodopa ER tablets (Sinemet CR, Rytary) can be taken as whole tablets or half tablets but should not be chewed or crushed. ER tablets are less bioavailable than IR tablets and patients may require up to a 30% dose ↑ to attain similar efficacy.

- Rotigotine patch should be worn continuously for 24 hours. Heat may ↑ absorption.

Patient Education Pearls

- Avoid concomitant alcohol with any antiparkinsonian agent.

- Rotigotine patch should be worn continuously for 24 hours. Heat may ↑ absorption. Patients should not take a hot bath or sauna or apply a heated pad while wearing patch.

- Hallucinations, delusions, strange dreams, or impulse control disorders (e.g., hypersexuality, excessive gambling/shopping, binge eating) should be immediately reported to a physician.
- Duopa is administered via PEG-J tube.

MIGRAINE HEADACHE

Definitions

Migraine headaches are defined as recurring headaches of moderate to severe intensity and are associated with gastrointestinal, neurological, and autonomic symptoms. Migraine headaches may or may not be preceded by an aura.

Diagnosis

Diagnostic criteria are established by the International Headache Society (IHS) and consist of distinct criteria for migraine with aura and migraine without aura.

Migraine with aura:

- ≥2 attacks
- Aura symptoms that do not last more than 60 minutes
- Organic disorder ruled out or headaches do not relate temporally to organic disorder

Migraine without aura:

- ≥5 attacks
- Headache lasts 4–72 hours
- Unilateral, pulsating, moderate/severe intensity, or aggravated by physical activity
- N/V, photophobia, or phonophobia
- Organic disorder ruled out or headaches do not relate temporally to organic disorder

Signs and Symptoms

Pain is the primary symptom of migraine headache. The pain is generally gradual in onset, peaks in intensity over minutes to hours, and lasts 4–72 hours if untreated. Intensity is often described as moderate to severe and generally stated as a ≥5 on a 0–10 pain scale. Most commonly, pain occurs in the frontotemporal region and is most often unilateral and pulsating. Other symptoms that may accompany the pain include gastrointestinal symptoms of N/V and neurological symptoms of photo- or phonophobia.

Guidelines

Evidence-based guideline update: Pharmacologic treatment for episodic migraine prevention in adults. Report of the Quality Standards Subcommittee of the American Academy of Neurology and the American Headache Society. *Neurology* 2012;78: 1337–1345.

Summary of Treatment Recommendations

- Migraine treatment is divided into abortive treatment, rescue treatment, and prophylactic treatment. Most patients will respond to abortive treatment and can be controlled without the addition of rescue or prophylactic therapy.

- Abortive treatment options include analgesics (over-the-counter [OTC] and prescription), NSAIDs (detailed in bone and joint chapter), ergotamine and dihydroergotamine, serotonin agonists, and butorphanol. Over-the-counter analgesics, prescription non-opioid analgesics, and NSAIDs are reserved for patients with mild symptoms.

- The serotonin agonists are the mainstay of abortive therapy options for patients with moderate to severe symptoms. Various dosage forms are available and there is only slight variability between the efficacy and safety of available agents. Patients may respond to one agent in this class and not to another; therefore, trial and error is often the approach taken.

- For patients who have >2 headaches/week or >8 headaches/month, or who do not have an adequate response to abortive therapy, prophylactic therapy may be warranted.

- Available prophylactic agents include antihypertensive medications such as propranolol, atenolol, and metoprolol (detailed in cardiovascular chapter); antidepressant medications such as amitriptyline, paroxetine, fluoxetine, and sertraline (detailed in psychiatric disorders chapter); and anticonvulsant medications such valproic acid, gabapentin, tiagabine, and topiramate (detailed earlier in this chapter). In general, migraine prophylactic doses are low compared to normal doses of these medications.

Medications for Migraine

Generic • Brand • Dose/Dosage Forms	Contraindications	Primary Side Effects	Key Monitoring Parameters	Pertinent Drug Interactions	Med Pearls
Analgesics					
Acetaminophen, aspirin, caffeine • Excedrin Migraine, Anacin • 2 tabs at onset, then every 6 hr PRN • Tabs	• Hypersensitivity to any component • Pregnancy	Minimal	• Response to therapy • Presence of side effects	Other acetaminophen-containing meds (do not exceed 4 g/day)	Available OTC
Aspirin or acetaminophen with butalbital and caffeine ☆ • Fiorinal, Fioricet • 1–2 tabs every 4–6 hrs PRN (max = 6 doses/day)	• Hypersensitivity to any component • Pregnancy	• Tachycardia • Dizziness • Drowsiness • Insomnia • Orthostatic hypotension	• Response to therapy • Presence of side effects	Alcohol ↑ CNS depression with butalbital	• Limit to 4 tabs/day and use max of 2 days/wk • Dependence may develop with continued use
Isometheptene/dichloral-phenazone/APAP • Nodolor • 2 caps at onset, then 1 cap every hr PRN (max = 6 capsules/24 hr)	• Glaucoma • Severe renal disease • Hypertension • Cardiovascular disease • Cerebrovascular accident • MAOI use	• Dizziness • Skin rash	• Response to therapy • Presence of side effects	Use with MAOIs may ↑ risk for hypertensive crisis	Max 6 caps/day; 20 caps/mo
Mechanism of action – exert serotonergic agonist activity, resulting in vasoconstriction					
Ergotamine tartrate • Ergomar • 1 tab at onset, then 1 tab every 30 min PRN • Not to exceed 3 tabs/day or 5 tabs/wk • SL tabs	• Hypersensitivity • Peripheral arterial disease • Coronary artery disease • Hypertension • Hepatic or renal impairment • Concurrent use of strong 3A4 inhibitors • Pregnancy	• Chest pain • Myocardial infarction • Hypertension • Tachycardia • Nausea • Valvular fibrosis	• Response to therapy • Presence of side effects • BP • HR	• CYP3A4 substrate • CYP3A4 inhibitors may ↑ effects/toxicity • CYP3A4 inducers may ↓ effects	Potential for dependence with long-term use
Dihydroergotamine • DHE 45, Migranal • IV, IM, or subcut: 1 mg at onset, repeated at 1-hr intervals (max = 2 mg/day IV or 3 mg/day subcut or IM) • Nasal: 1 spray (0.5 mg) in each nostril; repeat in 15 min with spray in each nostril (max = 3 mg/day)	• Hypersensitivity • Peripheral arterial disease • Coronary artery disease • Hypertension • Hepatic or renal impairment • Concurrent use of strong 3A4 inhibitors • Pregnancy • Within 24 hr of triptan product • Within 2 wk of MAOI				

Medications for Migraine *(cont'd)*

Generic • Brand • Dose/Dosage Forms	Contraindications	Primary Side Effects	Key Monitoring Parameters	Pertinent Drug Interactions	Med Pearls
Mechanism of action – serotonin agonists (triptans): serotonin 5HT1 receptor agonists, resulting in vasoconstriction in the cerebral vasculature					
Sumatriptan ☆ • Imitrex oral tablets • 25–100 mg at onset, may redose at >2 hr (max = 200 mg/day) • Imitrex or Alsuma subcut injection • 4–6 mg subcut; may repeat in 1 hr (max = 2 doses/day) • Imitrex nasal spray • 10–20-mg spray in 1 nostril at onset; may repeat after 2 hr (max = 40 mg/day) • Sumavel Dosepro, needle-free, subcut injection • 6 mg subcut; may repeat in 1 hr (max = 12 mg/day) • Zembrace SymTouch subcut injection • 3 mg subcut; may repeat in 1 hr (max = 12 mg/day) • Onzetra Xsail powder for nasal inhalation • 22 mg, delivered by one nosepiece (11 mg in each nostril); may repeat in 2 hr (max = 44 mg/day)	• Coronary artery disease • Wolff-Parkinson-White syndrome • Stroke or transient ischemic attack • Peripheral arterial disease • Ischemic bowel disease • Uncontrolled hypertension • Within 24 hr of an ergot product • Within 2 wks of MAOI • Within 24 hr of strong 3A4 inhibitor (eletriptan) • Severe hepatic impairment (sumatriptan) • Severe renal or hepatic impairment (naratriptan)	• Fatigue • Dizziness • Flushing • Chest/neck/throat pressure • Unpleasant taste • Hypertension	• Response to therapy • Presence of side effects • BP	Use with meperidine, dextromethorphan, tramadol, SSRIs, SNRIs, TCAs, MAOIs, triptans, or St. John's wort may ↑ risk of serotonin syndrome	Onset: 30 min (PO); 15–30 min (intranasal); 10 min (subcut)
Zolmitriptan • Zomig, Zomig ZMT • Tabs: 1.25–2.5 at onset; may repeat in >2 hr if needed (max = 10 mg/day) • ODTs: 2.5 mg at onset; may repeat in >2 hr if needed (max = 10 mg/day) • Nasal spray: 2.5-mg spray in 1 nostril at onset; may repeat in >2 hr if needed (max = 10 mg/day)					Onset: 45 min

Medications for Migraine *(cont'd)*

Generic • Brand • Dose/Dosage Forms	Contraindications	Primary Side Effects	Key Monitoring Parameters	Pertinent Drug Interactions	Med Pearls
Naratriptan • Amerge • Tabs: 1–2.5 mg at onset; may repeat in >4 hr if needed (max = 5 mg/day)	[Same as above]	[Same as above]	[Same as above]	[Same as above]	Onset: 1–2 hr
Rizatriptan ☆ • Maxalt, Maxalt MLT • Tabs, ODTs: 5–10 mg at onset; repeat in >2 hr if needed (max = 30 mg/day)					Onset: Within 2 hr
Almotriptan • Axert • Tabs: 6.25–12.5 mg at onset; repeat in >2 hr if needed (max = 2 doses/day)					Onset: 30 min
Eletriptan • Relpax • Tabs: 20–40 mg at onset; repeat in >2 hr if needed (max = 80 mg/day)					Onset: 30 min
Frovatriptan • Frova • Tabs: 2.5 mg at onset; repeat in >2 hr if needed (max = 7.5 mg/day)					Onset: 3 hr
Combination product: Sumatriptan/naproxen (Treximet)					
Mechanism of action – butorphanol: mixed opioid agonist/antagonist with opioid analgesic properties					
Butorphanol • Only available generically • Nasal spray: 1 mg (1 spray) in 1 nostril at onset; may repeat in >1 hour; may then repeat in 3–4 hr after last dose if needed	• Hypersensitivity • Patients with a history of narcotic dependenc	• Somnolence • Dizziness • Nausea • Nasal congestion • Insomnia	• Response to therapy • Presence of adverse effects	Concurrent use of other CNS depressants will have additive adverse effects and should be avoided	• Schedule IV controlled substance • Not routinely used for migraines • High addiction potential

Storage and Administration Pearls

- Store all preparations between 2–30°C (36–86°F). Protect from light.
- Place ODTs directly on tongue and allow them to dissolve.
- Sumatriptan, zolmitripan, and butorphanol nasal sprays are sprayed into one nostril only.
- Sumatriptan injection is self-administered subcutaneously using prefilled syringes and an autoinjector.

Patient Education Pearls

- Follow dosing recommendations carefully to decrease risk of adverse effects or dependence.

ALZHEIMER'S DISEASE

Definition

Alzheimer's disease (AD) is a dementia of progressive nature that affects, in the early stages, primarily cognition and in later stages, behavior and functional status. The pathophysiology is not fully understood but is known to involve destruction of neurons and synapses and cortical atrophy.

Diagnosis

The *Diagnostic and Statistical Manual of Mental Disorders, Fifth Edition* (DSM 5) criteria describe an insidious onset of memory impairment plus one additional cognitive defect. The diagnosis is based upon evidence of progressive cognitive decline from baseline that has reached the point of impacting social or occupational functioning along with the ruling out of reversible causes such as thyroid abnormalities, vitamin deficiencies, medication side effects, and infections.

Signs and Symptoms

Problems with memory, difficulty performing familiar tasks, forgetting information that was recently acquired, poor judgment, difficulty with abstract concepts, mood changes, and loss of interest in usual activities include some of the most common elements of the clinical presentation. The Folstein Mini-Mental State Examination (MMSE) is often used to provide staging and clinical guidance. MMSE scores of ≥20 are considered mild AD, scores of 10–19 indicate moderate disease, and scores <10 indicate severe cases.

Guidelines

American College of Physicians/American Academy of Family Physicians (ACP/AAFP). Current pharmacologic treatment of dementia: a clinical practice guideline from the American College of Physicians and the American Academy of Family Physicians. *Ann Intern Med.* 2008;148:370–8.

Guidelines Summary

- Goals of treatment include preservation of function and symptomatic slowing of cognitive decline. A commonly used benchmark is the change in MMSE within one year. Without therapy, MMSE would be expected to ↓ approximately 2–4 points per year. Therapeutic efficacy is often determined if MMSE ↓ by ≤2 points per year. None of the available therapies has an impact on halting disease progression or reversing pathophysiology.

- Cholinesterase inhibitors are the treatment of choice in mild to moderate AD. Although slight differences exist in the mechanism of action of these agents, there is no evidence to indicate greater efficacy with one agent over another. Agent selection is typically made based upon patient preference, cost, and potential for drug interactions. There is insufficient evidence to support a dose-response relationship within this class. It is currently recommended that patients be started on the lowest dose and titrated slowly to the typical maintenance dose.

- Memantine is the only currently available N-methyl-D-aspartate (NMDA) receptor antagonist and has been studied and approved in moderate to severe AD as either monotherapy or an adjunct to a cholinesterase inhibitor.

- The most widely accepted approach to treatment is to initiate a low dose of a cholinesterase inhibitor at the time of diagnosis with slow titration to a typical maintenance dose. After 6 months to 1 year, efficacy is assessed. If this therapy is not efficacious, the patient can be switched to an alternate cholinesterase inhibitor or memantine can be added (in moderate to severe disease).

Cholinesterase Inhibitors

Generic • Brand • Dose/Dosage Forms	Contraindications	Primary Side Effects	Key Monitoring Parameters	Pertinent Drug Interactions	Med Pearls
Mechanism of action – inhibit the activity of the cholinesterase enzyme, thereby allowing ↑ acetylcholine activity					
Donepezil ☆ • Aricept • 5 mg daily, then ↑ to 10 mg daily after 4–6 wk (max = 23 mg daily in moderate–severe AD) • ODTs, tabs	Hypersensitivity	• N/V/D • Peptic ulcer disease • Weight loss • Urinary incontinence • Dizziness • Headache • Syncope • Salivation • Sweating • Bradycardia • AV block • Rash (Stevens-Johnson syndrome possible)	• Presence of side effects • ECG • HR • MMSE (at 6–12 mo intervals)	• May ↑ neuromuscular blockade with succinylcholine • Anticholinergic drugs ↓ efficacy • Cholinergic drugs ↑ toxicity	Slow titration can ↑ tolerability
Galantamine • Razadyne, Razadyne ER • IR: 4 mg BID × 4 wk, then 8 mg BID × ≥4 wk, then 12 mg BID • ER: 8 mg daily × 4 wk, then 16 mg daily × ≥4 wk, then 24 mg daily • ER caps, solution, tabs					
Rivastigmine • Exelon • Caps: 1.5–6 mg BID • Patch: 4.6–13.3 mg daily • Caps, transdermal patch				• May ↑ neuromuscular blockade with succinylcholine • Anticholinergic drugs ↓ efficacy • Cholinergic drugs ↑ toxicity • Metoclopramide: ↑ risk of extrapyramidal symptoms	• Capsules should be administered with meals • Also indicated for Parkinson-related dementia

NMDA Receptor Antagonist

Generic • Brand • Dose/Dosage Forms	Contraindications	Primary Side Effects	Key Monitoring Parameters	Pertinent Drug Interactions	Med Pearls
Mechanism of action – NMDA receptor antagonist, preventing detrimental effects of glutamate					
Memantine ☆ • Namenda, Namenda XR • IR: 5 mg daily × ≥1 wk, then 5 mg BID × ≥1 wk, then 5 mg AM and 10 mg PM × ≥1 wk, then 10 mg BID • ER: 7–28 mg daily • ER caps, solution, tabs	Hypersensitivity	• Confusion • Constipation • Dizziness • Headache • D/V • Hypertension	• Presence of side effects • BP • MMSE at 6–12 month intervals	Carbonic anhydrase inhibitors and sodium bicarbonate may ↑ effects/ toxicity	• Indicated for moderate–severe AD as monotherapy or in combination with cholinesterase inhibitor • Adjust dose in renal impairment
Combination product: Donepezil/memantine (Namzaric)					

Storage and Administration Pearls

- Donepezil: Take in evening prior to bed with or without food. Allow ODTs to dissolve on tongue and then follow with glass of water.

- Galantamine: Ensure adequate fluid intake while on therapy, and take with food. Do not crush, break, or chew ER capsules.

- Rivastigmine: Apply patch to a dry, hairless area of skin (preferably upper back) and rotate site of application daily.

Patient Education Pearls

- The most common side effects of cholinesterase inhibitors are N/V/D and dizziness.

- Abrupt discontinuation of therapy may cause worsening of symptoms.

- The expected outcome is that the medications will slow progression. Significant improvement is not likely to be observed.

LEARNING POINTS

- Disease-modifying drugs are the agents of choice in treating MS.

- First-line choice of AED is based on seizure classification. Options include carbamazepine, phenytoin, lamotrigine, valproic acid, levetiracetam, and oxcarbazepine.

- Many AEDs have a significant number of drug-drug interactions due to their impact on and metabolism by the cytochrome P450 enzyme system.

- Carbidopa/levodopa is the mainstay of therapy for PD and is available in numerous dosage forms. CR and IR tablets are often prescribed simultaneously.

- Anticholinergic agents should be avoided in elderly patients.

- Agents affecting dopamine, including dopamine agonists and carbidopa/levodopa, may elicit psychiatric side effects.

- Serotonin agonists are the mainstay of treatment for migraine headache and are available in numerous dosage forms.

- Acetylcholinesterase inhibitors are generally first-line treatment for AD, and memantine may be added for those with severe disease.

PRACTICE QUESTIONS

1. What is recommended first-line for newly diagnosed multiple sclerosis?

   (A) Oral prednisone
   (B) Betaseron
   (C) Methylprednisolone
   (D) Natalizumab
   (E) Rebif + mitoxantrone

2. What patient counseling should be provided when dispensing an interferon injectable prescription for multiple sclerosis?

   (A) If the medication cannot be used within 1 month, freeze the syringe to allow beyond-date use.
   (B) Apply heat to the injection site before and after the injection.
   (C) Try to use the same injection site each time.
   (D) If the medication reaches room temperature, it is no longer usable and must be discarded.
   (E) NSAIDs may decrease the flu-like symptoms.

3. Which of the following is associated with the use of divalproex?

   (A) Hepatotoxicity
   (B) Hirsutism
   (C) Hypoglycemia
   (D) Renal dysfunction
   (E) Thrombocytosis

4. Which of the following medications is a contraindication to using sumatriptan?

   (A) Ibuprofen
   (B) Lisinopril
   (C) Phenelzine
   (D) Sertraline
   (E) Zolpidem

5. Which of the following is a contraindication to the use of rizatriptan? (Select ALL that apply.)

   (A) Uncontrolled hypertension
   (B) History of a stroke
   (C) Peripheral arterial disease (PAD)
   (D) Concomitant use of phenelzine
   (E) Concomitant use of naproxen

6. Which of the following medications should be AVOIDED with the use of donepezil? (Select ALL that apply.)

    (A) Diphenhydramine
    (B) Memantine
    (C) Amlodipine
    (D) Rivastigmine

7. Which of the following is a dopamine agonist?

    (A) Artane
    (B) Comtan
    (C) Mirapex
    (D) Sinemet

8. Which of the following medications, if added to a regimen containing apixaban, may cause a reduction in the efficacy of apixaban? (Select ALL that apply.)

    (A) Depakote
    (B) Dilantin
    (C) Keppra
    (D) Tegretol

9. Which of the following medications used to treat Parkinson's disease is formulated for PEG-J tube administration?

    (A) Duopa
    (B) Rytary
    (C) Sinemet CR

10. Which of the following disease states may memantine be used to treat?

    (A) Alzheimer's disease
    (B) Multiple sclerosis
    (C) Migraine
    (D) Parkinson's disease

ANSWERS AND EXPLANATIONS

1. **B**

Interferon agents (such as Betaseron, Avonex, and Rebif) and glatiramer acetate (Copaxone) are considered first-line disease-modifying drugs (DMDs) for the treatment of MS. Therefore, (B) is correct. Natalizumab (D) is reserved for patients who do not respond to traditional therapy. Treatment is usually initiated one agent at a time and, as the disease progresses, treatment with DMD + mitoxantrone pulse therapy (E) may be used. Corticosteroids (A and C) are the cornerstone of acute exacerbations but will play no role in treating the disease itself.

2. **E**

Acetaminophen or NSAIDs can reduce the flu-like symptoms associated with the interferon injections. The injectables for multiple sclerosis should never be frozen (A) and should always be protected from light. To ease the discomfort of the injections, ice—not heat (B)—can be applied to the injection site prior to the injection, and the injection site should be rotated each time (making choice C incorrect). It is perfectly fine and recommended to allow the injectable to reach room temperature prior to the injection (D), but it should otherwise be stored in the refrigerator.

3. **A**

Divalproex is associated with elevations in AST and ALT with potential hepatotoxicity. Hirsutism (B) is not correct as divalproex is associated with alopecia. Divalproex is not associated with hypoglycemia (C) and may be associated with hyperglycemia in rare instances. Divalproex does not cause renal dysfunction (D), and thrombocytosis (E) is not correct as divalproex is associated with thrombocytopenia.

4. **C**

The triptans are contraindicated if a patient has taken an MAOI within 2 weeks of using the triptan, as there is a risk of serotonin syndrome. NSAIDs may be taken with triptans; therefore, ibuprofen (A) is not a contraindication. Patients with uncontrolled HTN may not take triptans, but antihypertensive medications such as lisinopril (B) can be used. Sertraline (D) and zolpidem (E) may be used with triptans, but sertraline should be used with caution as there is a risk of serotonin syndrome with concomitant use.

5. **A, B, C, D**

Triptans cause vasoconstriction and cannot be used with ischemic heart or cerebrovascular disease. Patients with uncontrolled hypertension (A), history of a cerebrovascular accident or transient ischemic attack (B), PAD (C), or vasospastic condition should avoid the use of any triptan. Triptans also may cause serotonin syndrome if used within 2 weeks on an MAOI such as phenelzine (D), so the combination should be avoided. NSAIDs can be used with rizatriptan, so E is not correct.

6. **A, D**

Diphenhydramine is an anticholinergic agent that should not be used concomitantly with any acetylcholinesterase inhibitor, which may decrease the efficacy of the acetylcholinesterase inhibitor. Rivastigmine is also an acetylcholinesterase inhibitor; it should not be used together with any acetylcholinesterase inhibitor, as that would be a therapeutic duplication. Memantine (B) is an NMDA receptor antagonist and can be used in combination with acetylcholinesterase inhibitors. Amlodipine (C) may be used with acetylcholinesterase inhibitors.

7. **C**

Mirapex (ropinirole) is a dopamine agonist used for the treatment of Parkinson's disease. Artane (trihexphenidyl) (A) is an anticholinergic agent. Comtan (entacapone) (B) is a COMT inhibitor. Sinemet (carbidopa/levodopa) (D) is a decarboxylase inhibtor (carbidopa) combined with a dopamine precursor (levodopa). All agents can be used for the treatment of Parkinson's disease.

8. **B, D**

Dilantin (phenytoin) and Tegretol (carbamazepine) are both strong CYP3A4 inducers that will increase the metabolism of apixaban, possibly causing its therapeutic failure.

9. **A**

All 3 medications are formulations of carbidopa/levodopa. Duopa is an enteral suspension administered via continuous infusion through a PEG-J tube. Rytary (B) and Sinemet CR (C) are both long-acting formulations intended for oral administration.

10. **A**

Memantine (Namenda, Namenda XR) is an NMDA receptor antagonist that is use to treat moderate to severe Alzheimer's disease.

Gastrointestinal Disorders

6

This chapter covers the following diseases:

- **Gastroesophageal reflux disease/peptic ulcer disease**
- **Inflammatory bowel disease**

 Suggested Study Time: **45 minutes**

GASTROESOPHAGEAL REFLUX DISEASE/PEPTIC ULCER DISEASE

Definitions

Gastroesophageal reflux disease (GERD) is a condition in which patients have symptoms or mucosal damage resulting from the abnormal reflux of stomach contents into the esophagus. If the esophagus is chronically exposed to these contents, inflammation of the esophagus can develop which is termed reflux esophagitis, and/or the esophageal mucosa can become ulcerated, leading to erosive esophagitis. Often, GERD results because of reduced lower esophageal sphincter (LES) pressures; however, this condition may also arise because of a delay in gastric emptying, use of certain medications or foods, or a hiatal hernia. Various medications may precipitate GERD symptoms either by decreasing LES pressure (e.g., anticholinergics, benzodiazepines, β-agonists, calcium channel blockers, dopamine agonists, estrogen, opioid narcotics, nicotine, nitrates, progesterone, theophylline) or by irritating the esophageal mucosa (e.g., nonsteroidal anti-inflammatory drugs [NSAIDs], bisphosphonates, salicylates, iron, potassium chloride).

Peptic ulcer disease (PUD) refers to the development of duodenal or gastric ulcers. The majority of PUD cases are caused by either *Helicobacter pylori* (*H. pylori*) infection or the use of NSAIDs, but can also be induced by stress. A number of risk factors exist that may predispose patients to NSAID-induced ulcers, including a prior gastrointestinal

(GI) ulcer or hemorrhage; age >65 years; concurrent use of corticosteroids, antiplatelets, or anticoagulants; and chronic debilitating disorders, especially cardiovascular (CV) disease.

Patients taking NSAIDs can be categorized as being at high risk, moderate risk, or low risk for GI injury:

- High risk
  - History of previously complicated ulcer (especially recent)
  - Multiple (>2 risk factors)
- Moderate risk (1–2 risk factors)
  - Age >65 years
  - High-dose NSAID therapy
  - Previous history of uncomplicated ulcer
  - Concurrent use of aspirin (including low dose), corticosteroids, or anticoagulants
- Low risk
  - No risk factors

Diagnosis

Gastroesophageal Reflux Disease

- Diagnosis of uncomplicated cases is based primarily on description of symptoms and potential risk factors. Response to treatment can also be used as a diagnostic strategy.
- Endoscopy is recommended for the following patients:
  - Age >45 years
  - Presenting with atypical or alarm symptoms
  - Refractory to initial treatment
- Ambulatory pH testing can also be used if patients continue to have symptoms despite either normal endoscopic findings or appropriate therapy.

Peptic Ulcer Disease

- Clinical history (including symptoms and history of medication use) can be helpful in arriving at a preliminary diagnosis (not important to differentiate between duodenal and gastric ulcers).
- All patients with a suspected diagnosis of PUD should be tested for *H. pylori*.
  - Invasive tests (endoscopy): rapid urease tests (80–95% sensitive, 95–100% specific; false negatives can occur if patients previously on proton pump inhibitors [PPIs], H_2 receptor antagonists (H2RAs), or bismuth therapy; patient needs to be off these drugs for at least 1 week before performing this test)

- Noninvasive tests:
  - » Serological: 85% sensitive, 79% specific; not influenced by prior acid-suppressive therapy; can be used to confirm diagnosis but will not be helpful in determining eradication of infection
  - » Urea breath test: 97% sensitive, 95% specific; influenced by prior acid-suppressive and antibiotic therapy (increased risk of false negative); can be used to confirm diagnosis and eradication
  - » Stool antigen test: 88–92% sensitive, 87% specific; influenced by prior acid-suppressive therapy; can be used to confirm diagnosis and eradication

Signs and Symptoms

Gastroesophageal Reflux Disease

- Typical symptoms: Heartburn (pyrosis), regurgitation, belching, water brash (increased salivation)
- Atypical symptoms: Noncardiac chest pain, hoarseness, nausea, asthma-like symptoms, chronic cough, sore throat, dental erosions
- Alarm symptoms (indicate need for immediate evaluation): Dysphagia (difficulty swallowing), odynophagia (painful swallowing), bleeding, weight loss
- Long-term complications: Esophageal strictures, Barrett's esophagus, esophageal cancer

Peptic Ulcer Disease

- Abdominal pain (usually epigastric): The most common symptom
  - Can be described as burning, discomfort, or fullness
  - Duodenal ulcer: Pain often occurs 1–3 hours after a meal and is relieved with food
  - Gastric ulcer: Pain brought on by food
- Other symptoms: Heartburn, belching, bloating, nausea, anorexia
- Long-term complications: Upper GI bleeding, perforation

Guidelines

Gastroesophageal Reflux Disease

Katz PO, Gerson LB, Vela MF. Guidelines for the diagnosis and management of gastroesophageal reflux disease. *Am J Gastroenterol* 2013;108:308–28.

Peptic Ulcer Disease

Chey WD, Wong BC; Practice Parameters Committee of the American College of Gastroenterology. American College of Gastroenterology guideline on the management of *Helicobacter pylori* infection. *Am J Gastroenterol* 2007;102:1808–25.

Lanza FL, Chan FK, Quigley EM; Practice Parameters Committee of the American College of Gastroenterology. Guidelines for prevention of NSAID-related ulcer complications. *Am J Gastroenterol* 2009;104:728–38.

Lanza FL; Parameters of the American College of Gastroenterology. A guideline for the treatment and prevention of NSAID-induced ulcers. Members of the Ad Hoc Committee on Practice. *Am J Gastroenterol* 1998;93:2037–46.

Guidelines Summary

Gastroesophageal Reflux Disease

The goals of therapy are to relieve symptoms, promote healing of esophageal mucosa, prevent recurrence, and prevent complications.

- **Lifestyle modifications**
  - Unlikely to control symptoms, when used alone, in most patients
  - Dietary changes: Avoid foods that can worsen symptoms (alcohol, caffeine, chocolate, citrus juices, peppermint/spearmint, coffee, spicy foods, tomatoes, high-fatty meals, garlic, onions); avoid eating before bedtime; remain upright after meals
  - Weight loss
  - Smoking cessation
  - Head elevated off the bed by 6–8 inches
  - No tight-fitting clothes
  - No medications that can worsen symptoms
- **Pharmacological therapy**
  - Step 1: Antacids and over-the-counter (OTC) acid suppressants (H2RAs, omeprazole, lansoprazole, esomeprazole) can be used initially on an as-needed basis for intermittent or mild symptoms. If symptoms persist after 2 weeks, proceed to Step 2.
  - Step 2: PPI or H2RA (can be used at higher prescription doses).
    - » PPIs are considered more effective than H2RAs.
  - A promotility agent (e.g., metoclopramide) can be used as adjunctive therapy, if needed.

Peptic Ulcer Disease

The goals of therapy are to relieve symptoms, promote healing of the ulcer, eradicate *H. pylori* (if present), prevent recurrence, and prevent complications.

- **Lifestyle modifications:** Reduce stress, smoking cessation, discontinue NSAID use, avoid foods that can worsen symptoms

- **Pharmacological therapy**
  - *H. pylori*-associated ulcers: PPI + two antibiotics (usually clarithromycin and amoxicillin); duration = 10–14 days. If this therapy fails, four-drug therapy should be used (PPI + bismuth + metronidazole + tetracycline); duration = 14 days.
  - NSAID-induced ulcers
    - » Treatment:
      - – First-line therapy: PPI (duration of therapy = 6–8 weeks; may be longer if recurrent symptoms, heavy smoker, or continued NSAID use)
      - – Second-line therapies: Misoprostol or H2RA
    - » Primary prevention:
      - – Recommendations based on whether patient is at low, moderate, or high risk for NSAID GI toxicity (see Definitions) and the patient's risk for CV disease; high CV risk is defined by the patient's need for low-dose aspirin to prevent future CV events

	Low GI Risk	Moderate GI Risk	High GI Risk
Low CV Risk	NSAID alone	NSAID + PPI/misoprostol	Alternative therapy, if possible; or, cyclooxygenase-2 inhibitor + PPI/misoprostol
High CV Risk	Naproxen + PPI/ misoprostol	Naproxen + PPI/ misoprostol	Avoid NSAIDs or cyclooxygenase-2 inhibitors; use alternative therapy

Antacids

Generic • Brand • Dose	Contraindications	Primary Side Effects	Key Monitoring	Pertinent Drug Interactions	Med Pearl
Mechanism of action – neutralize stomach acid and ↑ gastric pH					
Magnesium hydroxide/ aluminum hydroxide • Mag-Al • 15 mL with meals and at bedtime	None	• Diarrhea (from magnesium [Mg^{2+}]) • Constipation (from aluminum [Al^{3+}] or calcium [Ca^{2+}])	S/S of GERD	• May bind to numerous drugs (separate from other drugs by at least 2 hrs) • May ↓ absorption of drugs whose absorption is pH-dependent (e.g., itraconazole, ketoconazole, iron, atazanavir, nelfinavir, rilpivirine, mycophenolate mofetil, and erlotinib)	Use Mg^{2+}- and Al^{3+}- containing products with caution in patients with renal impairment
Calcium carbonate • Tums, Maalox Chewables • 1–2 tabs q2h as needed					

H$_2$ Receptor Antagonists

Generic • Brand • Dose	Dosage Forms	Primary Side Effects	Key Monitoring	Pertinent Drug Interactions	Med Pearl
Mechanism of action – reversibly inhibit histamine (H$_2$) receptors in the gastric parietal cells, which inhibits secretion of gastric acid					
Cimetidine • Tagamet HB • 200–1,600 mg/day	• Rx: Solution, tabs • OTC: Tabs	• Headache • Fatigue • Dizziness • Confusion • Gynecomastia (cimetidine)	S/S of GERD/PUD	• Cimetidine inhibits cytochrome P450 (CYP) enzymes to greater extent than the other drugs (inhibits CYP1A2, CYP2C19, CYP2D6, and CYP3A4) • May ↓ absorption of drugs whose absorption is pH-dependent (e.g., itraconazole, ketoconazole, iron, atazanavir, nelfinavir, rilpivirine, mycophenolate mofetil, and erlotinib)	Adjust dose of all H2RAs in renal impairment
Famotidine ☆ • Pepcid • 20–80 mg/day	• Rx: Injection, suspension, tabs • OTC: Tabs				
Nizatidine • Axid • 150–300 mg/day	• Rx: Caps, solution				
Ranitidine ☆ • Zantac • 75–300 mg/day	• Rx: Caps, injection, syrup, tabs • OTC: Tabs				
Combination product: Famotidine/calcium carbonate/magnesium hydroxide (Pepcid Complete)					

Proton Pump Inhibitors

Generic • Brand • Dose	Dosage Forms	Primary Side Effects	Key Monitoring	Pertinent Drug Interactions	Med Pearl
Mechanism of action – irreversibly inhibit H$^+$/K$^+$-ATPase in gastric parietal cells, which inhibits secretion of gastric acid					
Dexlansoprazole ☆ • Dexilant • 30–60 mg/day	Caps, tabs	• Diarrhea • Headache	S/S of GERD/PUD	• May ↓ absorption of drugs whose absorption is pH-dependent (e.g., itraconazole, ketoconazole, iron, atazanavir, nelfinavir, rilpivirine, mycophenolate mofetil, and erlotinib) • May ↓ antiplatelet effects of clopidogrel • May ↑ effects/ toxicity of methotrexate	May be associated with: • Osteoporosis-related fractures • ↓ Mg^{2+} • *Clostridium difficile* • Vitamin B$_{12}$ deficiency • Acute interstitial nephritis
Esomeprazole ☆ • Nexium, Nexium 24 hr • 20–40 mg/day	• Rx: Caps, granules for suspension, injection • OTC: Caps, tabs				
Lansoprazole ☆ • Prevacid • 15–30 mg/day	• Rx: Caps, tabs • OTC: Caps				
Omeprazole ☆ • Prilosec • 20 mg/day	• Rx: Caps, granules for suspension • OTC: Tabs				
Pantoprazole ☆ • Protonix • 20–40 mg/day	Granules for suspension, injection, tabs				
Rabeprazole ☆ • Aciphex • 20 mg/day	Sprinkle capsules, tabs				
Combination products: Esomeprazole/naproxen (Vimovo)　　　Omeprazole/sodium bicarbonate (Zegerid)　　　Omeprazole/aspirin (Yosprala)					

Promotility Drug

Generic • Brand • Dose/Dosage Forms	Contraindications	Primary Side Effects	Key Monitoring	Pertinent Drug Interactions	Med Pearl
Mechanism of action – dopamine antagonist; ↑ LES pressure and accelerates gastric emptying					
Metoclopramide ☆ • Reglan, Metozolv ODT • 40–60 mg/day • Injection, solution, tabs	Seizures	• Dizziness • Sedation • Diarrhea • Extrapyramidal symptoms (EPS)	• S/S of GERD • EPS	Use with antipsychotic agents may ↑ risk of EPS	• Can also be used for diabetic gastroparesis; erythromycin is an alternative • Adjust dose in renal impairment

Mucosal Protectant Drug

Generic • Brand • Dose/Dosage Forms	Contraindications	Primary Side Effects	Key Monitoring	Pertinent Drug Interactions	Med Pearl
Mechanism of action – nonabsorbable aluminum salt that forms bonds with damaged and normal GI tissue; complex forms protective cover over ulcerated area					
Sucralfate ☆ • Carafate • 4 g/day • Suspension, tabs	None	Constipation	S/S of PUD	May bind to numerous drugs (separate from other drugs by at least 2 hrs)	• Limited value in treatment of GERD; more useful in treatment of PUD • Use cautiously in patients with chronic kidney disease (↑ risk of Al^{3+} toxicity)

Prostaglandin Analog

Generic • Brand • Dose/Dosage Forms	Contraindications	Primary Side Effects	Key Monitoring	Pertinent Drug Interactions	Med Pearl
Mechanism of action – prostaglandin E1 analog; replaces protective prostaglandins inhibited by NSAID therapy					
Misoprostol • Cytotec • 400–800 mcg/day • Tabs	Pregnancy (abortifacient)	Diarrhea	S/S of PUD	None	• Women of childbearing age should have pregnancy test before initiating therapy; educate regarding appropriate use of contraception • Can also be used for medical termination of pregnancy
Combination product: Misoprostol/diclofenac (Arthrotec)					

Helicobacter pylori Treatment Regimens (for PUD)

Proton Pump Inhibitor	Drug #2	Drug #3	Drug #4	Comments
Three-Drug Regimen (PPI + two antibiotics; duration of therapy = 10–14 days; 14 days preferred)				
Esomeprazole 40 mg daily **OR** lansoprazole 30 mg BID **OR** omeprazole 20 mg BID **OR** pantoprazole 40 mg BID **OR** rabeprazole 20 mg BID	Amoxicillin 1,000 mg BID	Clarithromycin 500 mg BID		• Metronidazole (500 mg BID) can be used instead of amoxicillin or clarithromycin in patients with penicillin or macrolide allergy, respectively • Rabeprazole regimen should be given for 7 days • Prevpac is a compliance package that contains individual units of lansoprazole, amoxicillin, and clarithromycin • Omeclamox-Pak is a compliance package that contains individual units of omeprazole, amoxicillin, and clarithromycin
Four-Drug Regimen (PPI + bismuth subsalicylate + metronidazole + tetracycline; duration of therapy = 14 days)				
Esomeprazole 40 mg daily **OR** lansoprazole 30 mg BID **OR** omeprazole 20 mg BID **OR** pantoprazole 40 mg BID **OR** rabeprazole 20 mg BID	Bismuth subsalicylate 525 mg 4 × daily	Metronidazole 250 mg 4 × daily	Tetracycline 500 mg 4 × daily	• Pylera contains bismuth, metronidazole, and tetracycline in each capsule • Can alternatively use H_2RA instead of PPI (4-drug regimen given for 2 wk and then H_2RA alone continued for additional 2 wk)

Storage and Administration Pearls

- Dexlansoprazole
  - Capsules can be opened and mixed with applesauce (eat immediately)
  - Capsules and orally disintegrating tablets (ODTs) can be mixed in water to be given via oral syringe
  - May be administered via nasogastric (NG) tube
    - » Capsules: Open the capsule and mix with water
    - » ODTs: Dilute tablet in water
- Esomeprazole
  - Capsules can be opened and mixed with applesauce (eat immediately)

- Mix granules for oral suspension in water
- May be administered via NG tube
  - » Capsules: Open the capsule and mix with water
  - » Granules for oral suspension: Dilute granules in water
- May be administered via gastric tube
  - » Granules for oral suspension: Dilute granules in water

- Lansoprazole
  - Capsules can be opened and mixed with applesauce, Ensure pudding, cottage cheese, yogurt, or strained pears (swallow immediately); can also mix in orange, apple, or tomato juice (swallow immediately)
  - ODTs can be mixed in water to be given via oral syringe
  - May be administered via NG tube
    - » Capsules: Open the capsule and mix with apple juice
    - » ODTs: Dilute tablet in water

- Omeprazole
  - Capsules can be opened and mixed with applesauce (eat immediately); **cannot** be given via NG or gastric tube
  - Mix granules for oral suspension in water
  - Tablets should **not** be crushed; **cannot** be given via NG or gastric tube
  - Granules for oral suspension may be administered via NG or gastric tube (dilute granules in water)

- Pantoprazole
  - Tablets: Should **not** be crushed; **cannot** be given via NG or gastric tube
  - Granules for oral suspension can be mixed in apple juice or sprinkled on applesauce
  - Granules for oral suspension may be administered via NG or gastric tube (dilute in apple juice)

- Rabeprazole
  - Tablets should **not** be crushed; **cannot** be given via NG or OG tube
  - Sprinkle capsules can be opened and sprinkled on applesauce, baby food (fruit or vegetable-based), or yogurt or mixed in apple juice, infant formula, or pediatric electrolyte solution; **cannot** be given via NG or gastric tube

- Misoprostol should be administered with meals
- Sucralfate should be administered 1 hour before meals

Patient Education Pearls

- Lifestyle changes should be continued throughout the course of therapy.
- Patient should separate the administration of antacids from other medications by at least 2 hours.

- PPIs should be taken 15–30 minutes before breakfast; if patient is taking two daily doses, final dose should be taken before dinner (not at bedtime).
- A patient who is being treated for *H. pylori* should complete the entire course of therapy to facilitate eradication of the infection.

INFLAMMATORY BOWEL DISEASE

Definitions

Inflammatory bowel disease (IBD) is a broad term used to describe two conditions: ulcerative colitis (UC) and Crohn's disease (CD). UC is a chronic inflammatory disease that consists of superficial mucosal lesions localized to the colon and rectum. CD is also a chronic inflammatory disease, but is characterized by transmural lesions that can occur anywhere along the GI tract. The etiology of both of these disorders is thought to be due to immunologic or infectious causes; however, environmental, psychological, or genetic factors may also contribute to the development of these diseases.

Diagnosis

Diagnosis is suspected on the basis of clinical presentation, but is confirmed through various studies, including sigmoidoscopy, colonoscopy, barium enema, and stool examination. A biopsy of the lesions is usually performed during the sigmoidoscopy or colonoscopy.

Signs and Symptoms

The following symptoms can occur with both UC and CD: fever, diarrhea, weight loss, rectal bleeding, and abdominal pain.

Clinical Findings Associated with Ulcerative Colitis or Crohn's Disease

Clinical Finding	Ulcerative Colitis	Crohn's Disease
Abdominal mass	No	Yes
Fistulas/strictures	No	Yes
Bowel involvement	Rectum/colon	Can affect anywhere from mouth to anus (often affects ileum)
Systemic complications (i.e., extraintestinal involvement)	Yes	Yes
Toxic megacolon	Yes	No
At risk for colorectal cancer	Yes	Rare
Pattern of inflammation	Continuous	Segmented ("cobblestone" appearance)

Severity of Disease: Ulcerative Colitis

- Mild: >4 stools/day (with or without blood), no systemic signs of toxicity, and normal erythrocyte sedimentation rate (ESR)
- Moderate: >4 stools/day and minimal signs of toxicity
- Severe: >6 stools/day (with blood) and evidence of toxicity (e.g., fever, tachycardia, anemia, or elevated ESR)

Severity of Disease: Crohn's Disease

- Mild-moderate: Ambulatory and able to tolerate oral intake without evidence of dehydration, systemic toxicity, abdominal tenderness, painful mass, intestinal obstruction, or >10% weight loss
- Moderate-severe: Fail to respond to treatment for mild-moderate disease or have fever, significant weight loss (>10%), abdominal mass/tenderness, intermittent nausea/vomiting (N/V) (without findings of obstruction), or significant anemia
- Severe/fulminant: Persistent symptoms despite the initiation of treatment with corticosteroids or biologic agents as outpatients or presenting with high fevers, persistent vomiting, evidence of intestinal obstruction, significant peritoneal signs (e.g., rebound tenderness, cachexia, or evidence of abscess)

Guidelines

Kornbluth A, Sachar DB; Practice Parameters Committee of the American College of Gastroenterology. Ulcerative colitis practice guidelines in adults: American College of Gastroenterology, Practice Parameters Committee. *Am J Gastroenterol* 2010;105:501–23.

Lichtenstein GR, Hanauer SB, Sandborn WJ; Practice Parameters Committee of American College of Gastroenterology. Management of Crohn's disease in adults. *Am J Gastroenterol* 2009;104:465–83.

Guidelines Summary

The goals of therapy are to induce and maintain remission, to prevent and resolve complications and systemic symptoms, and to maintain quality of life. There is no pharmacologic cure for these diseases; therefore, treatment focuses on management of symptoms.

- **Nonpharmacologic therapy**
  - Lifestyle changes/diet: Avoid foods that may worsen disease symptoms
  - Possible surgery when complications (e.g., fistulas, strictures, perforation) develop or to manage refractory disease

- **Pharmacologic therapy**
  - Adjunctive therapies: antidiarrheals (e.g., loperamide), antispasmodics (e.g., dicyclomine, propantheline, hyoscyamine)
  - Ulcerative colitis:
    » Treatment based upon whether inflammation is distal (below the splenic flexure; topical therapy appropriate) or extensive (proximal to the splenic flexure; requires systemic therapy)
    » Mild/moderate distal disease:
      - Active disease: Topical mesalamine (enema or suppository preferred), oral aminosalicylate, or topical corticosteroid
      - Maintenance of remission: Topical mesalamine or oral aminosalicylate
    » Mild/moderate extensive disease:
      - Active disease: Oral aminosalicylate (first-line), oral corticosteroids, azathioprine, 6-mercaptopurine, infliximab, adalimumab, golimumab, or vedolizumab
      - Maintenance of remission: Oral aminosalicylate (first-line), azathioprine, 6-mercaptopurine, infliximab, adalimumab, golimumab, or vedolizumab
    » Severe disease:
      - Infliximab (if urgent hospitalization not needed), intravenous (IV) corticosteroids (if urgent hospitalization needed), IV cyclosporine
  - Crohn's disease:
    » Mild/moderate active disease:
      - First-line: Oral aminosalicylate, budesonide (disease localized to ileum and/or right colon)
      - Second-line: Metronidazole, ciprofloxacin
    » Moderate/severe disease:
      - First-line: Prednisone
      - Second-line: Infliximab, adalimumab, certolizumab pegol, vedolizumab, natalizumab, methotrexate (IM or subcut)
    » Severe/fulminant disease:
      - First-line: IV corticosteroids
      - Second-line: IV cyclosporine or IV tacrolimus
    » Maintenance therapy:
      - First line: Azathioprine, 6-mercaptopurine, methotrexate, infliximab, adalimumab, certolizumab pegol, vedolizumab, or natalizumab

Aminosalicylates

Generic • Brand • Dose	Dosage Forms	Contraindications	Primary Side Effects	Key Monitoring	Med Pearl
Mechanism of action – ↓ inflammation in GI tract by inhibiting prostaglandin synthesis and subsequent production of various immune mediators; sulfasalazine is cleaved in colon to mesalamine (responsible for therapeutic effect) + sulfapyridine (causes side effects); olsalazine and balsalazide also contain mesalamine					
Sulfasalazine • Azulfidine, Azulfidine EN • Induction: 3–4 g/day • Maintenance: 2 g/day	Tabs, delayed-release (DR) (enteric-coated) tabs	• Aspirin allergy • Sulfa allergy • Glucose-6-phosphate dehydrogenase (G6PD) deficiency • Pregnancy (near term)	• Stevens-Johnson syndrome • Photosensitivity • N/V • Headache • Folate deficiency • Hemolytic anemia • Agranulocytosis • Hepatitis • Orange discoloration of bodily fluids	• S/S of IBD • Liver function tests (LFTs) (with sulfasalazine) • Complete blood count (CBC) (with sulfasalazine)	• Mesalamine, olsalazine, and balsalazide are not sulfa derivatives; are poorly absorbed from GI tract (better tolerated than sulfasalazine) • Folic acid should be given to patients on sulfasalazine • Sulfasalazine may ↑ effects of warfarin and oral hypoglycemics • All may ↓ absorption of digoxin
Mesalamine • Apriso, Asacol HD, Canasa, Delzicol, Lialda, Pentasa, Rowasa • Oral: *Induction* 2.4–4.8 g/day; *Maintenance*, 1.5–4 g/day • Rectal enema (Rowasa): 4 g at bedtime • Rectal suppository (Canasa): 1 g at bedtime	Extended-release (ER) caps, DR tabs, rectal enema, rectal suppository	• Aspirin allergy • G6PD deficiency	• Nausea • Diarrhea • Headache • Malaise		
Olsalazine • Dipentum • 1–3 g/day	Caps				
Balsalazide • Colazal, Giazo • 1.5–6.75 g/day	Caps, tabs				

Corticosteroids

Generic • Brand • Dose	Dosage Forms	Contraindications	Primary Side Effects	Key Monitoring	Med Pearl
Mechanism of action – quickly ↓ inflammation during acute exacerbations of IBD					
Budesonide • Entocort EC, Uceris • Entocort EC: *Initial*: 9 mg daily for up to 2 mo; *Maintenance*: 6 mg daily for up to 3 mo • Uceris (PO): 9 mg daily for up to 2 mo • Uceris (rectal foam): 1 metered dose (2 mg) BID for 2 wk, then 1 metered dose (2 mg) daily for 4 wk	DR caps, ER tabs, rectal foam	None	• Hyperglycemia • ↑ appetite • Insomnia • Hypertension • Edema • Adrenal suppression • Osteoporosis • Cataracts • Delayed wound healing	• S/S of IBD • Blood glucose • Blood pressure (BP) • Electrolytes	• Methylprednisolone and prednisone should only be used to treat acute exacerbation (4–8 wk) and then tapered • IV therapy given for severe exacerbations for 7–10 days, then switched to PO therapy • Budesonide has localized effect; has minimal systemic side effects • Entocort EC indicated for CD • Uceris indicated for UC
Methylprednisolone ☆ • Solu-Medrol • 10–100 mg/day	Injection, tabs				
Prednisone ☆ • Sterapred • 20–60 mg/day	Tabs				

Immunosuppressants

Generic • **Brand** • **Dose**	Contraindications	Primary Side Effects	Key Monitoring	Pertinent Drug Interactions	Med Pearl
Mechanism of action – ↓ production of inflammatory mediators (e.g., interleukins) through various mechanisms					
Azathioprine • Azasan, Imuran • 75–150 mg/day 6-Mercaptopurine • Purixan • 50–100 mg/day	• Pregnancy • Bone marrow suppression • Hepatic impairment	• Pancreatitis • Arthralgias • Nausea • Diarrhea • Rash • Bone marrow suppression • Hepatotoxicity	• Amylase/lipase (if symptoms) • CBC with differential • LFTs	• Allopurinol and febuxostat may ↑ risk of side effects (↓ azathioprine dose by 75% when used with allopurinol; avoid concomitant use with febuxostat) • Aminosalicylates may ↑ risk of side effects • May ↓ effects of warfarin	• 6-mercaptopurine is active metabolite of azathioprine • Adjust dose in renal impairment
Cyclosporine • Sandimmune • 4–8 mg/kg/day IV	Renal failure	• Hypertension • Nephrotoxicity • Hypomagnesemia • Infection • Anaphylaxis	• BP • Blood urea nitrogen (BUN)/serum creatinine (SCr) • Electrolytes • S/S of infection • Cyclosporine levels	• CYP3A4 substrate and inhibitor • CYP3A4 inhibitors may ↑ levels/toxicity • CYP3A4 inducers may ↓ effects • May ↑ effects of other CYP3A4 substrates	• Used only for severe disease that has not responded to corticosteroids • Used only for 7–10 days
Methotrexate☆ • Rheumatrex • 15–25 mg/wk IM or subcut	• Pregnancy • Bone marrow suppression • Severe renal or hepatic impairment	• Hepatotoxicity • Bone marrow suppression • Pneumonitis • Rash • N/V • Diarrhea	• LFTs • CBC with differential • Chest x-ray (if symptoms)	• NSAIDs and salicylates ↑ risk of toxicity • Penicillins, sulfonamides, and tetracyclines may ↑ risk of toxicity	• Only effective for CD (useful for steroid-dependent and steroid-refractory CD) • Adjust dose in renal impairment

Biological Agents

Generic • Brand • Dose	Contraindications	Primary Side Effects	Key Monitoring	Pertinent Drug Interactions	Med Pearl
Mechanism of action – inhibit tumor necrosis factor (TNF)					
Adalimumab • Humira • 160 mg subcut on day 1 or over 2 days, then 80 mg 2 wk later (day 15), then 40 mg every other wk beginning day 29	None	• Headache • Rash • Injection site reactions • Anaphylaxis • Infection (especially tuberculosis [TB], fungal infections and hepatitis B virus [HBV] reactivation) • Lymphoma • Heart failure (HF) exacerbation • Bone marrow suppression • Lupus-like syndrome • Demyelinating disorders	• S/S of infection • S/S of HF • CBC with differential	Do not administer live vaccines	• PPD and HBV screening should be done before initiating treatment • Approved for moderately to severely active CD or UC in patients who have not responded despite adequate therapy with a corticosteroid or immunosuppressant
Certolizumab pegol • Cimzia • 400 mg subcut at 0, 2, and 4 wks; then 400 mg every 4 wk	None				• PPD and HBV screening should be done before initiating treatment • Only approved for moderately to severely active CD in patients who have not responded despite adequate therapy with a corticosteroid or immunosuppressant
Golimumab • Simponi • 200 mg subcut at wk 0, then 100 mg at wk 2, then 100 mg every 4 wk	None				• PPD and HBV screening should be done before initiating treatment • Only approved for moderately to severely active UC in patients who have not responded despite adequate therapy with a corticosteroid or immunosuppressant
Infliximab • Inflectra, Remicade • 5 mg/kg IV at 0, 2, and 6 wk; then every 8 wk	New York Heart Association class III or IV HF (for doses >5 mg/kg)	• Infusion reactions (hypotension, dyspnea, urticaria) • Delayed hypersensitivity reactions (fever, rash, myalgia, headache, sore throat, hand/facial edema, dysphagia, arthralgias) • Infection (especially TB, fungal infections, or HBV reactivation) • HF exacerbation • Bone marrow suppression • Lymphoma • Hepatotoxicity	• BP • LFTs • S/S of infection • S/S of HF • CBC with differential		• Delayed hypersensitivity reaction may occur as early as after 2nd dose • Premedicate with H_1 antagonist, H2RA, acetaminophen, and/or corticosteroid • PPD and HBV screening should be done before initiating treatment • Approved for moderately to severely active CD or UC in patients who have not responded despite adequate therapy with a corticosteroid or immunosuppressant

Biological Agents *(cont'd)*

Generic • Brand • Dose	Contraindications	Primary Side Effects	Key Monitoring	Pertinent Drug Interactions	Med Pearl
Mechanism of action − ↓ inflammation by binding to α4-subunit of integrins					
Natalizumab • Tysabri • 300 mg IV every 4 wk; discontinue if no response by wk 12	• Progressive multifocal leuko-encephalopathy (PML) • Concurrent use of TNF inhibitors or immunosuppressants	• PML (may be fatal) • Headache • Fatigue • Depression • Rash • Nausea • Arthralgia • Hypersensitivity reactions (hypotension, urticaria, fever, rash, rigors, nausea, flushing, dizziness, chest pain) • Anaphylaxis • Infection (especially opportunistic infections or herpes encephalitis meningitis) • Hepatotoxicity	• S/S of PML • Brain MRI (at baseline) • S/S of infection • LFTs	Do not administer live vaccines	• Patients need to be enrolled in CD-TOUCH program • Must be administered as monotherapy • Only approved for moderate to severely active CD in patients who are refractory to or unable to tolerate conventional therapies and TNF inhibitors
Mechanism of action − ↓ inflammation by binding to α4β7-subunit of integrins					
Vedolizumab • Entyvio • 300 mg IV at 0, 2, and 6 wk; then every 8 wk; discontinue if no response by wk 14	None	• Hypersensitivity reactions • Anaphylaxis • Infusion reactions • Infection (especially TB) • PML • Hepatotoxicity	• S/S of infection • S/S of PML • LFTs	Do not administer live vaccines	• Consider performing PPD before treatment • Approved for moderately to severely active CD or UC in patients who are refractory to or unable to tolerate TNF blocker or corticosteroid therapy

Storage and Administration Pearls

- Patients receiving infliximab should be pretreated with antihistamines (H_1 and H_2 blockers), acetaminophen, and/or corticosteroid to prevent infusion-related reaction.
- Infliximab should be administered as an IV infusion over at least 2 hours.
- Natalizumab should be administered as an IV infusion over 1 hour.
- Vedolizumab should be administered as an IV infusion over 30 minutes.
- If switching from prednisone to budesonide, prednisone should be tapered over a two-week period.

Patient Education Pearls

- Adherence to medication is very important as disease exacerbations can have a significant impact on quality of life.
- Mesalamine enemas and suppositories should be administered at bedtime to allow for direct contact of the drug with the rectal mucosa for at least 8 hours.
- Live vaccines should not be administered if a patient is receiving biological agents.
- Patients receiving azathioprine, 6-mercaptopurine, methotrexate, infliximab, adalimumab, certolizumab pegol, golimumab, natalizumab or vedolizumab are at ↑ risk for infection. They should wash their hands frequently and avoid crowds or other persons who are sick.
- Patients taking sulfasalazine should wear sunscreen and protective clothing. Sulfasalazine should be taken with meals to minimize GI effects. Patients taking sulfasalazine should take folic acid (1 mg/day) to prevent folate deficiency. Sulfasalazine may cause an orange discoloration of body fluids (urine, tears), which may stain clothing and contact lenses.
- Women receiving azathioprine, 6-mercaptopurine, or methotrexate should be counseled on using appropriate contraceptive methods.
- NSAIDs and high-dose salicylates (not the doses of aspirin used for prevention of CV diseases) may ↑ risk of methotrexate toxicity and should be avoided if the patient is receiving this immunosuppressant.

LEARNING POINTS

- **GERD/PUD**

  - Antacids should be separated from other medications by at least 2 hours because of the risk for binding and ↓ the absorption of these drugs.

  - The majority of PUD cases are caused by either *H. pylori* infection or NSAIDs.

  - Three-drug regimen (PPI + two antibiotics [usually clarithromycin and amoxicillin]) is recommended for treatment of *H. pylori* infection.

  - The dosage of all H_2RAs needs to be adjusted in patients with renal impairment.

  - Of all the H_2RAs, cimetidine is the most likely to be involved with drug interactions involving the CYP450 system.

  - Of all the PPIs, only esomeprazole and pantoprazole are available as IV injection; also be familiar with the various dosage forms of the PPIs.

- **IBD**

  - Sulfasalazine should not be used in patients with sulfa allergies. The other aminosalicylates—mesalamine, olsalazine, and balsalazide—can be used in these patients.

  - Folic acid should be administered to patients receiving sulfasalazine to prevent folate deficiency.

  - Know the various dosage forms of the aminosalicylates.

  - Be familiar with the side effects of systemic corticosteroids.

  - Methotrexate is only effective for CD.

  - PPD should be performed prior to starting adalimumab, certolizumab pegol, golimumab, infliximab, or vedolizumab.

  - Patients receiving infliximab need to be pretreated with antihistamine, acetaminophen, and/or corticosteroid.

  - Natalizumab and vedolizumab are associated with PML.

PRACTICE QUESTIONS

1. Remicade is the brand name for which of the following medications?

    (A) Azathioprine
    (B) Balsalazide
    (C) Budesonide
    (D) Cyclosporine
    (E) Infliximab

2. Which of the following is a contraindication for the use of metoclopramide?

    (A) Hyperkalemia
    (B) Myasthenia gravis
    (C) Porphyria
    (D) Seizure disorder
    (E) Sulfa allergy

3. A patient using NSAIDs for chronic pain develops a bleeding ulcer. Which of the following medications would be MOST appropriate to treat his condition?

    (A) Aluminum hydroxide
    (B) Bismuth subsalicylate
    (C) Calcium carbonate
    (D) Metoclopramide
    (E) Misoprostol

4. A patient who is taking warfarin for chronic atrial fibrillation develops GERD. Which of the following medications would MOST likely interact with the warfarin and increase this patient's risk for bleeding?

    (A) Cimetidine
    (B) Magnesium hydroxide
    (C) Misoprostol
    (D) Pantoprazole
    (E) Sucralfate

5. Which of the following reasons MOST likely explains why the plasma levels of ketoconazole are decreased in patients taking lansoprazole?

    (A) Lansoprazole induces the CYP450 enzymes that metabolize ketoconazole.
    (B) Ketoconazole requires an acidic environment for its oral absorption.
    (C) Lansoprazole binds acidic drugs in the GI tract.
    (D) Lansoprazole has prokinetic effects, which decrease GI transit time.
    (E) There is a competition for transport mechanisms in the GI tract.

6. Which of the following medications needs to be dose-adjusted in patients with renal impairment? (Select ALL that apply.)

    (A) Adalimumab
    (B) Budesonide
    (C) Esomeprazole
    (D) Metoclopramide
    (E) Ranitidine

7. A patient with UC has a history of anaphylaxis when taking trimethoprim/ sulfamethoxazole. Which of the following medications would be safe to use for the treatment of UC in this patient? (Select ALL that apply.)

    (A) Asacol HD
    (B) Azulfidine
    (C) Dipentum
    (D) Simponi
    (E) Uceris

8. Which of the following characteristics is more likely to occur with UC than CD?

    (A) Confinement of the disease to the colon and rectum
    (B) Fistula formation
    (C) Cobblestone pattern of inflammation
    (D) Transmural lesion in the GI tract
    (E) Systemic complications

9. Which of the following supplements may be needed in a patient taking chronic sulfasalazine therapy for IBD?

    (A) Calcium carbonate
    (B) Folic acid
    (C) Iron
    (D) Vitamin B_{12}
    (E) Vitamin C

10. Which of the following baseline tests should be performed before a patient begins certolizumab pegol therapy for CD?

    (A) Brain MRI
    (B) LFTs
    (C) PPD
    (D) Serum creatinine
    (E) Uric acid

ANSWERS AND EXPLANATIONS

1. **E**

Remicade is the brand name for infliximab. Imuran is the brand name for azathioprine (A). Colazal is the brand name for balsalazide (B). Entocort EC or Uceris are brand names for oral budesonide (C). Sandimmune, Gengraf, and Neoral are brand names for cyclosporine (D).

2. **D**

Seizure disorder is a contraindication for the use of metoclopramide; therefore, choice (D) is correct.

3. **E**

The first-line therapy for an NSAID-induced ulcer is a PPI. However, no PPIs are listed as answer choices. Appropriate second-line therapies for an NSAID-induced ulcer are either misoprostol or an H_2RA. Misoprostol is a prostaglandin E1 analog that acts to replace protective prostaglandins that have been inhibited by NSAID therapy. Aluminum hydroxide (A), bismuth subsalicylate (B), calcium carbonate (C), and metoclopramide (D) would not be appropriate treatments for a NSAID-induced ulcer.

4. **A**

Cimetidine is a strong inhibitor of CYP3A4 and a moderate inhibitor of CYP1A2. It is also a weak inhibitor of CYP2C9. (R)-warfarin is a substrate of CYP3A4 and CYP1A2, while (S)-warfarin is a substrate of CYP2C9. Therefore, cimetidine has the potential to inhibit the metabolism of both the (S)- and (R)-enantiomers of warfarin, which could lead to an increased risk of bleeding. Magnesium hydroxide (B), misoprostol (C), pantoprazole (D), and sucralfate (E) do not inhibit the CYP450 system and therefore should not increase the risk of bleeding with warfarin.

5. **B**

The absorption of ketoconazole is pH-dependent; this antifungal drug requires an acidic environment to be adequately absorbed; therefore, the bioavailability of this drug decreases as gastric pH increases. By increasing gastric pH, lansoprazole may reduce the absorption of ketoconazole, which would lead to decreased plasma concentrations. Lansoprazole is not known to be an inducer of the CYP450 isoenzymes (A). If anything, it may be a weak inhibitor of CYP2C19; however, this inhibition would not have any effect on ketoconazole plasma concentrations. Lansoprazole does not bind to acidic drugs in the GI tract (C). Lansoprazole also does not have prokinetic effects in the GI tract (D); metoclopramide has these properties. Lansoprazole does not compete with ketoconazole for transport mechanisms in the GI tract (E).

6. **D, E**

Both metoclopramide (D) and ranitidine (E) are primarily excreted in the urine as unchanged drug. Therefore, the doses of these drugs need to be adjusted in patients with renal impairment. In fact, the dose of all H_2RAs needs to be adjusted in this patient population. None of the PPIs (C) needs to be dose adjusted in patients with renal impairment. Also, neither adalimumab (A) nor budesonide (B) needs to be dose-adjusted in these patients.

7. **A, C, D, E**

Sulfasalazine (Azulfidine) (B) is a sulfa derivative and should be avoided in patients with a history of anaphylaxis to sulfa products (e.g., trimethoprim/sulfamethoxazole). Mesalamine (Asacol HD) (A), olsalazine (Dipentum) (C), golimumab (Simponi) (D), and budesonide (Uceris) (E) are not sulfa derivatives and could be safely used in this patient with UC.

8. **A**

UC is more likely to be confined to the colon and rectum, whereas CD can affect anywhere in the GI tract from the mouth to the anus. Fistulas (B) are more likely to develop in patients with CD as opposed to those with UC. The inflammation in CD occurs in a segmented or cobblestone pattern (C), while it occurs in a more continuous fashion in UC. The mucosal lesions in UC are more superficial than those in CD, which are more transmural (D). Systemic complications can occur with either UC or CD (E).

9. **B**

Sulfasalazine can impair folate absorption. Therefore, patients taking chronic sulfasalazine therapy are at risk for developing folate deficiency and should supplement with folic acid to prevent this adverse effect. Sulfasalazine does not impair the absorption of calcium (A), iron (C), vitamin B_{12} (D), or vitamin C (E). Therefore, routine supplementation of these vitamins/minerals during sulfasalazine is not necessary.

10. **C**

Before starting therapy with certolizumab pegol, patients should be evaluated for tuberculosis risk factors and latent tuberculosis infection with a PPD. Cases of reactivation of tuberculosis or new tuberculosis infections have been reported in patients receiving therapy with TNF-inhibitors, including certolizumab pegol; patients who are receiving these drugs are at increased risk for developing serious infections. Certolizumab pegol has not been associated with PML (life-threatening), so there is no need to perform a brain MRI (A) before starting therapy with this drug; a baseline brain MRI should be performed prior to initiating therapy with natalizumab. Certolizumab pegol is not associated with hepatotoxicity or nephrotoxicity, so there is no need to monitor baseline LFTs (B) or SCr (D). Finally, certolizumab pegol does not affect uric acid levels, so this parameter does not need to be monitored at baseline.

Viral Hepatitis

7

This chapter covers the following diseases:

- **Hepatitis B**
- **Hepatitis C**

There are 5 different types of viral hepatitis: hepatitis A, hepatitis B, hepatitis C, hepatitis D, and hepatitis E. While all 5 of these viruses can cause acute hepatitis, hepatitis B, C, D are most likely to cause chronic hepatitis. Chronic viral hepatitis may lead to cirrhosis, which may result in complications such as end-stage liver disease and/or hepatocellular carcinoma. This overview will focus on hepatitis B and hepatitis C, as these are the most common types of viral hepatitis.

 Suggested study time: **30 minutes**

HEPATITIS B

Definitions

Hepatitis B virus (HBV) is a DNA virus. HBV is primarily transmitted through perinatal, sexual, or percutaneous exposure to infectious blood or bodily fluids (e.g., semen).

Individuals who are at high risk for acquiring HBV include those who are household or sexual contacts of the hepatitis B surface antigen (HBsAg); those who have used injectable drugs; those with multiple sexual partners or a history of sexually transmitted diseases; men who have sex with men; inmates of correctional facilities; those who are infected with human immunodeficiency virus (HIV) or hepatitis C virus (HCV); patients undergoing dialysis; pregnant women; patients receiving immunosuppressive therapy; healthcare workers in contact with contaminated needles or with mucosal exposure; and individuals born in areas that have a high/intermediate prevalence of HBV. These patients should be screened for HBV infection.

Diagnosis

Hepatitis B is diagnosed when HBsAg is detectable in the serum. The following laboratory serologies can be used to differentiate acute from chronic HBV:

Laboratory Test	Result	Interpretation
HBsAg IgG anti-HBc IgM anti-HBc Anti-HBs HBV DNA	Positive Positive Positive Negative High	Acutely infected
HBsAg IgG anti-HBc IgM anti-HBc Anti-HBs HBV DNA	Positive Positive Negative Negative High or low	Chronically infected

Anti-HBc = antibodies against hepatitis B core antigen; anti-HBs = antibodies against hepatitis B surface antigen

Chronic HBV is diagnosed when the following criteria are present:

- HBsAg-positive for longer than 6 months
- Serum HBV DNA >20,000 IU/mL (10^5 copies/mL)
- Persistent or intermittent elevation in alanine aminotransferase (ALT)/aspartate aminotransferase (AST) levels
- Liver biopsy demonstrates chronic hepatitis with moderate/severe necroinflammation

Signs and Symptoms

Most patients with any type of viral hepatitis have no symptoms. If signs/symptoms do occur, they may include the following:

- Symptoms: Flu-like symptoms, fever, fatigue, anorexia, nausea, vomiting, diarrhea, pruritus, abdominal pain, dark urine, pale-color stools
- Signs: Jaundice, hepatomegaly, ascites, variceal bleeding, asterixis

Guidelines

Terrault NA, Bzowej NH, Chang KM, et al. AASLD guidelines for treatment of chronic hepatitis B. *Hepatology*. 2016;63:261-83.

Guidelines Summary

Preferred Regimens for Patients with Chronic HBV

Phase	HBeAg Status	HBV DNA	ALT	Treatment and Duration
Immune-tolerant	Positive	<1,000,000 IU/mL	Normal	No treatment; monitor ALT q4-6 mo
Immune-tolerant (>40 yo with liver biopsy showing significant necroinflammation or fibrosis)	Positive	>1,000,000 IU/mL	Normal	Peginterferon (peg-IFN) alfa-2a x 48 wk **OR** Entecavir **OR** Tenofovir
Immune-active	Positive or negative	>20,000 IU/mL	≥2× ULN	Peginterferon (peg-IFN) alfa-2a × 48 wk **OR** Entecavir **OR** Tenofovir
Inactive carrier	Negative	≤2,000 IU/mL	Normal	Observe/monitor (no treatment)

Interferons

Generic • Brand • Dose/Dosage Forms	Contraindications	Primary Side Effects	Key Monitoring	Pertinent Drug Interactions	Med Pearl
Mechanism of action – induces the innate antiviral immune response					
Peginterferon alfa-2a • Pegasys • 180 mcg subcut 1×/wk • Injection	• Autoimmune hepatitis • Hepatic decompensation before treatment • Neonates/infants (contains benzyl alcohol)	• Flu-like symptoms • Fatigue • Depression • Hallucinations • Aggression • Insomnia • Suicidal ideation • Neutropenia • Thrombocytopenia • Anemia • Hypo-/hyperthyroidism • Visual disturbances • Hepatic decompensation/failure • Hypersensitivity reactions • Hypotension • Arrhythmia • Tachycardia	• Liver function tests (LFTs) • Electrocardiogram (ECG) • Complete blood count (CBC) with differential • Thyroid function tests (TFTs) • Blood urea nitrogen (BUN)/serum creatinine (SCr) • CD4+ cell counts (in patients with HIV) • HBV RNA levels	• May ↑ theophylline and methadone levels • ↑ risk of bone marrow suppression with zidovudine	• Inject into abdomen or thigh • Adjust dose in renal impairment

Nucleoside/Nucleotide Analogs

Generic • Brand • Dose/Dosage Forms	Contraindications	Primary Side Effects	Key Monitoring	Pertinent Drug Interactions	Med Pearl
Mechanism of action – inhibit HBV replication by interfering with HBV viral DNA polymerase					
Adefovir • Hepsera • 10 mg PO daily • Tabs	None	• Renal impairment • Nausea/diarrhea • Headache • Lactic acidosis • Hepatomegaly with steatosis	• BUN/SCr • LFTs • HIV status • HBV DNA levels • HBeAg and anti-HBe	• ↑ risk of nephrotoxicity when used with amphotericin B, loop diuretics, tacrolimus, cyclosporine, or cisplatin • Not to be used with tenofovir-containing products	• Adjust dose in renal impairment • Considered 2nd-line oral therapy for HBV
Entecavir • Baraclude • Treatment-naïve: 0.5 mg PO daily • Lamivudine-resistant viremia (or known lamivudine- or telbivudine-resistant mutations): 1 mg PO daily • Decompensated liver disease: 1 mg PO daily • Solution, tabs	None	• Nausea • Headache • Fatigue • Dizziness • Lactic acidosis • Hepatomegaly with steatosis		Nephrotoxic drugs may ↑ levels	• Adjust dose in renal impairment • Give on an empty stomach (2 hr before or after a meal)
Lamivudine • Epivir HBV • 100 mg PO daily • Solution, tabs	None	• Diarrhea • Lactic acidosis • Hepatomegaly with steatosis		Not to be used with lamivudine- or emtricitabine-containing products	• Adjust dose in renal impairment • Lamivudine + tenofovir one of the preferred regimens in patients coinfected with HBV and HIV; cannot use Epivir HBV formulation for this use (must use Epivir 150 mg BID or 300 mg PO daily)
Telbivudine • Tyzeka • 600 mg PO daily • Tabs	Concurrent use with Peg-IFN alfa-2a	• Myalgias/myopathy • Peripheral neuropathy • Lactic acidosis • Hepatomegaly with steatosis	• BUN/SCr • LFTs • Creatine kinase • S/S of myopathy or peripheral neuropathy • HIV status • HBV DNA levels • HBeAg and anti-HBe	Concurrent use with peg-IFN alfa-2a ↑ risk of peripheral neuropathy	• Adjust dose in renal impairment • Associated with high rate of resistance

Nucleoside/Nucleotide Analogs (cont'd)

Generic • Brand • Dose/Dosage Forms	Contraindications	Primary Side Effects	Key Monitoring	Pertinent Drug Interactions	Med Pearl
Tenofovir disoproxil fumarate • Viread • 300 mg PO daily • Powder, tabs	None	• Renal impairment • Fanconi syndrome • ↓ bone mineral density • Lactic acidosis • Hepatomegaly with steatosis	• BUN/SCr • LFTs • HIV status • HBV DNA levels • HBeAg and anti-HBe	• ↓ atazanavir levels • ↑ didanosine levels (↓ didanosine dose) • Lopinavir/ritonavir, atazanavir/ritonavir, darunavir/ritonavir, acyclovir, valacyclovir, ganciclovir, valganciclovir, aminoglycosides, ledipasvir/sofosbuvir, and nonsteroidal anti-inflammatory drugs ↑ levels • Not to be used with tenofovir-containing products	• Adjust dose in renal impairment • Oral powder can be used if patient unable to swallow tabs • Lamivudine + tenofovir **OR** tenofovir + emtricitabine preferred regimens in patients coinfected with HBV and HIV

HEPATITIS C

Definitions

HCV is an RNA virus. Like HBV, HCV is primarily transmitted through perinatal, sexual, or percutaneous exposure to infectious blood or bodily fluids (e.g., semen).

Individuals who are at high risk for acquiring HCV include those who have used injectable drugs (or illicit intranasal drugs); those who are infected with HIV; patients who received blood transfusions or organ transplants before 1992; patients who received clotting factors before 1987; patients undergoing hemodialysis; healthcare workers in contact with contaminated needles or with mucosal exposure; children born to HCV-positive mothers; sexual partners of HCV-positive individuals; those receiving tattoos under nonsterile settings; and individuals born between 1945 and 1965. These patients should be screened for HCV infection.

Diagnosis

Hepatitis C is diagnosed by testing for antibodies against HCV (anti-HCV). If the anti-HCV test is positive, current (active) infection should be confirmed by a sensitive HCV RNA test. HCV RNA is detectable within 1–2 weeks of exposure. Once current (active) infection is confirmed, the HCV genotype (1–6) should be determined. Genotype 1 is most common in United States; it has also been the most difficult genotype to treat.

Signs and Symptoms

Most patients with any type of viral hepatitis have no symptoms. If signs/symptoms do occur, they may include the following:

- Symptoms: Flu-like symptoms, fever, fatigue, anorexia, nausea, vomiting, diarrhea, pruritus abdominal pain, dark urine, pale-color stools
- Signs: Jaundice, hepatomegaly, ascites, variceal bleeding, asterixis

Guidelines

AASLD/IDSA. Initial treatment of HCV infection. HCV Guidance: Recommendations for testing, managing, and treating hepatitis C. http://www.hcvguidelines.org/full-report/hcv-testing-and-linkage-care. Accessed July 17, 2016.

Guidelines Summary

Recommended Regimens for Treatment-Naïve Patients with HCV

Genotype	Treatment and Duration	
	Without Cirrhosis	*With Cirrhosis*
1a	Elbasvir/grazoprevir × 12 wk **OR** Ledipasvir/sofosbuvir × 12 wk **OR** Ombitasvir/paritaprevir/ritonavir + dasabuvir + ribavirin (RBV) × 12 wk **OR** Simeprevir + sofosbuvir × 12 wk **OR** Sofosbuvir/velpatasvir × 12 wk **OR** Daclatasvir + sofosbuvir × 12 wk	Elbasvir/grazoprevir × 12 wk **OR** Ledipasvir/sofosbuvir × 12 wk **OR** Sofosbuvir/velpatasvir × 12 wk
1b	Elbasvir/grazoprevir × 12 wk **OR** Ledipasvir/sofosbuvir × 12 wk **OR** Ombitasvir/paritaprevir/ritonavir + dasabuvir × 12 wk **OR** Simeprevir + sofosbuvir × 12 wk **OR** Sofosbuvir/velpatasvir × 12 wk **OR** Daclatasvir + sofosbuvir × 12 wk	Elbasvir/grazoprevir × 12 wk **OR** Ledipasvir/sofosbuvir × 12 wk **OR** Ombitasvir/paritaprevir/ritonavir + dasabuvir × 12 wk **OR** Sofosbuvir/velpatasvir × 12 wk
2	Sofosbuvir/velpatasvir × 12 wk	Sofosbuvir/velpatasvir × 12 wk

Recommended Regimens for Treatment-Naïve Patients with HCV *(cont'd)*

Genotype	Treatment and Duration	
	Without Cirrhosis	*With Cirrhosis*
3	Daclatasvir + sofosbuvir × 12 wk **OR** Sofosbuvir/velpatasvir × 12 wk	Sofosbuvir/velpatasvir × 12 wk **OR** Daclatasvir + sofosbuvir +/− RBV × 24 wk
4	Ombitasvir/paritaprevir/ritonavir + RBV × 12 wk **OR** Sofosbuvir/velpatasvir × 12 wk **OR** Elbasvir/grazoprevir × 12 wk **OR** Ledipasvir/sofosbuvir × 12 wk	
5 or 6	Sofosbuvir/velpatasvir × 12 wk **OR** Ledipasvir/sofosbuvir × 12 wk	

Ribavirin

Generic • Brand • Dose/Dosage Forms	Contraindications	Primary Side Effects	Key Monitoring	Pertinent Drug Interactions	Med Pearl
Mechanism of action – inhibits replication of DNA (HBV) and RNA (HCV) viruses					
Ribavirin • Copegus (with peg-IFN alfa-2a), Rebetol (with peg-IFN alfa-2b) • Copegus: Genotypes 1, 4: <75 kg: 500 mg PO BID, ≥75 kg: 600 mg PO BID; Genotypes 2,3 or HIV coinfection: 400 mg PO BID • Rebetol: 800–1,400 mg/day (in divided doses, based on weight) • Caps, solution, tabs	• Pregnancy and men with partners who are pregnant • Hemoglobinopathy (including sickle-cell disease) • Concurrent use with didanosine • Creatinine clearance (CrCl) <50 mL/min (Rebetol only)	• Rash • Fatigue • Nausea/vomiting (N/V) • Anemia	• LFTs • CBC with differential • Pregnancy test	• ↑ risk of hepatic failure, peripheral neuropathy, and pancreatitis with didanosine (contraindicated) • ↑ risk of bone marrow suppression with azathioprine and zidovudine	• Patients must use ≥2 forms of contraception during treatment and for 6 mo after discontinuation • Adjust dose in renal impairment • Give with food

Protease Inhibitor

Generic • Brand • Dose/ Dosage Forms	Contraindications	Primary Side Effects	Key Monitoring	Pertinent Drug Interactions	Med Pearl
Mechanism of action – inhibits HCV replication by blocking the NS3/4A protease enzyme from cleaving the HCV polyprotein					
Simeprevir • Olysio • 150 mg daily • Caps	None	• Photosensitivity • Rash • Nausea • Myalgia • Dyspnea	• LFTs • HCV RNA levels • NS3 Q80K polymorphism (before treatment)	• Cytochrome P450, CYP3A4 and P-glycoprotein (P-gp) substrate • CYP1A2 inhibitor • Concurrent use of simeprevir/sofosbuvir with amiodarone ↑ risk of bradycardia (avoid concurrent use)	• Must be used with other antiviral drugs (peg-IFN alfa/RBV or sofosbuvir) • ↓ efficacy in patients with NS3 Q80K polymorphism • Use with caution in patients with sulfa allergy • Discontinue simeprevir, peg-IFN alfa, and RBV if HCV RNA ≥25 IU/mL at wk 4 or wk 12; discontinue peg-IFN alfa and RBV if HCV RNA ≥25 IU/mL at wk 24

NS5A Inhibitor

Generic • Brand • Dose/Dosage Forms	Contraindications	Primary Side Effects	Key Monitoring	Pertinent Drug Interactions	Med Pearl
Mechanism of action – inhibits HCV replication by inhibiting the NS5A protein					
Daclatasvir • Daklinza • 60 mg daily • Concurrent use of strong CYP3A inhibitors: ↓ dose to 30 mg daily • Concurrent use of moderate CYP3A inducers: ↑ dose to 90 mg daily • Tabs	Concurrent use with phenytoin, carbamazepine, rifampin, or St. John's wort	• Headache • Fatigue • Nausea • Diarrhea	• LFTs • HCV RNA levels • NS5A polymorphism (before treatment in genotype 1a)	• CYP3A4 substrate • P-gp inhibitor • Concurrent use of daclatasvir/ sofosbuvir with amiodarone ↑ risk of bradycardia (avoid concurrent use)	Must be used with sofosbuvir

NS5B Inhibitor

Generic • Brand • Dose/Dosage Forms	Contraindications	Primary Side Effects	Key Monitoring	Pertinent Drug Interactions	Med Pearl
Mechanism of action – inhibits HCV replication by inhibiting HCV NS5B RNA-dependent RNA polymerase					
Sofosbuvir • Sovaldi • 400 mg daily • Tabs	None	• Fatigue • Headache • Nausea	• LFTs • HCV RNA levels	• P-gp substrate • Concurrent use with another HCV direct acting antiviral and amiodarone ↑ risk of bradycardia (avoid concurrent use)	Must be used with RBV or peg-IFN alfa + RBV

Combination Therapy

Generic • Brand • Dose/Dosage Forms	Pertinent Drug Interactions	Med Pearl
Elbasvir/grazoprevir • Zepatier • 1 tab = elbasvir 50 mg/grazoprevir 100 mg • 1 tab daily	• Elbasvir: CYP3A4 and P-gp substrate • Grazoprevir: CYP3A4 and P-gp substrate	• Elbasvir - NS5A inhibitor • Grazoprevir = protease inhibitor
Ledipasvir/sofosbuvir • Harvoni • 1 tab = ledipasvir 90 mg/sofosbuvir 400 mg • 1 tab daily	• Ledipasvir: P-gp substrate and inhibitor • Sofosbuvir: P-gp substrate • Concurrent use with amiodarone ↑ risk of bradycardia (avoid concurrent use)	• Ledipasvir = NS5A inhibitor • Sofosbuvir = NS5B inhibitor
Ombitasvir/paritaprevir/ritonavir • Technivie • 1 tab = ombitasvir 12.5 mg/paritaprevir 75 mg/ritonavir 50 mg • 2 tabs daily	• Ombitasvir: P-gp substrate • Paritaprevir: CYP3A4 and P-gp substrate; P-gp inhibitor • Ritonavir: CYP3A4 and P-gp substrate; CYP3A4 and P-gp inhibitor	• Ombitasvir = NS5A inhibitor • Paritaprevir = protease inhibitor • Ritonavir = CYP3A4 inhibitor • Give with food
Ombitasvir/paritaprevir/ritonavir + dasabuvir • Viekira Pak • Contains ombitasvir 12.5 mg/paritaprevir 75 mg/ritonavir 50 mg combination tablet + dasabuvir 250-mg tablet) • 2 ombitasvir/paritaprevir/ritonavir tabs daily + 1 dasabuvir tab BID • Viekira XR • 1 tab = dasabuvir 200 mg/ombitasvir 8.33 mg/paritaprevir 50 mg/ritonavir 33.33 mg • 3 tabs daily	• Ombitasvir: P-gp substrate • Paritaprevir: CYP3A4 and P-gp substrate; P-gp inhibitor • Ritonavir: CYP3A4 and P-gp substrate; CYP3A4 and P-gp inhibitor • Dasabuvir: CYP2C8 substrate	• Ombitasvir = NS5A inhibitor • Paritaprevir = protease inhibitor • Ritonavir = CYP3A4 inhibitor • Dasabuvir = NS5B inhibitor • Give all tabs with food
Sofosbuvir/velpatasvir • Epclusa • 1 tab = sofosbuvir 400 mg/velpatasvir 100 mg • 1 tab daily	• Sofosbuvir: P-gp substrate • Velpatasvir: CYP2B6, CYP2C8, CYP3A4, and P-gp substrate	• Sofosbuvir: NS5B inhibitor • Velpatasvir: NS5A inhibitor

Renal Disorders

8

This chapter covers the following:

- **Renal disorders**

 Suggested Study Time: **20 minutes**

RENAL DISORDERS

Definition

Chronic kidney disease (CKD) is defined as either kidney damage (albuminuria ≥30 mcg:mg creatinine) and/or decreased glomerular filtration rate (GFR) (<60 mL/min) for ≥3 months.

Diagnosis

Among individuals meeting the criteria for CKD just listed, staging is based upon GFR, with higher stages indicating worsening renal function (lower GFR).

Stage	GFR (mL/min/1.73m²)
1	>90 (+ kidney damage)
2	60–89 (+ kidney damage)
3	30–59
4	15–29
5	<15 (or dialysis)

Signs and Symptoms

The earliest detectable sign of kidney damage is microalbuminuria. The majority of signs and symptoms do not become apparent until later in the course of disease. Symptoms may include sequelae of hypervolemia including edema, weight gain, and fatigue. Signs may include anemia, hyperkalemia, vitamin D deficiency, hyperparathyroidism, hypocalcemia, and hyperphosphatemia.

Albuminuria is a helpful measure of disease progression. It is classified according to the criteria listed in the following table:

Collection	Normal (A_1)	Microalbuminuria (A_2)	Macroalbuminuria (A_3)
Spot collection albumin:creatinine ratio	<30 mcg/mg Cr	30–300 mcg/mg Cr	>300 mcg/mg Cr
24-hr collection (mg of albumin/24 hr)	<30 mg/24 hr	30–300 mg/24 hr	>300 mg/24 hr
Timed collection (mcg of protein/min)	<20 mcg/min	20–200 mcg/min	>200 mcg/min

Guidelines

National Kidney Foundation. K/DOQI clinical practice guidelines for chronic kidney disease: evaluation, classification, and stratification. *Am J Kidney Dis* 2002;39(2 Suppl 1): S1–266.

Guidelines Summary

- Goals of therapy:
  - Slow the progression of the disease, ↓ proteinuria, prevent complications, correct and manage reversible risk factors
  - Blood pressure (BP) <130/80 mmHg for CKD + any degree of proteinuria (A_2, A_3)
  - BP <140/90 mmHg for CKD with A_1 proteinuria (<30 mcg/mg)
- Pharmacologic therapy for CKD
  - CKD and hypertension
    - » Patient with any degree of proteinuria (A_2, A_3) should be initiated on an angiotensin-converting enzyme inhibitor (ACEI) or an angiotensin II receptor blocker (ARB).
    - » Patient with A_1 proteinuria (<30 mcg/mg) should be initiated on diuretic therapy (thiazide if creatinine clearance [CrCl] >30 mL/min or loop if <30 mL/min).
    - » Patients with BP that is elevated >20/10 mmHg above goal should be initiated on ACEI + diuretic.

- CKD without hypertension
  - » Patient with macroalbuminuria should be initiated on ACEI or ARB.
  - » Patient with microalbuminuria and DM should be initiated on ACEI or ARB.
  - » Patient with microalbuminuria without DM should not be initiated on pharmacologic therapy.
- With initiation of ACEI or ARB, up to 30% increase in serum creatinine is acceptable/expected.

- Pharmacologic therapy for complications of CKD
  - Edema: loop diuretics
    - » Hyperkalemia: loop diuretics, sodium polystyrene sulfonate, calcium, regular insulin, dialysis
    - » Anemia
      - When hemoglobin falls below 10 g/dL, erythropoietin stimulating agents (ESAs) are indicated. Iron indices should also be monitored and appropriately supplemented.
    - » Renal osteodystrophy
      - Hyperphosphatemia (phosphate goals: 2.7–4.6 mg/dL for stages 3 and 4; 3.5–5.5 mg/dL for stage 5)
        - ◦ Calcium-containing phosphate binders are the treatment of choice as long as corrected calcium <10.2 mg/dL and calcium phosphate product <55 mg^2/dL^2.
        - ◦ Non–calcium containing phosphate binders such as sevelamer and lanthanum are appropriate for patients with corrected calcium >10.2 mg/dL or calcium phosphate product >55 mg^2/dL^2.
        - ◦ Aluminum-containing phosphate binders are only indicated in severe hyperphosphatemia (serum phosphate >7 mg/dL) because they are associated with an ↑ risk for side effects.
      - Secondary hyperparathyroidism (intact parathyroid hormone [iPTH] goals: 35–70 pg/mL for stage 3; 70–110 pg/mL for stage 4; and 150–300 pg/mL for stage 5)
        - ◦ Phosphate should be at goal before treating elevated iPTH.
        - ◦ Activated vitamin D analogs are paricalcitol, calcitriol, doxercalciferol.
      - Vitamin D insufficiency/deficiency (goal 25(OH) vitamin D >30 ng/mL)
        - ◦ Insufficiency 16–30 ng/mL
        - ◦ Deficiency ≤15 ng/mL
        - ◦ Treatment: loading dose (ergocalciferol) followed by maintenance dose
        - ◦ Treatment timeframe determined by severity of deficiency

Medications for Chronic Kidney Disease

Generic • Brand • Dose/Dosage Forms	Contraindications	Primary Side Effects	Key Monitoring	Pertinent Drug Interactions	Med Pearl
Calcium-containing phosphate binders					
Calcium carbonate • Tums • 1,000 mg of elemental calcium/day (max should not exceed 2,000 mg/day)	Hypercalcemia	• Constipation • Flatulence • Hypercalcemia	• Serum calcium concentrations • Serum phosphorus concentrations • Intact parathyroid hormone (iPTH) concentrations	May ↓ absorption of tetracyclines, fluoroquinolones, levothyroxine, ketoconazole, and atazanavir (separate by 2–4 hr)	• For females ≥51 yr, recommended daily allowance is 1,200 mg of elemental calcium/ day • Take with meals • Take in doses <500 mg of elemental calcium at a time for greatest absorption
Calcium acetate ☆ • Eliphos, PhosLo, Phoslyra • Initial: 1,334 mg with each meal; can be ↑ every 2–3 wk to usual dose of 2,001–2,668 mg with each meal					Do not give additional calcium supplements
Non–calcium-containing phosphate binders					
Sevelamer • Renagel, Renvela • 800–1,600 mg TID with meals; initial dose may be based on serum phosphorus concentrations	Bowel obstruction	• Nausea/ vomiting/ diarrhea (N/V/D) • Dyspepsia • Abdominal pain • Constipation	• Serum calcium concentrations • Serum phosphorus concentrations • Bicarbonate concentrations • Chloride concentrations • iPTH concentrations	May ↓ absorption of ciprofloxacin and mycophenolate	Initial dose may be based on serum phosphorus
Lanthanum • Fosrenol • 500 mg TID with meals; can ↑ by up to 750 mg/day every 2–3 wk (max = 3,000 mg/day)	• Bowel obstruction • Fecal impaction • Ileus	• N/V • Abdominal pain • Constipation	• Serum calcium concentrations • Serum phosphorus concentrations • iPTH concentrations	May ↓ absorption of tetracyclines, fluoroquinolones, and levothyroxine, (separate by 2–4 hr)	• Do not swallow intact tablets (chew them) • Sprinkle oral powder over applesauce (not to be dissolved in liquid)

Medications for Chronic Kidney Disease (cont'd)

Generic • Brand • Dose/Dosage Forms	Contraindications	Primary Side Effects	Key Monitoring	Pertinent Drug Interactions	Med Pearl
Ferric citrate • Auryxia • 2 tabs (420 mg ferric iron) TID with meals; adjust dose based on serum phosphorus concentrations (max = 12 tabs [2,520 mg ferric iron] daily)	Hemochromatosis	• N/V/D • Discolored stools	• Serum phosphorus concentrations • iPTH concentrations • Serum iron concentrations • Ferritin • Transferrin saturation	May ↓ absorption of doxycycline and ciprofloxacin (separate by 1–2 hr)	None
Sucroferric oxyhydroxide • Velphoro • 500 mg TID with meals; can by 500 mg of iron/day every wk (max = 3,000 mg iron/day)	None	• N/D • Discolored stools	• Serum phosphorus concentrations • iPTH concentrations	May ↓ absorption of doxycycline and levothyroxine, (separate from doxycycline by >1 hr; avoid use with levothyroxine)	Do not swallow intact tablets (chew them)
Aluminum-containing phosphate binders					
Aluminum hydroxide • 300–600 mg TID with meals	Hypersensitivity	• Hypomagnesemia • Hypophosphatemia • Constipation • Neurotoxicity	• Serum calcium concentrations • Serum phosphorus concentrations • Serum magnesium concentrations • iPTH concentrations	• May ↓ absorption of tetracyclines, fluoroquinolones, levothyroxine, ketoconazole, and atazanavir (separate by 2–4 hr)	
Calcimimetic					
Cinacalcet • Sensipar • Secondary hyperparathyroidism: initial: 30 mg daily; adjust dose based on iPTH concentration (max = 180 mg daily) • Parathyroid carcinoma or primary hyperparathyroidism: initial: 30 mg BID; adjust dose based on serum calcium concentrations (max = 90 mg 3–4 × /day)	Hypocalcemia	• QTc interval prolongation • Seizures • Hypotension • Worsening heart failure • Bone fracture • N/V • Paresthesia	• Serum calcium concentrations • Serum phosphorus concentrations • iPTH concentrations • Electrocardiogram • Bone mineral density • BP	• CYP3A4 substrate • CYP2D6 inhibitor • CYP3A4 inhibitors may ↑ effects/toxicity • CYP3A4 inducers may ↓ effects • May ↑ effects/toxicity of CYP2D6 substrates	• For patients with secondary hyperparathyroidism on dialysis • Titrate every 2–4 wk • May require dosage adjustment if used with strong 3A4 inhibitors • Take with food • Do not crush, chew, or divide tabs

Medications for Chronic Kidney Disease *(cont'd)*

Generic • Brand • Dose/Dosage Forms	Contraindications	Primary Side Effects	Key Monitoring	Pertinent Drug Interactions	Med Pearl
Vitamin D analogs					
Paricalcitol • Zemplar • Stages 3 and 4 CKD: iPTH ≤500 pg/mL: 1 mcg PO daily or 2 mcg PO 3 × /wk; iPTH >500 pg/mL: 2 mcg PO daily or 4 mcg PO 3 × /wk • Stage 5 CKD: 0.04–0.1 mcg/kg IV during dialysis	• Hypercalcemia • Vitamin D toxicity	• Hypercalcemia • Calciphylaxis • N/D • Edema	• Serum calcium concentrations • Serum phosphorus concentrations • Serum 25(OH)D concentrations • iPTH concentrations	• CYP3A4 substrate • CYP3A4 inhibitors may ↑ effects/toxicity • CYP3A4 inducers may ↓ effects • Thiazide diuretics may ↑ hypercalcemic effects Thiazide diuretics may ↑ hypercalcemic effects	• Paricalcitol and doxercalciferol are synthetic forms of vitamin D that have less effect on calcium and phosphate • Calcitriol is active form of vitamin D (1,25-dihydroxyvitamin D) • Doxercalciferol needs to be metabolized to active form of vitamin D
Calcitriol ☆ • Rocaltrol • Stages 3 and 4 CKD: 0.25–0.5 mcg PO daily • Stage 5 CKD: 0.5–1 mcg PO daily or 1–2 mcg IV 3 × /wk					
Doxercalciferol • Hectorol • Stages 3 and 4 CKD: 1–3.5 mcg PO daily • Stage 5 CKD: 10 mcg PO 3 × /wk or 4 mcg IV 3 × /wk					
Ergocalciferol • Calcidol, Calciferol, Drisdol • 50,000 units weekly for 8–12 wk	• Hypercalcemia • Malabsorption syndrome	• Constipation • Nausea/vomiting (N/V) • Hypercalcemia	• Serum calcium concentrations • Serum phosphorus concentrations • Serum 25(OH)D concentrations	Thiazide diuretics may ↑ hypercalcemic effects	• Dosing may differ depending on level of vitamin D deficiency • Needs to be converted into active form (1,25-dihydroxyvitamin D)
Calcifediol • Rayaldee • Stages 3 and 4 CKD: 30–60 mcg PO daily	None	• Hypercalcemia • ↑ serum creatinine • Dyspnea	• Serum calcium concentrations • Serum phosphorus concentrations • Serum 25(OH)D concentrations • iPTH concentrations	• CYP3A4 substrate • CYP3A4 inhibitors may ↑ effects/toxicity • CYP3A4 inducers may ↓ effects • Thiazide diuretics may ↑ hypercalcemic effects	Synthetic form of vitamin D

Medications for Chronic Kidney Disease *(cont'd)*

Generic • Brand • Dose/Dosage Forms	Contraindications	Primary Side Effects	Key Monitoring	Pertinent Drug Interactions	Med Pearl
Erythropoiesis stimulating agents					
Epoetin alfa • Epogen, Procrit • 50–100 U/kg IV or subcut 3×/wk	• Hypersensitivity • Uncontrolled hypertension • Pure red cell aplasia	• Hypertension • Seizures • Anaphylaxis • Thromboembolism	• Hemoglobin/ hematocrit • Ferritin • Transferrin saturation • BP	None	• Boxed warning: ↑ risk of death, myocardial infarction, stroke, and thrombosis in patients with CKD • Initiate treatment with hemoglobin <10 g/dL • Do NOT exceed hemoglobin of 11 g/dL
Darbepoetin alfa • Aranesp • 0.45 mcg/kg IV or subcut weekly or 0.75 mcg/kg IV or subcut every 2 wk					

Dosing Considerations in Patients with CKD

Estimating Renal Clearance

As serum creatinine increases, renal function declines. The Cockcroft-Gault equation is the most commonly used method of estimating creatinine clearance (CrCl). The CrCl serves as an approximation of the GFR when considering the renal clearance of medications.

$$Creatinine\ clearance\,(female)\,(mL/min) = \frac{(140 - age) \times IBW \times 0.85}{72 \times serum\ creatinine}$$

$$Creatinine\ clearance\,(male)\,(mL/min) = \frac{(140 - age) \times IBW}{72 \times serum\ creatinine}$$

This formula is not ideal for use in the very elderly, very young, or in end stage renal disease (ESRD). IBW is ideal body weight.

Medications Requiring Dose Adjustment in CKD

Medications that are primarily eliminated via renal excretion often require dose and/or interval adjustment in advanced stages of renal disease. Reducing medication doses results in reduced peak concentrations while trough concentrations are maintained. Extending dosing intervals results in reduced trough concentrations while peak concentrations are maintained. Certain renally eliminated medications should be avoided in the setting of advanced renal disease due to the risk of serious side effects related to accumulation. Examples of commonly used medications that should be avoided and that require renal dose adjustment are provided in the following list.

Commonly Used Medications Requiring Dose/Interval Adjustment in CKD

- Acyclovir
- Allopurinol
- Aminoglycosides
- Amphotericin B
- Aztreonam
- Beta-lactam antibiotics
- Clarithromycin
- Colchicine
- Dabigatran
- Didanosine
- Digoxin
- Enoxaparin
- Ethambutol
- Famotidine
- Fluoroquinolones
- Gabapentin
- Ganciclovir
- Lamivudine
- Metoclopramide
- Penicillins
- Pregabalin
- Sulfamethoxazole/trimethoprim
- Tramadol
- Valacyclovir
- Vancomycin
- Venlafaxine
- Zidovudine
- Zoledronic acid

Commonly Used Medications That Should Be Avoided or Discontinued in Advanced CKD

- Alendronate
- Chlorpropamide
- Cidofovir
- Dabigatran
- Dofetilide
- Duloxetine
- Eplerenone
- Fondaparinux
- Foscarnet
- Glyburide
- Lithium
- Meperidine
- Metformin
- Nitrofurantoin
- NSAIDs
- Rivaroxaban
- Sotalol
- Spironolactone
- Tadalafil
- Tenofovir

Dosing Considerations in Dialysis

Patients with ESRD who require dialysis also require careful consideration of medication regimens to determine if medications are removed during dialysis and if replacement dosing is necessary post-dialysis. Some factors affecting removal of a drug via dialysis include the drug's volume of distribution, molecular size, and degree of protein binding as well as the type of dialysis membrane. Drugs with larger volume of distribution, larger molecular size, and higher degree of protein binding will be less effectively cleared via dialysis. High-flux dialysis membranes remove more medication than low- or medium-flux membranes.

Storage and Administration Pearls

- Preferred route of administration for ESAs is subcutaneous, except when administered to patients undergoing hemodialysis, for whom intravenous administration is preferred.
- Phosphate binders should be administered with meals.

Patient Education Pearls

- Patients should report if they experience injection-site reactions with ESAs to their health care professional. Patients should seek emergency medical care for shortness of breath, wheezing, or swelling of the tongue.

PRACTICE QUESTIONS

1. A 66-year-old female (5′2″, 80 kg) has a stable serum creatinine of 1.5 mg/dL. Which is an accurate assessment of her renal function?

    (A) Stage 1 CKD
    (B) Stage 2 CKD
    (C) Stage 3 CKD
    (D) Stage 4 CKD

2. A 58-year-old man (5′10″, 92 kg) presents for routine follow-up. He has a medical history of hypertension. At last visit 4 months ago, BP was 148/96 mmHg, serum creatinine was 1.6 mg/dL, and urine albumin:creatinine was 10 mcg:mg. Data today includes BP 146/94 mmHg, HR 84 bpm, serum potassium 4.5 mEq/L, serum creatinine 1.5 mg/dL, and urine albumin:creatinine 10 mcg:mg. Which of the following is the best recommendation?

    (A) Initiate chlorthalidone
    (B) Initiate lisinopril
    (C) Initiate amlodipine
    (D) Non-pharmacological therapy only

3. A female patient with stage 3 CKD and hypertension presents for follow-up after a BP reading at last visit of 138/88 mmHg. She began non-pharmacological therapy for BP at that time. Vital signs today include BP 136/84 mmHg and HR 88 bpm. Serum labs include potassium 4.2 mEq/L, sCr 1.4 mg/dL, and urine albumin:creatinine ratio 100 mg:g. Which is the best recommendation?

    (A) Initiate chlorthalidone
    (B) Initiate lisinopril
    (C) Initiate amlodipine
    (D) Non-pharmacological therapy only

4. Which is the most appropriate therapy in a patient with stage 4 CKD and edema?

    (A) Indapamide
    (B) Spironolactone
    (C) Bumetanide
    (D) Chlorthalidone

5. A patient with stage 3 CKD presents for a routine follow-up and has the following serum lab results: 25(OH) vitamin D 40 ng/mL, PTH 115 pg/mL, phosphate 5.3 mg/dL, calcium 9.9 mg/dL, albumin 3 mg/dL. Which is the most appropriate therapy to recommend at this time?

   (A) Sevelamer
   (B) Calcitriol
   (C) Calcium carbonate
   (D) Ergocalciferol

6. A patient with stage 4 CKD presents for routine follow up with the following serum lab results: 25(OH) vitamin D 35 ng/mL, PTH 105 pg/mL, phosphate 5.3 mg/dL, calcium 9.2 mg/dL, albumin 3.8 mg/dL. Which is the most appropriate therapy to recommend?

   (A) Sevelamer
   (B) Calcitriol
   (C) Calcium carbonate
   (D) Ergocalciferol

ANSWERS AND EXPLANATIONS

1. D

$$\text{Creatinine clearance (female)(mL/min)} = \frac{(140 - \text{age}) \times \text{IBW} \times 0.85}{72 \times \text{serum creatinine}}$$

$$= \frac{(140 - 66) \times 50.1 \times 0.85}{72 \times 1.5} = 29 \, \text{mL/min}$$

This patient has an estimated creatinine clearance of 29 mL/min calculated via the Cockcroft-Gault equation. Stage 4 CKD includes estimated GFR (calculated CrCl) of 15–29 mL/min.

2. A

This patient's estimated GFR (calculated CrCl) is 52 mL/min placing him into stage 3 CKD (30–59 mL/min). His urine protein assessment is below the range considered positive for microalbuminuria (<30 mcg:mg). Patient's with non-proteinuric CKD have a BP goal of <140/90 mmHg and, therefore, pharmacotherapy is indicated making (D) incorrect. First line therapy per NKF is thiazide-type diuretic such as chlorthalidone (A). Lisinopril (B), an ACEI, would be an appropriate second line choice or would be appropriate first-line option for him if he had proteinuria. Calcium channel blockers are appropriate for add on therapy for hypertension.

3. B

Because this patient has CKD with proteinuria, her evidence-based BP goal is <130/80 mmHg and her BP readings require treatment. Therefore, option (D) is incorrect. First line therapy for hypertension in patients with CKD and proteinuria is an ACEI such as lisinopril (B) or an ARB per National Kidney Foundation (NKF) guidelines. Thiazide diuretics such as chlorthalidone (A) are appropriate first line therapy in a patient with non-proteinuric CKD or as second line therapy in a patient with proteinuric CKD per the NKF. Calcium channel blockers such as amlodipine (C) are appropriate add-on agents for BP reduction but are not first line treatment.

4. C

Patients with stage 4 CKD have an estimated glomerular filtration rate (GFR) of <30 mL/min. In this setting, loop diuretics (e.g., [C] bumetanide) maintain efficacy, whereas thiazide diuretics such as (A) indapamide and (D) chlorthalidone do not. Additionally, loop diuretics are more effective in treating edema as compared to aldosterone antagonists (B) spironolactone and thiazide diuretics.

5. **A**

This patient has complications of CKD including hyperphosphatemia and secondary hyperparathyroidism. Before treating hyperparathyroidism, the phosphate should be brought into the goal range. Both sevelamer (A) and calcium carbonate (C) are phosphate binders. The calcium-containing phosphate binder, calcium carbonate, should be avoided because the patient's corrected calcium is >10.2 mg/dL and the calcium × phosphate product is >55 mg^2/dL^2. Ergocalciferol (D) is incorrect because patient's 25(OH) vitamin D level is at goal of >30 ng/mL.

6. **C**

This patient has hyperphosphatemia as a complication of CKD. Because the patient's corrected calcium is <10.2 mg/dL (9.4 mg/dL) and calcium × phosphate product is <55 mg^2/dL^2, a calcium-containing phosphate binder such as calcium carbonate (C) is the best recommendation. Sevelamer (A) is reserved for hyperphosphatemia in the setting of elevated corrected calcium (>10.2 mg/dL) or elevated calcium × phosphate product (>55 mg^2/dL^2). Calcitriol (B) would not be indicated as the patient's intact PTH is within the stage 4 CKD range of 70–110 pg/mL. Ergocalciferol (D) is not indicated because 25(OH) vitamin D level is at goal of >30 ng/mL.

Oncology

9

This chapter covers the following topics:

- **Lymphoma**
- **Leukemia**
- **Lung cancer**
- **Colorectal cancer**
- **Breast cancer**
- **Prostate cancer**
- **Ovarian cancer**
- **Cancer chemotherapy drugs**
- **Target and biologic agents**
- **Supportive care**

 Suggested Study Time: **2 hours**

Since many of the drugs used in chemotherapy are indicated for multiple types of cancer, the background information for all of the hematologic malignancies and solid tumors will be discussed first, with the drug therapies described in charts at the end of the section. Because cancer therapy is generally protocol-driven, your focus should be mostly on drug toxicities and on certain cases where a specific drug is indicated on the basis of cell-surface markers such as CD20 or HER-2 overexpression. Supportive care (antiemetic agents and colony-stimulating factors) is covered at the end of this chapter.

LYMPHOMA

Definitions

Lymphomas are tumors of the lymphoid cells. Hodgkin's lymphoma (or Hodgkin's disease, HD) is less common than other types of lymphoma and is marked by the presence of Reed-Steinberg cells. HD may have a genetic component and, while HD is not contagious, certain infections (particularly Epstein-Barr and human immunodeficiency virus [HIV]) may increase the risk of acquiring the disease. HD is more common in young adults (15–35 years) and those over 55.

Non-Hodgkin's lymphomas (NHLs) are a group of related cancers including follicular, diffuse large B-cell, and Burkitt's lymphoma. NHL is the eighth leading cause of cancer in the United States, and the incidence increases with age (median age of diagnosis is 66 years). Immunodeficiency and infections are risk factors for NHL, as is prior chemotherapy. The various types of NHL are typified by proliferation of malignant B or T lymphocytes. The cancer may be classified as either aggressive (fast-growing) or indolent (slow-growing).

Diagnosis

HD

- Lymph node biopsy → Presence of Reed-Sternberg cells
- Computed tomography (CT) scan, magnetic resonance imaging (MRI), position emission tomography (PET) scan, or bone marrow biopsy to determine staging

NHL

- Lab values:
  - Elevated white blood cells (WBCs)
  - Lactate dehydrogenase levels may be high
- Lymph node or tissue biopsy
- Flow cytometry—cell surface marker analysis

Staging is the same for HD and NHL. Each stage is subdivided into A and B; B denotes the presence of systemic symptoms, specifically night sweats, weight loss, and fever:

- Stage 1: present in one lymph node or one part of tissue or organ
- Stage 2: present in ≥2 lymph nodes on the same side of the diaphragm
- Stage 3: present in lymph nodes above and below the diaphragm
- Stage 4: present in several parts of ≥1 tissue(s), or in an organ and distant lymph nodes
- Recurrent: disease returns after remission

Signs and Symptoms

HD

- Painless enlargement of lymph nodes, especially in the neck
- Fever, night sweats, and/or weight loss
- Malaise
- Possible bone pain

NHL

- Swollen lymph nodes on neck, underarms, and groin
- Fever, weight loss, and night sweats
- Fatigue
- Weakness

LEUKEMIA

Definitions

The leukemias are a group of blood malignancies characterized by unregulated growth of blood-forming cells in the bone marrow. These immature white cells crowd out normal cells in the bone marrow, leading to low red cell, white cell, and platelet counts. Four major types of leukemia exist: Acute lymphocytic (ALL), acute myeloid (AML), chronic lymphocytic (CLL), and chronic myeloid (CML) leukemias. Acute leukemias worsen rapidly; chronic leukemias worsen slowly. Exposure to radiation and chemicals (particularly benzene and formaldehyde) can increase leukemia risk.

Although the overall incidence of acute leukemias is low, they are the most common cancers in children, and ALL is the leading cause of cancer-related death in those under 35 years. AML occurs with increasing frequency in the elderly.

Virtually all patients with CML have a specific chromosomal abnormality (Philadelphia chromosome).

Diagnosis

- Bone marrow biopsy → Send for morphologic examination
- AML diagnosis requires 20% blasts

Signs and Symptoms

- Weight loss, fatigue, malaise
- Palpitations and dyspnea on exertion
- Fever and chills; night sweats
- Bruising
- Bone pain

LUNG CANCER

Definitions

Lung cancer is the leading cause of cancer death in men and women. Most lung cancers are non-small cell (NSCLC); while this type of cancer is slow-growing, it does not respond well to chemotherapy and only about 14% of patients can be cured. Small-cell lung cancer (SCLC) is very aggressive and, though it is chemotherapy-sensitive, most patients die within 2 years of diagnosis. Smoking is the primary risk factor for lung cancer; over 80% of patients have a history of smoking. Occupational exposure to asbestos, radon, and other agents may also increase risk, as can certain genetic abnormalities and family history of the disease.

Diagnosis

- Chest x-ray, CT scans, and PET scan to detect lesions and determine extent of disease
- Pathological confirmation by sputum cytology or tumor biopsy

Signs and Symptoms

- Cough—most common
- Other lung-related symptoms (sputum production, dyspnea, wheezing); often misattributed to concomitant pulmonary conditions
- Weight loss, fever, bone pain
- Paraneoplastic syndromes:
  - Occur in 10% of cases; may be first sign or symptom
  - Inappropriate secretion of antidiuretic hormone (SIADH)
  - Hypercalcemia
  - Eaton-Lambert myasthenic syndrome: muscle weakness and autonomic dysfunction

COLORECTAL CANCER

Definitions

Colorectal cancer is the third leading cause of cancer death in the United States. Incidence is highest in industrialized countries and may be linked to a higher-fat, lower-fiber diet in such locations. Genetic predisposition also plays a role in 5–10% of cases. Primary prevention strategies involve dietary change (increase calcium, fiber, and antioxidants and decrease fat).

Diagnosis

- Fecal occult blood testing (FOBT) may decrease cancer mortality by one-third, but has a high false-negative rate as many early stage tumors do not bleed.
- FOBT plus immunochemical assays lead to improved specificity and sensitivity.
- Flexible sigmoidoscopy can detect lesions in distal and sigmoid colon; early detection and excision can decrease mortality by 60%.
- Colonoscopy is preferred screening method as it shows entire colon, but it requires more bowel preparation.
- Double-contrast barium enema plus flexible sigmoidoscopy may be used instead of colonoscopy.

Signs and Symptoms

- Change in bowel habits (diarrhea, constipation, stools narrower than usual)
- Rectal bleeding/blood in the stool
- Nausea, vomiting, and abdominal discomfort (gas pains or cramps, bloating)
- Fatigue (generally related to anemia)
- Weight loss
- Leg edema (result of lymph node involvement)
- Hepatomegaly and jaundice

BREAST CANCER

Definitions

Breast cancer is the most common cancer in women and is second only to lung cancer as a cause of cancer death in women. Family history plays a large role in the development of breast cancer, with mutations in the *BRCA1/BRCA2* tumor suppressor genes leading to high risk. Long-term progestin use and other endocrine factors (early menarche, late menopause, advanced age at first pregnancy) and lifestyle factors (high fat intake, alcohol consumption, obesity) also increase risk of developing breast cancer. Prognosis is poor in younger (<35 years) and premenopausal patients, African Americans, and those with *HER2/neu* overexpression.

Diagnosis

- Palpable mass on physical examination
- Breast imaging techniques: mammography and/or ultrasound
- Biopsy if mass or cluster of calcifications is detected

Signs and Symptoms

- May be asymptomatic
- Painless lump: Initial sign in 90% of patients
- Stabbing or aching pain is initial sign in remaining 10%
- Nipple discharge, retraction, dimpling
- Scaly, red, or swollen skin of breast or nipple
- Advanced disease: Bone pain, difficulty breathing, jaundice, abdominal enlargement, mental status changes

PROSTATE CANCER

Definitions

Prostate cancer is the most common cancer in men, and the second most common cause of cancer death in men. One-third to one-half of men present with advanced disease, for which there is no cure. High-fat diet and hormonal factors are two of the primary risk factors; as prostate cancer is androgen-dependent, high levels of testosterone can fuel tumor growth. This may explain the increased incidence in African-American men, who generally have testosterone levels 15% higher than Caucasian men.

Diagnosis

- Transrectal ultrasound or cystoscopy
- Biopsy: Only sure method of diagnosis

Signs and Symptoms

- Elevated prostate-specific antigen (PSA)
- Nodule on digital rectal exam of the prostate

- Localized disease: Generally asymptomatic; symptoms of prostatic enlargement may indicate cancer, benign prostatic hyperplasia, or infection; further investigation warranted
  - Urinary difficulty
  - Difficulty in having an erection
  - Blood in the urine or semen
- Advanced disease:
  - Bone pain
  - Anemia and fatigue
  - Weight loss
  - Back pain
  - Leg edema

OVARIAN CANCER

Definitions

Ovarian cancer typically occurs postmenopause. Risk factors include family history of ovarian or breast cancer, personal history of other types of cancer, nulliparity, and long-term estrogen therapy (without progesterone). Genetics also play a role; breast cancer and ovarian cancer are linked to mutation in *BRCA1/BRCA2*, along with other genetic alterations.

Diagnosis

- Ovarian size/contour on pelvic exam
- Elevation of CA-125 (antigen common to most ovarian cancers)
- Pelvic ultrasound
- Biopsy

Signs and Symptoms

Symptoms may be vague and nonspecific, but may include:

- Fatigue
- Back pain
- Bloating, constipation, abdominal pain
- Palpable abdominal mass, abdominal distention
- Hepatic and renal function abnormalities

Cancer Chemotherapy Drugs

Alkylating Agents

Generic • Brand • Dosage Forms	Contraindications	Primary Side Effects	Key Monitoring	Pertinent Drug Interactions	Med Pearl
Mechanism of action – alkylate DNA, making it more prone to breakage; most effective against rapidly dividing cells					
Cyclophosphamide • Only available generically • Caps, injection (IV), tabs	Hypersensitivity to any alkylating agent	• Alopecia • Hemorrhagic cystitis • Infertility • Nausea, vomiting (N/V), mucositis, stomatitis • Bone marrow suppression	• Complete blood count (CBC) with differential • Blood urea nitrogen (BUN)/serum creatinine (SCr) • Uric acid (UA)	CYP3A4 inducers may ↑ levels of active metabolite (acrolein)	• Maintain adequate hydration to avoid hemorrhagic cystitis; can also use mesna • High emetogenic potential
Chlorambucil • Leukeran • Tabs		• Bone marrow suppression • Infertility • Secondary leukemias • Seizures • Stevens-Johnson syndrome • Hepatotoxicity	• CBC with differential • Liver function tests (LFTs)	None	Take on empty stomach
Carmustine • BiCNU, Gliadel • Injection (IV), intracranial implant		• Bone marrow suppression • Pulmonary fibrosis • Severe N/V • Hypotension (IV) • Secondary leukemias (with long-term use) • Reversible elevation of LFTs	• CBC with differential • Pulmonary function tests • LFTs • Blood pressure (BP) (during IV administration)	IV solution contains ethanol; do not give aldehyde-dehydrogenase inhibitors	Very high emetogenic potential

Platinum-Based Agents

Generic • Brand • Dosage Forms	Contraindications	Primary Side Effects	Key Monitoring	Pertinent Drug Interactions	Med Pearl
Mechanism of action – crosslink DNA, causing it to break					
Cisplatin • Only available generically • Injection (IV)	• Hypersensitivity to any platinum-containing compounds • Renal impairment • Pre-existing hearing impairment (cisplatin)	• Anaphylaxis • Dose-related myelosuppression • N/V • Ototoxicity (cisplatin) • Nephrotoxicity with cumulative doses (esp. cisplatin) • Peripheral neuropathy • QT interval prolongation (oxaliplatin) • Rhabdomyolysis (oxaliplatin)	• BUN/SCr • Electrolytes • Neurologic exam • CBC with differential • Urine output	Administration with taxane derivatives may ↑ myelosuppression and ↓ efficacy of platinum agents	• Do not administer doses exceeding 100 mg/m^2 every 3 wks • High emetogenic potential
Carboplatin • Only available generically • Injection (IV)					• Moderate emetogenic potential • Dose often calculated by target AUC using Calvert formula (total dose [mg] = Target AUC × [GFR + 25]) • Adjust dose in renal impairment
Oxaliplatin • Eloxatin • Injection (IV)					• Moderate emetogenic potential • Warn patients to wear a scarf if being treated during cold weather • Adjust dose in renal impairment

Enzyme Inhibitors

Generic • Brand • Dosage Forms	Contraindications	Primary Side Effects	Key Monitoring	Pertinent Drug Interactions	Med Pearl
Mechanism of action – target enzymes responsible for DNA replication and repair					
Irinotecan • Camptosar • Injection (IV)	Concurrent therapy with strong CYP3A4 inhibitors	• Bone marrow suppression • Severe, life-threatening diarrhea	• CBC with differential • Electrolytes (esp. if diarrhea)	CYP3A4 substrate	• Diarrhea may be early or late onset • Moderate emetogenic potential • Atropine can be used to treat early-onset diarrhea; loperamide for late-onset diarrhea
Irinotecan liposomal • Onivyde • Injection (IV)	None	• Bone marrow suppression • Severe, life-threatening diarrhea • Interstitial lung disease (ILD) • Hypersensitivity reactions	• CBC with differential • Electrolytes (esp. if diarrhea) • S/S of ILD	CYP3A4 substrate	• Diarrhea may be early or late onset • Atropine can be used to treat early-onset diarrhea; loperamide for late-onset diarrhea

Enzyme Inhibitors *(cont'd)*

Generic • Brand • Dosage Forms	Contraindications	Primary Side Effects	Key Monitoring	Pertinent Drug Interactions	Med Pearl
Etoposide • Only available generically • Caps, injection (IV)	None	• Bone marrow suppression • Hypersensitivity reactions	• CBC with differential • LFTs	CYP3A4 substrate	• Do NOT give IV push (may cause hypotension) • Do NOT give IM (necrosis) • Adjust dose in renal impairment

Antimitotic Agents

Generic • Brand • Dosage Forms	Contraindications	Primary Side Effects	Key Monitoring	Pertinent Drug Interactions	Med Pearl
Mechanism of action – spindle poisons; interfere with mitotic spindle; prevent chromosome segregation and lead to cell death					
Vincristine • Only available generically • Injection (IV)	None	• Peripheral neuropathy (dose-limiting) • Constipation • Paralytic ileus (secondary to neurologic toxicity)	• Neurologic exam • Change in frequency of bowel movements	CYP3A4 substrate	• Do NOT give intrathecally (IT) (fatal) • All patients should be on a prophylactic bowel management regimen • Avoid extravasation (vesicant) • Should NOT exceed 2 mg/dose
Vinblastine • Only available generically • Injection (IV)	None	• Peripheral neuropathy • Bone marrow suppression (dose-limiting)	• CBC with differential • Neurologic exam	CYP3A4 substrate	• Do not give IT (fatal) • Avoid extravasation (vesicant)
Paclitaxel • Only available generically • Injection (IV)	• Hypersensitivity to Cremophor • Baseline neutrophils <1,500/mm³ (ovarian, lung, or breast cancer) • ANC <1,000/mm³ (Kaposi's sarcoma)	• Bone marrow suppression (dose-limiting) • Hypersensitivity reactions • Peripheral neuropathy • Cardiac rhythm abnormalities • Mucositis, stomatitis (severe)	• CBC with differential • Electrocardiogram (ECG) • Neurologic exam	• CYP2C8 and CYP3A4 substrate • Administer prior to platinum derivatives to limit myelosuppression and enhance efficacy	• Premedicate with dexamethasone, diphenhydramine, and H₂-receptor antagonist • Adjust dose in hepatic impairment
Paclitaxel protein-bound particles • Abraxane • Injection (IV)	Baseline neutrophils <1,500/mm³				• No need for premedication • Adjust dose in hepatic impairment

Antimitotic Agents *(cont'd)*

Generic • Brand • Dosage Forms	Contraindications	Primary Side Effects	Key Monitoring	Pertinent Drug Interactions	Med Pearl
Docetaxel • Taxotere, Docefrez • Injection (IV)	• Hypersensitivity to polysorbate 80 • Baseline neutrophils <1,500/mm^3 • Severe hepatic impairment	• Significant, dose-dependent fluid retention • Bone marrow suppression • Hypersensitivity reactions • Erythema (with edema) • Peripheral neuropathy	• CBC with differential • LFTs • Weight, signs of edema	CYP3A4 substrate	• Avoid doses >100 mg/m^2 • Premedicate with corticosteroids for 3 days (starting 1 day before docetaxel administration) to prevent fluid retention and hypersensitivity reactions • Contains ethanol • Adjust dose in hepatic impairment

Antimetabolites

Generic • Brand • Dosage Forms	Contraindications	Primary Side Effects	Key Monitoring	Pertinent Drug Interactions	Med Pearl
Mechanism of action — nucleoside analogs					
Cytarabine • Cytosar-U • Injection (IV)	None	• Severe bone marrow suppression • Cytarabine syndrome: myalgia, bone pain, rash, conjunctivitis, and fever • Sudden respiratory distress syndrome • Tumor lysis syndrome	CBC with differential	None	• Premedicate with corticosteroid; may prevent cytarabine syndrome • May be administered IV, IT or subcut • Moderate emetogenic potential
Cytarabine liposomal • DepoCyt • Injection (IT)	Active meningeal infection	• Chemical arachnoiditis (N/V, headache, and fever) • Neurotoxicity	Monitor closely for signs of immediate reactions and neurotoxicity	None	• Coadminister dexamethasone to lessen chemical arachnoiditis • Moderate emetogenic potential
5-Fluorouracil • Only available generically • Injection (IV)	Dihydropyrimidine dehydrogenase (DPD) deficiency	• Hand-and-foot syndrome • N/V/D • Mucositis • Stomatitis • Bone marrow suppression	CBC with differential	• CYP2C9 inhibitor • May ↑ risk of bleeding with warfarin	Leucovorin ↑ effectiveness and toxicity; dose of fluorouracil may need to be ↓

Antimetabolites (cont'd)

Generic • Brand • Dosage Forms	Contraindications	Primary Side Effects	Key Monitoring	Pertinent Drug Interactions	Med Pearl
Mechanism of action – folic acid antagonist					
Methotrexate ☆ • Trexall (PO) • Injection (IM, IT, IV), tabs	None	• Nephrotoxicity • Bone marrow suppression • Stevens-Johnson syndrome • Severe diarrhea and ulcerative stomatitis • Neurotoxicity • Hepatotoxicity • Pneumonitis • Tumor lysis syndrome	• CBC with differential • SCr • LFTs • Chest x-ray	Diuretics and NSAIDs may ↑ risk of toxicity	• Give leucovorin rescue 24 hrs after dosing to limit toxicity; do not administer concurrently • Can be given IT for leukemias • Also used subcut or PO as DMARD for rheumatoid arthritis

Anthracyclines

Generic • Brand • Dosage Forms	Contraindications	Primary Side Effects	Key Monitoring	Pertinent Drug Interactions	Med Pearl
Mechanism of action – intercalate DNA and generate reactive oxygen species					
Daunorubicin • Cerubidine • Injection (IV) Doxorubicin • Only available generically • Injection (IV) Doxorubicin liposomal • Doxil • Injection (IV)	• Pre-existing severe myocardial insufficiency or arrhythmia • Baseline neutrophils <1,500/mm^3 • Severe hepatic impairment	• Dose-related cardiotoxicity • Severe bone marrow suppression • Secondary leukemias • Red coloration of body fluids	• CBC with differential • ECG • Left ventricular ejection fraction (LVEF)	↑ risk of cardiotoxiocity with trastuzumab, pertuzumab, cyclophosphamide, and taxane derivatives	• Greatest risk of irreversible myocardial damage at cumulative dose >550 mg/m^2 • Moderate emetogenic potential • Avoid extravasation (vesicant) • Dexrazoxane can be used to prevent doxorubicin-induced cardiotoxicity or to treat anthracycline-induced extravasation • Liposomal doxorubicin used for Kaposi's sarcoma, multiple myeloma, and ovarian cancer

Hormonal Agents

Generic • Brand • Dosage Forms	Contraindications	Primary Side Effects	Key Monitoring	Pertinent Drug Interactions	Med Pearl
Mechanism of action – treat cancers in which growth is accelerated by hormones					
Leuprolide • Eligard, Lupron Depot • Injection (subcut, IM/subcut depot)	• Spinal cord compression • Undiagnosed abnormal vaginal bleeding	• Abnormal menses • Exacerbation of endometriosis • Hot flashes/sweats • ↓ bone mineral density (if used >6 mo) • Spinal cord compression and urinary tract obstruction in prostate cancer • Tumor flare • Depression, mood disturbances	• Leutinizing hormone (LH) and follicle-stimulating hormone (FSH) levels • Serum testosterone (males), estradiol (females) • Bone mineral density	None	• Subcut injection administered daily • Rotate injection sites • Subcut/IM depot injection administered every 1–6 mo depending on dosage
Tamoxifen ☆ • Soltamox • Solution, tabs (PO)	• Concurrent warfarin therapy • History of deep vein thrombosis (DVT) or pulmonary embolism	• Thromboembolic events • ↑ risk of endometrial cancer • Hot flashes • Altered menses • Mood disturbances, depression • ↓ bone mineral density	Annual gynecologic exams	• CYP3A4 substrate • May ↑ risk of bleeding with warfarin • Selective serotonin reuptake inhibitors may ↓ effects	• Bone pain may indicate a good therapeutic response; manage with mild analgesia • Duration of treatment = 5-10 yr (depending on menopausal status)
Anastrozole ☆ • Arimidex • Tabs (PO)	None	• ↓ bone mineral density • Hyperlipidemia • Mood disturbances • Hot flashes • Insomnia	• Bone mineral density • Low-density lipoprotein (LDL) and total cholesterol	None	• Aromatase inhibitor • Indicated for postmenopausal women with breast cancer • Duration of treatment = 5 yr
Exemestane • Aromasin • Tabs (PO)	None	• ↓ bone mineral density • Hot flashes • Insomnia	• Bone mineral density	CYP3A4 substrate	• Aromatase inhibitor • Indicated for postmenopausal women with breast cancer • Duration of treatment = 5 yr
Letrozole • Femara • Tabs (PO)	None	• ↓ bone mineral density • Hyperlipidemia • Hot flashes	• Bone mineral density • LDL and total cholesterol	None	• Aromatase inhibitor • Indicated for postmenopausal women with breast cancer • Duration of treatment = 5 yr • Adjust dose in hepatic impairment

Chemotherapy Agents: Common Adverse Effects

- Cardiotoxicity
  - Doxorubicin
  - Daunorubicin
  - Idarubicin
  - Lapatinib
  - Mitoxantrone
  - Pertuzumab
  - Trastuzumab
- N/V
  - Cisplatin
  - Carboplatin
  - Cytarabine
  - Doxorubicin
  - Cyclophosphamide
- Mucositis
  - Cytarabine
  - Cyclophosphamide
  - 5-Fluorouracil
  - Methotrexate
- Neuropathy
  - Vincristine
  - Vinblastine
  - Oxaliplatin
  - Paclitaxel
- Renal impairment
  - Cisplatin
  - Cyclophosphamide
  - Ifosfamide
- Pulmonary fibrosis
  - Bleomycin
  - Busulfan
- Infusion reactions
  - Monoclonal antibodies
  - Paclitaxel

Targeted and Biologic Agents

Monoclonal Antibodies

Generic • Brand • Dosage Forms	Contraindications	Primary Side Effects	Key Monitoring	Pertinent Drug Interactions	Med Pearl
Mechanism of action – target the CD20 antigen					
Ibritumomab tiuxetan • Zevalin • Injection (IV)	None	• Infusion-related reactions • Myelosuppression (prolonged) • Secondary leukemia • Myelodysplastic syndrome • Rash (can be severe)	• CBC with differential • S/S of infusion reactions • S/S of dermatologic reactions	Do not administer live vaccines	• Used for CD20-positive, B-cell NHL • Linked to a radioisotope that targets B cells • Used in combination with rituximab as part of a 2-step process • Premedicate with diphenhydramine and acetaminophen (to prevent infusion reactions)
Obinutuzumab • Gazyva • Injection (IV)		• Infusion-related reactions • Tumor lysis syndrome • Myelosuppression (prolonged) • Infection (esp. bacterial, fungal, or hepatitis B virus [HBV] reactivation) • Progressive multifocal leukoencephalopathy (PML)	• CBC with differential • S/S of infusion reactions • S/S of infection • S/S of PML		• Used for CLL • HBV screening should be done before initiating treatment • Premedicate with diphenhydramine, acetaminophen, and glucocorticoid (to prevent infusion reactions) • Premedicate with antihyperuricemics and hydration in patients at ↑ risk for tumor lysis syndrome
Ofatumumab • Arzerra • Injection (IV)		• Infusion-related reactions • Tumor lysis syndrome • Myelosuppression (prolonged) • HBV reactivation • PML	• CBC with differential • S/S of infusion reactions • S/S of HBV • S/S of PML		

Monoclonal Antibodies *(cont'd)*

Generic • Brand • Dosage Forms	Contraindications	Primary Side Effects	Key Monitoring	Pertinent Drug Interactions	Med Pearl
Rituximab • Rituxan • Injection (IV)	None	• Infusion-related reactions • Tumor lysis syndrome • Rash (can be severe) • PML • Arrhythmias • Infection (esp. bacterial, fungal, or HBV reactivation) • Nephrotoxicity • Bowel obstruction/perforation	• CBC with differential • S/S of infusion reactions • S/S of infection • S/S of PML • BUN/SCr • Electrolytes • ECG • S/S of abdominal pain • S/S of dermatologic reactions	Do not administer live vaccines	• Used for CD20-positive, B-cell NHL, and CD20-positive CLL • Also used for rheumatoid arthritis • HBV screening should be done before initiating treatment • Premedicate with diphenhydramine and acetaminophen (to prevent infusion reactions) • Premedicate with antihyperuricemics and hydration in patients at ↑ risk for tumor lysis syndrome

Epidermal Growth Factor Receptor (EGFR) Inhibitors

Generic • Brand • Dosage Forms	Contraindications	Primary Side Effects	Key Monitoring	Pertinent Drug Interactions	Med Pearl
Mechanism of action – prevent tumor growth by inhibiting the various EGFR receptors					
Afatinib • Gilotrif • Tabs (PO)	None	• Diarrhea • Rash (can be severe) • ILD • Hepatotoxicity • Keratitis	• EGFR mutation status • LFTs • S/S of dermatologic reactions • S/S of dehydration • Electrolytes • S/S of ILD • S/S of eye inflammation/visual abnormalities	P-glycoprotein (P-gp) substrate	• Used for metastatic NSCLC with EGFR exon 19 deletions or exon 21 substitution mutations • Adjust dose in renal impairment • Take 1 hr before or 2 hr after a meal
Cetuximab • Erbitux • Injection (IV)	None	• Infusion-related reactions • Rash (can be severe) • ILD • Sudden cardiac death • Electrolyte abnormalities ($\downarrow Mg^{2+}$, $\downarrow K^+$, $\downarrow Ca^{2+}$)	• EGFR and *K-Ras* status (for colorectal cancer) • S/S of infusion reactions • S/S of dermatologic reactions • S/S of ILD • Electrolytes	None	• Used for squamous cell cancer of head and neck and *K-Ras* wild type, EGFR expressing colorectal cancer • Premedicate with diphenhydramine (to prevent infusion reactions)

Epidermal Growth Factor Receptor (EGFR) Inhibitors *(cont'd)*

Generic • Brand • Dosage Forms	Contraindications	Primary Side Effects	Key Monitoring	Pertinent Drug Interactions	Med Pearl
Erlotinib • Tarceva • Tabs (PO)	None	• Rash (can be severe) • Diarrhea • ILD • Renal failure • Hepatotoxicity • Gastrointestinal (GI) perforation • Myocardial ischemia/infarction • Stroke • Keratitis	• EGFR mutation status • S/S of dermatologic reactions • S/S of dehydration • S/S of ILD • BUN/SCr • Electrolytes • LFTs • S/S of GI perforation • S/S of eye inflammation/visual abnormalities	• CYP1A2 and CYP3A4 substrate • CYP3A4 inducers and cigarette smoking ↓ levels (↑ erlotinib dose) • May ↑ risk of bleeding with warfarin • H$_2$-antagonists, proton pump inhibitors (PPIs), and antacids may ↓ absorption (space apart)	• Used for locally advanced/metastatic NSCLC with EGFR exon 19 deletions or exon 21 substitution mutations • Also used for locally advanced, surgically unresectable, or metastatic pancreatic cancer
Gefitinib • Iressa • Tabs (PO)	None	• Rash (can be severe) • Diarrhea • ILD • Hepatotoxicity • GI perforation • Keratitis	• EGFR mutation status • S/S of dermatologic reactions • S/S of dehydration • BUN/SCr • Electrolytes • S/S of ILD • LFTs • S/S of GI perforation • S/S of eye inflammation/visual abnormalities	• CYP3A4 substrate • Strong CYP3A4 inducers ↓ levels (↑ gefitinib dose) • May ↑ risk of bleeding with warfarin • H$_2$-antagonists, PPIs, and antacids may ↓ absorption (avoid concomitant use of PPIs; may use H$_2$-antagonists or antacids [need to space administration])	Used for metastatic NSCLC with EGFR exon 19 deletions or exon 21 substitution mutations
Lapatinib • Tykerb • Tabs (PO)	None	• Cardiotoxicity • Diarrhea • Hepatotoxicity • Rash (can be severe) • QT interval prolongation • ILD	• HER2 status • LVEF • S/S of dehydration • Electrolytes • LFTs • S/S of dermatologic reactions • ECG • S/S of ILD	• CYP3A4 and P-gp substrate • CYP2C8, CYP3A4, and P-gp inhibitor • Avoid concomitant use of strong CYP3A4 inhibitors and inducers • May ↑ digoxin levels • ↑ risk of torsade de pointes (TdP) with other drugs that prolong QT interval	• Used for HER2-positive metastatic breast cancer • Adjust dose in hepatic imparment
Necitumumab • Portrazza • Injection (IV)	None	• Cardiopulmonary arrest • ↓ Mg^{2+} • Thromboembolic events • Rash (can be severe) • Infusion-related reactions	• Electrolytes • S/S of thromboembolism • S/S of dermatologic reactions • S/S of infusion reactions	None	Used for metastatic NSCLC

Epidermal Growth Factor Receptor (EGFR) Inhibitors (cont'd)

Generic • Brand • Dosage Forms	Contraindications	Primary Side Effects	Key Monitoring	Pertinent Drug Interactions	Med Pearl
Osimertinib • Tagrisso • Tabs (PO)	None	• ILD • QT interval prolongation • Cardiotoxicity	• EGFR mutation status • S/S of ILD • ECG • LVEF	• CYP3A4 substrate and inhibitor • CYP1A2 and CYP3A4 inducer • Avoid concomitant use of strong CYP3A4 inhibitors and inducers • ↑ risk of TdP with other drugs that prolong QT interval	Used for metastatic NSCLC with EGFR T790M mutation
Panitumumab • Vectibix • Injection (IV)	None	• Diarrhea • Rash (can be severe) • Infusion-related reactions • ILD • Electrolyte abnormalities ($\downarrow$ Mg^{2+}, $\downarrow$ K$^+$, $\downarrow$ Ca^{2+}) • Keratitis • Photosensitivity	• *K-Ras* status • S/S of dehydration • Electrolytes • S/S of dermatologic reactions • S/S of infusion reactions • S/S of ILD • S/S of eye inflammation/ visual abnormalities	None	• Used for wild-type *K-Ras* metastatic colorectal cancer • Advise patients to wear sunscreen
Pertuzumab • Perjeta • Injection (IV)	None	• Cardiotoxicity • Infusion-related reactions • Anaphylaxis	• HER2 status • LVEF • S/S of infusion reactions/ anaphylaxis	↑ risk of cardiotoxicity with anthracyclines	Used for HER2-positive metastatic breast cancer
Trastuzumab • Herceptin • Injection (IV)	None	• Cardiotoxicity • Infusion-related reactions • Myelosuppression • ILD	• HER2 status • LVEF • S/S of infusion reactions • CBC with differential • S/S of ILD	↑ risk of cardiotoxicity with anthracyclines	Used for HER2-positive metastatic breast cancer and gastric cancer
Ado-trastuzumab emtansine • Kadcyla • Injection (IV)	None	• Hepatotoxicity • Cardiotoxicity • Infusion-related reactions • ILD • Myelosuppression • Peripheral neuropathy • Hemorrhage	• HER2 status • LFTs • LVEF • S/S of infusion reactions • S/S of ILD • CBC with differential • S/S of neuropathy • S/S of bleeding	• CYP3A4 substrate • Avoid concomitant use of strong CYP3A4 inhibitors or inducers • ↑ risk of cardiotoxicity with anthracyclines	Used for HER2-positive metastatic breast cancer

Vascular Endothelial Growth Factor (VEGF) Inhibitors

Generic • Brand • Dosage Forms	Contraindications	Primary Side Effects	Key Monitoring	Pertinent Drug Interactions	Med Pearl
Mechanism of action – block angiogenesis and tumor growth by inhibiting VEGF receptors					
Axitinib • Inlyta • Tabs (PO)	None	• Thromboembolic events • Hypertension • Hemorrhage • Heart failure • GI perforation/fistula formation • Hypo-/hyperthyroidism • Proteinuria • ↑ LFTs • Impaired wound healing • Reversible posterior leuko-encephalopathy syndrome (RPLS)	• S/S of thromboembolism • BP • S/S of bleeding • S/S of heart failure • Thyroid function tests (TFTs) • Urinalysis • LFTs • S/S of GI perforation/fistula formation • S/S of RPLS	• CYP3A4 substrate • Avoid concomitant use of strong CYP3A4 inhibitors or inducers	• Used for metastatic renal cell carcinoma • Reduce dose in hepatic impairment
Bevacizumab • Avastin • Injection (IV)	None	• Thromboembolic events • Hypertension • Hemorrhage • GI perforation/fistula formation • Proteinuria • ↑ LFTs • Impaired wound healing • Infusion-related reactions • RPLS	• S/S of thromboembolism • BP • S/S of bleeding • Urinalysis • LFTs • S/S of GI perforation/fistula formation • S/S of infusion reactions • S/S of RPLS	None	Used for metastatic colorectal cancer; locally advanced, recurrent, or metastatic non-squamous NSCLC; glioblastoma; metastatic renal cell carcinoma; persistent, recurrent, or metastatic cervical cancer; or recurrent epithelial ovarian, fallopian tube, or primary peritoneal cancer
Cabozantinib • Cabometyx • Injection (IV)	None	• Thromboembolic events • Hypertension • Hemorrhage • GI perforation/fistula formation • Diarrhea • Palmar-plantar erythro-dysesthesia syndrome • RPLS	• S/S of thromboembolism • BP • S/S of bleeding • S/S of GI perforation/fistula formation • S/S of dehydration • Electrolytes • S/S of RPLS	• CYP3A4 substrate • Avoid concomitant use of strong CYP3A4 inhibitors or inducers	• Used for advanced renal cell carcinoma • Reduce dose in hepatic impairment

Vascular Endothelial Growth Factor (VEGF) Inhibitors *(cont'd)*

Generic • Brand • Dosage Forms	Contraindications	Primary Side Effects	Key Monitoring	Pertinent Drug Interactions	Med Pearl
Ramucirumab • Cyramza • Injection (IV)	None	• Thromboembolic events • Hypertension • Hemorrhage • GI perforation • Hypo-/hyperthyroidism • Proteinuria • ↑ LFTs • Impaired wound healing • Infusion-related reactions • RPLS	• S/S of thromboembolism • BP • S/S of bleeding • TFTs • Urinalysis • LFTs • S/S of GI perforation • S/S of infusion reactions • S/S of RPLS	None	• Used for advanced gastric cancer, metastatic NSCLC, and metastatic colorectal cancer • Premedicate with diphenhydramine
Sorafenib • Nexavar • Tabs (PO)	None	• Myocardial ischemia/infarction • Hepatotoxicity • Diarrhea • Rash (can be severe) • Hand-foot syndrome • Hypertension • QT interval prolongation • Hemorrhage • Hypo-/hyperthyroidism • Impaired wound healing • GI perforation	• LFTs • S/S of dehydration • Electrolytes • S/S of dermatologic reactions • BP • ECG • S/S of bleeding • TFTs • S/S of GI perforation	• CYP3A4 substrate • Avoid concomitant use of strong CYP3A4 inducers • May ↑ risk of bleeding with warfarin • ↑ risk of TdP with other drugs that prolong QT interval	Used for advanced renal cell carcinoma; unresectable hepatocellular carcinoma; and locally recurrent or metastatic, progressive differentiated thyroid cancer
Sunitinib • Sutent • Tabs (PO)	None	• Hepatotoxicity • Diarrhea • Rash (can be severe) • Hypertension • Heart failure • QT interval prolongation • Hemorrhage • Tumor lysis syndrome • Hypo-/hyperthyroidism • Proteinuria • Hypoglycemia • Impaired wound healing	• LFTs • S/S of dehydration • Electrolytes • S/S of dermatologic reactions • BP • LVEF • S/S of heart failure • ECG • S/S of bleeding • TFTs • Urinalysis • Glucose	• CYP3A4 substrate • Avoid concomitant use of strong CYP3A4 inhibitors or inducers	Used for gastrointestinal stromal tumor (GIST), advanced renal cell carcinoma, and locally advanced or unresectable or metastatic pancreatic neuroendocrine tumors

Tyrosine Kinase Inhibitors

Generic • Brand • Dosage Forms	Contraindications	Primary Side Effects	Key Monitoring	Pertinent Drug Interactions	Med Pearl
Mechanism of action – halt proliferation of tumor cells by inhibiting tyrosine kinase					
Bosutinib • Bosulif • Tabs (PO)	None	• N/V/D • Myelosuppression • Hepatotoxicity • Renal impairment • Fluid retention	• S/S of dehydration • Electrolytes • CBC with differential • LFTs • BUN/SCr • S/S of peripheral/ pulmonary edema	• CYP3A4 and P-gp substrate • P-gp inhibitor • Avoid concomitant use of strong or moderate CYP3A4 inhibitors or inducers • H_2-antagonists, PPIs, and antacids may ↓ absorption (avoid concomitant use of PPIs; may use H_2-antagonists or antacids [need to space administration])	• Used for Philadel- phia-positive (Ph+) CML and Ph+ ALL • Adjust dose in hepatic or renal impair- ment
Dasatinib • Sprycel • Tabs (PO)	None	• Myelosuppression • Hemorrhage • Fluid retention • Pulmonary arterial hypertension • Rash (can be severe) • Tumor lysis syndrome • QT interval prolongation	• CBC with differential • S/S of bleeding • S/S of peripheral/ pulmonary edema • S/S of pulmonary arterial hypertension • S/S of dermatologic reactions • ECG	• CYP3A4 substrate and inhibitor • Avoid concomitant use of strong 3A4 inhibitors or inducers • H_2-antagonists, PPIs, and antacids may ↓ absorption (avoid concomitant use of H_2-antagonists and PPIs; may use ant- acids [need to space administration]) • ↑ risk of TdP with other drugs that prolong QT interval	Used for Ph+ CML and Ph+ ALL
Imatinib • Gleevec • Tabs (PO)	None	• Myelosuppression • Hemorrhage • Fluid retention • Rash (can be severe) • Tumor lysis syndrome • Heart failure • Hepatotoxicity • Hypothyroidism	• CBC with differential • S/S of bleeding • S/S of peripheral/ pulmonary edema • S/S of dermatologic reactions • S/S of heart failure • LFTs • TFTs	• CYP3A4 substrate and inhibitor • CYP2D6 inhibitor • Avoid concomitant use of strong CYP3A4 inhibitors or inducers	• Used for Ph+ CML, Ph+ ALL, Kit (CD117)- positive GIST, and a variety of other disorders • Adjust dose in hepatic or renal impair- ment

Tyrosine Kinase Inhibitors *(cont'd)*

Generic • Brand • Dosage Forms	Contraindications	Primary Side Effects	Key Monitoring	Pertinent Drug Interactions	Med Pearl
Lenvatinib • Lenvima • Caps (PO)	None	• Thromboembolic events • Hypertension • Hemorrhage • Heart failure • Hepatotoxicity • Proteinuria • Renal failure • GI perforation/fistula formation • QT interval prolongation • Hypocalcemia • RPLS • Hypothyroidism	• S/S of thromboembolism • BP • S/S of bleeding • LVEF • S/S of heart failure • LFTs • Urinalysis • BUN/SCr • S/S of GI perforation/fistula formation • ECG • Electrolytes • S/S of RPLS • TFTs	↑ risk of TdP with other drugs that prolong QT interval	• Used for locally recurrent or metastatic, progressive radioactive iodine-refractory differentiated thyroid cancer and renal cell carcinoma • Adjust dose in hepatic or renal impairment
Nilotinib • Tasigna • Caps (PO)	• Hypokalemia • Hypomagnesemia • Long QT syndrome	• Myelosuppression • Hemorrhage • Fluid retention • QT interval prolongation • Cardiovascular events • Pancreatitis • Hepatotoxicity • Electrolyte abnormalities ($\downarrow PO_4$, $\downarrow/\uparrow K^+$, $\downarrow Na^+$) • Tumor lysis syndrome	• CBC with differential • S/S of bleeding • S/S of peripheral/pulmonary edema • ECG • S/S of cardiovascular events • Amylase/lipase • Glucose • LFTs • Electrolytes	• CYP3A4 substrate and inhibitor • CYP2C8, CYP2C9, CYP2D6, and P-gp inhibitor • CYP2C9 inducer • Avoid concomitant use of strong CYP3A4 inhibitors or inducers • H_2-antagonists, PPIs, and antacids may ↓ absorption (avoid concomitant use of PPIs; may use antacids and H_2-antagonists [need to space administration]) • ↑ risk of TdP with other drugs that prolong QT interval	• Used for Ph+ CML • Take on empty stomach • Adjust dose in hepatic impairment

Anaplastic Lymphoma Kinase (ALK) Inhibitors

Generic • Brand • Dosage Forms	Contraindications	Primary Side Effects	Key Monitoring	Pertinent Drug Interactions	Med Pearl
Mechanism of action – reduce proliferation of tumor cells by inhibiting ALK					
Alectinib • Alecensa • Caps (PO)	None	• Hepatotoxicity • ILD • Bradycardia • Myalgias	• ALK status • S/S of ILD • ECG • Heart rate (HR) • Creatine kinase	None	Used for ALK-positive, metastatic NSCLC
Ceritinib • Zykadia • Caps (PO)	None	• N/V/D • Hepatotoxicity • ILD • QT interval prolongation • Hyperglycemia • Bradycardia • Pancreatitis	• ALK status • S/S of dehydration • Electrolytes • LFTs • S/S of ILD • ECG • Glucose • HR • Amylase/lipase	• CYP3A4 substrate • CYP2C9 and CYP3A4 inhibitor • Avoid concomitant use of strong CYP3A4 inhibitors or inducers	Used for ALK-positive, metastatic NSCLC
Crizotinib • Xalkori • Caps (PO)	None	• N/V/D • Hepatotoxicity • ILD • QT interval prolongation • Bradycardia • Vision loss	• ALK status • ROS-1 status • S/S of dehydration • Electrolytes • LFTs • S/S of ILD • ECG • HR	• CYP3A4 substrate and inhibitor • Avoid concomitant use of strong CYP3A4 inhibitors or inducers • Avoid concomitant use of CYP3A4 substrates with narrow therapeutic range • ↑ risk of TdP with other drugs that prolong QT interval	• Used for ALK-positive, metastatic NSCLC and ROS-1-positive NSCLC • Adjust dose in renal impairment

Storage and Administration Pearls

- Do not administer live vaccines during chemotherapy cycles.

Patient Education Pearls

- Patient should not breastfeed or attempt to become pregnant while taking chemotherapy.
- Because Zevalin contains radioactive isotopes, patients should be instructed on proper handwashing, special disposal of bodily waste, and other ways to limit exposure to family members postdischarge.

SUPPORTIVE CARE

Nausea and Vomiting

About 55% of cancer patients experience nausea and vomiting during the first week of chemotherapy. 5HT3 antagonists are useful in most cases, but should be used only for prevention of nausea and vomiting. Corticosteroids should be given unless contraindicated, as they are synergistic with the 5HT3 antagonists; other drug therapies depend on the type of nausea and vomiting experienced.

- Benzodiazepines: Treatment of choice for anticipatory nausea and vomiting (caused by the sights and smells of the chemotherapy environment)
- Aprepitant: Useful for delayed nausea and vomiting caused by drugs with high emetic potential (cisplatin, cyclophosphamide, doxorubicin)
- Prochlorperazine or metoclopramide: May be used in less severe cases

Management of Neutropenia and Anemia

Neutropenia and its major complication, neutropenic fever, are major concerns in many types of cancer. The nadir, or lowest, concentration of WBCs in the peripheral blood usually occurs 1–2 weeks following the administration of chemotherapy and is typically proportional to the dose. Subsequent chemotherapy is delayed until the ANC recovers, which explains the 3- to 4-week cycle length of most chemotherapy regimens. Classification of ANC is:

- Normal: 3,000–7,000 neutrophils/mm^3
- Mild neutropenia: 500–1,000/mm^3
- Moderate neutropenia: 100–500/mm^3
- Severe neutropenia: <100/mm^3

Colony-stimulating factors (CSF) such as filgrastim have been shown to shorten the duration of neutropenia, but they have little effect on mortality and are very expensive. CSFs do decrease hospitalizations, however, and clinical judgment should be used to determine which patients are most likely to benefit. Because infection leads to death in a large percentage of neutropenic patients (possibly up to 30%), anti-infective therapy is frequently needed. Broad-spectrum bactericidal antibiotics are generally used (third- and fourth-generation cephalosporins, carbapenems, or fluoroquinolones with or without aminoglycosides or β-lactams), with antipseudomonal activity being particularly important. If antifungal therapy is needed, amphotericin B is the drug of choice.

Anemia is also common in cancer patients. Treatment of anemia is currently the subject of much controversy; use of erythropoiesis-stimulating agents, including erythropoietin and darbepoetin, is no longer supported in myeloid malignancies (these agents have been associated with increase in mortality compared to patients not receiving erythropoietin).

The hypothesis is that the drug may be stimulating cancer growth. These drugs should NOT be used in patients with myeloid malignancies who are receiving chemotherapy when the anticipated outcome is a cure. This finding may not apply to solid tumors; more information is needed. Refer to Chapter 8 for discussion of the erythropoiesis-stimulating agents.

Antiemetic Drugs

Generic • Brand • Dose • Dosage Forms	Contraindications	Primary Side Effects	Key Monitoring	Pertinent Drug Interactions	Med Pearl
Mechanism of action – 5HT₃ antagonists; prevent release of serotonin in GI mucosa					
Ondansetron ☆ • Zofran, Zuplenz • 16–24 mg PO or 8–12 mg IV • Films, injection, solution, tabs Granisetron • Sancuso • 2 mg PO or 1 mg IV • Injection, tabs, transdermal patch Dolasetron • Anzemet • 100 mg PO • Tabs Palonosetron • Aloxi • 0.25 mg IV • Injection	Current N/V (useful only for prevention)	• Headache • Constipation or diarrhea • Fatigue • Dry mouth • Transient ↑ LFTs • QT interval prolongation	None	• CYP3A4 substrate • Use with serotonergic agents may ↑ risk of serotonin syndrome • ↑ risk of TdP with other drugs that prolong QT interval	• Single dose prior to chemotherapy; repeat doses do not ↑ effect • Palonosetron effective in preventing acute and delayed N/V
Mechanism of action – neurokinin-1 (NK-1) antagonist; block substance P from NK-1 receptor					
Aprepitant • Emend • PO: 125 mg on day 1, then 80 mg daily on days 2 and 3 • IV: 150 mg on day 1 • Caps, injection, suspension	None	• Asthenia • Fatigue • Diarrhea • Hiccups • Dizziness • Dehydration	Monitor levels of chemotherapy agents metabolized by CYP3A4	• CYP3A4 substrate • Inhibits CYP3A4 • Induces CYP2C9	• Use in combination with 5HT₃ antagonist and dexamethasone • Prevents acute and delayed N/V
Rolapitant • Varubi • 180 mg PO on day 1 • Tabs	Concurrent therapy with thioridazine	• Neutropenia • Hiccups • Anorexia • Dizziness • Dyspepsia	CBC with differential	CYP2D6 and P-gp inhibitor	• Used in combination with 5HT₃ antagonist and dexamethasone • Prevents delayed N/V

Antiemetic Drugs *(cont'd)*

Generic • **Brand** • **Dose** • **Dosage Forms**	**Contraindications**	**Primary Side Effects**	**Key Monitoring**	**Pertinent Drug Interactions**	**Med Pearl**
Netupitant/palonosetron • Akynzeo • 1 capsule (300 mg netupitant/0.5 mg palonosetron) PO on day 1 • Caps	None	• Dyspepsia • Fatigue • Constipation • Headache • Asthenia	Monitor levels of chemo-therapy agents metabolized by CYP3A4	• CYP3A4 substrate and inhibitor • Use with serotonergic agents may ↑ risk of serotonin syndrome	• Netupitant is NK-1 antagonist; palonosetron is 5HT$_3$ antagonist • Used in combination with dexamethasone • Prevents acute and delayed N/V
Mechanism of action – corticosteroids; potentiate antiemetic properties of 5HT$_3$ antagonists					
Dexamethasone • Decadron • 8–40 mg daily PO/IV • Injection, solution, tabs	Systemic fungal infections	• Hyperglycemia • Immunosuppression • Adrenal suppression • Insomnia • Mood changes, anxiety • GI irritation • Weight gain	• Hemoglobin/ hematocrit • Serum potassium • Glucose	CYP3A4 substrate	• Synergistic with 5HT$_3$ antagonists • Can use as single agents for mild chemotherapy-induced N/V
Methylprednisolone ☆ • Solu-Medrol • 40–125 mg daily IV • Injection					
Mechanism of action – dopamine-2 antagonists					
Metoclopramide ☆ • Reglan • 10–20 mg PO/IV q4–6h PRN • Injection, solution, tabs	Seizures	• Dizziness • Sedation • Diarrhea • Extrapyramidal symptoms (EPS)	EPS	Antipsychotic agents may ↑ risk of EPS	Should not drive or operate heavy machinery while taking this drug

Colony-Stimulating Factors

Generic • Brand • Dose	Contraindications	Primary Side Effects	Key Monitoring	Pertinent Drug Interactions	Med Pearl
Mechanism of action – stimulate production of WBCs					
Filgrastim • Granix, Neupogen, Zarxio • 5 mcg/kg subcut daily	Hypersensitivity to *E. coli*	• Bone pain • Hypertension • Swelling • Redness • Hypersensitivity reactions	CBC with differential	Use lithium with caution, as it can potentiate neutrophil release	• Requires daily administration • Neutrophil-specific
PEG-Filgrastim • Neulasta • 6 mg subcut with each chemotherapy cycle					• PEG unit ↑ half-life; can give once per chemotherapy cycle • Neutrophil-specific
Sargramostim • Leukine • 250–500 mcg/m^2/day subcut	• Hypersensitivity to yeast • Excessive leukemic myeloid blasts in bone marrow	• Fever, chills • Bone pain • Myalgia • Hypertension • Hypersensitivity reactions			• Requires daily administration • Stimulates formation of all WBCs except lymphocytes

Storage and Administration Pearls

- Zofran ODT contains phenylalanine.

Patient Education Pearls

- Patient should not take echinacea if taking corticosteroids.

LEARNING POINTS

- Chemotherapy protocols vary tremendously; do NOT spend your time memorizing drugs of choice for the various cancers (pharmacists usually do not play a role in selecting drug therapies as treatment is usually protocol driven).
  - Focus more on the toxicity profile of the most commonly used drugs and less on dosing and specific drug combinations.
- Because of the increasing importance of pharmacogenomics, you should know which drugs target specific receptors (e.g., Trastuzumab, HER2 receptor; Cetuximab, EGFR; Rituximab, CD20 cell surface protein, etc.).
- Leucovorin is used as a rescue agent in patients receiving methotrexate but enhances the effect of 5-fluorouracil.
- To treat N/V, most patients should receive a corticosteroid, a 5HT3 antagonist, and possibly a benzodiazepine. For severe cases, an NK-1 antagonist should be added.

PRACTICE QUESTIONS

1. Which of the following chemotherapeutic agents may cause left ventricular systolic dysfunction as a toxicity? (Select ALL that apply.)

    (A) Cetuximab
    (B) Cisplatin
    (C) Doxorubicin
    (D) Trastuzumab
    (E) Vincristine

2. Which of the following chemotherapeutic agents is associated with profound acute- and late-onset diarrhea?

    (A) Daunorubicin
    (B) Doxorubicin
    (C) Irinotecan
    (D) Methotrexate
    (E) Trastuzumab

3. The mechanism of action of Emend is

    (A) $5HT_3$ receptor antagonist.
    (B) neurokinin-1 receptor antagonist.
    (C) D_2 receptor antagonist.
    (D) benzodiazepine receptor agonist.
    (E) histamine receptor antagonist.

4. A patient with NHL is to be started on cyclophosphamide, doxorubicin, vincristine, and prednisone. Which of the following medications is MOST likely to be protective against the toxicity of doxorubicin?

    (A) Amifostine
    (B) Dexrazoxane
    (C) Folic acid
    (D) Leucovorin
    (E) Mesna

5. A patient receiving cancer chemotherapy presents to the emergency department complaining of an increase in urinary frequency and dysuria. No significant findings are apparent on physical examination. This patient's urinalysis reveals (–) WBC, (+) blood, (–) bacteria, (–) casts. If the symptoms experienced by the patient are related to the cancer chemotherapy, which of the following medications is MOST likely the cause?

   (A) Cyclophosphamide
   (B) Irinotecan
   (C) Methotrexate
   (D) Paclitaxel
   (E) Tamoxifen

6. Which of the following BEST describes the mechanism of action of Zofran?

   (A) It competes for the binding sites of serotonin receptors.
   (B) It inhibits the substance P/neurokinin-1 receptor.
   (C) It inhibits histamine H_1 receptors.
   (D) It stimulates dopamine-2 receptors.
   (E) It stimulates cannabinoid receptors.

7. Etoposide should not be administered via intravenous push because of the increased risk of which of the following adverse effects?

   (A) Diarrhea
   (B) Hepatotoxicity
   (C) Hypotension
   (D) Pulmonary fibrosis
   (E) Seizure

8. Pulmonary fibrosis is MOST likely to occur as a toxicity of which of the following chemotherapy drugs?

   (A) Bleomycin
   (B) Cisplatin
   (C) Daunorubicin
   (D) Trastuzumab
   (E) Vincristine

9. Which of the following antiemetic drugs is available as a transdermal patch?

   (A) Aprepitant
   (B) Dexamethasone
   (C) Granisetron
   (D) Metoclopramide
   (E) Prochlorperazine

10 Which of the following drugs is/are considered VEGF inhibitors? (Select ALL that apply.)

   (A) Bevacizumab
   (B) Ceritinib
   (C) Erlotinib
   (D) Rituximab
   (E) Trastuzumab

ANSWERS AND EXPLANATIONS

1. **C, D**

Cardiotoxicity is a major adverse effect associated with both doxorubicin (C) and trastuzumab (D). Cetuximab (A), cisplatin (B), and vincristine (E) do not cause cardiotoxicity. Instead, cetuximab is associated with severe rash and interstitial lung disease; cisplatin is associated with nephrotoxicity; ;and vincristine is associated with neurotoxicity.

2. **C**

Of the drugs listed, only irinotecan (C) exhibits major gastrointestinal adverse effects. The other drugs are more likely to lead to cardiomyopathy (trastuzumab [E], daunorubicin [A], and doxorubicin [B]) or neuro-, nephro-, and hepatotoxicity (methotrexate [D]).

3. **B**

Emend (aprepitant) is a highly selective emetogenic agent that works against the neurokinin-1 receptor. It has little to no affinity for the other receptor targets listed.

4. **B**

Dexrazoxane can be used to reduce the incidence and severity of cardiomyopathy associated with doxorubicin administration (cumulative doses >300 mg/m^2). Amifostine (A) is used to reduce the cumulative renal toxicity associated with repeated administration of cisplatin. The use of methotrexate can lead to folate deficiency; folic acid (C) can be administered to patients receiving methotrexate to prevent side effects. Leucovorin (D) can be given after administration of methotrexate to limit its toxicity. Mesna (E) is used to prevent hemorrhagic cystitis associated with cyclophosphamide or ifosfamide.

5. **A**

This patient is most likely exhibiting signs of chemotherapy-induced hemorrhagic cystitis. This adverse effect is most commonly associated with cyclophosphamide (A) and ifosfamide. The major toxicity associated with irinotecan (B) is diarrhea. Methotrexate (C) can cause numerous organ toxicities, including nephrotoxicity (acute renal failure), neurotoxicity, and hepatotoxicity. Paclitaxel (D) can be associated with peripheral neuropathy. The major adverse effect associated with tamoxifen (E) is thromboembolic events.

6. **A**

The antiemetic Zofran (ondansetron) is a selective serotonin ($5HT_3$) receptor antagonist. The antiemetics, aprepitant (Emend) and rolapitant (Varubi), inhibit the substance P/neurokinin-1 receptor (B). By inhibiting dopamine-2 receptors—not stimulating them (D)—metoclopramide (Reglan) also acts as an antiemetic.

7. **C**

Administering etoposide via intravenous (IV) push may lead to hypotension. Etoposide should be administered over 30–60 minutes to minimize the risk of this adverse effect.

8. **A**

Pulmonary fibrosis is a significant adverse effects associated with bleomycin (A) and busulfan. The major toxicity associated with cisplatin (B) is nephrotoxicity. Daunorubicin (C) and trastuzumab (D) are associated with cardiotoxicity. Vincristine (E) is associated with dose-limiting peripheral neuropathy.

9. **C**

Of the listed antiemetic drugs, only granisetron, a $5HT_3$ antagonist, is available as a transdermal patch (Sancuso). Aprepitant (A) is available as a capsule, oral suspension, and IV injection. Dexamethasone (B) is available as a tablet, oral solution, and IV injection. Metoclopramide (D) is available as a tablet, orally disintegrating tablet, oral solution, and IV injection. Prochlorperazine (E) is available as a tablet, rectal suppository, and IV injection.

10. **A**

Only bevacizumab (A) is considered a VEGF inhibitor. Ceritinib (B) is an anaplastic lymphoma kinase (ALK) inhibitor. Erlotinib (C) is an epidermal growth factor receptor (EGFR) inhibitor. Rituximab (D) is a monoclonal antibody directed against the CD20 antigen on B-lymphocytes. Trastuzumab (E) is a monoclonal antibody targeted against the HER2 receptor.

Psychiatric Disorders

10

This chapter covers the following disease states:

- **Depression**
- **Anxiety**
- **Bipolar disorder**
- **Schizophrenia**
- **Sleep disorders**
- **Attention-deficit/hyperactivity disorder (ADHD)**

 Suggested Study Time: **60 minutes**

DEPRESSION

Definition

Depression, or major depressive disorder, is a complex mood disorder that has many subtypes and is due to multiple etiologies. Depression can be classified as single-episode, recurrent, or chronic and as depression with or without psychotic features, with typical or atypical symptoms, and so on.

Diagnosis

The diagnosis of depression is based on the *Diagnostic and Statistical Manual of Mental Disorders*, 5th Edition (DSM-5). Criteria for diagnosis are based primarily on symptoms. Five or more of the following symptoms must have been present during the same 2-week period and must represent a change from previous functioning; at least one of the symptoms is either (1) depressed mood or (2) loss of interest or pleasure.

- Depressed mood most of the day, nearly every day
- Markedly diminished interest or pleasure in all, or almost all, activities
- Significant weight loss when not dieting, or weight gain
- Insomnia or hypersomnia nearly every day
- Psychomotor agitation or retardation nearly every day
- Fatigue or loss of energy nearly every day
- Feelings of worthlessness or of excessive or inappropriate guilt
- Diminished ability to think or concentrate, or indecisiveness
- Recurrent thoughts of death (not just fear of dying), recurrent suicidal ideation without a specific plan, or a suicide attempt or a specific plan for committing suicide

Signs and Symptoms

Signs and symptoms are detailed in the diagnostic criteria.

Guidelines

American Psychiatric Association. *Practice Guideline for the Treatment of Patients with Major Depressive Disorder*, 3rd ed. Arlington, VA: American Psychiatric Association; 2010:1-152. http://psychiatryonline.org/pb/assets/raw/sitewide/practice_guidelines/guidelines/mdd.pdf.

Guidelines Summary

- The primary goal of therapy is remission of symptoms.
- There are various antidepressant medications available. Clinical evidence indicates that, in general, efficacy is similar between classes.
- Initial choice of pharmacotherapy agent is based on anticipated side effects, tolerability of these side effects for an individual patient, patient preference, quantity and quality of clinical evidence, and cost.
- First-line options for most patients include selective serotonin reuptake inhibitors (SSRIs), serotonin norepinephrine reuptake inhibitors (SNRIs), bupropion, and mirtazapine. Because of the potential for serious side effects and drug interactions, monoamine oxidase inhibitors (MAOIs) should be reserved for patients who do not respond to other therapies.
- An adequate therapy trial requires at least 6–8 weeks. Dose adjustments or treatment changes are made at 6- to 8-week intervals at the earliest.
- There is significant interpatient variability in response to antidepressants. Patients may respond to classes/agents that have been effective in the past or that have been effective for family members.

- Bupropion has a lower incidence of sexual side effects and may be preferred in patients presenting with this complaint related to therapy.
- In 2005, the Food and Drug Administration required that all product labeling for antidepressants include a boxed warning regarding the potential for ↑ risk of clinical worsening and suicidality in children, adolescents, and young adults taking these agents.

Antidepressants

Generic • Brand • Dose/Dosage Forms	Contraindications	Primary Side Effects	Key Monitoring Parameters	Pertinent Drug Interactions	Med Pearls
Mechanism of action – SSRIs: inhibit reuptake of serotonin, allowing more serotonin availability in synapses					
Citalopram☆ • Celexa • 10–40 mg daily • Age >60 yr: max = 20 mg daily • Solution, tabs	• Hypersensitivity • Use of MAOI within 2 wk (5 wk for fluoxetine) • Concurrent use of pimozide • Within 5 wk of thioridazine (fluoxetine) • Concurrent use of linezolid or methylene blue	• Lightheadedness • Syncope • Sweating • N/D • Xerostomia • Confusion • Dizziness • Somnolence • Tremor • Hallucinations • Ejaculation disorders • Impotence • Fatigue • Female sexual disorder • QT interval prolongation (citalopram) • Serotonin syndrome	• Reduction or resolution of symptoms • Withdrawal symptoms from abrupt discontinuation • Abnormal bleeding • Worsening of depression, suicidality, or unusual behavior at initiation of therapy or when changing dose	• CYP2C19 and CYP3A4 substrate • CYP2C19 or CYP3A4 inhibitors may ↑ effects/toxicity; max dose = 20 mg/day when used with CYP2C19 inhibitors due to risk of QTc interval prolongation • CYP2C19 or CYP3A4 inducers may ↓ effects • ↑ risk of serotonin syndrome with MAOIs, SNRIs, triptans, tricyclic antidepressants (TCAs), fentanyl, lithium, dextromethorphan, meperidine, buspirone, linezolid, methylene blue, St. John's wort, and tramadol • ↑ risk of bleeding with used with aspirin, nonsteroidal anti-inflammatory drugs (NSAIDs), or anticoagulants	• Racemic mixture of R- and S- isomers • QTc interval prolongation may occur with doses >40 mg • Max dose of 20 mg/day in severe hepatic impairment
Escitalopram☆ • Lexapro • 10–20 mg daily • Solution, tabs					• Contains only the S-isomer of citalopram • Adjust dose in hepatic impairment

Antidepressants *(cont'd)*

Generic • Brand • Dose/Dosage Forms	Contraindications	Primary Side Effects	Key Monitoring Parameters	Pertinent Drug Interactions	Med Pearls
Fluoxetine ☆ • Prozac, Prozac Weekly, Sarafem • 20–80 mg daily or 90 mg weekly • Caps, ER caps, solution, tabs	[Same as above]	[Same as above]	[Same as above]	• CYP2C9 and CYP2D6 substrate • CYP2D6 inhibitor • CYP2C9 or CYP2D6 inhibitors may ↑ effects/toxicity • CYP2C9 inducers may ↓ effects • May ↑ effects/toxicity of CYP2D6 substrates • ↑ risk of serotonin syndrome with MAOIs, SNRIs, triptans, TCAs, fentanyl, lithium, dextromethorphan, meperidine, buspirone, linezolid, methylene blue, St. John's wort, and tramadol • ↑ risk of bleeding with used with aspirin, NSAIDs, or anticoagulants	• Allow 5 wk washout prior to using MAOI due to long half-life • Does not require taper due to long half-life • Also indicated for premenstrual dysphoric disorder (PMDD)
Fluvoxamine • Luvox, Luvox CR • 50–300 mg daily • ER caps, tabs	• Hypersensitivity • Concurrent use of tizanidine, thioridazine, alosetron, or pimozide • Use of MAOI within 2 wk • Concurrent use of linezolid or methylene blue			• CYP1A2 and CYP2D6 substrate • CYP1A2 and CYP2C19 inhibitor • CYP1A2 or CYP2D6 inhibitors may ↑ effects/toxicity • CYP1A2 inducers may ↓ effects • May ↑ effects/toxicity of CYP1A2 or CYP2C19 substrates • ↑ risk of serotonin syndrome with MAOIs, SNRIs, triptans, TCAs, fentanyl, lithium, dextromethorphan, meperidine, buspirone, linezolid, methylene blue, St. John's wort, and tramadol • ↑ risk of bleeding with used with aspirin, NSAIDs, or anticoagulants	Only approved to treat obsessive-compulsive disorder (OCD)
Paroxetine ☆ • Paxil, Paxil CR, Pexeva • IR: 20–50 mg daily • ER: 25–62.5 mg daily • Suspension, tabs	• Hypersensitivity • Concurrent use of thioridazine or pimozide • Use of MAOI within 2 wk • Concurrent use of linezolid or methylene blue			• CYP2D6 substrate and inhibitor • CYP2D6 inhibitors may ↑ effects/toxicity • May ↑ effects/toxicity of CYP2D6 substrates • ↑ risk of serotonin syndrome with MAOIs, SNRIs, triptans, TCAs, fentanyl, lithium, dextromethorphan, meperidine, buspirone, linezolid, methylene blue, St. John's wort, and tramadol • ↑ risk of bleeding with used with aspirin, NSAIDs, or anticoagulants	• Brisdelle approved to treat vasomotor symptoms of menopause • Paxil CR also approved for PMDD • Adjust dose in renal impairment

Antidepressants *(cont'd)*

Generic • Brand • Dose/Dosage Forms	Contraindications	Primary Side Effects	Key Monitoring Parameters	Pertinent Drug Interactions	Med Pearls
Sertraline ☆ • Zoloft • 50–200 mg daily • Solution, tabs	• Hypersensitivity • Use of MAOI within 2 wk • Concurrent use of pimozide • Concurrent use of disulfiram-like products (oral concentrate contains alcohol) • Concurrent use of linezolid or methylene blue	[Same as above]	[Same as above]	• CPY2C19 and CPY206 substrate • ↑ risk of serotonin syndrome with MAOIs, SNRIs, triptans, TCAs, fentanyl, lithium, dextromethorphan, meperidine, buspirone, linezolid, methylene blue, St. John's wort, and tramadol • ↑ risk of bleeding with used with aspirin, NSAIDs, or anticoagulants • ↓ effectiveness of tamoxifen	• Oral concentrate contains alcohol • Also indicated for PMDD
Vortioxetine • Trintellix • 5–20 mg daily • Tabs	• Hypersensitivity • Use of MAOI within 2–3 wk • Concurrent use of linezolid or methylene blue			• CYP2D6 and CYP3A4 substrate • CYP2D6 or CYP3A4 inhibitors may ↑ effects/toxicity; ↓ dose by 50% when used with strong CYP2D6 inhibitor • CYP3A4 inducers may ↓ effects • ↑ risk of serotonin syndrome with MAOIs, SNRIs, triptans, TCAs, fentanyl, lithium, dextromethorphan, meperidine, buspirone, linezolid, methylene blue, St. John's wort, and tramadol • ↑ risk of bleeding with used with aspirin, NSAIDs, or anticoagulants	
Mechanism of action – SSRI, partial 5HT1A receptor agonist					
Vilazodone • Viibryd • 10–40 mg daily • Tabs	Use of MAOI within 2 wk	• N/D • Xerostomia • Dizziness • Insomnia • Serotonin syndrome	• Reduction or resolution of symptoms • Withdrawal symptoms from abrupt discontinuation • Abnormal bleeding • Worsening of depression, suicidality, or unusual behavior at initiation of therapy or when changing dose	• CYP3A4 substrate • CYP3A4 inhibitors may ↑ effects/toxicity; max dose = 20 mg/day when used with strong CYP3A4 inhibitors • CYP3A4 inducers may ↓ effects; consider ↑ dose when used with strong CYP3A4 inducers (max dose = 80 mg/day) • ↑ risk of serotonin syndrome with MAOIs, SNRIs, triptans, TCAs, fentanyl, lithium, dextromethorphan, meperidine, buspirone, linezolid, methylene blue, St. John's wort, and tramadol • ↑ risk of bleeding with used with aspirin, NSAIDs, or anticoagulants	Take with food

Antidepressants *(cont'd)*

Generic • Brand • Dose/Dosage Forms	Contraindications	Primary Side Effects	Key Monitoring Parameters	Pertinent Drug Interactions	Med Pearls
Mechanism of action – TCAs: $\uparrow$ synaptic concentration of norepinephrine and serotonin					
Amitriptyline☆ • Only available generically • 25–300 mg/day in 1–3 divided doses • Tabs Amoxapine • Only available generically • 50–600 mg/day in 2–3 divided doses • Tabs Clomipramine • Anafranil • 25–250 mg/day in 3 divided doses • Caps Desipramine • Norpramin • 25–300 mg/day in 1–2 divided doses • Tabs Doxepin☆ • Only available generically • 25–300 mg/day in 1–3 divided doses • Caps, solution Imipramine☆ • Tofranil • 75–300 mg/day in 1–2 divided doses • Caps, tabs Nortriptyline☆ • Pamelor • 75–150 mg/day in 3–4 divided doses • Caps, solution Protriptyline • Vivactil • 10–60 mg/day in 3–4 divided doses • Tabs	• Hypersensitivity • Use of MAOI within 2 wk • Concurrent use of linezolid or methylene blue • Acute recovery period post-myocardial infarction (MI)	• Anticholinergic symptoms • Weight gain • Bloating • Blurred vision • Xerostomia • Constipation • Dizziness • Somnolence • Headache • Fatigue • Serotonin syndrome	• Reduction or resolution of symptoms • Withdrawal symptoms from abrupt discontinuation • Worsening of depression, suicidality, or unusual behavior at initiation of therapy or when changing dose • Blood pressure (BP) • Electrocardiogram (ECG) (in patients with cardiac disease or hyperthyroidism)	• CYP2D6 substrate • CYP2D6 inhibitors may $\uparrow$ effects/toxicity • $\uparrow$ risk of serotonin syndrome with MAOIs, SSRIs, SNRIs, triptans, fentanyl, lithium, dextromethorphan, meperidine, buspirone, linezolid, methylene blue, St. John's wort, and tramadol	• Dangerous in overdose situations • Avoid in patients with high suicidality • Avoid dispensing large quantities • Also used for sleep disorders • Clomipramine indicated only for OCD

Antidepressants *(cont'd)*

Generic • Brand • Dose/Dosage Forms	Contraindications	Primary Side Effects	Key Monitoring Parameters	Pertinent Drug Interactions	Med Pearls
Trimipramine • Surmontil • 25–300 mg/day in 1–3 divided doses • Caps	[Same as above]	[Same as above]	[Same as above]	[Same as above]	[Same as above]
Mechanism of action – SNRIs: inhibit the reuptake of serotonin and norepinephrine to allow higher available synaptic concentrations					
Duloxetine ☆ • Cymbalta • 30–120 mg/day in 1–2 divided doses • DR caps	• Hypersensitivity • Use of MAOI within 2 wk • Concurrent use of linezolid or methylene blue	• Hepatotoxicity • Orthostatic hypotension • Rash (Stevens-Johnson syndrome possible) • Palpitations • Diaphoresis • Constipation • ↓ appetite • N/D • Xerostomia • Asthenia • Dizziness • Insomnia or somnolence • Vertigo • Blurred vision • Polyuria • ↓ libido • Serotonin syndrome	• Liver function tests (LFTs) • BP • Reduction or resolution of symptoms • Withdrawal symptoms from abrupt discontinuation • Abnormal bleeding • Worsening of depression, suicidality, or unusual behavior at initiation of therapy or when changing dose	• CYP1A2 and CYP2D6 substrate • CYP1A2 or CYP2D6 inhibitors may ↑ effects/toxicity; avoid concomitant use with strong CYP1A2 inhibitors • CYP1A2 inducers may ↓ effects • ↑ risk of serotonin syndrome with MAOIs, SSRIs, triptans, TCAs, fentanyl, lithium, dextromethorphan, meperidine, buspirone, linezolid, methylene blue, St. John's wort, and tramadol • ↑ risk of bleeding with used with aspirin, NSAIDs, or anticoagulants	• Doses >60 mg/day do not provide additional benefit • May also be used to treat neuropathic and musculo-skeletal pain and fibromyalgia • Avoid use if creatinine clearance <30 mL/min
Venlafaxine ☆ • Effexor XR • 37.5–375 mg/day in 1–3 divided doses • ER caps/tabs, tabs		• Hypertension • Sweating • Weight loss • Constipation • ↓ appetite • Nausea • Xerostomia • Insomnia or somnolence • Erectile dysfunction • Serotonin syndrome	• BP • Reduction or resolution of symptoms • Withdrawal symptoms from abrupt discontinuation • Abnormal bleeding • Worsening of depression, suicidality, or unusual behavior at initiation of therapy or when changing dose	• CYP2D6 and CYP3A4 substrate • CYP2D6 or CYP3A4 inhibitors may ↑ effects/toxicity • CYP3A4 inducers may ↓ effects • ↑ risk of serotonin syndrome with MAOIs, SSRIs, triptans, TCAs, fentanyl, lithium, dextromethorphan, meperidine, buspirone, linezolid, methylene blue, St. John's wort, and tramadol • ↑ risk of bleeding with used with aspirin, NSAIDs, or anticoagulants	Adjust dose in renal or hepatic impairment

Antidepressants *(cont'd)*

Generic • Brand • Dose/Dosage Forms	Contraindications	Primary Side Effects	Key Monitoring Parameters	Pertinent Drug Interactions	Med Pearls
Levomilnacipran • Fetzima • 20–120 mg daily • ER caps	[Same as above]	• Nausea • Orthostasis • Constipation • ↑ sweating • Tachycardia • Serotonin syndrome • Hypertension • Urinary retention	• BP • Heart rate • Reduction or resolution of symptoms • Withdrawal symptoms from abrupt discontinuation • Abnormal bleeding • Worsening of depression, suicidality, or unusual behavior at initiation of therapy or when changing dose	• CYP3A4 substrate • CYP3A4 inhibitors may ↑ effects/toxicity; max dose = 80 mg/day when used with strong CYP3A4 inhibitors • CYP3A4 inducers may ↓ effects • ↑ risk of serotonin syndrome with MAOIs, SSRIs, triptans, TCAs, fentanyl, lithium, dextromethorphan, meperidine, buspirone, linezolid, methylene blue, St. John's wort, and tramadol • ↑ risk of bleeding with used with aspirin, NSAIDs, or anticoagulants	Adjust dose in renal impairment
Desvenlafaxine ☆ • Khedezla, Pristiq • 50 mg daily • ER tabs		• Hypertension • Nausea • Dizziness • Insomnia or somnolence • ↑ sweating • Constipation • ↓ appetite • Anxiety • Male sexual dysfunction • Serotonin syndrome	• BP • Reduction or resolution of symptoms • Withdrawal symptoms from abrupt discontinuation • Abnormal bleeding • Worsening of depression, suicidality, or unusual behavior at initiation of therapy or when changing dose	• ↑ risk of serotonin syndrome with MAOIs, SSRIs, triptans, TCAs, fentanyl, lithium, dextromethorphan, meperidine, buspirone, linezolid, methylene blue, St. John's wort, and tramadol • ↑ risk of bleeding with used with aspirin, NSAIDs, or anticoagulants	Adjust dose in renal or hepatic impairment

Antidepressants *(cont'd)*

Generic • Brand • Dose/Dosage Forms	Contraindications	Primary Side Effects	Key Monitoring Parameters	Pertinent Drug Interactions	Med Pearls
Nefazodone • Only available generically • 100–600 mg/day in 1–2 divided doses • Tabs	• Hypersensitivity • Previous nefazodone-induced hepatic damage • Liver disease • Use of MAOI within 2 wk • Concurrent use with carbamazepine, triazolam, or pimozide	• Hepatotoxicity • Lightheadedness • Constipation • Nausea • Xerostomia • Urinary retention • Blurred vision • Confusion • Dizziness • Insomnia or somnolence • Sexual dysfunction • Serotonin syndrome	• LFTs • Reduction or resolution of symptoms • Withdrawal symptoms from abrupt discontinuation • Abnormal bleeding • Worsening of depression, suicidality, or unusual behavior at initiation of therapy or when changing dose	• CYP2D6 and CYP3A4 substrate • CYP2D6 or CYP3A4 inhibitors may ↑ effects/toxicity • CYP3A4 inducers may ↓ effects • ↑ risk of serotonin syndrome with MAOIs, SSRIs, triptans, TCAs, fentanyl, lithium, dextromethorphan, meperidine, buspirone, linezolid, methylene blue, St. John's wort, and tramadol • ↑ risk of bleeding with used with aspirin, NSAIDs, or anticoagulants	Black box warning for hepatotoxicity
Mechanism of action – MAOIs: ↑ epinephrine, norepinephrine, dopamine, and serotonin through inhibition of monoamine oxidase					
Isocarboxazid • Marplan • 10–60 mg/day in 2–4 divided doses • Tabs	• Hypersensitivity • Concurrent use of sympathomimetics, SSRIs, SNRIs, TCAs, central nervous system depressants, buproprion, meperidine, buspirone, dextromethorphan, anesthetics, or high-tyramine foods • Cardiovascular disease • Hypertension • Cerebrovascular disease • History of headache • Pheochromocytoma • Liver disease • Severe renal impairment	• Weight gain • Orthostatic hypotension • Constipation • Xerostomia • Dizziness • Headache • Insomnia or somnolence • Blurred vision • Anxiety • Serotonin syndrome	• BP • LFTs • Reduction or resolution of symptoms • Withdrawal symptoms from abrupt discontinuation • Abnormal bleeding • Worsening of depression, suicidality, or unusual behavior at initiation of therapy or when changing dose	• ↑ risk of serotonin syndrome with SSRIs, SNRIs, triptans, TCAs, fentanyl, lithium, dextromethorphan, meperidine, buspirone, linezolid, methylene blue, St. John's wort, and tramadol • ↑ risk of hypertensive crises with sympathomimetics and high-tyramine foods	Used very infrequently due to poor side effect profile and risk of drug interactions

Antidepressants *(cont'd)*

Generic • Brand • Dose/Dosage Forms	Contraindications	Primary Side Effects	Key Monitoring Parameters	Pertinent Drug Interactions	Med Pearls
Phenelzine • Nardil • 45–90 mg daily (TID–QID) Tranylcypromine • Parnate • 30–60 mg daily (divided doses)	• Cardiovascular disorder • Hypertension • Cerebrovascular disorder • Concurrent administration of interacting medications • General anesthesia • History of headache • Hypersensitivity • Pheochromocytoma • Severe renal function impairment	[Same as above]	[Same as above]	[Same as above]	[Same as above]
Selegiline • Emsam • 6–12 mg daily transdermal patch (max = 12 mg/24 hrs)	• Concurrent use of sympathomimetics, SSRIs, SNRIs, TCAs, buproprion, meperidine, tramadol, methadone, buspirone, dextromethorphan, carbamazepine, or high-tyramine foods • <12 yr old • Pheochromocytoma				• Apply patch once daily • Patch indicated for depression, not Parkinson's disease

Antidepressants *(cont'd)*

Generic • Brand • Dose/Dosage Forms	Contraindications	Primary Side Effects	Key Monitoring Parameters	Pertinent Drug Interactions	Med Pearls
Mechanism of action — weak inhibitor of dopamine and norepinephrine reuptake					
Bupropion ☆ • Aplenzin, Forfivo XL, Wellbutrin, Wellbutrin SR, Wellbutrin XL • IR: 200–450 mg/day in 2–4 divided doses • ER: 150–450 mg daily • ER tabs, tabs	• Hypersensitivity • Bulimia or anorexia • Abrupt discontinuation of alcohol, benzodiazepines, barbiturates, or AEDs • Seizure disorders • Use of MAOI within 2 wk • Concurrent use of linezolid or methylene blue	• Taste disturbance • Agitation • ↑ seizure activity • Hypertension • Psychotic symptoms • Anaphylaxis • Headache • Tachycardia • Weight loss	• Reduction or resolution of symptoms • Withdrawal symptoms from abrupt discontinuation • Worsening of depression, suicidality, or unusual behavior at initiation of therapy or when changing dose • Seizure activity	• CYP2B6 substrate • CYP2D6 inhibitor • CYP2B6 inhibitors may ↑ effects/toxicity • CYP2B6 inducers may ↓ effects • May ↑ effects/toxicity of CYP2D6 substrates • ↑ risk of hypertensive crises with MAOIs	• Also used for smoking cessation (Zyban) • Mostly dopamine reuptake activity
Mechanism of action — tetracyclic antidepressants: ↑ available synaptic concentrations of norepinephrine and/or serotonin					
Maprotiline • Only available generically • 25–225 mg/day in 2–3 divided doses • Tabs	• Hypersensitivity • Seizure disorder • Use of MAOI within 2 wk • Acute recovery period post-MI	• ↑ seizure activity • Somnolence • Constipation • Nausea • Xerostomia	• Reduction or resolution of symptoms • Withdrawal symptoms from abrupt discontinuation	• CYP2D6 substrate • CYP2D6 inhibitors may ↑ effects/toxicity	
Mirtazapine ☆ • Remeron, Remeron Solutab • 15–45 mg at bedtime	• Hypersensitivity • Use of MAOI within 2 wk	• ↑ appetite • Hyperlipidemia • Weight gain • Constipation • Somnolence • LFTs • Agranulocytosis • Serotonin syndrome	• Worsening of depression, suicidality, or unusual behavior at initiation of therapy or when changing dose • Seizure activity • LFTs	• CYP1A2, CYP2D6, and CYP3A4 substrate • CYP1A2, CYP2D6, or CYP3A4 inhibitors may ↑ effects/toxicity • CYP1A2 or CYP3A4 inducers may ↓ effects	• Dosed at bedtime due to somnolence • Off-label use for appetite stimulation

Medications That May Exacerbate Depression

- Beta-blockers
- Clonidine
- Corticosteroids
- Efavirenz
- GnRH agonsits
- Hormonal contraceptives
- Interferons
- Isotretinoin
- Levetiracetam
- Mefloquine
- Methyldopa
- Montelukast
- Non-nucleoside reverse transcriptase inibitors
- Phenobarbital
- Phenytoin
- Tamoxifen
- Tiagabine
- Topiramate
- Triptans
- Varenicline
- Vigabatrin

Patient Education Pearls

- It may take several weeks for medication to demonstrate maximal efficacy. Allow adequate trial before determining effectiveness of medication.
- Patients should not abruptly discontinue their medication. They should consult with a healthcare professional to determine appropriate tapering procedures.
- Patients on MAOIs should avoid excessive caffeine intake, chocolate, and foods containing high levels of tyramine, including red wine, aged cheeses, avocado, eggplant, figs, and soy-based foods.

ANXIETY

Definition

Anxiety disorders consist of a number of conditions, including generalized anxiety disorder (GAD) and panic disorder. This chapter focuses on these two most common subtypes of anxiety disorders. The pathophysiology of anxiety is poorly understood but is theoretically linked to abnormal function of several neurotransmitters, including GABA, serotonin, and norepinephrine.

While OCD and post-traumatic stress disorder (PTSD) are not considered as subtypes of anxiety (i.e., they are considered disorders separate from anxiety in the DSM-5), medications that are indicated to treat these conditions will be outlined in this section.

Diagnosis

GAD diagnosis is based on the presence of anxiety or excessive worry (1) that has been present on most days over at least 6 months, and (2) over which the patient feels a lack of control. Three or more subjective symptoms must be present in order to make the diagnosis.

Panic disorder is a complex disorder characterized by panic attacks. During a panic attack, at least four psychic and somatic symptoms will be present. To be diagnosed with panic disorder, a patient must have a history of recurrent panic attacks

Signs and Symptoms

- Subjective symptoms of GAD include restlessness, feeling easily fatigued, difficulty concentrating, irritability, muscle tension, and sleep difficulties.
- Symptoms of panic disorder include depersonalization, fear of dying, derealization, fear of losing control, and fear of going "crazy."
- Somatic symptoms of panic disorder include sweating, trembling, shaking, choking, chest pain, nausea, abdominal pain, palpitations, tachycardia, shortness of breath, dizziness, lightheadedness, chills, and hot flashes.

Summary of Treatment Recommendations

- Goals of therapy include improvement in overall functionality and quality of life through reduction of symptom frequency and intensity. Complete remission of illness is the long-term treatment goal.

- Treatment options are detailed in the medication charts and no consensus exists as to the preferred initial therapy or order of options thereafter.

- Many clinicians prefer antidepressants (SSRIs, venlafaxine, duloxetine) as initial therapy due to their favorable side-effect profile as compared to other therapies. Benzodiazepines are commonly used, especially in acute situations. Although efficacious, these agents lend themselves to issues related to dependence, ↑ fall risk in the elderly, and potential for negative cognitive effects in general. Buspirone is a unique treatment option that is effective but requires 2 to 3 wk to reach efficacy; thus, it is not useful in acute situations.

- Benzodiazepine selection should take into account varying pharmacokinetic profiles of agents. In elderly patients, preference is given to those agents that are shorter acting (less accumulation) and those metabolized by glucoronidation (e.g., lorazepam, oxazepam) versus oxidation (e.g., alprazolam, diazepam). Agents with a rapid onset have a greater potential for dependence.

Anxiolytics

Generic • Brand • Dose/Dosage Forms	Contraindications	Primary Side Effects	Key Monitoring Parameters	Pertinent Drug Interactions	Med Pearls
Mechanism of action – Benzodiazepines: bind to GABA receptors, causing an influx of chloride which results in hyperpolarization and a less excitable state					
Alprazolam☆ • Xanax, Xanax XR • IR: 0.75–4 mg/day in 2–3 divided doses • ER: 0.5–6 mg daily • ER tabs, ODTs, solution, tabs	• Hypersensitivity • Narrow-angle glaucoma • Concurrent use with ketoconazole or itraconazole (alprazolam) • Significant liver disease (clonazepam) • Myasthenia gravis, severe respiratory impairment, severe liver disease, or sleep apnea (diazepam)	• Somnolence • Ataxia • Dizziness • Changes in appetite • ↓ libido • Confusion • Constipation • Blurred vision • Dependence	• BP • Excessive sedation • Signs of withdrawal • LFTs (for chronic therapy)	• CYP3A4 substrates • CYP3A4 inhibitors may ↑ effects/toxicity • CYP3A4 inducers may ↓ effects • Other CNS depressants, including alcohol, may ↑ CNS depressant effects	• Schedule IV controlled substance • Adjust dose in severe hepatic impairment • Avoid use in pregnancy • Smoking ↓ concentration by up to 50% • Rapid onset, short-acting
Chlordiazepoxide • Librium • 5–25 mg 3–4×/day • Caps					• Schedule IV controlled substance • Avoid in elderly • Avoid use in pregnancy • Slower-onset, long-acting
Clonazepam☆ • Klonopin • 0.25–2 mg BID • ODTs, tabs					• Schedule IV controlled substance • Avoid use in pregnancy • Rapid-onset, long-acting
Clorazepate • Tranxene T-Tab • IR: 3.75–15 mg 2–4×/day • Tabs					• Schedule IV controlled substance • Avoid in elderly • Avoid use in pregnancy • Rapid-onset, long-acting
Diazepam☆ • Diastat, Valium • 2–10 mg PO 2–4×/day • 2–10 mg IV/IM every 3–4 hr PRN • Injection, rectal gel, solution, tabs					• Schedule IV controlled substance • Avoid use in pregnancy • Rapid-onset, long-acting
Lorazepam☆ • Ativan • 0.5–2 mg 2–3×/day (max = 10 mg/day) • Injection, solution, tabs					• Schedule IV controlled substance • Avoid use in pregnancy • Medium-onset, short-acting
Oxazepam • Only availably generically • 10–30 mg 3–4×/day • Caps					• Schedule IV controlled substance • Avoid use in pregnancy • Medium-onset, short-acting

Anxiolytics *(cont'd)*

Generic • Brand • Dose/Dosage Forms	Contraindications	Primary Side Effects	Key Monitoring Parameters	Pertinent Drug Interactions	Med Pearls
Mechanism of action – SSRIs: selectively inhibit the reuptake of serotonin by presynaptic neuronal membranes with little to no effect on norepinephrine or dopamine reuptake					
Citalopram☆ • Celexa • Details in antidepressants table	[See Antidepressants table]		Unlabeled use for panic disorder, GAD, posttraumatic stress disorder (PTSD), and OCD		
Escitalopram☆ • Lexapro • Details in antidepressants table			Indicated for GAD		
Fluoxetine☆ • Prozac, Sarafem • Details in antidepressants table			Indicated for OCD, panic disorder		
Paroxetine☆ • Paxil, Paxil CR • Details in antidepressants table			Indicated for panic disorder, PTSD, GAD, OCD, social anxiety disorder (SAD)		
Sertraline☆ • Zoloft • Details in antidepressants table			Indicated for OCD, panic disorder, SAD, PTSD		
Fluvoxamine • Luvox • Details in antidepressants table			Indicated for OCD		
Mechanism of action – nonselective beta-adrenergic blocker which competitively blocks response to β_1- and β_2-adrenergic stimulation in the heart muscle, vascular smooth muscle, and bronchial muscles					
Propranolol☆ (nonselective) • Inderal, Inderal LA, InnoPran XL • 10–80 mg 1 hr prior to anxiogenic event	• Hypersensitivity • Severe bradycardia • Heart block • Acute decompensated failure • Severe chronic obstructive pulmonary disease (COPD) or asthma	• Dizziness • Fatigue • Bradycardia • Gastrointesinal upset • Hypotension	• HR • BP	Use with other negative chronotropes (e.g., digoxin, verapamil, diltiazem, clonidine, or ivabradine) may ↑ risk of bradycardia	Unlabeled for situational anxiety, acute panic attack

Anxiolytics *(cont'd)*

Generic • Brand • Dose/Dosage Forms	Contraindications	Primary Side Effects	Key Monitoring Parameters	Pertinent Drug Interactions	Med Pearls
Mechanism of action – exact mechanism is unknown; high affinity for 5-HT$_{1A}$ and 5-HT$_2$ receptors, mild affinity for dopamine (D$_2$) receptors					
Buspirone ☆ • Only available generically • 7.5–30 mg BID • Tabs	• Hypersensitivity • Concurrent use with MAOI	• Headache • Dizziness • Nausea • Hostility • Confusion • Drowsiness • Restlessness	• Mental status • Symptoms of anxiety • Pseudo-parkinsonism	• CYP3A4 substrate • CYP3A4 inhibitors may ↑ effects/ toxicity • CYP3A4 inducers may ↓ effects	• Avoid use in severe renal or hepatic impairment • Takes 2–3 wk to reach efficacy
Mechanism of action – SNRIs: inhibit reuptake of neuronal serotonin and norepinephrine; may have weak inhibitory effect on reuptake of dopamine					
Venlafaxine XR ☆ • Effexor XR • Details in antidepressants table	[See Antidepressants table]		Indicated for GAD, panic disorder, SAD; unlabeled use for PTSD and OCD		
Duloxetine • Cymbalta • Details in antidepressants table			Indicated for GAD		
Mechanism of action – competes with histamine for H$_1$-receptor sites on effector cells in GI, blood vessels, and respiratory tract					
Hydroxyzine ☆ • Vistaril • 50–100 mg PO 4×/day • 50–100 mg IM every 4–6 hr PRN • Caps, injection, solution, tabs	• Hypersensitivity • Early pregnancy	• Dizziness • Drowsiness • Fatigue • Xerostomia • Blurry vision • Urinary retention	• BP • Mental status	Other CNS depressants, including alcohol, may ↑ CNS depressant effects	• Use with caution in benign prostatic hyperplasia, respiratory disease, or glaucoma • Avoid in elderly • Adjust dose in renal impairment

Storage and Administration Pearls

- Tablets and capsules should all be stored at room temperature, in dry area out of direct sunlight.
- Keep liquid preparations from freezing or overheating. Do not expose to temperatures >77°F (25°C).

Patient Education Pearls

- Take as directed by physician.
- Patients should *not* abruptly discontinue any anxiety medication.
- Antidepressants may take up to several weeks (2–4 wk) to see effect.
- Patients should avoid alcohol when taking any of these medications.
- Patients should avoid driving or operating heavy machinery while taking benzodiazepines until they know how they respond to the medication.

BIPOLAR DISORDER

Definition

Bipolar disorder is an episodic, lifelong illness with symptoms of depression alternating with symptoms of mania or hypomania. Bipolar disorder is classified on the basis of the frequency of alternating symptoms and the subtype of manic symptoms demonstrated. Bipolar I disorder is defined as one or more manic episodes plus one or more major depressive episodes. Bipolar II disorder is defined as one or more episodes of major depression and one or more hypomanic episodes with no history of a full manic or mixed episode.

Diagnosis

The diagnosis of bipolar disorder is based on the DSM-5 criteria for each of the subtype mood disorders (mania, hypomania, depression, mixed episode). Bipolar disorder diagnosis requires that a patient exhibits diagnosed episodes of both major depression plus manic, hypomanic, or mixed episodes. Acute manic symptoms are hallmarks of the disorder and consist of elevated, expansive, or irritable mood lasting for at least 1 week or requiring hospitalization. Hypomania is defined as symptoms of mania that do not meet the criteria for a manic episode and last for at least 4 days. A mixed episode is one that meets criteria for major depression and a manic episode for at least 1 week.

Signs and Symptoms

Acute mania requires that three of the following symptoms must be present: flight of ideas or racing thoughts, ↓ need for sleep, inflated self-esteem or grandiosity, more talkative than usual or pressured speech, distractibility, psychomotor agitation, and excessive involvement in pleasurable activities with high potential for negative consequences.

Major depressive symptoms are detailed in the Depression section of this chapter.

Guidelines

Texas Implementation of Medication Algorithms: update to the algorithms for the treatment of bipolar disorder. *J Clin Psychiatry.* 2005;66: 870–86.

Guidelines Summary

- First-line treatment options for patient with acute manic episodes include lithium, valproate, aripiprazole, quetiapine, risperidone, ziprasidone, olanzapine, or carbamazepine. Antipsychotic medications are detailed in medication charts later in the Schizophrenia section of this chapter.

- First-line treatment options for acute depressive episodes include lamotrigine monotherapy or lamotrigine in combination with antimania therapy.
- Maintenance therapy generally consists of continuation of therapy used in acute phases. Lithium and valproate have a long history of clinical success in maintenance therapy.

Mood Stabilizers

Generic • Brand • Dose/Dosage Forms	Contraindications	Primary Side Effects	Key Monitoring Parameters	Med Pearls
Mechanism of action – lithium: altered sodium transport leads to a shift toward intraneuronal metabolism of catecholamines; the specific mechanism in mania is not fully understood				
Lithium ☆ • Lithobid • IR: 300–1,800 mg/day in 3–4 divided doses • ER: 450–900 mg BID • Caps, ER tabs, solution, tabs	• Severe renal or cardiovascular disease • Dehydration	• D/V • Drowsiness • Muscle weakness • Lack of coordination • Ataxia • Blurred vision • Tinnitus	Serum drug concentration 0.6–1.2 mEq/L	• Angiotensin-converting enzyme inhibitors, angiotensin II receptor blockers, diuretics, and nonsteroidal anti-inflammtory drugs may ↑ levels and risk of toxicity • Sodium depletion ↑ risk of toxicity
Mechanism of action – valproic acid: not fully understood; thought to ↑ GABA concentrations in the brain				
Valproic acid (divalproex sodium) ☆ • Depakote, Depakote ER, Depakene, Depacon • 10–60 mg/kg/day • Caps, delayed-release caps/tabs, ER tabs, injection, solution, sprinkle caps	[Specific drug details outlined in Epilepsy section of Neurological Disorders chapter]			
Mechanism of action – carbamazepine: inhibits voltage-gated sodium channels, thereby depressing electrical transmission in the nucleus ventralis anterior of the thalamus				
Carbamazepine ☆ • Equetro • 200–1,600 mg/day in 2 divided doses • ER caps	[Specific drug details outlined in Epilepsy section of Neurological Disorders chapter]			
Mechanism of action – lamotrigine: affects sodium channels stabilizing neuronal membranes; the exact mechanism in bipolar disorder is unknown				
Lamotrigine ☆ • Lamictal • 25–700 mg/day in 1–2 divided doses • Chewable tabs, ODTs, tabs	[Specific drug details outlined in Epilepsy section of Neurological Disorders chapter]			

Storage and Administration Pearls

- All medications should be stored at room temperature in a dry area away from direct sunlight.
- Patient may take medications with food if gastrointestinal upset occurs.

Patient Education Pearls

- It is important that medications be continued once the symptoms have resolved.
- Patients should discuss any new medications with a healthcare professional prior to use due to risk of drug interactions.

SCHIZOPHRENIA

Definition

Schizophrenia is a psychiatric disorder that manifests as symptoms including hallucinations or delusions, and has a dramatic impact on the affected individual's functionality and quality of life. The pathophysiology is not fully understood, but theories suggest an excessive firing of dopamine and potential activity of additional neurotransmitters such as norepinephrine, serotonin, and glutamate.

Diagnosis

Persistent disturbances in social, occupational, and self-care functioning must be present for at least 6 months, with 1 month of symptoms including at least two of the following: hallucinations, delusions, disorganized speech, disorganized behavior, or negative symptoms.

Signs and Symptoms

There are multiple subtypes of schizophrenia and symptoms vary widely between them, ranging from catalepsy or stupor to disorganized speech. Potential symptoms include auditory or visual hallucinations, delusions, disorganized speech or behavior, flat or inappropriate affect, and catatonic behavior.

Guidelines

American Psychiatric Association. *Practice Guideline for the Treatment of Patients with Schizophrenia*, 2nd ed. Arlington, VA: American Psychiatric Association; 2004: 1–114. http://psychiatryonline.org/pb/assets/raw/sitewide/practice_guidelines/guidelines/schizophrenia.pdf

Guidelines Summary

For many years, atypical antipsychotics were considered the obvious first-line choice because of significantly reduced incidence of extrapyramidal side effects (EPS). Considerable controversy has surfaced, because of the ability of these medications to ↑ the risk of the metabolic syndrome. Choice of either a typical or atypical antipsychotic is appropriate as first-line therapy. It should be considered, however, that atypical agents have better efficacy in treating negative symptoms associated with schizophrenia.

- Goals of therapy include: Reduce or eliminate symptoms, minimize side effects of pharmacological treatment, and prevent relapse.

- Atypical and typical antipsychotics have similar efficacy profiles. Decision on first-line therapy is based on consideration of side-effect profiles, adherence issues, history of response, and cost.

- EPS are more likely to occur with typical antipsychotics, but may be seen with atypical antipsychotics depending on the agent and dose.

- Neuroleptic malignant syndrome (NMS) is a rare side effect associated with antipsychotic use that presents in less than 1% of patients but may be life threatening if left untreated. NMS is characterized by rigidity, hyperthermia, and autonomic instability; however, elevation of serum creatinine may also been seen. The onset of NMS is generally within a week of starting treatment with an antipsychotic, but may also occur with an ↑ in dose of the antipsychotic. If NMS occurs, antipsychotics should be discontinued and supportive care can be implemented to target hydration as well as cardiovascular and renal symptoms.

Antipsychotics

Generic • Brand • Dose/Dosage Forms	Contraindications	Primary Side Effects	Key Monitoring Parameters	Pertinent Drug Interactions	Med Pearls
Typical Antipsychotics					
Mechanism of action – phenothiazines: block postsynaptic mesolimbic dopaminergic receptors in the brain					
Chlorpromazine • Only available generically • 30–800 mg/day PO in 2–4 divided doses • 25–100 mg IM every 4–6 hr PRN • Injection, tabs	• Hypersensitivity • Severe CNS depression • Coma	• Orthostatic hypotension • Drowsiness • Xerostomia • Constipation • Nausea • Urinary retention • Blurred vision • Photosensitivity • EPS • NMS • QT interval prolongation • Neutropenia	• BP • HR • Mental status • Lipid profile • Fasting blood glucose • Severity of EPS • Complete blood count (CBC) • LFTs • Involuntary movement • S/S of NMS • ECG	• CYP2D6 substrate (all but trifluoperazine and prochlorperazine) • CYP2D6 inhibitors may ↑ effects/toxicity • CYP1A2 substrate (trifluoperazine only) • CYP1A2 inhibitors may ↑ effects/ toxicity • CYP1A2 inducers may ↓ effects • CYP2D6 inhibitor (thioridazine only) • May ↑ effects/ toxicity of CYP2D6 substrates • All may ↑ risk of torsades de pointes (TdP) with other drugs that prolong QT interval	May produce false-positive phenylketonuria and pregnancy test results
Fluphenazine • Only available generically • 2.5–10 mg/day PO in 3–4 divided doses • 1.25–2.5 mg IM every 6–8 hr PRN • Decanoate (long-acting): 12.5–100 mg IM/subcut every 2–4 wk • Injection, injection (long-acting), solution, tabs	• Hypersensitivity • Severe CNS depression • Coma • Subcortical brain damage • Blood dyscrasias • Liver disease				
Perphenazine • Only available generically • 4–16 mg 2–4×/day • Tabs					
Trifluoperazine • Only avaialble generically • 2–20 mg BID • Tabs					May produce false-positive phenylketonuria test results
Prochlorperazine☆ • Compro • 15–150 mg/day PO in 3–4 divided doses • 10–20 mg IM every 4–6 hr PRN • Injection, rectal suppository, tabs					May produce false-positive phenylketonuria and pregnancy test results
Thioridazine • Only available generically • 300–800 mg/day in 2–4 divided doses • Tabs					May produce false-positive methadone and phencyclidine results

Antipsychotics *(cont'd)*

Generic • Brand • Dose/Dosage Forms	Contraindications	Primary Side Effects	Key Monitoring Parameters	Pertinent Drug Interactions	Med Pearls
Mechanism of action – not well established; thought to block postsynaptic mesolimbic dopaminergic D_2 receptors in the brain					
Haloperidol ☆ • Haldol, Haldol Deconoate • 0.5–5 mg PO 2–3×/day • 2–5 mg IM every 4–8 hr PRN • Decanoate (long-acting): 10–15× the daily PO dose (max = 200 mg) IM every 4 wk • Injection, injection (long-acting), solution, tabs	• Hypersensitivity • Parkinson's disease • Severe CNS depression • Coma	• Xerostomia • Drowsiness • Constipation • Nausea • Urinary retention • Blurred vision • EPS • Priapism • QT interval prolongation • NMS • Neutropenia	• BP • HR • CBC • Mental status • ECG • EPS • Involuntary movement • S/S of NMS • LFTs	• CYP2D6 and CYP3A4 substrate • CYP2D6 or CYP3A4 inhibitors may ↑ effects/ toxicity • CYP3A4 inducers may ↓ effects • May ↑ risk of TdP with other drugs that prolong QT interval	• IM decanoate form uses sesame oil • Immediate-release injection may also be given IV in ICU setting for treatment of delirium
Mechanism of action – a potent, centrally acting dopamine-receptor antagonist					
Pimozide • Orap • 1–2 mg/day in divided doses (max = 0.2 mg/kg/day or 10 mg/ day, whichever is less) • Tabs	• Severe CNS depression • Coma • History of arrhythmias • Congenital long QT syndrome • Concurrent use with other QT in-terval prolonging medications • Hypokalemia or hypomagnesemia • Concurrent use with 3A4 inhibi-tors • Concurrent use with citalopram, escitalopram, or sertraline	• Somnolence • Drowsiness • Rash • Xerostomia • Constipation • Diarrhea • ↑ appetite • Taste disturbance • Impotence • Weakness • Visual disturbances • Speech disorder • Hypotension • QT interval prolongation • EPS • NMS • Neutropenia	• BP • HR • CBC • Mental status • ECG • EPS • Involuntary movement • S/S of NMS • LFTs	• CYP1A2, CYP2D6, and CYP3A4 substrate • CYP1A2, CYP2D6 or CYP3A4 inhibitors may ↑ effects/ toxicity • CYP1A2 or CYP3A4 inducers may ↓ effects • May ↑ risk of TdP with other drugs that prolong QT interval	FDA-labeled for Tourette's disorder

Antipsychotics (cont'd)

Generic • Brand • Dose/Dosage Forms	Contraindications	Primary Side Effects	Key Monitoring Parameters	Pertinent Drug Interactions	Med Pearls
Mechanism of action – blocks postsynaptic mesolimbic D_1 and D_2 receptors in the brain, and also possesses serotonin 5-HT$_2$ blocking activity					
Loxapine • Adasuve • 20–250 mg/day PO in 2–4 divided doses • 10 mg via inhalation daily • Caps, inhalation	*PO:* • Hypersensitivity • Severe CNS depression • Coma *Inhalation:* • Hypersensitivity • Asthma, COPD, or other bronchospastic disease • Acute wheezing	• Hypotension • N/V • Constipation • Xerostomia • Weakness • Sexual dysfunction • Dizziness • EPS • NMS • Seizures	• BP • HR • Mental status • EPS • S/S of NMS • CBC • Involuntary movement • S/S of bronchospasm (with inhalation)	No significant CYP450 interactions	May produce false-positive phenylketonuria test results
Mechanism of action – exerts effect on the ascending reticular activating system					
Molindone • Only available generically • 30–100 mg/day in 3–4 divided doses • Tabs	• Hypersensitivity • Severe CNS depression • Coma	• Drowsiness • Xerostomia • Constipation • Hypotension • Tachycardia • EPS • NMS	• BP • HR • Mental status • EPS • Involuntary movement • S/S of NMS • CBC	No significant CYP450 interactions	
Mechanism of action – blocks postsynaptic dopamine receptors, resulting in inhibition of dopamine-mediated effects; also has alpha-adrenergic blocking activity					
Thiothixene • Navane • 6–60 mg/day in 2–3 divided doses • Caps	• Hypersensitivity • Severe CNS depression • Coma • Blood dyscrasias	• Hypotension • Dizziness • N/V • Constipation • Sexual dysfunction • Tachycardia • Insomnia • EPS • NMS	• BP • HR • CBC • Mental status • EPS • Involuntary movement • S/S of NMS	• CYP1A2 substrate • CYP1A2 inhibitors may ↑ effects/toxicity • CYP1A2 inducers may ↓ effects	May cause false-positive pregnancy test results

Antipsychotics *(cont'd)*

Generic • Brand • Dose/Dosage Forms	Contraindications	Primary Side Effects	Key Monitoring Parameters	Pertinent Drug Interactions	Med Pearls
Atypical Antipsychotics					
Mechanism of action – mixed and varied (per agent) D_2/5-HT_2 antagonist activity					
Aripiprazole ☆ Abilify (PO): • 10–30 mg PO daily • ODTs, solution, tabs Abilify Maintena (ER IM injection): • 400 mg IM monthly (doses must be ≥26 days apart) Aristada (ER IM injection): • 441–882 mg IM every 4–6 wk	• Hypersensitivity • Severe hepatic impairment (asenapine)	• Weight gain • Constipation • N/V/D • Akathisia • Hyperglyce-mia • Hyperlipid-emia • Anxiety • Sedation • QT interval prolongation • Orthostatic hypotension • Tachycardia • Neutropenia • Hyperpro-lactinemia (rare) • EPS (rare) • NMS	• Fasting plasma glucose • Fasting lipid panel • CBC • BP • HR • ECG • Weight/body mass index • Mental status • EPS • S/S of NMS	Aripiprazole and brexpiprazole: • CYP2D6 and CYP3A4 substrate • CYP2D6 or CYP3A4 inhibi-tors may ↑ ef-fects/toxicity • CYP3A4 inducers may ↓ effects Olanzapine, asenapine, and clozapine: • CYP1A2 substrate • CYP1A2 inhibi-tors may ↑ ef-fects/toxicity • CYP1A2 inducers may ↓ effects Quetiapine, lurasidone, and cariprazine: • CYP3A4 substrate • CYP3A4 inhibi-tors may ↑ ef-fects/toxicity • CYP3A4 inducers may ↓ effects Iloperidone and risperidone: • CYP2D6 substrate • CYP2D6 inhibitors may ↑ effects/ toxicity • All may ↑ risk of TdP with other drugs that prolong QT interval	• Among the lowest risk of metabolic syndrome • Also indicated to treat acute manic and mixed episodes associated with bipolar I disorder, major depressive disorder (as adjunctive therapy), irritabilty with autistic disorder, and Tourette's disorder

Antipsychotics *(cont'd)*

Generic • Brand • Dose/Dosage Forms	Contraindications	Primary Side Effects	Key Monitoring Parameters	Pertinent Drug Interactions	Med Pearls
Olanzapine ☆ Zyprexa (PO, immediate-release IM injection), Zyprexa Zydis (ODT): • 5–20 mg PO daily • 10–30 mg/dose IM • IM (immediate release), ODTs, tabs Zyprexa Relprevv (ER IM injection): • 150–405 mg IM (max = 300 mg every 2 wk or 405 mg every 4 wk)	[Same as above]	[Same as above]	[Same as above]	[Same as above]	• Higher degree of weight gain than some other atypicals • Oral formulations also indicated to treat acute and chronic manic and mixed episodes associated with bipolar I disorder • Immediate-release IM injection indicated to treat acute agitation associated with schizophrenia and bipolar I mania
Paliperidone ☆ Invega (ER tabs): • 3–12 mg PO daily Invega Sustenna (monthly ER IM injection): • 39–234 mg IM monthly Invega Trinza (every 3 mo ER IM injection): • 273–819 mg IM every 3 mo					• Major active metabolite of risperidone • Invega Trinza should only be used in patients who have been stabilized with Invega Sustenna for ≥4 mo
Quetiapine ☆ • Seroquel, Seroquel XR • IR: 50–750 mg/day in 2–3 divided doses • ER: 300–800 mg daily • ER tabs, tabs					• ER tabs usually dosed at bed time due to somnolence • Also indicated for manic and depressive episodes associated with bipolar I disorder
Iloperidone • Fanapt • 1–12 mg BID • Tabs					• Lower risk of weight gain than many atypicals • Low risk of somnolence • May improve cognitive function
Asenapine • Saphris • 5–10 mg BID • SL tabs					• Very low incidence of EPS • Also indicated to treat acute manic and mixed episodes associated with bipolar I disorder
Risperidone ☆ Risperdal, Risperdal M-Tab: • 2–16 mg/day PO in 1–2 divided doses • ODTs, solution, tabs Risperdal Consta (ER IM injection) • 25–50 mg IM every 2 wk					• Sedation often leads to bed time dosing • Oral formulations also indicated to treat acute manic and mixed episodes associated with bipolar I disorder and irritabilty with autistic disorder • ER IM injection also indicated for maintenance treatment of bipolar I disorder

Antipsychotics (cont'd)

Generic • Brand • Dose/Dosage Forms	Contraindications	Primary Side Effects	Key Monitoring Parameters	Pertinent Drug Interactions	Med Pearls
Ziprasidone ☆ • Geodon • 20–100 mg PO BID • 10 mg IM every 2 hr or 20 mg IM every 4 hr • Caps, injection	• Hypersensitivity • Decompensated heart failure • Recent MI • History of QT interval prolongation • Concurrent use of QT interval prolonging medications	[Same as above]	[Same as above]	[Same as above]	• Lower risk of metabolic syndrome when compared to other atypicals • Oral formulation also indicated to treat acute manic and mixed episodes associated with bipolar I disorder and for maintenance treatment of bipolar I disorder • IM injection indicated to treat acute agitation associated with schizophrenia
Lurasidone • Latuda • 40–160 mg daily • Tabs	• Hypersensitivity • Concurrent use with strong 3A4 inhibitors or inducers				Also indicated for treatment of depressive episodes associated with bipolar I disorder
Brexpiprazole • Rexulti • 1–4 mg daily • Tabs	Hypersensitivity				Also indicated as adjunctive therapy for major depressive disorder
Cariprazine • Vraylar • 1.5–6 mg daily • Caps					Also indicated to treat acute manic and mixed episodes associated with bipolar I disorder
Clozapine ☆ • Clozaril, FazaClo, Versacloz • 12.5–900 mg/day in 1–3 divided doses • ODTs, suspension, tabs		• Orthostatic hypotension • Bradycardia • QT interval prolongation • Hyperglycemia • Hyperlipidemia • Weight gain • Agranulocytosis • NMS	• WBC and absolute neutrophil count weekly for 6 mo, then every 2 wk for 6 mo, then every 4 wk • Fasting plasma glucose • Fasting lipid panel • BP • HR • ECG • Weight/body mass index • Mental status • S/S of NMS		• Used less frequently than other atypicals due to requirement for frequent monitoring • Effective in treatment of refractory cases and in patients at high risk for suicide

Storage and Administration Pearls

- All medications should be stored at room temperature in a dry area away from direct sunlight.
- Patient may take medications with food if gastrointestinal upset occurs.

Patient Education Pearls

- Grapefruit juice should be avoided when taking medications that are 3A4 substrates.
- Alcohol should be avoided due to excessive CNS depression.
- Driving or operating heavy machinery should be avoided until patients know how they respond to medication.
- All medications can take up to several weeks (2–4 weeks) to see full effect.
- Medications should *not* be abruptly discontinued.
- Patients should not self-adjust dose.
- Patients should report to a physician any side effects that disrupt their daily life (i.e., EPS).

SLEEP DISORDERS

Insomnia

Definition

According to the American Academy of Sleep Medicine, insomnia is the subjective perception of difficulty with sleep initiation, duration, consolidation, or quality that occurs despite adequate opportunity for sleep that results in some form of daytime impairment.

Diagnosis

The diagnosis of insomnia is made primarily based upon patient history with assessment of complaints, pre-sleep conditions, sleep-wake patterns, other symptoms, and daytime consequences. Some instruments that may aid in diagnosis include patient questionnaires, sleep diaries, polysomnography, symptom checklists, and psychological assessments. Diagnostic criteria include:

- Complaint of difficulty initiating sleep, maintaining sleep, waking too early, or sleep that is of nonrestorative/poor quality. This difficulty occurs despite adequate opportunity and circumstances for sleep.

- At least one form of daytime impairment is reported: fatigue, impairment in concentration/attention/memory, social/vocational impairment, poor school performance, mood disturbance/irritability, daytime sleepiness, ↓ motivation/energy/initiation, proneness for errors/accidents, tension, headaches, or gastrointestinal symptoms in response to sleep loss, concerns, or worries about sleep.

Signs and Symptoms

Detailed in the diagnostic description, most patients complain of difficulty with falling asleep, staying asleep, or with chronically nonrestorative/quality sleep. These common complaints may also be accompanied by other nocturnal symptoms including snoring, coughing, kicking, restlessness, walking/movement, vocalization, pain, or anxiety.

Guidelines

Schutte-Rodin S, Broch L, Buysse D, Dorsey C, Sateia M. Clinical guideline for the evaluation and management of chronic insomnia in adults. *J Clin Sleep Med.* 2008;4:487–504.

Guideline Summary

- Goals of therapy: Improve quality and quantity of sleep and improve daytime sleep-related impairment.

- All patients should be educated about good sleep hygiene. Nonpharmacological measures are the preferred initial treatment.

- Pharmacological therapy should be combined with behavioral therapy to achieve the best results.

- Medication selection is based upon the following patient-specific elements: (1) symptom pattern, (2) patient preference, (3) availability, (4) cost, (5) prior response, (6) comorbid conditions, (7) contraindications, (8) concurrent medications, (9) side effect profile, and (10) treatment goals.

- Pharmacological classes for insomnia include benzodiazepines, benzodiazepine receptor agonists (BzRA), melatonin receptor agonists, and sedating antidepressants.

- Short-intermediate acting BzRAs, benzodiazepines, or melatonin receptor agonists are first-line therapy options for most patients. BzRAs and benzodiazepines ideally should be limited to short-term use (7–10 days); however, there is limited evidence to support use extended to 6–12 months.

- Inadequate response after an initial trial of the above agents can be followed with a trial on a second agent from within these therapeutic class options.

- Third-line options include sedating antidepressants or off-label combination therapy or self-care therapies such as antihistamines.

Treatment Algorithm

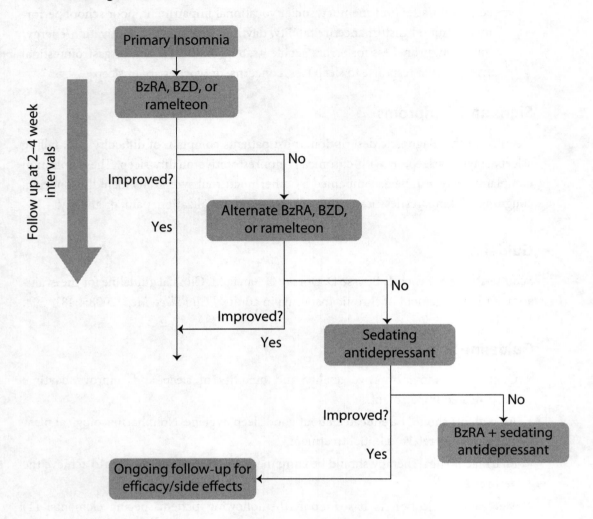

Medications for Insomnia

Generic • Brand • Dose/Dosage Forms	Contra-indications	Primary Side Effects	Key Monitoring	Pertinent Drug Interactions	Med Pearl
Benzodiazepine receptor agonists (schedule IV controlled substances)					
Mechanism of action – enhances GABA through stimulation of the benzodiazepine 1 receptor, which results in hyperpolarization and a ↓ in neuronal excitabilty with sedative and hypnotic effects					
Eszopiclone☆ • Lunesta • 1–3 mg at bedtime • Tabs	Hypersensitivity	• Headache • Taste disturbance • Xerostomia • Dizziness • Nausea • Somnolence • Sleep-related activities: hazardous activities such as sleep-driving and cooking have been reported (rare), incidence ↑ with alcohol use or using above max doses • Behavior changes such as ↓ inhibition, aggression, agitation, hallucinations, and depersonalization (rare)	• Improvement in sleep quality/ quantity • Presence of side effects	• CYP3A4 substrate • CYP3A4 inhibitors may ↑ effects/ toxicity • CYP3A4 inducers may ↓ effects • Other CNS depressants, including alcohol, may ↑ CNS depressant effects	High-fat/heavy meal will delay absorption; administer on an empty stomach
Zolpidem☆ • Ambien, Ambien CR, Zolpimist • IR or oral spray: 5–10 mg PO at bedtime (max = 5 mg for females) • CR: 6.25–12.5 mg PO at bedtime (max = 6.25 mg for females) • ER tabs, oral spray, tabs • Edluar, Intermezzo (SL tabs) • Edluar: 5–10 mg/night SL (max = 5 mg for females) • Intermezzo: 1.75–3.5 mg/ night SL (max = 1.75 mg for females)					• Take IR tabs, ER tabs, oral spray, and SL tabs (Edluar only) immediately before bedtime • SL tabs (Intermezzo only) helpful for nighttime awakenings; take in bed if patient awakes in the middle of the night (only if ≥4 hr remain before waking) and there is difficulty in returning to sleep • Place SL tabs under the tongue and allow to disintegrate; do not chew or swallow • Heavy/high-fat meal will delay absorption; administer on an empty stomach
Zaleplon • Sonata • 5–20 mg PO at bedtime • Caps					• Heavy/high-fat meal will delay absorption; administer on an empty stomach • Headache incidence = 30–40%

Medications for Insomnia *(cont'd)*

Generic • Brand • Dose/Dosage Forms	Contra-indications	Primary Side Effects	Key Monitoring	Pertinent Drug Interactions	Med Pearl
Benzodiazepines (schedule IV controlled substances)					
Mechanism of action – bind to GABA A receptors to enhance inhibitory effect of GABA on neuronal excitability					
Estazolam • Only available generically • 1–2 mg PO at bedtime • Tabs	• Pregnancy • Narrow-angle glaucoma • Concurrent use with itraconazole or ketoconazole	• Somnolence • Dizziness • Hypokinesia • Hangover effect • Abnormal coordination • Confusion • Xerostomia • Constipation	• Improvement in sleep quality/ quantity • Presence of side effects	• CYP3A4 substrate • CYP3A4 inhibitors may ↑ effects/ toxicity • CYP3A4 inducers may ↓ effects • Other CNS depressants, including alcohol, may ↑ CNS depressant effects	• Time to peak 0.5–6 hr; $T_{1/2}$ 10–24 hr • Administer on an empty stomach
Temazepam ☆ • Restoril • 7.5–30 mg PO at bedtime • Caps	• Pregnancy • Narrow-angle glaucoma				Time to peak 1.2–1.6 hr; $T_{1/2}$ 3.5–18 hr
Triazolam • Halcion • 0.125–0.5 mg PO at bedtime • Tabs	• Pregnancy • Narrow-angle glaucoma • Concurrent use with itraconazole, ketoconazole, nefazodone, or protease inhibitors				• Time to peak 1–2 hr; $T_{1/2}$ 1.5–5.5 hr • Administer on an empty stomach
Flurazepam • Only available generically • 15–30 mg PO at bedtime (max = 15 mg for females) • Caps	• Pregnancy • Narrow-angle glaucoma				Time to peak 3–6 hr; $T_{1/2}$ 2.5 hr (active metabolite ~70 hr)

Medications for Insomnia *(cont'd)*

Generic • Brand • Dose/Dosage Forms	Contra-indications	Primary Side Effects	Key Monitoring	Pertinent Drug Interactions	Med Pearl
Melatonin Receptor Agonists					
Mechanism of action – MT1 and MT2 receptor agonist					
Ramelteon • Rozerem • 8 mg within 30 min of bedtime • Tabs	• Angioedema with prior use • Concurrent use with fluvoxamine	• Anaphylaxis/angioedema • Dizziness • Fatigue • Depression • Sleep-related activities: hazardous activities such as sleep-driving and cooking have been reported (rare), incidence ↑ with alcohol use • Behavior changes such as agitation, hallucinations, and mania	• Improvement in sleep quality/quantity • Presence of side effects	• CYP1A2 substrate • CYP1A2 inhibitors may ↑ effects/toxicity • CYP1A2 inducers may ↓ effects • Other CNS depressants, including alcohol, may ↑ CNS depressant effects	• Not a scheduled/controlled substance • Heavy/high-fat meal will delay absorption; administer on an empty stomach
Tasimelteon • Hetlioz • 20 mg PO at bedtime • Caps	None	• Drowsiness • Headache • Abnormal dreams • ↑ LFTs	• Improvement in sleep quality/quantity • Presence of side effects • LFTs	• CYP1A2 and CYP3A4 substrate • CYP1A2 and CYP3A4 inhibitors may ↑ effects/toxicity • CYP1A2 and CYP3A4 inducers may ↓ effects • Other CNS depressants, including alcohol, may ↑ CNS depressant effects	• Indicated for non-24-hour sleep-wake disorder • Should be taken at the same time each night • Not a scheduled/controlled substance • May take weeks to months to see effect • Administer on an empty stomach

Medications for Insomnia *(cont'd)*

Generic • Brand • Dose/Dosage Forms	Contra-indications	Primary Side Effects	Key Monitoring	Pertinent Drug Interactions	Med Pearl
Orexin Receptor Antagonist					
Mechanism of action – antagonizes OX1R and OX2R which blocks the binding of wake-promoting compounds orexin A and orexin B					
Suvorexant • Belsomra • 10–20 mg PO at bedtime	Narcolepsy	• Drowsiness • Headache • Dizziness • Sleep-related activities: hazardous activities such as sleep-driving and cooking have been reported (rare), incidence ↑ with alcohol or other CNS depressant use or using above max doses • Depression • Abnormal dreams	• Improvement in sleep quality/quantity • Presence of side effects	• CYP3A4 substrate • CYP3A4 inhibitors may ↑ effects/toxicity • CYP3A4 inducers may ↓ effects	• Schedule IV controlled substance • Should be taken with ≥7 hr remaining before planned time of awakening • Heavy/high-fat meal will delay absorption; administer on an empty stomach

Storage and Administration Pearls

- Intermezzo should be taken in bed if patient wakes in the middle of the night (i.e., if ≥ 4 hours left before desired wake time) and has difficulty returning to sleep.
- Zolpidem CR tablets should be swallowed whole; do not divide, crush, or chew.
- Zolpidem SL tablets should be placed under the tongue and allowed to disintegrate; do not swallow or administer with water.
- Zolpidem oral spray should be sprayed directly into the mouth over the tongue. Prior to initial use, pump should be primed by spraying 5 times. If pump is not used for at least 14 days, reprime pump with 1 spray.

Patient Education Pearls

- Proper sleep hygiene is essential for effective insomnia management.
  - Avoid daytime naps.
  - Keep the bedroom dark, comfortable, and free from noise/distractions.
  - Stay on a routine sleep schedule.
  - Avoid heavy meals and exercise prior to bedtime.

- Avoid caffeine in the evening.
- Limit liquid consumption in the evening.

■ Benzodiazepines and BzRAs should be reserved for short-term use in most instances. Some patients may require use for longer periods; however, need should be re-evaluated every 6 months.

■ Benzodiazepines and BzRAs should not be abruptly discontinued following long-term use due to the potential for withdrawal. Patient should work with their health care provider to determine an appropriate dosage taper.

■ BzRAs, melatonin receptor agonists, and the orexin receptor antagonist should not be taken with heavy/high-fat meal due to the potential for delayed absorption; therefore, take on an empty stomach.

Restless Leg Syndrome

Definition

Restless leg syndrome (RLS) is disorder of the nervous system that causes a need for leg movement. Patients generally experience uncomfortable sensations that produce the urge to move the legs to resolve the sensations.

Diagnosis

Four main features are associated with RLS:

■ There is an urge to move the limb that is associated with paresthesias or dysesthesias.
■ Symptoms are worse with rest.
■ Relief of symptoms may be seen with physical activity.
■ Symptoms worsen at night.

Signs and Symptoms

Symptoms include unpleasant sensations of aching, burning, tingling, itching, pins and needles, or a creepy-crawly feeling that produces the need to move the legs. Rest generally causes worsening of symptoms, while physical activity produces relief of symptoms. Patients may complain of poor sleep or report kicking their bed partner.

Guidelines

Aurora RN, Kristo DA, Bista SR, et al. The treatment of restless legs syndrome and periodic limb movement disorder in adults—an update for 2012: practice parameters with an evidence-based systematic review and meta-analyses: an American Academy of Sleep Medicine Clinical Practice Guideline. *Sleep.* 2012;35:1039–62.

Guidelines Summary

- First-line options for the treatment of RLS include ropinirole and pramipexole.
- Other treatment options include carbidopa/levodopa, opioids, gabapentin enacarbil, gabapentin, and pregabalin.

Drug Treatment

Please see the medication chart in the Parkinson's Disease section of the Neurological Disorders chapter for more specific information on ropinirole, pramipexole, and carbidopa/levodopa. Please see the medication chart in the Epilepsy section of the Neurological Disorders chapter for more specific information on gabapentin and pregabalin.

Storage and Administration

- Medications should be stored in a dry place and protected from light.

Patient Education Pearls

- Hallucinations, delusions, or strange dreams should be immediately reported to a physician.

Narcolepsy

Definition

Narcolepsy is a condition marked by excessive daytime drowsiness and intermittent periods of rapid eye movement (REM) sleep while awake.

Diagnosis

Diagnosis of narcolepsy starts with assessment of symptoms. The diagnosis is often delayed due to vague symptoms of sleepiness which could be attributed to other causes. Tests such as a polysomnogram or a sleep latency test may be administered for a definitive diagnosis.

Signs and Symptoms

Common symptoms of narcolepsy include excessive daytime sedation and cataplexy (sudden, transient periods of muscle weakness in full consciousness, often evoked by periods of emotion). Other symptoms include hallucinations, sleep paralysis, brief periods of sleep while still functioning, nighttime wakefulness, and REM sleep upon falling asleep.

Guidelines

Morgenthaler TI, Kapur VK, Brown T, et al. Practice parameters for the treatment of narcolepsy and other hypersomnias of central origin. *Sleep*. 2007;30:1705–11.

Guidelines Summary

- First-line treatment options for excessive daytime sedation include modafinil, sodium oxybate, stimulants (amphetamine, methamphetamine, dextroamphetamine, methylphenidate) and selegiline. For information on the stimulants, please see the Attention-Deficit Hyperactivity Disorder (ADHD) section in this chapter. For information on selegiline, please see the Parkinson's Disease section in the Neurological Disorders chapter.

- TCAs and fluoxetine may be used for the treatment of cataplexy. Please see the Depression section of this chapter for more information regarding these medications.

- Nonpharmacologic treatment includes scheduled naps.

Medications for Narcolepsy

Generic • Brand • Dose/Dosage Forms	Contraindications	Primary Side Effects	Key Monitoring	Pertinent Drug Interactions	Med Pearl
Mechanism of action – binds to the dopamine receptor and inhibits dopamine reuptake					
Modafinil • Provigil • 200 mg daily • Tabs	Hypersensitivity	• Rash (Stevens-Johnson syndrome possible) • Angioedema • Headache • Nervousness • Anxiety • Dizziness • Insomnia • Hypertension • N/D	• Level of alertness • BP • Exacerbation of agitation, anxiety, depression	• CYP3A4 substrate and inducer • CYP2C19 inhibitor • CYP3A4 inhibitors may ↑ effects/ toxicity • CYP3A4 inducers may ↓ effects • May ↑ effects/ toxicity of CYP2C19 substrates • May ↓ effects of CYP3A4 substrates • May ↓ effects of hormonal contraceptives during and for 1 mo after discontinuing treatment	• Schedule IV controlled substance • If used for narcolepsy or obstructive sleep apnea/ hypopnea, administer dose in the morning • If used for shift work sleep disorder, administer dose 1 hr before work
Armodafinil • Nuvigil • 150–250 mg daily • Tabs					• R-enantiomer of modafinil • Schedule IV controlled substance • If used for narcolepsy or obstructive sleep apnea, administer dose in the morning • If used for shift work sleep disorder, administer dose 1 hr before work
Mechanism of action – derivative of GABA that serves as an inhibitory transmitter					
Sodium oxybate • Xyrem • Initial: 2.25 g at bedtime after patient in bed, then 2.25 g 2.5–4 hr later; titrate dose to usual effective dose of 6–9 g per night • Solution	Concurrent use with alcohol or sedative hypnotic agents	• Dizziness • N/V • Somnolence • Enuresis • Tremor • Confusion • Anxiety • Sleepwalking • Depression	• Drug abuse • Depression or suicidality • Mental status	• CNS depressants, including alcohol, may ↑ CNS depressant effects • Divalproex sodium may ↑ effects/ toxicity; ↓ sodium oxybate dose by 20%	• Schedule III controlled substance • 1.1 g Na^+ in 6 g nightly dose • Administer on an empty stomach

Storage and Administration

- Medications should be stored in a dry place and protected from light.

Patient Education Pearls

- Modafinil and armodafinil should be taken in the morning for narcolepsy or obstructive sleep apnea.

- Sodium oxybate should be taken at night and patients should avoid alcohol or use of sedatives and hypnotics.

ATTENTION DEFICIT HYPERACTIVITY DISORDER (ADHD)

Definition

ADHD is a chronic illness that often initially presents in childhood and may persist into adulthood. Patients affected exhibit core symptoms include inattention, hyperactivity and/or impulsivity.

Diagnosis

The diagnosis of ADHD is based upon the DSM-5. Criteria provide examples of inattention and hyperactivity/impulsivity and require a persistent pattern of at least six symptoms of either inattention or hyperactivity/impulsivity that have been present for at least 6 mo and that interfere with functioning or development. Criteria further specify that several symptoms were present prior to age 12 and in two or more settings.

Signs and Symptoms

- Inattention:
  - Failure to pay attention
  - Trouble holding attention
  - Lack of follow-through on instructions
  - Failure to finish schoolwork
  - Difficulty organizing tasks
  - Avoidance/dislike of tasks requiring mental effort
  - Loss of things/demonstrates forgetfulness
  - Easy distractibility
- Hyperactivity/impulsivity:
  - Fidgets/squirms
  - Leaves seat unexpectedly
  - Inability to play quietly
  - Excessive talking
  - Trouble waiting
  - Interrupts/intrudes
  - Blurts out answer/responses
  - Runs around when not appropriate
  - Inability to keep still

Guidelines

Subcommittee on Attention-Deficit/Hyperactivity Disorder; Steering Committee on Quality Improvement and Management. Wolraich M, Brown L, Brown RT, et al. ADHD: clinical practice guideline for the diagnosis, evaluation, and treatment of attention-deficit/hyperactivity disorder in children and adolescents. *Pediatrics* 2011;128:1007–22.

Guideline Summary

- First-line pharmacologic therapy for ADHD includes stimulant medications. Approved options included methylphenidate, dexmethylphenidate, dextroamphetamine, dextroamphetamine + amphetamine, and lisdexamfetamine.

- Nonstimulant options approved for ADHD are generally reserved for one of the following: concerns related to abuse/diversion, strong family/patient preference for nonstimulant medications, or as adjunctive therapy to stimulants. Options include atomoxetine, guanfacine, and clonidine. Of these options, atomoxetine monotherapy is preferred to guanfacine and clonidine, which are generally reserved for adjunctive therapy.

- When selecting a stimulant, patient-specific factors such as ability to swallow tablets/capsules, affordability, number of daily doses required, and presence of a tic disorder are considerations.

- Interpatient variability in efficacy is recognized and alternate stimulant agents are recommended as second- and third-line options after appropriate titration to maximal effective/tolerated dose of initial stimulant selected.

Medications for Attention Deficit Hyperactivity Disorder

Generic • Brand • Dose & Max	Contraindications	Primary Side Effects	Key Monitoring	Pertinent Drug Interactions	Med Pearl
Stimulants					
Methylphenidate IR☆ • Ritalin, Methylin • 10–60 mg/day in 2–3 divided doses • Chewable tabs, solution, tabs **Methylphenidate ER** • Aptensio XR: 10–60 mg daily • Concerta: 18–72 mg every morning • Metadate CD: 10–60 mg daily • Quillichew ER: 10–60 mg every morning • Quillivant XR: 10–60 mg every morning • Ritalin LA: 10–60 mg daily • Ritalin SR: 10–60 mg/day in 2–3 divided doses • ER Caps, ER chewable tabs, ER suspension, ER tabs **Methylphenidate transdermal patch** • Daytrana • Initial: 10-mg patch daily; titrate to effect	• Anxiety • Tension • Agitation • Glaucoma • Motor tics • Recent MAOI use (within 14 days) • Family history or diagnosis of Tourette's syndrome	General • Anorexia • Nausea • Weight loss • Insomnia • Dizziness • Lightheadedness • Irritability • ↑ sweating • Blurred vision • Priapism • Growth suppression • Peripheral vasculopathy (Raynaud's) • Dependence Cardiovascular • ↑ BP • Tachycardia Psychiatric • May exacerbate anxiety, mania, aggression, hostility, or depression • Use with caution in patients with pre-existing psychiatric conditions	• Resolution of symptoms • BP • HR • Height/weight • ECG at baseline and if chest pain or syncope • Signs of misuse/ abuse	MAOIs require 14-day washout period prior to stimulant initiation	• Schedule II controlled substance • Black box: Potential for dependency • Generally taken every morning to avoid insomnia • Remove patch after 9 hr of wear; alternate application site (hips) • Withdrawal potential; titrate slowly and taper upon discontinuation • Also indicated for narcolepsy
Dexmethylphenidate IR • Focalin, Focalin XR • IR: 2.5–10 mg BID • ER: 5–40 mg every morning • ER caps, tabs					• Schedule II controlled substance (prescriptions issued 1 mo at a time) • Black box: Potential for dependency • ER generally taken q A.M. to avoid insomnia • For IR, 1st dose given q A.M., 2nd dose given at least 4 hr later • Withdrawal potential; titrate slowly and taper upon discontinuation

Medications for Attention Deficit Hyperactivity Disorder *(cont'd)*

Generic • Brand • Dose & Max	Contraindications	Primary Side Effects	Key Monitoring	Pertinent Drug Interactions	Med Pearl
Dextroamphetamine and amphetamine ☆ • IR only available generically, Adderall XR • IR: 5–40 mg/day in 1-3 divided doses • ER: 5–30 mg every morning • ER caps, tabs	[Same as above]	[Same as above]	[Same as above]	[Same as above]	• Schedule II controlled substance • Black box: Potential for dependency • ER generally taken q A.M. to avoid insomnia • Withdrawal potential; titrate slowly and taper upon discontinuation • IR also indicated for narcolepsy
Dextroamphetamine • IR only available generically, Dexedrine Spansules (ER) • IR: 2.5–40 mg/day in 1–2 divided doses • ER: 5-40 mg/day in 1–2 divided doses • ER caps, solution, tabs					• Schedule II controlled substance • Black box: Potential for dependency • ER generally taken q A.M. to avoid insomnia • For IR, 1st dose given q A.M., 2nd dose given 4–6 hr later • Withdrawal potential; titrate slowly and taper upon discontinuation • Also indicated for narcolepsy
Lisdexamfetamine ☆ • Vyvanse • 30–70 mg every morning • Caps					• Schedule II controlled substance • Black box: Potential for dependency • Prodrug of dextro-amphetamine; rapid effect muted if injected or snorted (designed to decrease abuse potential) • Contents can be mixed with water—drink immediately • Withdrawal potential; titrate slowly and taper upon discontinuation • Also indicated for binge eating disorder

Medications for Attention Deficit Hyperactivity Disorder *(cont'd)*

Generic • Brand • Dose & Max	Contraindications	Primary Side Effects	Key Monitoring	Pertinent Drug Interactions	Med Pearl
Nonstimulants					
Atomoxetine ☆ • Strattera • 40–100 mg/ day in 1–2 divided doses • Caps	• Narrow-angle glaucoma • Pheochromocytoma • Recent MAOI use (within 14 days) • Cardiovascular conditions that may worsen with ↑ BP or HR	• Headache • Insomnia • Nausea • Anorexia • Somnolence • Xerostomia • Menstrual changes • Orthostasis • Urinary hesitancy/ retention • Growth suppression • Can exacerbate pre-existing psychiatric illness, including hallucinations/mania • Priapism • Suicidal ideation • Liver injury (rare)	• Resolution of symptoms • S/S liver injury (fatigue, abdominal pain, yellowed skin, darkened urine) • LFTs • BP • HR • Height/weight • ECG at baseline and if chest pain or syncope • Signs of misuse/ abuse	• CYP2D6 substrate • CYP2D6 inhibitors may ↑ effects/ toxicity; ↓ dose in patients who are CYP2D6 poor metabolizers if taking strong CYP2D6 inhibitor (paroxetine, fluoxetine, quinidine) • MAOIs require 14 day washout period prior to stimulant initiation	• Risk of suicidal ideation in children • Capsules cannot be opened
Guanfacine ☆ • Intuniv • 1–7 mg daily • ER tabs	Hypersensitivity	• Dizziness • Fatigue • Somnolence • Nausea • Xerostomia • Constipation • Bradycardia • Atrioventricular block • Headache • Hypotension • Syncope	• Resolution of symptoms • BP • HR • ECG	• CYP3A4 substrate • ↓ daily dose by 50% if used with strong or moderate 3A4 inhibitors; double daily dose if used with strong or moderate CYP3A4 inducers • Additive CNS depressant effects with other CNS depressants • Additive BP lowering with other antihypertensives	• High-fat meals ↑ medication absorption; administer on an empty stomach • Can be used as monotherapy or as adjunctive to stimulant therapy • Also used for hypertension (formulations not interchangeable) • Do not crush
Clonidine • Kapvay • 0.1–0.4 mg at bedtime	Hypersensitivity	• Headache • Irritability • Nightmares • Insomnia • Constipation • Xerostomia • Somnolence • Bradycardia • Atrioventricular block • Hypotension • Rebound hypertension (if abruptly discontinue)	• Resolution of symptoms • BP • HR • ECG	• Additive CNS depressant effects with other CNS depressants • Additive BP lowering with other antihypertensives	• Do not crush • Do not stop abruptly

Storage and Administration Pearls

- Store stimulants where they cannot be accessed by others or stolen.
- Some of the formulations including Focalin XR, Ritalin LA, Metadate CD, and Adderall XR can be mixed with room temperature or cool applesauce and eaten right away if patient has difficulty swallowing capsules.
- Vyvanse can be mixed with water but must be taken immediately once mixed.
- Daytrana patches are applied to the hip approximately 2 hours prior to desire effect and rotated to alternate hip every morning. Remove after 9 hours of wear. Patient can bathe/swim while wearing the patch. Dispose of used patches in a place that is not accessible to small children or pets.
- Do not crush guanfacine or clonidine tablets.
- ER formulations can be used to avoid the need for doses delivered during school day.

Patient Education Pearls

- Most side effects to stimulant medications are minor and many subside with continued use. Lack of appetite or trouble sleeping may occur initially or with ↑ in dose but often resolve with continued use. If these side effects persist, patient should discuss with prescriber.
- Report any significant chest pain, shortness of breath, or fainting to a health care professional immediately.
- Report any hallucinations or changes in personality to a health care professional immediately.
- Store stimulant medications where they cannot be accessed by others or stolen.
- Stimulant medications should not be abruptly discontinued due to the potential for withdrawal.
- Clonidine should not be abruptly discontinued due to the potential for rebound hypertension.

LEARNING POINTS

- The most commonly used antidepressants are the SSRIs. These agents may take several weeks to reach maximal efficacy.

- Bupropion is the antidepressant of choice in patients with sexual side effects resulting from other classes of antidepressants.

- The treatment of anxiety and panic disorder may include acute therapies such as benzodiazepines but may also include chronic prophylactic therapies with antidepressants.

- Mood stabilizer therapy is the mainstay of treatment for bipolar disorder. Lithium has a narrow therapeutic window and requires therapeutic serum monitoring.

- While atypical antipsychotic medications exhibit fewer extrapyramidal side effects than typical agents, they do carry a greater risk of metabolic side effects such as weight gain, hyperglycemia, and hyperlipidemia. Atypical antipsychotics are more effective in treating the negative symptoms of schizophrenia.

- Sleep hygiene is preferred for insomnia, but medications can be used for short periods of time.

PRACTICE QUESTIONS

1. Which of the following is first-line in the treatment of acute depressive episode in a patient with bipolar disorder?

   (A) Lithium
   (B) Valproic acid
   (C) Oxcarbazepine
   (D) Lamictal
   (E) Carbamazepine

2. A 48-year-old woman is newly diagnosed with depression. She has a medical history significant for type 2 diabetes and hypertension. Current medications include metformin 1,000 mg PO BID and lisinopril 40 mg PO daily. Her blood pressure remains elevated at today's visit. Which antidepressant has the greatest potential to worsen this patient's hypertension?

   (A) Citalopram
   (B) Desipramine
   (C) Venlafaxine
   (D) Vilazodone

3. To avoid withdrawal symptoms, most antidepressants require tapering upon discontinuation. Which SSRI does not require a taper upon discontinuation due to its long elimination half-life?

   (A) Escitalopram
   (B) Fluoxetine
   (C) Paroxetine
   (D) Sertraline

4. Antidepressants with serotonergic activity should be avoided in combination with which of the following antibiotics due to the clinically significant risk of serotonin syndrome?

   (A) Cefazolin
   (B) Meropenem
   (C) Vancomycin
   (D) Linezolid

5. A 36-year-old woman with bipolar disorder is on lithium 300 mg PO TID with a serum drug concentration of 0.9 mEq/L. She is diagnosed with hypertension and her physician is considering therapy initiation. Which of the following medications would result in a significant drug interaction with the patient's lithium, increasing the risk for lithium toxicity? (Select ALL that apply.)

   (A) Chlorthalidone
   (B) Metoprolol
   (C) Lisinopril
   (D) Amlodipine

6. Which of the following antipsychotics would have the greatest risk of extrapyramidal side effects?

   (A) Olanzapine
   (B) Risperidone
   (C) Clozapine
   (D) Asenapine

7. Coadministration with a high-fat meal would result in delayed absorption of which of the following medications?

   (A) Eszopiclone
   (B) Triazolam
   (C) Ramelteon
   (D) Melatonin

8. HC is a 34-year-old man recently diagnosed with GAD. Given HC's past history of substance abuse, which of the following medications would be best to treat his GAD?

   (A) Buspirone
   (B) Diazepam
   (C) Chlordiazepoxide
   (D) Alprazolam

9. Which of the following is indicated to treat non-24-hour sleep-wake cycle disorder?

   (A) Belsomra
   (B) Hetlioz
   (C) Ambien
   (D) Sonata

10. An 11-year-old boy is diagnosed with attention deficit hyperactivity disorder (ADHD). He has an older brother (18 years) with ADHD and opioid dependence. The patient wants to avoid pharmacological treatment options with potential for dependency. Which of the following would be the most appropriate first-line pharmacological therapy for this patient's ADHD?

    (A) Methylphenidate
    (B) Atomoxetine
    (C) Guanfacine
    (D) Clonidine

ANSWERS AND EXPLANATIONS

1. D

According to the guidelines, first-line treatment options for acute depression episodes include lamotrigine as monotherapy or in combination with antimania agents. Lithium (A) and valproic acid (B) are used as first-line treatment options for acute manic episodes. Oxcarbazepine (C) and carbamazepine (E) would also be used as first-line treatment options of acute manic episodes. Maintenance therapy may consist of a combination of medications for both depression and manic episodes.

2. C

Serotonin, norepinephrine reuptake inhibitors, specifically venlafaxine, can increase blood pressure due the impact on norepinephrine. SSRIs such as citalopram (A) and vilazodone (D) are not associated with increasing blood pressure. Tricyclic antidepressants such as desipramine (B) can result in orthostatic hypotension due to anticholinergic side effects.

3. B

Fluoxetine's terminal half-life is measured in days (4–16) rather than hours; this pharmacokinetic principle allows the medication to slowly eliminate thereby diminishing the need for tapering upon discontinuation. The other drugs' half-lives are escitalopram (A) about 28 hours, paroxetine (C) 21 hours, and sertraline (D) 26 hours.

4. D

Linezolid is a reversible, nonselective inhibitor of monoamine oxidase, and coadministration with serotonergic agents such as SSRIs should be avoided due to the significant risk of serotonin syndrome.

5. A, C

Both thiazide diuretics such as chlorthalidone (A) and ACEIs such as lisinopril (C) decrease the clearance of lithium and increase the risk of lithium toxicity. Although these medications may be used in combination with lithium, the concomitant administration should be monitored very closely. Beta blockers such as metoprolol (B) and calcium channel blockers such as amlodipine (D) do not interact with lithium.

6. **B**

Risperidone has a relatively low risk of EPS among the first-generation (typical) antipsychotics. Its risk is greater, however, compared with the atypical antipsychotics such as olanzapine (A), asenapine (C), and clozapine (D).

7. **A**

BzRAs such as eszopiclone have demonstrated delayed absorption when co-administered with high-fat/heavy meals. The same precaution does not apply to benzodiazepines such as triazolam (B), melatonin receptor agonists such as ramelteon (C), or melatonin (D).

8. **A**

Buspirone (A) would be the best choice as it is not a controlled substance and can be used to treat GAD. Diazepam, chlordiazepoxide and alprazolam are all benzodiazepines and could place a patient at risk for substance abuse.

9. **B**

Hetlioz (B) (tasimelteon) is a melatonin receptor agonist used to treat non-24-hour sleep-wake disorder, which affects primarily patients with total blindness. Belsomra is an aorexin receptor antagonist used to treat insomnia. Ambien and Sonata are nonbenzodiazepine benzodiazepine receptor agonists that are used in the treatment of insomnia.

10. **B**

Atomoxetine is a nonstimulant option that is not a scheduled/controlled substance. Methylphenidate (A) is a stimulant option and would not address the family's concerns related to dependence. For patients/families with concerns regarding dependence, atomoxetine is considered the first-line option, while other nonstimulants such as guanfacine (C) and clonidine (D) are reserved for second-line/adjunctive therapy.

Pain Management

11

This chapter covers the following drug classes:

- **Nonsteroidal anti-inflammatory drugs (NSAIDs)**
- **Nonopioid pain management**
- **Opioid pain management**

The text also provides an overview of basic treatment and management of pain.

 Suggested Study Time: **30 minutes**

PAIN MANAGEMENT

Definitions

Managing pain can be very challenging, as providers must rely on patient report rather than objective measures like tachycardia. Because of the subjective nature of pain, strategies to manage pain must be individualized. An important consideration when choosing appropriate therapy is the type and duration of pain the patient is experiencing. **Nociceptive pain** arises from damage to tissue or bone and can also be classified as somatic or visceral pain; it is most likely to be treated as acute pain. **Somatic pain** comes from damage to bone or joint tissue, whereas **visceral pain** originates in organs. **Neuropathic pain** is attributable to nerve damage and is frequently characterized as a burning or tingling sensation. Successful treatment of neuropathic pain is often achieved with anticonvulsants and antidepressants (also known as coanalgesics).

By definition, **acute pain** usually requires only temporary therapy, usually fewer than 30 days. In some situations, however, treatment may last up to 3 months or for the duration required for a wound or condition to resolve. Unlike acute pain, **chronic pain** is persistent, lasting beyond 3 months or the expected healing time, and adversely affects the patient's function or well-being. Nociceptive, neuropathic, psychologically based pain syndromes, and mixed or undetermined pathophysiologic pain may all manifest as chronic pain. Similarly, **chronic cancer pain** occurs in 60–90% of patients with cancer and may present similarly to chronic nonmalignant pain. When possible, nonnarcotic therapies should be used. As chronic pain progresses and intensifies, however, more complex regimens and combination therapy with narcotics and nonnarcotics will be required. Finally, **breakthrough pain** describes intermittent peaks of more intense pain that occur in the presence of baseline chronic pain.

Diagnosis

Because pain is identified principally through self-reports and is very much subjective, it is challenging for a clinician to accurately assess and is virtually impossible to diagnose.

- Pain is always subjective.
- No neurophysiological or laboratory test can measure pain directly.
- The clinician should conduct a thorough history to fully understand the patient's pain.

Signs and Symptoms

- Objective observations such as grimacing, limping, or tachycardia may be helpful in assessing patients, but theses signs are often absent in patients with chronic pain.
- Pain intensity scales help patients communicate the signs and symptoms and pain intensity. This assessment can help guide treatments.
- Most adults and children above the age of 7 can score their pain intensity on a verbal numerical rating scale: 0 = no pain; 10 = the worst pain imaginable.

Guidelines

- Chou R, Fanciullo GJ, Fine PG, et al; American Pain Society-American Academy of Pain Medicine Opioids Guidelines Panel. Clinical guidelines for the use of chronic opioid therapy in chronic noncancer pain. *J Pain* 2009;10:113–30.
- NCCN Clinical Practice Guidelines in Oncology Adult Cancer Pain. Version 2.2016. National Comprehensive Cancer Network, Inc. 2016.
- Dowell D, Haegerich TM, Chou R. CDC Guideline for Prescribing Opioids for Chronic Pain - United States 2016. *MMWR Recomm Rep.*2016;65:1-49.
- See S, Ginzburg R. Choosing a skeletal muscle relaxant. *Am Fam Physician.* 2008;78(3):365-70.

Guidelines Summary

- Drug therapy is the mainstay of management for acute pain. The drugs discussed in this review are classified into three categories: Nonopioid analgesics, including acetaminophen and nonsteroidal anti-inflammatory drugs (NSAIDs); opioid pain management; and co-analgesics. The drug classes can be used in monotherapy and combination for pain.

- As the pain ↑, so does the dose of medications, the migration to stronger medications, and the use of combinations of medications with different mechanisms of actions.
- Acetaminophen and NSAIDs are useful for acute and chronic pain arising from a variety of causes, including surgery, trauma, arthritis, and cancer.
- NSAIDs are indicated for pain involving inflammation because acetaminophen lacks clinically effective anti-inflammatory properties.
- NSAIDs differ from opioid analgesic by the following mechanisms:
    - NSAIDs are both analgesics and anti-inflammatory in nature and have some antipyretic effect.
    - NSAIDs have a dose ceiling of effect in relationship with adverse effects.
    - NSAIDs do not produce physical or psychological dependence.
- Initiation of opioid analgesics should be based on a pain-directed history and physical that includes repeated pain assessment.
    - Opioid analgesics should be added to nonopioids to manage acute pain and cancer-related pain that does not respond to nonopioids alone.
    - There is enormous variability in doses of opioids required to provide pain relief, even among opioid-naïve patients.
    - It is important to give each analgesic an adequate trial. As a result, a clinician will ↑ the opioid dose until unacceptable side effects appear before changing to another opioid.
    - It is recommended to administer analgesics on a regular schedule if pain is present most of the day. This approach allows the patient to stay ahead of the pain.
        - » For chronic pain, consider having a scheduled long-acting agent on board and a short-acting agent for times of breakthrough pain.
- Patient-controlled analgesia (PCA) using an IV opioid for acute pain is a commonly used technique for pain control.
    - PCA is used with a microprocessor-controlled infusion pump.
    - PCA is most often used for the IV administration of opioids for acute pain.
    - PCA allows patients considerable control over the treatment of pain.
    - PCA is not recommended in situations in which oral opioids could readily manage pain.
- Skeletal muscle relaxants (SMRs) are classified as either antispastic agents (baclofen, dantrolene, tizanidine), which are used to treat cerebral palsy or multiple sclerosis, or as antispasmodic agents (carisoprodol, chlorzoxazone, cyclobenzaprine, metaxolone, methocarbamol, orphenadrine) which are used for the treatment of musculoskeletal conditions such as lower back pain.
- SMRs should not be used as first-line agents in the treatment of musculoskeletal pain. SMRs should be used only for the short-term treatment of acute low back pain if the patient is unable to tolerate or is unresponsive to NSAIDs or acetaminophen.

Nonnarcotic Oral and Nonsteroidal Anti-inflammatory Drugs (NSAIDs)

Generic • Brand • Dose & Max mg (frequency)	Contraindications	Primary Side Effects	Key Monitoring Parameters	Pertinent Drug Interactions	Med Pearls
Mechanism of action – ↓ pain through inhibition of central cyclooxygenase, which in turn inhibits prostaglandin synthesis					
Acetaminophen • Tylenol Ofirmev (injection) • Oral: 325–1,000 mg TID–QID (max = 4,000 mg/day) • IV: < 50 kg: 15 mg/kg every 6 hr (max = 3.75 g/day)	• Hepatic disease • Alcoholism	Hepatotoxicity	Pain relief	Alcohol	• Over-the-counter (OTC) • Best if taken on scheduled basis vs. as needed (PRN)
Mechanism of action – NSAIDs: decrease pain and inflammation by inhibition of prostaglandin synthesis through inhibition of cyclooxygenase enzymes					
Aspirin • Various • Immediate release (IR): 325–3,600 mg/day in 4–6 divided doses • Extended release (ER) product: 650–1,300 mg TID (max = 5.4 g/day)	• Allergy to aspirin • Active bleeding • Age <16 years	• Gastrointestinal (GI) (dyspepsia, GI ulceration) • Bleeding	• Pain relief • GI symptoms	• Warfarin • Other NSAIDs • Angiotensin-converting enzyme inhibitors (ACEIs) • Anticoagulants	• OTC • Anti-inflammatory only at high doses (>3 g/day)
Nonacetylated Salicylates					
Salsalate • None • 500–3,000 mg/day in 2–3 divided doses (max = 3 g/day)	• Hypersensitivity • Allergy to aspirin or NSAIDs	• GI (upset stomach, bleeding) • Rash • Diminished renal function • Edema	• Pain relief • GI symptoms	• Other salicylates • Warfarin • ACEIs	• Monitor serum salicylate levels with chronic use or very high doses • Desired range 10–30 mg/100 mL
Diflunisal • None • 250–750 mg BID	Hypersensitivity				Administer with food

Nonnarcotic Oral and Nonsteroidal Anti-inflammatory Drugs (NSAIDs) *(cont'd)*

Generic • Brand • Dose & Max mg (frequency)	Contraindications	Primary Side Effects	Key Monitoring Parameters	Pertinent Drug Interactions	Med Pearls
Acetic Acids					
Etodolac • None • 200–1,200 mg/day in 3–4 divided doses	Hypersensitivity	• GI (upset stomach, bleeding) • Rash • Diminished renal function • ↑ blood pressure (BP) • Edema	• Pain relief • GI symptoms • Renal function • BP	• Other salicylates • Warfarin • Lithium • ACEIs	Administer with food
Diclofenac☆ • Cataflam, Voltaren-XR • 50–150 mg/day in 2–3 divided doses • Zipsor • 25 mg QID • Cambia (oral solution) • 50 mg at onset of migraine • Flector • 1.3% patch: apply 1 patch BID • Pennsaid • 1.5% or 2% solution: apply 2 sprays BID • Dyloject (IV) • 37.5 mg IV every 6 hr		• GI (upset stomach, bleeding) • Rash • Diminished renal function • ↑ BP • Edema	• Pain relief • GI symptoms • Renal function • BP	• Other salicylates • Warfarin • Lithium • ACEIs	• Administer with food • Cambia packet should be mixed in 1-2 oz of water
Indomethacin☆ • Indocin, Tivorbex • IR: 25–200 mg/day in 2–3 divided doses • ER: 75 mg BID		• GI (upset stomach, bleeding) • Rash • Diminished renal function • ↑ BP • Edema • Central nervous system (CNS) disturbances	• Pain relief • GI symptoms • Renal function • BP	• Other salicylates • Warfarin • Lithium • ACEIs	• Most commonly used for treatment of gout • Fat-soluble, crosses blood-brain barrier • Administer with food

Nonnarcotic Oral and Nonsteroidal Anti-inflammatory Drugs (NSAIDs) *(cont'd)*

Generic • Brand • Dose & Max mg (frequency)	Contraindications	Primary Side Effects	Key Monitoring Parameters	Pertinent Drug Interactions	Med Pearls
Ketorolac • Toradol • 10 mg PO every 4–6 hr • 30 mg IV/IM every 6 hr	• Active peptic ulcer disease (PUD) or bleeding • History of GI bleeding • Severe renal impairment • Labor and delivery	• GI (upset stomach, bleeding) • Rash • Diminished renal function • ↑ BP	• Pain relief • GI symptoms • Renal function • BP	• Other salicylates • Warfarin • Lithium • ACEIs	Only approved for moderate-severe pain for ≤5 days' duration, due to risk of renal and GI dysfunction
Nabumetone • Relafen • 500–2,000 mg/day in 1–2 divided doses	Hypersensitivity				Administer with food
Propionic Acids					
Fenoprofen • Nalfon • 200–3,200 mg/day in 3–4 divided doses	Hypersensitivity	• GI (upset stomach, bleeding) • Rash • Diminished renal function • ↑ BP	• Pain relief • GI symptoms • Renal function • BP	• Other salicylates • Warfarin • Lithium • ACEIs	Administer with food
Flurbiprofen • Ansaid • 50–300 mg/day in 2–4 divided doses					Administer with food
Ibuprofen ☆ • Motrin, Advil, Caldolor • 200–3,200 mg/day in 3–4 divided doses					• Available OTC and Rx (400–800 mg tabs) • Administer with food • Available in pediatric preparations
Ketoprofen • Nexcede, Orudis Nexcede • IR: 50–300 mg/day in 3–4 divided doses • SR: 75–200 mg daily					Administer with food
Naproxen ☆ • Naprosyn, Naprelan • IR: 1,000 mg/day in 2–3 divided doses • ER: 750–1,500 mg daily					• Available OTC and Rx • Administer with food
Naproxen sodium ☆ • Anaprox, Aleve • 200 mg every 8–12 hr					• Available OTC and Rx • Administer with food

Nonnarcotic Oral and Nonsteroidal Anti-inflammatory Drugs (NSAIDs) *(cont'd)*

Generic • Brand • Dose & Max mg (frequency)	Contraindications	Primary Side Effects	Key Monitoring Parameters	Pertinent Drug Interactions	Med Pearls
Oxaprozin • Daypro • 600–1,200 mg daily					Administer with food
Fenamates					
Meclofenamate • Meclomen • 50–400 mg/day in 4–6 divided doses	Hypersensitivity	• GI (upset stomach, bleeding) • Rash • Diminished renal function • ↑ BP	• Pain relief • GI symptoms • Renal function • BP	• Other salicylates • Warfarin • Lithium • ACEIs	Administer with food
Oxicams					
Piroxicam ☆ • Feldene • 10–20 mg/day in 1–2 divided doses	Hypersensitivity	• GI (upset stomach, bleeding) • Rash • Diminished renal function • ↑ BP	• Pain relief • GI symptoms • Renal function • BP	• Other salicylates • Warfarin • Lithium • ACEIs	• More COX-2 selectivity than traditional NSAIDs • Slightly less GI symptoms
Meloxicam ☆ • Mobic, Vivlodex • Mobic: 7.5–15 mg daily • Vivlodex: 5–10 mg daily					
Selective COX-2 Inhibitors					
Celecoxib ☆ • Celebrex • 50–200 mg/day in 1–2 divided doses	• Hypersensitivity • Sulfa allergy	• GI (upset stomach, bleeding; less than other NSAIDs) • Rash • Diminished renal function • ↑ BP • Edema	• Pain relief • GI symptoms • Renal function • BP	• Other salicylates (including aspirin) • Warfarin • Lithium • ACEIs	• Lower incidence of GI toxicity than with NSAIDs • Concern about cardiovascular adverse effects prompted withdrawal of similar drug from market (rofecoxib)

Opioid Analgesics

Generic • Brand • Dose/Dosage Forms	Contraindications	Primary Side Effects	Key Monitoring Parameters	Pertinent Drug Interactions	Med Pearls
Mechanism of action – stimulate opioid receptors in the brain					
Hydrocodone • Hysingla ER (tablet), Zohydro ER (capsule) • Initial: 10 mg every 12 hr • ER caps, ER tabs	• Hypersensitivity • Respiratory depression • Paralytic ileus • Severe or acute asthma • Gastrointestinal (GI) obstruction	• Constipation • Nausea/vomiting (N/V) • Central nervous system (CNS) depression • Confusion • Sedation • Respiratory depression • Hypotension • Bradycardia	• Pain relief • Respiratory rate (RR) • Blood pressure (BP) • Heart rate (HR)	• Hydrocodone is CYP3A4 substrate • CYP3A4 inhibitors may ↑ effects/toxicity • CYP3A4 inducers may ↓ effects • Other CNS depressants, including alcohol, may ↑ CNS depressant effects • MAOIs may ↑ effects; avoid use if MAOIs have been used within past 2 wk	• Schedule II controlled substances • May take with food if nausea occurs • Adjust dose of hydrocodone ER in renal or hepatic impairment • Often need a laxative for constipation • High abuse potential
Hydrocodone/ Acetaminophen (APAP) ☆ • Norco • 5–10 mg/325 mg APAP every 4–6 hr • Dose is limited by APAP component • Do not exceed 4 g/day of APAP • Tabs					
Codeine ☆ • Only available generically • 15–60 mg every 4 hr (max = 360 mg/day) • Tabs	• Hypersensitivity • Respiratory depression • Acute or severe bronchial asthma • Paralytic ileus			• Codeine is CYP2D6 substrate • CYP2D6 inhibitors may ↓ effects • Other CNS depressants, including alcohol, may ↑ CNS depressant effects • MAOIs may ↑ effects; avoid use if MAOIs have been used within past 2 wk	• Schedule II controlled substances • Codeine has good antitussive properties • Must be metabolized by 2D6 to morphine for analgesic effect
Codeine/APAP • Tylenol with Codeine #3, Tylenol with Codeine #4 • 15–60 mg codeine every 4–6 hr (max = 360 mg/day of codeine and 4 g/day of APAP) • Tabs					

Opioid Analgesics *(cont'd)*

Generic • Brand • Dose/Dosage Forms	Contraindications	Primary Side Effects	Key Monitoring Parameters	Pertinent Drug Interactions	Med Pearls
Morphine☆ • Astramorph, Duramorph, Infumorph, Kadian, Morphabond, MS Contin • IR: 10–30 mg every 4 hr • IV: 2.5–5 mg every 3–4 hr • IV continuous infusion: 0.8–10 mg/hr • Rectal: 10–20 mg every 3–4 hr • No max dose; max dose of generic ER capsules = 1,600 mg/day • ER caps, ER tabs, injection (IV, IT, epidural), rectal suppository, solution, tabs	[Same as above]	[Same as above]	[Same as above]	• Other CNS depressants, including alcohol, may ↑ CNS depressant effects • MAOIs may ↑ effects; avoid use if MAOIs have been used within past 2 wk	• Schedule II controlled substance • May take with food if nausea occurs • Often need a laxative for constipation • High abuse potential • Most often started on IR then switched to ER • Kadian administered every 12 hr or every 24 hr • MS Contin administered every 8 hr or every 12 hr • Morphabond administered every 12 hr • Generic ER caps administered every 24 hr
Morphine sulfate and naltrexone • Embeda • 20 mg/0.8–100 mg/ 4 mg daily • ER caps					• Schedule II controlled substance • Abuse deterrent formulation of morphine with combination of naltrexone
Oxycodone☆ • Oxaydo, OxyContin, Roxicodone, Xtampza ER • IR: 5–15 mg every 4–6 hr • ER: Initiate oxycodone ER at a dose of 50% of the total daily oral oxycodone daily dose (mg/day) and administer every 12 hr. • No max dose • Caps, ER caps, ER tabs, solution, tabs	• Hypersensitivty • Respiratory depression • Paralytic ileus • Severe or acute asthma • GI obstruction			• Oxycodone is CYP3A4 substrate • CYP3A4 inhibitors may ↑ effects/toxicity • CYP3A4 inducers may ↓ effects • Other CNS depressants, including alcohol, may ↑ CNS depressant effects • MAOIs may ↑ effects; avoid use if MAOIs have been used within past 2 wk	• Schedule II controlled substances • Oxaydo and OxyContin are abuse deterrent formulations • May take with food if nausea occurs • Often need a laxative for constipation • High abuse potential • ER oxycodone caps are NOT bioequivalent to ER oxycodone tabs

Opioid Analgesics *(cont'd)*

Generic • Brand • Dose/Dosage Forms	Contraindications	Primary Side Effects	Key Monitoring Parameters	Pertinent Drug Interactions	Med Pearls
Oxycodone/APAP ☆ • Endocet, Percocet, Roxicet, Xartemis XR • IR: 2.5–10 mg/325 mg APAP every 6 hr • ER: 2 tabs (oxycodone 15 mg/APAP 650 mg) every 12 hr • Dose is limited by APAP component • Do not exceed 4 g/day of APAP • ER tabs, solution, tabs	[Same as above]	[Same as above]	[Same as above]	[Same as above]	[Same as above]
Fentanyl ☆ • Duragesic (transdermal patch) • 25–100 mcg/hr applied every 72 hr • Actiq (transmucosal lozenge) • 200 mcg per episode (limit to ≤4 units/day) • Fentora (buccal tab) • 100–200 mcg per episode (limit to ≤4 units/day) • Subsys (sublingual spray) • 100 mcg per episode (limit to ≤4 units/day) • Abstral (sublingual tablet) • 100–200 mcg per episode (limit to ≤4 units/day) • Lazanda (nasal spray) • 100–200 mcg per episode (limit to ≤4 episodes/day) • IV: 25–35 mcg every 1–2 hr • IV continuous infusion: 50–700 mcg/hr	• Hypersensitivity • Respiratory depression • Paralytic ileus • Severe or acute asthma • GI obstruction • Short-term treatment • Opioid-nontolerant patients			• CYP3A4 substrate • CYP3A4 inhibitors may ↑ effects/toxicity • CYP3A4 inducers may ↓ effects • Other CNS depressants, including alcohol, may ↑ CNS depressant effects • MAOIs may ↑ effects; avoid use if MAOIs have been used within past 2 wk	• Schedule II controlled substance • Patch takes 24 hr to begin working • Fentanyl remains in patch at 72 hr; fold in half to avoid diversion • Actiq, Fentora, Lazanda, Abstral, and Subsys should only be used for breakthrough pain; they are not interchangeable • Transdermal patch used to treat chronic, NOT acute pain

Opioid Analgesics *(cont'd)*

Generic • Brand • Dose/Dosage Forms	Contraindications	Primary Side Effects	Key Monitoring Parameters	Pertinent Drug Interactions	Med Pearls
Hydromorphone ☆ • Dilaudid, Dilaudid-HP, Exalgo • IR: 2–4 mg every 4–6 hr (tabs) or 2.5–10 mg every 3–6 hr (solution) • IV: 0.2–1 mg every 2–3 hr • IV continuous infusion: 0.5–3 mg/hr • Rectal: 3 mg every 6–8 hr • ER: Initiate hydromorphone ER at the same total daily dose of oral hydromorphone and administer every 24 hr • No max dose • ER tabs, injection (IV, epidural), rectal suppository, solution, tabs	• Hypersensitivity • Respiratory depression • Paralytic ileus • Severe or acute asthma • GI obstruction • Opioid-nontolerant patients	[Same as above]	[Same as above]	• Other CNS depressants, including alcohol, may ↑ CNS depressant effects • MAOIs may ↑ effects; avoid use if MAOIs have been used within past 2 wk	• Schedule II controlled substance • High potential for abuse • Dilaudid-HP is highly concentrated
Meperidine • Demerol • 50–150 mg PO/IM/subcut every 3–4 hr • Injection, tabs	• Hypersensitivity • Use of MAOI within 2 wk • Respiratory depression	• Constipation • N/V • CNS depression • Confusion • Sedation • Respiratory depression • Hypotension • Bradycardia • Seizures	• Pain relief • RR • BP • HR • Seizures	• Other CNS depressants, including alcohol, may ↑ CNS depressant effects • ↑ risk of serotonin syndrome with MAOIs, selective serotonin reuptake inhibitors (SSRIs) serotonin norepinephrine reuptake inhibitors (SNRIs), triptans, tricyclic antidepressants (TCAs), lithium, dextromethorphan, buspirone, linezolid, methylene blue, St. John's wort, and tramadol	• Schedule II controlled substance • NOT recommended as an analgesic • Accumulation of active metabolite, normeperidine, can ↑ risk of seizures • Renal or hepatic impairment can lead to accumulation of normeperidine • Treatment duration should be limited to ≤48 hr and doses should not exceed 600 mg/day

Opioid Analgesics *(cont'd)*

Generic • Brand • Dose/Dosage Forms	Contraindications	Primary Side Effects	Key Monitoring Parameters	Pertinent Drug Interactions	Med Pearls
Methadone☆ • Dolophine, Methadose • Initial opioid naïve: 2.5 mg PO every 8–12 hr or 2.5–10 mg IV every 8–12 hr • Injection, solution, tabs	• Hypersensitivty • Respiratory depression • Paralytic ileus • Severe or acute asthma	• Constipation • N/V • CNS depression • Confusion • Sedation • Respiratory depression • Hypotension • Bradycardia • QT interval prolongation	• Pain relief • RR • BP • HR • Electrocardiogram (ECG)	• CYP3A4 substrate • CYP3A4 inhibitors may ↑ effects/toxicity • CYP3A4 inducers may ↓ effects • Other CNS depressants, including alcohol, may ↑ CNS depressant effects • MAOIs may ↑ effects; avoid use if MAOIs have been used within past 2 wk • May ↑ risk of torsades de pointes with other drugs that prolong QT interval	• Schedule II controlled substance • Long half-life and difficult to titrate • NOT to be used for acute pain
Tapentadol • Nucynta, Nucynta ER • IR: 50–100 mg every 4–6 hr (max = 600 mg/day) • ER: Initiate tapentadol ER at the same total daily dose of oral hydromorphone but divide into 2 doses and administer every 12 hr (max = 500 mg/day) • ER tabs, solution, tabs	• Hypersensitivty • Respiratory depression • Paralytic ileus • Severe or acute asthma • Use of MAOI within 2 wk	• Constipation • N/V • CNS depression • Confusion • Dizziness • Sedation • Respiratory depression • Hypotension • Bradycardia	• Pain relief • RR • BP • HR	• Other CNS depressants, including alcohol, may ↑ CNS depressant effects • MAOIs may ↑ effects; avoid use if MAOIs have been used within past 2 wk • ↑ risk of serotonin syndrome with MAOIs, SSRIs, SNRIs, triptans, TCAs, meperidine, lithium, dextromethorphan, buspirone, linezolid, methylene blue, St. John's wort, and tramadol	• Schedule II controlled substance • Avoid use in severe renal impairment
Mechanism of action – binds to μ-opiate receptors in the CNS, causing inhibition of ascending pain pathways					
Tramadol☆ • Ultram, Ultram ER • IR: 50–100 mg every 4–6 hr (max = 400 mg/day) • ER: 100–300 mg daily • ER tabs, tabs Tramadol/APAP • Utracet • 2 tabs (tramadol 75 mg/APAP 650 mg) every 4–6 hr • Max = 8 tablets/day • Treatment duration should not exceed 5 days • Tabs	Hypersensitivity	• Confusion • Sedation • Suicidal thoughts • Rash • Nausea • Orthostatic hypotension • Seizures • Serotonin syndrome	• Pain relief • BP • Suicidality	• CYP2D6 and CYP3A4 substrate • CYP2D6 or CYP3A4 inhibitors may ↑ effects/toxicity • CYP3A4 inducers may ↓ effects • ↑ risk of serotonin syndrome with MAOIs, SSRIs, SNRIs, triptans, TCAs, fentanyl, lithium, dextromethorphan, meperidine, buspirone, linezolid, methylene blue, and St. John's wort • Other CNS depressants, including alcohol, may ↑ CNS depressant effects	• Schedule IV controlled substance • Adjust dose in renal impairment

Analgesic Adjuncts

Generic • Brand • Dose/Dosage Forms	Contraindications	Primary Side Effects	Key Monitoring Parameters	Pertinent Drug Interactions	Med Pearls
Mechanism of action – ↑ synaptic concentration of norepinephrine, desensitization of adenyl cyclase, and downregulation of serotonin receptors					
Desipramine • Norpramin • Initial: 10–25 mg/day (max = 150 mg) • Tabs Amitriptyline☆ • Only available generically • Initial: 25–50 mg/day (max = 150 mg) • Tabs	• Hypersensitivity • Use of MAOI within 2 wk • Concurrent use of linezolid or methylene blue • Acute recovery period post-myocardial infarction (MI)	• Anticholinergic symptoms • Weight gain • Bloating • Blurred vision • Xerostomia • Constipation • Dizziness • Somnolence • Headache • Fatigue • Serotonin syndrome	• Pain relief • Withdrawal symptoms from abrupt discontinuation • Worsening of depression, suicidality, or unusual behavior at initiation of therapy or when changing dose • BP • ECG (in patients with cardiac disease or hyperthyroidism)	• CYP2D6 substrate • CYP2D6 inhibitors may ↑ effects/toxicity • ↑ risk of serotonin syndrome with MAOIs, SSRIs, SNRIs, triptans, fentanyl, lithium, dextromethorphan, meperidine, buspirone, linezolid, methylene blue, St. John's wort, and tramadol	• Dangerous in overdose situations • Avoid in patients with high suicidality • Avoid dispensing large quantities • Neuropathic pain is an unlabeled indication • Taper off when medication is discontinued
Mechanism of action – induces the release of substance P, the principal chemomediator of pain impulses from the periphery					
Gabapentin☆ • Neurontin • Initial 300 mg TID (max = 3,600 mg) • Caps, solution, tabs • Gralise • 300 mg daily on Day 1, then 600 mg daily on Day 2, then 900 mg daily on Days 3–6, then 1,200 mg daily on Days 7–10, then 1,500 mg daily on Days 11–14, then 1,800 mg daily • ER tabs • Horizant • 600 mg in AM. × 3 days, then 600 mg every 12 hr • ER tabs	Hypersensitivity	• Dizziness • Fatigue • Somnolence • Ataxia • Weight gain • Angioedema • Behavioral disturbances (aggression, agitation, anger, anxiety, depression, hostility, nervousness) • Difficulty concentrating • Restlessness	• Pain relief • Suicidality	Other CNS depressants, including alcohol, may ↑ CNS depressant effects	• Adjust dose in renal impairment • Chronic neuropathic pain is not a labeled indication for IR product • Gralise and Horizant indicated to treat post-herpetic neuralgia • Gralise and Horizant are NOT interchangeable with other gabapentin products

Analgesic Adjuncts *(cont'd)*

Generic • Brand • Dose/Dosage Forms	Contraindications	Primary Side Effects	Key Monitoring Parameters	Pertinent Drug Interactions	Med Pearls
Pregabalin ☆ • Lyrica • Initial: 150 mg/day in 2–3 divided doses (max = 300–600 mg/day based on indication) • Caps, solution	[Same as above]	• Angioedema • Peripheral edema • Dizziness • Somnolence • Weight gain • Blurred vision • ↑ creatine kinase • Thrombocytopenia • PR interval prolongation	[Same as above]	[Same as above]	• Schedule V controlled substance • Adjust dose in renal impairment • Indicated for neuropathic pain associated with diabetes or spinal cord injury, fibromylagia, and postherpetic neuralgia
Duloxetine ☆ • Cymbalta • 30–60 mg/day in 1–2 divided doses (max = 60 mg/day) • ER caps	• Hypersensitivity • Use of MAOI within 2 wk • Concurrent use of linezolid or methylene blue	• Hepatotoxicity • Orthostatic hypotension • Rash (Stevens-Johnson syndrome possible) • Palpitations • Diaphoresis • Constipation • ↓ appetite • N/D • Xerostomia • Asthenia • Dizziness • Insomnia or somnolence • Vertigo • Blurred vision • Polyuria • ↓ libido • Serotonin syndrome	• Pain relief • Liver function tests (LFTs) • BP • Withdrawal symptoms from abrupt discontinuation • Abnormal bleeding • Worsening of depression, suicidality, or unusual behavior at initiation of therapy or when changing dose	• CYP1A2 and CYP2D6 substrate • CYP1A2 or CYP2D6 inhibitors may ↑ effects/toxicity; avoid concomitant use with strong CYP1A2 inhibitors • CYP1A2 inducers may ↓ effects • ↑ risk of serotonin syndrome with MAOIs, SSRIs, triptans, TCAs, fentanyl, lithium, dextromethorphan, meperidine, buspirone, linezolid, methylene blue, St. John's wort, and tramadol • ↑ risk of bleeding with used with aspirin, NSAIDs, or anticoagulants	• Indicated to treat diabetic neuropathy, fibromyalgia, and chronic musculoskeletal pain • Avoid use if creatinine clearance <30 mL/min

Mechanism of action – induces the release of substance P, the principal chemomediator of pain impulses from the periphery

Capsaicin • Salonpas, Zostrix-HP • Cream, gel, lotion: 0.025–0.1% applied 3–4 × daily • Patch: apply to affected area 3–4 ×/day	Do not apply to wounds or damaged skin	Localized stinging	Pain relief	None	• Over-the-counter • Must be used regularly for ≥2 wk for maximal efficacy

Skeletal Muscle Relaxants

Generic • **Brand** • **Dose & Max mg** **(frequency)**	Contraindications	Primary Side Effects	Key Monitoring Parameters	Pertinent Drug Interactions	Med Pearls
Mechanism of action – inhibits reflexes at the level of the spinal cord by hyperpolarization of afferent fibers					
Baclofen • Gablofen, Lioresal • 5–20 mg PO TID–QID (max = 80 mg/day) • IT administration via infusion/ implanted pump 300–800 mcg/day	• Hypersensitivy • IV, IM, subcut, or epidural adminsi-tration (for IT use)	• Hypotonia • Drowsiness • Confusion • Headache • N/V • Hypotension • Seizures • Dizziness	• Pain relief • Presence of side effects	Other CNS depressants, including alcohol, may ↑ CNS depressant effects	Antispastic agent
Mechanism of action – depresses polysynaptic neuronal transmission in the spinal cord and reticular formation					
Carisoprodol • Soma • 250–350 mg 4 × /day • Tabs	• Hypersenstivity • Acute intermittent porphyria	• Drowsiness • Dizziness • Headache	• Pain relief • Presence of side effects • Signs of abuse/ misuse/ addic-tion	• CYP2C19 substrate • CYP2C19 inhibitors may ↑ effects/toxicity • CYP2C19 inducers may ↓ effects • Other CNS depres-sants, including alcohol, may ↑ CNS depressant effects	• Schedule IV controlled substance • Antispasmodic agent • Metabolized to meprobamate
Mechanism of action – inhibits polysynaptic reflexes					
Chlorzoxazone • Only available generically • 250–750 mg 3–4 × /day • Tabs	Hypersensitivity	• Dizziness • Drowsiness • N/V/D • Urine discoloration • Hepatotoxicity	• Pain relief • LFTs	Other CNS depressants, including alcohol, may ↑ CNS depressant effects	Antispasmodic

Skeletal Muscle Relaxants *(cont'd)*

Generic • Brand • Dose & Max mg (frequency)	Contraindications	Primary Side Effects	Key Monitoring Parameters	Pertinent Drug Interactions	Med Pearls
Mechanism of action – reduces tonic somatic motor activity by altering alpha and gamma motor neurons					
Cyclobenzaprine • Amrix • IR: 5–10 mg TID • ER: 15–30 mg daily • ER caps, tabs	• Hypersensitivity • Use of MAOI within 2 wk • Hyperthyroidism • Heart failure • Arrhythmias • Atrioventricular block or conduction disturbance • Acute recovery of MI	• Drowsiness • Dizziness • Xerostomia • Fatigue • Constipation • Confusion • Weakness • Blurred vision • Irritabilty • Serotonin syndrome	• Pain relief • Presence of side effects	• CYP1A2 substrate • CYP1A2 inhibitors may ↑ effects/toxicity • CYP1A2 inducers may ↓ effects • Other CNS depressants, including alcohol, may ↑ CNS depressant effects • ↑ risk of serotonin syndrome with MAOIs, SSRIs, SNRIs, triptans, TCAs, fentanyl, lithium, dextromethorphan, meperidine, buspirone, linezolid, methylene blue, St. John's wort, and tramadol	• Antispasmodic • ER formulation should not be used in older adults (>65 yr) or patients with hepatic impairment
Mechanism of action – inhibits the release of calcium from sarcoplasmic reticulum					
Dantrolene • Dantrium • 25 mg daily × 7days, then 25 mg TID × 7 days, then 50 mg TID × 7 days, then 100 mg TID (max= 400 mg/day) • Caps	• Hypersensitivity • Active liver disease • If spasticity is used to maintain upright posture/ balance or function	• Hepatotoxicity • Drowsiness • Dizziness • Headache • Weakness • Diarrhea	• Pain relief • LFTs	• CYP3A4 substrate • CYP3A4 inhibitors may ↑ effects/toxicity • CYP3A4 inducers may ↓ effects • Concurrent use with estrogen may ↑ risk of hepatotoxicity • Other CNS depressants, including alcohol, may ↑ CNS depressant effects	• Antispastic agent • Females and patients older than 35 yr at ↑ risk for hepatotoxicity • Can also be used to treat malignant hyperthermia (IV)
Mechanism of action – general depression of the CNS					
Metaxalone • Skelaxin • 800 mg 3–4 × /day • Tabs	• Hypersensitivity • Severe renal or hepatic impairment • Predisposition to drug-induced, hemolytic, or other anemias	• Dizziness • Drowsiness • Headache • N/V • Hemolytic anemia • Jaundice • Rash	• Pain relief • Complete blood count	Other CNS depressants, including alcohol, may ↑ CNS depressant effects	Antispasmodic

Skeletal Muscle Relaxants *(cont'd)*

Generic • Brand • Dose & Max mg (frequency)	Contraindications	Primary Side Effects	Key Monitoring Parameters	Pertinent Drug Interactions	Med Pearls
Mechanism of action – general depression of the CNS					
Methocarbamol • Robaxin • 4–6 g/day PO in 3–6 divided doses • 1 g IV/IM every 8 hr for no more than 3 consecutive days • Injection, tabs	• Hypersensitivity • Renal impairment (IV use because of polyethylene glycol in vehicle)	• Confusion • Impaired coordination • Headache • Sedation	• Pain relief • Presence of side effects	Other CNS depressants, including alcohol, may ↑ CNS depressant effects	Antispasmodic
Mechanism of action – central atropine-like effects for indirect skeletal muscle relaxation					
Orphenadrine • Norflex • 100 mg PO BID • 60 mg IV/IM every 12 hr • ER tabs, injection	• Hypersensitivity • Glaucoma • GI obstruction • Peptic ulcer disease • Benign prostatic hyperplasia • Bladder obstruction • Cardiospasm • Myasthenia gravis	• Tachycardia • Palpitation • Dizziness • Syncope • Anaphylaxis • Drowsiness • Confusion • Constipation • N/V • Xerostomia • Urinary retention • Tremor • Blurred vision	• Pain relief • HR	• Additive effects with other anticholinergic medications • Other CNS depressants, including alcohol, may ↑ CNS depressant effects	Antispasmodic
Mechanism of action – alpha-2 receptor agonist					
Tizanidine • Zanaflex • 2–12 mg TID • Caps, tabs	Concurrent use with strong 1A2 inhibitors	• Somnolence • Hypotension • Syncope • Hepatotoxicity • Hallucinations • Anaphylaxis • Xerostomia • Weakness • Dizziness	• Pain relief • LFTs • BP • Renal function	• CYP1A2 substrate • CYP1A2 inhibitors may ↑ effects/toxicity • CYP1A2 inducers may ↓ effects • Oral contraceptives may ↑ effects/toxicity • Concurrent use with clonidine may ↑ risk of hypotension • CYP1A2 inhibitors/inducers • Other CNS depressants, including alcohol, may ↑ CNS depressant effects	Antispastic agent

Storage and Administration Pearls

- Do not freeze acetaminophen suppositories.

- Hydrolysis of aspirin occurs upon exposure to water or moist air, resulting in salicylate and acetate, which possess a vinegar-like odor. Do not use if a strong odor is present.

- Wash hands after application of capsaicin products.

- Do not crush ER morphine products; Kadian and generic ER capsules may be opened and sprinkled on applesauce (do not crush, chew, or dissolve the beads prior to swallowing as it may result in a fatal overdose of morphine). Kadian capsules may be opened and sprinkled over 10 mL of water and then administered through gastrostomy tube; do not administer through gastric or nasogastric (NG) tube.

- Embeda caps may be opened and sprinkled on applesauce (do not crush, chew, or dissolve the pellets prior to swallowing). Embeda capsules should not be administered via a gastric or NG tube.

- Do not moisten, dissolve, cut, crush, break, or chew ER oxycodone tabs (abuse deterrent). Do not moisten, crush, chew, or dissolve Oxaydo IR tabs (abuse deterrent).

- ER oxycodone caps may be opened and sprinkled on soft foods (e.g. applesauce, pudding, yogurt, ice cream, jam). Content of ER caps may also be administered via a gastrostomy or NG tube. Flush tube with water first, then pour capsule contents into tube (do not premix with water). Once contents are in tube, flush with 15 mL of milk, water, or liquid nutritional supplement, then repeat two additional times with 10 mL of the same liquid.

- Do not crush, break, chew, dissolve or inject ER hydromorphone tabs.

- Do not split, crush, break, chew, or dissolve ER tapentadol tabs.

- ER cyclobenzaprine caps may be opened and sprinkled on a tablespoon of applesauce.

Patient Education Pearls

- The patient should always take exactly what is prescribed. Never increase the dose without discussing with the prescriber

- The narcotic medications may cause physical and psychological dependence.

- While using pain medications, it is recommended not to use alcohol or other prescription or OTC medications.

LEARNING POINTS

- NSAIDs are both analgesics and anti-inflammatory in nature.

- No NSAID is any more effective than any other in the general population.

- Symptoms of overdose for narcotic medications include: CNS depression, bradycardia, hypotension, respiratory depression, miosis, apnea, pulmonary edema, and convulsions.

- Onset of action of most pain medication occurs within 45 minutes, with peak drug effect in 1 to 2 hours after oral administration for most immediate-release medications.

- PCA provides the important advantage of medication that is rapidly administered when needed, delaying pain exacerbation.

- In chronic pain, continuous opioid administration is recommended with controlled release medication, transdermal patch, or infusion. Short-acting medications should be available for breakthrough pain.

- SMRs should be used only for acute lower back pain for short periods of time.

PRACTICE QUESTIONS

1. Which of the following is a caution with the use of tramadol?

   (A) Bradycardia
   (B) GI bleed
   (C) HTN
   (D) Hyperglycemia
   (E) Seizures

2. Which of the following is a common effect of narcotic or opioid analgesics?

   (A) Constipation
   (B) Diarrhea
   (C) Hypertension
   (D) Tachypnea

3. Which of the following medications is contraindicated in a patient with a sulfa allergy?

   (A) Amitriptyline
   (B) Celecoxib
   (C) Gabapentin
   (D) Hydromorphone

4. Which of the following is TRUE regarding meperidine or the metabolite, normeperidine?

   (A) May be used for long-term analgesia
   (B) Normeperidine may cause seizures
   (C) Only available in oral formulation
   (D) Preferred agent for use in renal failure
   (E) Recommended first line for analgesia

5. Which of the following should be avoided in PUD? (Select ALL that apply.)

   (A) Ibuprofen
   (B) Indomethacin
   (C) Ketorolac
   (D) Naproxen
   (E) Cyclobenzaprine

6. Which of the following can be used to treat neuropathic pain?

    (A) Acetaminophen
    (B) Capsaicin
    (C) Gabapentin
    (D) Ibuprofen
    (E) Ketorolac

7. Which of the following formulations are available for oxycodone? (Select ALL that apply.)

    (A) ER tablet
    (B) IR tablet
    (C) IV injection
    (D) Oral solution

8. Which of the following is FDA approved for the treatment of fibromyalgia?

    (A) Gabapentin
    (B) Ketorolac
    (C) Morphine
    (D) Pregabalin

9. Which of the following NSAIDs is available as an IM injection formulation?

    (A) Celecoxib
    (B) Ibuprofen
    (C) Ketorolac
    (D) Naproxen

10. Which of the following is associated with methadone use?

    (A) Diarrhea
    (B) GI bleeding
    (C) Hyperkalemia
    (D) Hypertension
    (E) QTc prolongation

ANSWERS AND EXPLANATIONS

1. E

Tramadol is associated with a risk of seizures and should be used with caution in patients with epilepsy or a history of a seizure disorder. The risk of seizures is increased if given concomitantly with other agents that may lower the seizure threshold.

2. A

Constipation is a common side effect associated with opioid analgesics, which often needs to be treated with stimulant laxatives to provide relief to the patient. Opioid analgesics may also be associated with hypotension and bradypnea.

3. B

Use of celecoxib is contraindicated in a patient with a sulfa allergy. Amitriptyline (A), gabapentin (C), and hydromorphone (D) can all be used in a patient with a sulfa allergy.

4. B

Normeperidine is a toxic metabolite of meperidine that is known to cause seizures. Meperidine should not be used for >48 hours (A) and should be avoided in renal failure to prevent the accumulation of normeperidine (D). Meperidine is available in oral and IV formulations (C). Meperidine should not be used as a first-line agent (E) due to the risk associated with the medication.

5. A, B, C, D

A, B, C and D are NSAIDs and should not be used if a patient has PUD or a history of GI bleeding. If an NSAID must be used in a patient with PUD or a history of GI bleeding, a COX-2 selective inhibitor such as celecoxib would be preferred. E, cyclobenzaprine is a SMR and can be used in the presence of PUD.

6. C

Gabapentin may be used to treat neuropathic pain. Neuropathic pain does not respond well to acetaminophen (A) or NSAIDs such as ibuprofen (D) or ketorolac (E).

7. A, B, D

Oxycodone is available in IR and ER tablet formulations as well as a solution and oral concentrate. It is not available for IV, IM, or subcutaneous injection.

8. **D**

Pregabalin (Lyrica) is FDA approved for the treatment of fibromyalgia. Other FDA-approved medications for the treatment of fibromyalgia include duloxetine (Cymbalta) and milnacipran (Savella). Fibromyalgia is also treated off-label with various other agents.

9. **C**

Ketorolac is available as an IM formulation. It is also available in IV and oral formulations. Celecoxib (A) is available only in an oral formulation. Ibuprofen (B) is available in oral tablet, capsule, solution, suspension, and IV formulations, as well as a cream. Naproxen (D) is available as an oral tablet, a capsule, an oral suspension, and a topical cream.

10. **E**

Methadone is known to prolong the QTc interval and should not be used with other agents that prolong the QTc interval. Methadone is associated with constipation (not diarrhea, A), hypokalemia (not hyperkalemia, C), and hypotension (not hypertension, D). It is also not known to cause GI bleeding (B).

Bone and Joint Disorders

12

This chapter covers the following disease states:

- **Osteoarthritis**
- **Rheumatoid arthritis**
- **Osteoporosis**
- **Gout**

 Suggested Study Time: **45 minutes**

OSTEOARTHRITIS

Definition

Osteoarthritis (OA) is a disease of the cartilage resulting from an imbalance between cartilage destruction and formation with subsequent bony proliferation within the joint, which results in pain, potentially decreased range of motion, and local inflammation.

Diagnosis

The diagnosis of OA is based on history, physical exam, and radiographs. History and physical exam will reveal symptoms and signs consistent with OA (detailed in the next section) and should be used to rule out other potential conditions such as rheumatoid arthritis (RA). Radiologic changes may include joint space narrowing, osteophytes, or subchondral bone sclerosis.

Signs and Symptoms

- OA signs: Physical exam may reveal tenderness, crepitus, and/or enlargement of the affected joints. Radiologic evaluation is necessary to identify presence of OA and disease progression. Radiographic changes may not be easily identifiable in early, mild disease but with disease progression may include narrowing of the joint spaces, presence of osteophytes, subchondral bony sclerosis, and eventual subluxation and deformity.

- OA symptoms: Patients with OA present with pain, stiffness, and instability of joints that can be unilateral or bilateral. The pain is often worsened with weight-bearing activity and is described as deep and aching. Stiffness may resolve with motion but may limit physical activity. Commonly affected joints include the hands, knees, and hips.

Guidelines

Hochberg MC, Altman RD, April KT, et al. American College of Rheumatology 2012 recommendations for the use of nonpharmacologic and pharmacologic therapies in osteoarthritis of the hand, hip, and knee. *Arthritis Care Res* 2012;64:465–74.

Guidelines Summary

The goals of therapy are to ↓ pain and stiffness, maintain/improve joint mobility and limit functional impairment, and ↑ quality of life.

- OA of the hand:
  - First-line options: Topical capsaicin, topical nonsteroidal anti-inflammatory drugs (NSAIDs), oral NSAIDs, tramadol
  - Topical NSAIDs preferred over oral NSAIDs in patients ≥75 years of age
- OA of the knee or hip:
  - First-line option: Acetaminophen (scheduled, up to maximum of 4 g/day)
  - Second-line options: Topical or oral NSAIDs (topical preferred in patients ≥75 years of age) or intra-articular corticosteroid injections
  - Third-line options: Duloxetine, tramadol, or intra-articular hyaluronan injections

Treatment Algorithm

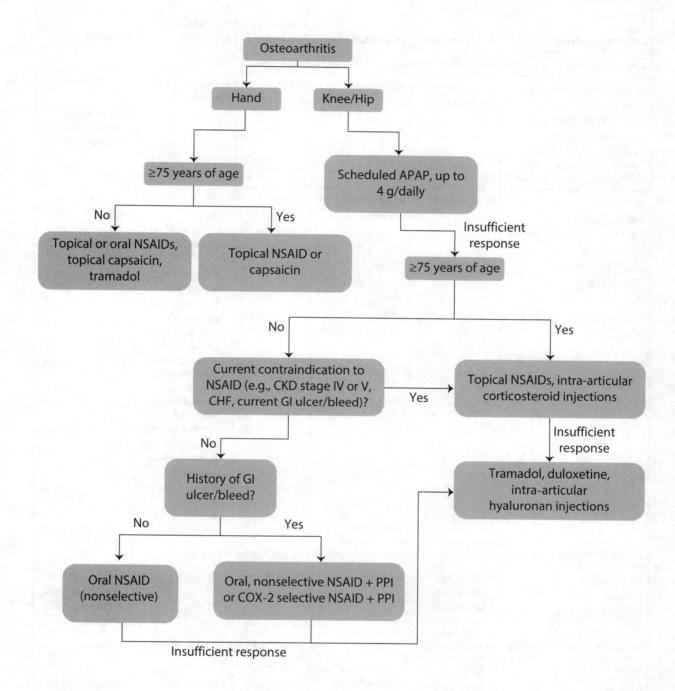

Drugs for Osteoarthritis

Generic • Brand • Dose/Dosage Forms	Contraindications	Primary Side Effects	Key Monitoring Parameters	Pertinent Drug Interactions	Med Pearls
Mechanism of action – ↓ pain through inhibition of central cyclo-oxygenase, which in turn inhibits prostaglandin synthesis					
Acetaminophen • Tylenol • 325–1,000 mg in 3–4 divided doses (max = 4 g/day) • Caps, chewable tabs, ER caps, injection, ODTs, rectal suppositoty, solution, suspension, tabs	• Hepatic disease • Alcoholism	Hepatotoxicity	Pain relief	Alcohol may ↑ risk of hepatotoxicity	• Over-the-counter (OTC) • Best if taken on scheduled basis vs. as needed (PRN)
Tramadol • Ultram, Ultram ER • IR: 50-100 mg every 4–6 hr (max = 400 mg/day) • ER: 100–300 mg daily • ER tabs, tabs	Hypersensitivity	• Confusion • Sedation • Suicidal thoughts • Rash • Nausea • Orthostatic hypotension • Seizures • Serotonin syndrome	• Pain relief • BP • Suicidality	• CYP2D6 and CYP3A4 substrate • CYP2D6 or CYP3A4 inhibitors may ↑ effects/toxicity • CYP3A4 inducers may ↓ effects • ↑ risk of serotonin syndrome with SSRIs, MAOIs, SNRIs, triptans, tricyclic antidepressants (TCAs), fentanyl, lithium, dextromethorphan, meperidine, buspirone, linezolid, methylene blue, and St. John's wort • Other CNS depressants, including alcohol, may ↑ CNS depressant effects	• Schedule IV controlled substance • Adjust dose in renal impairment
Mechanism of action – induces the release of substance P, the principal chemomediator of pain impulses from the periphery					
Capsaicin cream • Various • 0.025–0.1% applied 3–4 × daily	Do not apply to wounds or damaged skin	Localized stinging	Pain relief	None	• OTC • Must be used regularly for ≥2 wk for maximal efficacy
Mechanism of action – NSAIDs: ↓ pain and inflammation by inhibition of prostaglandin synthesis through inhibition of cyclooxygenase enzymes					
Aspirin • Various • IR: 325–3,600 mg/day in 4–6 divided doses • ER: 650–1,300 mg TID • Chewable tabs, ER tabs, rectal suppository, tabs	• Allergy • Fever in children • Active bleeding	• Gastrointestinal (GI) (upset stomach, bleeding) • Rash	• Pain relief • GI symptoms	↑ risk of bleeding when used with anticoagulants or other antiplatelets	• OTC • Anti-inflammatory only at high doses (>3 g/day)

Drugs for Osteoarthritis (cont'd)

Generic • Brand • Dose/Dosage Forms	Contraindications	Primary Side Effects	Key Monitoring Parameters	Pertinent Drug Interactions	Med Pearls
Nonacetylated Salicylates					
Salsalate • 500–3,000 mg/day in 2–3 divided doses • Tabs	Hypersensitivity	• GI (upset stomach, bleeding) • Rash • Renal impairment • Edema	• Pain relief • GI symptoms	↑ risk of bleeding when used with anticoagulants or other antiplatelets	Monitor serum salicylate levels with chronic use or very high doses; desired range 10–30 mg/100 mL
Diflunisal • Only available generically • 500 mg BID–TID • Tabs					Administer with food
Acetic Acids					
Etodolac • Only available generically • IR: 600–1,000 mg/day in 2–3 divided doses • ER: 400–1,000 mg daily • ER tabs, tabs	• Hypersensitivity • History of asthma, urticaria, or anaphylaxis after taking aspirin or other NSAID (allergic cross-reactivity can occur between NSAIDs) • During coronary artery bypass surgery	• GI (upset stomach, bleeding) • Rash • Renal impairment • ↑ Blood pressure (BP) • Edema • Myocardial infarction • Stroke • Hepatotoxicity (diclofenac, indomethacin)	• Pain relief • GI symptoms • Renal function • BP • Liver function tests (LFTs) (diclofenac, indomethacin)	• ↑ risk of bleeding when used with anticoagulants or other antiplatelets • May ↓ BP lowering effects of antihypertensives • May ↑ risk of lithium or methotrexate toxicity	• Administer with food • Dyloject injection indicated for mild–moderate pain • Zipsor indicated for mild–moderate acute pain • Flector patch indicated for acute pain
Diclofenac • Cambia, Dyloject, Flector, Voltaren, Zipsor, Zorvolex • IR: 150–200 mg/day in 3–4 divided doses • ER tab: 100–200 mg/day in 1–2 divided doses • IR cap (Zipsor): 25 mg 4 × /day • IR cap (Zorvolex): 18–35 mg TID • Injection: 37.5 mg IV q6 hr PRN • Topical gel: Apply 4 g of 1% gel to affected lower extremity 4 × /day or apply 2 g of 1% gel to affected upper extremity • Topical solution: Apply 40 drops of 1.5% solution to affected knee 4 × /day or apply 2 pump actuations of 2% solution to affected knee 4 × /day • Transdermal patch: Apply 1 patch BID to most painful areas • Caps, ER tabs, injection, solution, tabs, topical gel, topical solution, transdermal patch					

Drugs for Osteoarthritis (cont'd)

Generic • Brand • Dose/Dosage Forms	Contraindications	Primary Side Effects	Key Monitoring Parameters	Pertinent Drug Interactions	Med Pearls
Indomethacin • Indocin, Tivorbex • IR or rectal suppository: 50–200 mg/day in 2–3 divided doses • Tivorbex: 20–40 mg BID-TID • ER: 75–150 mg daily	[Same as above]	[Same as above]	[Same as above]	[Same as above]	• Most commonly used for treatment of gout • Fat-soluble; crosses blood-brain barrier • Administer with food • Tivorbex used for mild-moderate acute pain
Ketorolac • Toradol • IM/IV: 60 mg IM (30 mg if ≥65 yr) or 30 mg IV (15 mg if ≥65 yr) initially; then 30 mg IM/IV (15 mg if ≥65 yr) every 6 hr • PO: 20 mg initially, then 10 mg every 4–6 hr PRN • Intranasal (Sprix): 1 spray in each nostril every 6–8 hr (max = 4 sprays in each nostril/day); if ≥65 yr or <50 kg, give 1 spray in 1 nostril every 6–8 hr (max = 4 sprays in 1 nostril/day) • Injection, intranasal spray, tabs	• History of asthma, urticaria, or anaphylaxis after taking aspirin or other NSAID (allergic cross-reactivity can occur between NSAIDs) • During coronary artery bypass surgery • Active peptic ulcer disease or bleeding • History of GI bleeding • Severe renal impairment • Patients at risk for renal failure due to volume depletion • Labor and delivery • Concurrent use of aspirin, other NSAIDs, probenecid, or pentoxifylline				• All approved for moderate–severe pain for ≤5 days duration • Adjust dose in renal impairment
Nabumetone • Only available generically • 1,000–2,000 mg daily • Tabs	• Hypersensitivity • History of asthma, urticaria, or anaphylaxis after taking aspirin or other NSAID (allergic cross-reactivity can occur between NSAIDs) • During coronary artery bypass surgery				• Administer with food • Adjust dose in renal impairment

Drugs for Osteoarthritis *(cont'd)*

Generic • Brand • Dose/Dosage Forms	Contraindications	Primary Side Effects	Key Monitoring Parameters	Pertinent Drug Interactions	Med Pearls
Propionic acids					
Fenoprofen • Nalfon • 1,200–3,200 mg/day in 3–4 divided doses • Caps, tabs	• Hypersensitivity • History of asthma, urticaria, or anaphylaxis after taking aspirin or other NSAID (allergic cross-reactivity can occur between NSAIDs) • During coronary artery bypass surgery	• GI (upset stomach, bleeding) • Rash • Renal impairment • ↑ Blood pressure (BP) • Edema • Myocardial infarction • Stroke • Hepatotoxicity (fenoprofen, flurbiprofen, ibuprofen, naproxen, oxaprozin)	• Pain relief • GI symptoms • Renal function • BP • LFTs (fenoprofen, flurbiprofen, ibuprofen, naproxen, oxaprozin)	• ↑ risk of bleeding when used with anticoagulants or other antiplatelets • May ↓ BP lowering effects of antihypertensives • May ↑ risk of lithium or methotrexate toxicity	Administer with food
Flurbiprofen • Only available generically • 100–300 mg/day in 2–4 divided doses • Tabs					
Ibuprofen • Advil, Caldolor, Motrin • PO: 200–3,200 mg/day in 3–4 divided doses • IV: Caldolor: 400–800 mg IV every 6 hr PRN • Caps, chewable tabs, injection, suspension, tabs					• Available OTC and Rx (400–800 mg tabs) • Administer with food • Available in pediatric preparations • Neoprofen administered IV to close patent ductus arteriosus in premature infants
Ketoprofen • Only available generically • IR: 200–300 mg/day in 3–4 divided doses • ER: 200 mg daily • Caps, ER caps					• Administer with food • Adjust dose in renal impairment
Naproxen • Aleve, Anaprox DS, Naprelan, Naprosyn • IR: 500–1,500 mg/day in 2 divided doses • ER: 750–1,500 mg/day in 2 divided doses • Caps, ER tabs, suspension, tabs					• Available OTC and Rx • Administer with food
Oxaprozin • Daypro • 600–1800 mg daily • Tabs					Administer with food

Drugs for Osteoarthritis *(cont'd)*

Generic • Brand • Dose/Dosage Forms	Contraindications	Primary Side Effects	Key Monitoring Parameters	Pertinent Drug Interactions	Med Pearls
Fenamates					
Meclofenamate • Only available generically • 200–400 mg/day in 3–4 divided doses • Caps	• Hypersensitivity • History of asthma, urticaria, or anaphylaxis after taking aspirin or other NSAID (allergic cross-reactivity can occur between NSAIDs) • During coronary artery bypass surgery	• GI (upset stomach, bleeding) • Rash • Renal impairment • ↑ Blood pressure (BP) • Edema • Myocardial infarction • Stroke • Hepatotoxicity	• Pain relief • GI symptoms • Renal function • BP • LFTs	• ↑ risk of bleeding when used with anticoagulants or other antiplatelets • May ↓ BP lowering effects of antihypertensives • May ↑ risk of lithium or methotrexate toxicity	Administer with food
Oxicams					
Piroxicam • Feldene • 20 mg daily • Caps	• Hypersensitivity • History of asthma, urticaria, or anaphylaxis after taking aspirin or other NSAID (allergic cross-reactivity can occur between NSAIDs) • During coronary artery bypass surgery	• GI (upset stomach, bleeding) • Rash • Renal impairment • ↑ Blood pressure (BP) • Edema • Myocardial infarction • Stroke • Hepatotoxicity	• Pain relief • GI symptoms • Renal function • BP • LFTs	• ↑ risk of bleeding when used with anticoagulants or other antiplatelets • May ↓ BP lowering effects of antihypertensives • May ↑ risk of lithium or methotrexate toxicity	More COX-2 selectivity than traditional NSAIDs; slightly less GI symptoms
Meloxicam • Mobic (tabs, suspension), Vivlodex (caps) • Mobic: 7.5–15 mg daily • Vivlodex: 5–10 mg daily					
Selective COX-2 Inhibitors					
Celecoxib • Celebrex • 200 mg/day in 1–2 divided doses • Caps	• Hypersensitivity • History of asthma, urticaria, or anaphylaxis after taking aspirin or other NSAID (allergic cross-reactivity can occur between NSAIDs) • During coronary artery bypass surgery	• GI (upset stomach, bleeding–less than other NSAIDs) • Rash • Renal impairment • ↑ Blood pressure (BP) • Edema • Myocardial infarction • Stroke • Hepatotoxicity	• Pain relief • GI symptoms • Renal function • BP • LFTs	• CYP2C9 substrate • CYP2C8 and CYP2D6 inhibitor • CYP2C9 inhibitors may ↑ effects/toxicity • CYP2C9 inducers may ↓ effects • May ↑ effects/toxicity of CYP2C8 or CYP2D6 substrates • ↑ risk of bleeding when used with anticoagulants or other antiplatelets • May ↓ BP lowering effects of antihypertensives • May ↑ risk of lithium or methotrexate toxicity	• Lower incidence of GI toxicity than with nonselective NSAIDs • Concern about cardiovascular adverse effects prompted withdrawal of similar drug from market (rofecoxib)

Drugs for Osteoarthritis *(cont'd)*

Generic • Brand • Dose/Dosage Forms	Contraindications	Primary Side Effects	Key Monitoring Parameters	Pertinent Drug Interactions	Med Pearls
Adjunctive Therapies/Nutritional Supplements					
Glucosamine sulfate • Various • 500–1,500 mg/day in 1–2 divided doses daily	Unknown	• Itching • GI upset	• Pain relief • Presence of side effects	Unknown	• Nutritional supplement • Available OTC • Conflicting clinical trial data
Intra-Articular Injections					
Mechanism of action – serves as a lubricant for joint tissue					
Hyaluronate and derivates • Synvisc, Synvisc-One • Synvisc: Inject 16 mg (2 mL) once weekly for 3 wks (total of 3 injections) • Sinvisc-One: Inject 48 mg (6 mL) once per knee	Hypersensitivity	• Injection site reaction • Bruising • Erythema • Lumps • Pain • Swelling • Pruritus • Skin discoloration • Arthralgia • Infection	S/S of inflammation or infection	No known significant drug interactions	None

Storage and Administration Pearls

- NSAIDs should be administered with food to ↓ the risk of gastrointestinal side effects.

- Capsaicin cream may take several weeks for maximal efficacy to be demonstrated. Regular daily use, 2–4 times daily for 4 weeks, is considered an adequate trial.

Patient Education Pearls

- Take NSAIDs with food to avoid stomach upset.

- Avoid alcohol when taking acetaminophen due to the risk of liver damage.

- Capsaicin cream may take 2–4 weeks to become effective. Allow an adequate trial before determining efficacy.

- Wash your hands very thoroughly after capsaicin application.

- The Food and Drug Administration advises against use of NSAIDs in patients with history of coronary artery bypass graft surgery or high cardiovascular disease risk.

RHEUMATOID ARTHRITIS

Definition

RA is an autoimmune disease characterized by chronic inflammation of the synovial tissue lining the joint capsule. The erosive synovitis is generally symmetrical and extra-articular involvement may also occur, including rheumatoid nodules, cardiopulmonary disease, lymphadenopathy, splenomegaly, and neurological dysfunction.

Diagnosis

RA diagnosis is based on history and physical, laboratory evidence, and radiographic evaluation. History and physical will reveal consistent signs and symptoms of RA. Laboratory evidence will demonstrate the presence of rheumatoid factor (RF) in 60–70% of affected patients, ↑ erythrocyte sedimentation rate and C-reactive protein, and radiographic evidence of joint space narrowing or erosions. Level of disease activity and prior response to therapy guide treatment decisions.

- Disease activity: Categorized as low, moderate, or high via validated scales based upon clinical assessment.

Signs and Symptoms

- Symmetrical symptoms of joint pain and stiffness (especially in the morning) for > 6 weeks' duration
- Joint tenderness, erythema, swelling, and, potentially, rheumatoid nodules

Guidelines

Singh JA, Saag KG, Bridges SL, et al. 2015 American College of Rheumatology guideline for the treatment of rheumatoid arthritis. *Arthritis Rheumatol.* 2016;68:1-26.

Guidelines Summary

- Goals of therapy include achieving low disease activity or remission.

- A disease-modifying antirheumatic drug (DMARD) should be initiated within 3 months of diagnosis to retard disease progression.

- Leflunomide, sulfasalazine, hydroxychloroquine, and methotrexate are first-line DMARD options.

- In patients with moderate to severe disease activity, combination therapy may be considered initially.

- NSAIDs are useful for symptomatic relief during onset of DMARD and PRN otherwise. NSAIDs do not alter disease progression in RA.

- Corticosteroids are used as adjunctive therapy in patient with refractory symptoms.

- Biologic agents are used generally when initial DMARD therapy has been demonstrated to be ineffective as monotherapy. Additional DMARDs may be tried prior to use of biologics.

- Biologic therapies ↑ the risk of serious infections and should not be initiated in a patient with an active infection or in combination with live vaccines.

Treatment Algorithm

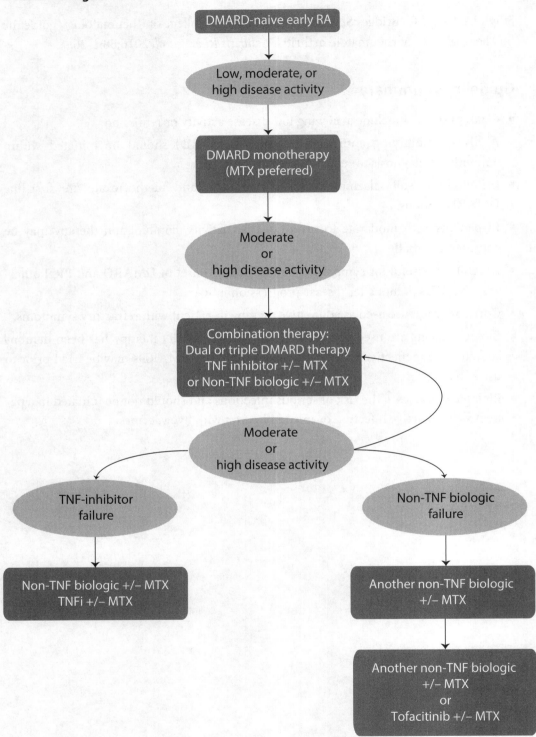

Medications for Rheumatoid Arthritis

Generic • Brand • Dose/Dosage Forms	Contraindications	Primary Side Effects	Key Monitoring Parameters	Pertinent Drug Interactions	Med Pearls
Mechanism of action – corticosteroids: exert anti-inflammatory and immunosuppressive effects by inhibiting prostaglandins and leukotrienes, which results in ↓ inflammation, ↓ pain, and a potential ↓ in joint destruction					
Prednisone ☆ • Only available generically • 5–60 mg daily initially; individualized • Solution, tabs	• Systemic fungal infection • Hypersensitivity	• Hyperglycemia • ↑ BP • ↓ bone mineral density (BMD) • Fluid retention • Impaired wound healing • Infection • Hyperglycemia • ↑ appetite • Irritability • Insomnia • Weight gain	• Blood sugar • BP • Electrolytes • BMD • Presence of edema/weight	May ↑ anti-coagulant effect of warfarin	Side effects generally present with chronic and/or long-term use
DMARDs					
Mechanism of action – inhibit cytokine production, inhibit purine biosynthesis, thereby ↓ inflammation in affected joints					
Methotrexate ☆ • Otrexup, Rasuvo, Rheumatrex, Trexall • 7.5 mg PO/subcut/IM weekly • Injection, tabs	• Hypersensitivity • Alcoholism • Liver disease • Immunodeficiency • Significant blood dyscrasias • Pregnancy • Lactation	• GI upset (nausea, diarrhea, abdominal pain) • Stomatitis • Thrombocytopenia • Leukopenia • Anemia • ↑ LFTs • Interstitial lung disease • Rash (Stevens-Johnson syndrome possible) • Malaise • Fatigue • Fever/chills • Infection	• Pain relief • LFTs • Complete blood count (CBC) with differential • Folate concentrations • S/S of infection	• NSAIDs and salicylates ↑ risk of toxicity • Penicillins, sulfonamides, and tetracyclines may ↑ risk of toxicity	• May supplement with folic acid to ↓ side effects and prevent folate deficiency • Myelosuppression is biggest concern • Should be taken with food
Mechanism of action – not fully understood; thought to be related to immunosuppressant properties					
Hydroxychloroquine ☆ • Plaquenil • 200–600 mg/day in 1–2 divided doses • Tabs	• Hypersensitivity • Retinal changes with agent in past • Children	• Macular damage • Corneal deposits • Retinopathy • Rash • Nausea • Diarrhea • Neutropenia • Thrombocytopenia • Anemia	• Ocular exams q 3 mo • CBC with differential	May ↑ serum digoxin concentrations	Hemolysis can occur in patients glucose-6-phosphate dehydrogenase deficiency

Medications for Rheumatoid Arthritis *(cont'd)*

Generic • Brand • Dose/Dosage Forms	Contraindications	Primary Side Effects	Key Monitoring Parameters	Pertinent Drug Interactions	Med Pearls
Mechanism of action – inhibits pyrimidine synthesis, thereby ↓ lymphocyte proliferation and inflammation					
Leflunomide • Arava • Loading dose of 100 mg daily × 3 days, then maintenance dose of 20 mg daily • Tabs	• Hypersensitivity • Severe hepatic impairment • Pregnancy	• Diarrhea • Hepatotoxicity • Alopecia • Rash (Stevens-Johnson syndrome possible) • Peripheral neuropathy • Interstitial lung disease • ↑ BP • Neutropenia • Thrombocytopenia • Anemia • Infection	• LFTs (monthly × 6 mo, then every 6–8 wk) • CBC with differential (monthly × 6 mo, then every 6–8 wk) • Pregnancy test (before therapy begins) • BP • S/S of infection	• CYP2C8 inhibitor • May ↑ effects/toxicity of CYP2C8 substrates • May ↓ effects of warfarin • May ↑ toxicity of rosuvastatin (max dose of rosuvastatin =10 mg/day)	• Highly teratogenic • Appropriate contraception should be used • After stopping therapy, accelerated drug elimination procedure should be used to rapidly ↓ concentrations of active metabolite (comprised of cholestyramine or activated charcoal)
Mechanism of action – not fully understood; related to anti-inflammatory properties					
Sulfasalazine • Azulfidine EN-tabs • 500–3,000 mg/day in 2 divided doses • ER tabs	• Hypersensitivity to any sulfa-containing drug or salicylates • Intestinal or urinary obstruction • Porphyria	• N/V/D • Rash (Stevens-Johnson syndrome possible) • Photosensitivity • Neutropenia • Anemia • Hepatotoxicity • Renal impairment • Alopecia • Stomatitis • Infection	• CBC with differential (every other wk × 3 mo, then every mo × 3 mo, then every 3 mo) • LFTs (every other wk × 3 mo, then every mo × 3 mo, then every 3 mo) • Renal function • Folate concentrations	• May ↑ effects of warfarin • May ↓ serum digoxin concentrations	• May supplement with folic acid to ↓ side effects and prevent folate deficiency • Preferred option in pregnant patients

Medications for Rheumatoid Arthritis *(cont'd)*

Generic • Brand • Dose/Dosage Forms	Contraindications	Primary Side Effects	Key Monitoring Parameters	Pertinent Drug Interactions	Med Pearls
Biologics					
Mechanism of action – binds to and inhibits the cytokine TNF, thereby inhibiting the subsequent inflammatory cascade					
Etanercept • Enbrel • 50 mg subcut weekly • Injection	Sepsis	• Injection site reactions • Anaphylaxis • Infection (especially latent tuberculosis [TB] reactivation, fungal infections and hepatitis B virus [HBV] reactivation) • Lymphoma • Leukemia • Skin cancer • Heart failure exacerbation • Bone marrow suppression • Lupus-like syndrome • Demyelinating disorders	• S/S of infection • S/S of heart failure • CBC with differential	Not to be given with live vaccines	• PPD and HBV screening should be done before initiating treatment • Refrigerate prior to use • Discontinue if serious infection occurs • Use with caution in patients with heart failure • Can be self-administered • Can be used alone or in combination with methotrexate
Infliximab • Inflectra, Remicade • 3 mg/kg IV infusion at initiation, wk 2 and wk 6, then every 8 wk • Injection	• Hypersensitivity • Doses >5 mg/kg in moderate-severe heart failure	• Infusion reactions (hypotension, dyspnea, urticaria) • Delayed hypersensitivity reactions (fever, rash, myalgia, headache, sore throat, hand/facial edema, dysphagia, arthralgias) • Infection (especially latent TB reactivation, fungal infections, or HBV reactivation) • Heart failure exacerbation • Bone marrow suppression • Lymphoma • Leukemia • Skin cancer • Hepatotoxicity	• BP • LFTs • S/S of infection • S/S of heart failure • CBC with differential	Not to be given with live vaccines	• Delayed hypersensitivity reaction may occur as early as after 2nd dose • Premedicate with H₁ antagonist, H₂ receptor antagonist, acetaminophen, and/or corticosteroid • PPD and HBV screening should be done before initiating treatment • *Always* used in combination with methotrexate • Dose limited to ≤5 mg/kg in patients with heart failure • Discontinue if serious infection occurs

Medications for Rheumatoid Arthritis *(cont'd)*

Generic • **Brand** • **Dose/Dosage Forms**	**Contraindications**	**Primary Side Effects**	**Key Monitoring Parameters**	**Pertinent Drug Interactions**	**Med Pearls**
Golimumab • Simponi, Simponi Aria • 50 mg subcut monthly or 2 mg/kg IV infusion at initiation and wk 4, then every 8 wk • Injection	None	• Injection site reactions • Anaphylaxis • Infection (especially latent TB reactivation, fungal infections and HBV reactivation) • Lymphoma • Leukemia • Skin cancer • Heart failure exacerbation • Bone marrow suppression • Lupus-like syndrome • Demyelinating disorders	• S/S of infection • S/S of heart failure • CBC with differential	Not to be given with live vaccines	• PPD and HBV screening should be done before initiating treatment • Indicated for use in combination with methotrexate • Use with caution in patients with heart failure • Discontinue if serious infection occurs • Subcut injection can be self-administered • Refrigerate subcut injection prior to use
Adalimumab • Humira • 40 mg subcut every other wk (if not taking methotrexate, may give weekly) • Injection					• PPD and HBV screening should be done before initiating treatment • Use with caution in patients with heart failure • Discontinue if serious infection occurs • Can be self-administered • Refrigerate prior to use • Can be used alone or in combination with methotrexate or other non-biological DMARDs
Certolizumab pegol • Cimzia • 400 mg subcut at initiation, wk 2, and wk 4, then 200 mg subcut every other wk • Injection					• PPD and HBV screening should be done before initiating treatment • Use with caution in patients with heart failure • Discontinue if serious infection occurs • Can be self-administered • Refrigerate prior to use • Can be used alone or in combination with other non-biological DMARDs

Medications for Rheumatoid Arthritis *(cont'd)*

Generic • Brand • Dose/Dosage Forms	Contraindications	Primary Side Effects	Key Monitoring Parameters	Pertinent Drug Interactions	Med Pearls
Mechanism of action – binds to interleukin-1 (IL-1) receptors on target cells, thereby preventing release of chemotactic factors and adhesion molecules and subsequently ↓ inflammation and connective tissue damage					
Anakinra • Kineret • 100 mg subcut daily • Injection	Hypersensitivity	• Injection-site reactions (inflammation, ecchymosis) • Infection (including latent TB reactivation) • Neutropenia • Anaphylaxis	• CBC with differential • S/S of infection	• Not to be given with TNF inhibitors • Not to be given with live vaccines	• Can be self-administered • Refrigerate prior to use • Can be used alone or in combination with other non-biological DMARDs
Mechanism of action – interleukin-6 (IL-6) receptor antagonist					
Tocilizumab • Actemra • IV: 4 mg/kg IV infusion every 4 wk; may be ↑ to 8 mg/kg based on clinical response (max = 800 mg per infusion) • Subcut: <100 kg: 162 mg subcut every other wk (may be ↑ to every wk based on clinical response); ≥100 kg: 162 mg subcut weekly • Injection	Hypersensitivity	• Infection (especially latent TB reactivation, fungal infections and viral reactivation) • GI perforation • Neutropenia • Thrombocytopenia • ↑ LFTs • Dyslipidemia • Anaphylaxis • Demyelinating disorders	• S/S of infection • CBC with differential • Lipid panel • LFTs	Not to be given with live vaccines	• PPD and HBV screening should be done before initiating treatment • Discontinue if serious infection occurs • Indicated for patients that have failed ≥1 TNF agent • Subcut injection can be self-administered • Refrigerate subcut injection prior to use • Can be used alone or in combination with methotrexate or other non-biological DMARDs
Mechanism of action – selective costimulation modulator; inhibits T-cell activation					
Abatacept • Orencia • IV dose based on body weight; administered at wk 0, wk 2, and wk 4, then every 4 wk IV weight-based dose: • <60 kg: 500 mg • 60–100 kg: 750 mg • >100 kg: 1,000 mg • Subcut: 125 mg subcut weekly (may be initiated with or with an IV loading dose)	None	• Anaphylaxis • Infection (especially latent TB reactivation, fungal infections and HBV reactivation) • Chronic obstructive pulmonary disease (COPD) exacerbations • Headache • Nausea	S/S of infection	• Not to be given with TNF inhibitors • Not to be given with live vaccines	• PPD and HBV screening should be done before initiating treatment • Discontinue if serious infection occurs • Use with caution in patients with COPD • Subcut injection can be self-administered • Refrigerate subcut injection prior to use • Can be used alone or in combination with other non-biological DMARDs

Medications for Rheumatoid Arthritis (cont'd)

Generic • Brand • Dose/Dosage Forms	Contraindications	Primary Side Effects	Key Monitoring Parameters	Pertinent Drug Interactions	Med Pearls
Mechanism of action – inhibits Janus kinase thereby reducing cytokine signaling					
Tofacitinib • Xeljanz, Xeljanz XR • IR: 5 mg BID • ER: 11 mg daily • ER tabs, tabs	None	• Infection (especially latent TB reactivation, fungal infections and HBV reactivation) • Malignancy • GI perforation • Lymphocytopenia • Neutropenia • Anemia • ↑ LFTs • Dyslipidemia • Headache • Diarrhea	• S/S of infection • CBC with differential • Lipid panel • LFTs	• CYP3A4 substrate • CYP3A4 inhibitors may ↑ effects/ toxicity; dose when used with strong CYP3A4 inhibitors • CYP3A4 inducers may ↓ effects • Not to be given with TNF inhibitors • Not to be given with live vaccines	• PPD and HBV screening should be done before initiating treatment • Can be used alone or in combination with methotrexate or other non-biological DMARDs • Oral therapy offers advantage over many available biologics

Storage and Administration Pearls

- NSAIDs should be administered with food to ↓ risk of GI side effects.

- Oral methotrexate should be administered with food to avoid stomach upset.

- The following medications should be refrigerated to 2–8°C (36–46°F): methotrexate injectable, etanercept, infliximab, adalimumab, anakinra, golimumab, certolizumab pegol, tocilizumab, and abatacept. These medications should *not* be frozen and should be protected from light.

- The following biologic DMARDs can be administered subcutaneously: etanercept, adalimumab, anakinra, golimumab, certolizumab pegol, tocilizumab, and abatacept.

- Methotrexate is administered orally, subcutaneously, or intramuscularly.

- Infliximab is the only biologic DMARD that must be administered via intravenous infusion (cannot be self-administered). Tocilizumab and abatacept can be administered either via intravenous infusion (cannot be self-administered) or subcutaneously (can be self-administered).

- The following medications are available in prefilled syringes and/or pen devices: etanercept, adalimumab, anakinra, golimumab, certolizumab pegol, tocilizumab, and abatacept.

Patient Education Pearls

- Promptly report any signs of infection to your physician. A temporary withdrawal of medication may be necessary during this time.
- Do not receive live vaccines while you are on biologic therapies.
- Appropriate administration of injectable therapies is as follows:
  - Visually inspect the products for particulate matter or discoloration. Do not use if either is present.
  - Rotate injection site.
  - Do not inject into tender, bruised, hard, or ulcerated skin.
  - Do not reuse needles or syringes.
  - Properly dispose of needles in a puncture-proof container.

OSTEOPOROSIS

Definition

Osteoporosis is a condition of low bone mass, which results in increased fragility of bone and subsequent increased risk of fracture. Potential etiologies of the decreased bone mass include age-related physiologic changes, disorders of estrogen or testosterone levels, or use of medications associated with drug-induced osteoporosis. Although more common in women, osteoporosis also occurs in men.

Normal bone physiology includes constant bone remodeling, which consists of bone formation via osteoblasts and bone resorption via osteoclasts. BMD reflects the balance between resorption and formation. Osteoporosis occurs when there is an imbalance between formation and resorption resulting in decreased BMD.

Diagnosis

The diagnosis of osteoporosis is most commonly based on the results of BMD measurement with dual energy x-ray absorptiometry (DXA) at the hip and spine. Results of the DXA are reported as the T-score. The T-score represents the number of standard deviations away from the mean BMD for a young, healthy individual. Normal BMD would be considered any T-score greater than −1, while osteopenia would be a T-score of −1 to −2.5; a T-score of less than −2.5 would be diagnostic for osteoporosis. Osteoporosis can also be diagnosed based on the occurrence of a nontraumatic fracture.

Signs and Symptoms

Typical signs of osteoporosis include kyphosis, shortened stature, and nontraumatic fractures of the vertebrae, hip, or forearm. Some patients may have symptoms of bone pain, and often vertebral fractures go undiagnosed as patients complain of chronic back pain. In a patient with risk factors for osteoporosis, radiographic investigation of back pain is warranted. Pain and physical changes associated with osteoporosis may lead to depression and lowered self-esteem. The FRAX® tool can be used to estimate 10-year fracture risk and guide treatment strategy.

Guidelines

Cosman F, de beur SJ, LeBoff MS, et al. Clinician's guide to prevention and treatment of osteoporosis. *Osteoporos Int.* 2014;25:2359-81.

Guidelines Summary

- Dietary and supplemental calcium and vitamin D are important prerequisites to pharmacological therapy. Without adequate calcium and vitamin D available, other therapies will be limited in their ability to improve bone architecture.

- Bisphosphonates are the first-line therapy for the prevention and treatment of osteoporosis in patients without contraindications.

- Oral bisphosphonates are approved for prevention and treatment of osteoporosis (including glucocorticoid-induced osteoporosis) in men and women.

- Efficacy of bisphosphonates beyond 5 years is limited, with rare but serious side effects such as osteonecrosis of the jaw (ONJ) and atypical femur fractures. It is reasonable to reassess fracture risk and consider therapy discontinuation after 3–5 years.

- Raloxifene is recommended as an alternative choice for the treatment of osteoporosis in patients with contraindications to bisphosphonates or in patients who are unable to comply with the appropriate bisphosphonate administration instructions.

- Calcitonin is reserved for third-line therapy because of a lack of compelling evidence indicating fracture reductions and lack of long-term data. Calcitonin is approved for the treatment of acute pain secondary to vertebral fractures and is well tolerated; therefore, this medication may have a specific role in certain situations.

- Teriparatide is approved for the treatment of osteoporosis and is indicated in patients with a history of fracture secondary to osteoporosis and in those with multiple risk factors for fracture who have not responded or are intolerant to bisphosphonate therapy, as well as for patients with glucocorticoid-induced osteoporosis.

- Denosumab is reserved for second-line therapy for the treatment of osteoporosis in postmenopausal females at high risk for fracture (previous osteoporotic fractures, multiple fracture risk factors, failed other therapies).

- Estrogens and tissue-selective estrogen complex (conjugated estrogens/bazedoxifene) are approved for the prevention of osteoporosis in postmenopausal women. Patients should consider potential risks (cardiovascular, breast cancer, venous thromboembolism) before initiating therapy with these agents. If the decision is made to initiate estrogen-based therapy for osteoporosis prevention, the lowest effective dose should be used for the shortest duration.

Osteoporosis Treatment Summary

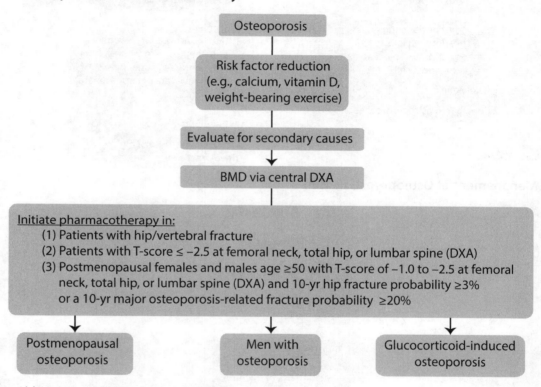

Abbreviations: BMD = bone mineral density

Management of Postmenopausal Osteoporosis

Postmenopausal Osteoporosis

Prevention

First-line: bisphosphonates
  alendronate
  ibandronate
  risedronate
  zoledronic acid

Estrogen/hormone therapy
  (FDA approved for prevention
  of osteoporosis associated
  with menopause)

Raloxifene

Conjugated estrogens/bazedoxifene

Treatment

First-line: bisphosphonates
  alendronate
  ibandronate
  risedronate
  zoledronic acid

Calcitonin
  (FDA approved for treatment
  of osteoporosis in women who
  are ≥5 years postmenopausal if
  alternatives are not appropriate)

Raloxifene

Teriparatide

Denosumab (those at high
risk of fracture)

Management of Osteoporosis in Men

Men with Osteoporosis

Treatment

First-line: bisphosphonates
  alendronate
  risedronate
  zoledronic acid

Teriparatide
  (FDA approved for men
  at high risk of fracture)

Denosumab (those at high
risk of fracture)

Management of Glucocorticoid-Induced Osteoporosis

Glucocorticoid-Induced Osteoporosis

Prevention

Bisphosphonates
  risedronate
  zoledronic acid

Treatment

Bisphosphonates
  alendronate
  risedronate
  zoledronic acid

Teriparatide
  (FDA approved for
  men at high risk of fracture)

Medications for Osteoporosis

Generic • Brand • Dose/Dosage Forms	Contraindications	Primary Side Effects	Key Monitoring Parameters	Pertinent Drug Interactions	Med Pearls
Mechanism of action – bisphosphonates: adsorb to bone apatite and inhibit osteoclast activity					
Alendronate ☆ • Binosto, Fosamax • 10 mg daily or 70 mg weekly (treatment) • 5 mg daily or 35 mg weekly (prevention) • Effervescent tabs, solution, tabs Risedronate ☆ • Actonel, Atelvia • IR: 5 mg daily or 35 mg weekly, or 150 mg monthly • ER: 35 mg weekly • ER tabs, tabs Ibandronate ☆ • Boniva • PO: 150 mg monthly • IV: 3 mg every 3 mo • Injection, tabs	• Esophageal stricture • Hypersensitivity • Inability to sit upright or stand for ≥30 min • Creatinine clearance (CrCl) <35 mL/min • Hypocalcemia	• Nausea • Dyspepsia • Esophageal irritation • Ulceration • Myalgia/arthralgia • ONJ • Atypical femur fractures	• BMD • Serum calcium concentrations • Serum 25(OH)D concentrations	• Absorption ↓ with antacids and products containing bi-or trivalent cations (e.g. iron, magnesium, aluminum, calcium, or zinc (separate by ≥30 min) • NSAIDs may ↑ risk of GI symptoms	• Tabs must be taken with 6–8 oz of water ≥30 minutes (60 min for ibandronate) prior to other medications/food • Alendronate oral solution should be followed by ≥2 oz of water; effervescent tabs should be dissolved in 4 oz of room-temperature water • Risedronate ER tabs must be taken ≥4 oz of water immediately after breakfast • Patient should remain upright for ≥30 min (60 min for ibandronate) (for alendronate, must also remain upright until after first food of day)
Zoledronic acid • Reclast • 5 mg IV infusion yearly (every 2 yr for prevention) • Injection	• Hypersensitivity • CrCl <35 mL/min • Hypocalcemia	• Renal impairment • ONJ • Atypical femur fractures • Hypocalcemia • Myalgia/arthralgia • Acute-phase reaction (fever, myalgia, flu-like symptoms)	• BMD • Renal function • Serum calcium concentrations • Serum 25(OH)D concentrations	• ↑ risk of hypocalcemia with loop diuretics • ↑ risk of nephrotoxicity with other nephrotoxic drugs (aminoglycosides, NSAIDs)	Acetaminophen may be given after drug is administered to minimize acute-phase reaction symptoms
Mechanism of action – selective estrogen receptor modulators: through selective binding to estrogen receptors, ↓ bone resorption and ↓ biochemical markers of bone turnover					
Raloxifene ☆ • Evista • 60 mg daily • Tabs	• History of pulmonary embolism, deep vein thrombosis, or retinal vein thrombosis • Pregnancy/lactation	• Hot flashes • Leg cramps • Thromboembolism • Peripheral edema • ↑ sweating	• BMD • S/S of thromboembolism	Absorption ↓ by bile acid sequestrants (avoid concurrent use)	Lipid effects include ↓ low-density lipoprotein cholesterol (LDL-C) with no effect on high-density lipoprotein cholesterol (HDL-C)/triglycerides

Medications for Osteoporosis *(cont'd)*

Generic • Brand • Dose/Dosage Forms	Contraindications	Primary Side Effects	Key Monitoring Parameters	Pertinent Drug Interactions	Med Pearls
Miscellaneous Agents					
Mechanism of action – inhibits bone resorption through inhibition of osteoclast activity, to a small degree, stimulates bone formation through stimulation of osteoblast activity					
Calcitonin • Fortical, Miacalcin • 1 spray (200 units) in 1 nostril daily intranasally • 100 units IM or subcut daily • Injection, nasal spray	Hypersensitivity	• Anaphylaxis • Hypocalcemia • Nasal irritation and dryness • Rhinitis • Malignancy	BMD	None	• Refrigerate injection and unopened nasal spray bottle; once opened, keep nasal spray at room temp while in use (<86°F/30°C) • Discard unused nasal spray after 30 days
Mechanism of action – acts as a parathyroid hormone (PTH) agonist; thereby ↑ bone formation by the stimulation of osteoblast activity and ↑ renal reabsorption of calcium					
Teriparatide • Forteo • 20 mcg subcut daily • Injection	• Hypersensitivity	• Orthostatic hypotension • Dizziness • Nausea • Hypercalcemia • Hyperuricemia • Hypercalciuria	• BMD • BP • Urinary calcium • Serum calcium concentrations • Serum 25(OH)D concentrations	May predispose to digoxin toxicity	• ↓ risk of vertebral and nonvertebral fractures • Should not use for >2 yr • Refrigerate
Mechanism of action – monoclonal antibody, bone-modifying agent					
Denosumab • Prolia • 60 mg subcut every 6 mo • Injection	• Hypersensitivity • Hypocalcemia • Pregnancy	• Anaphylaxis • Hypocalcemia • ONJ • Atypical femur fractures • Skin infections • Rash • Myalgia/ arthralgia • Hyperlipidemia	• BMD • Serum calcium concentrations • Serum 25(OH)D concentrations • Serum phosphorus concentrations • Serum magnesium concentrations	None	Refrigerate

Storage and Administration Pearls

- Oral bisphosphonates (tabs) should be taken on an empty stomach first thing in the morning with 6–8 oz of water. At least 30–60 min should pass prior to ingestion of any medication or food. Patient should remain upright for 30–60 min after taking dosage.

- Zoledronic acid solution for injection should be refrigerated prior to use. IV infusion should be administered only by healthcare professional.

- Calcitonin injection and nasal spray should be refrigerated at 2–8°C (36–46°F). Nasal spray can be kept at room temperature up 30°C to (86°F) during use.

- Nasal spray should be primed prior to use. Discard unused portion after 30 days.

- Calcitonin injection can be administered subcutaneously or intramuscularly.

- Teriparatide injection is available in a prefilled pen device and should be refrigerated at 2–8°C (36–46°F). The product should not be frozen, and any unused portion should be discarded after 28 days of use.

- Denosumab injection is available in a prefilled pen device and should be refrigerated at 2–8°C (36–46°F). The product should be brought to room temperature prior to injection (15–30 minutes) and injected by a health care professional. Once at room temperature it should be used within 14 days.

Patient Education Pearls

- Take oral bisphosphonates (tabs) on an empty stomach first thing in the morning with 6–8 oz of plain water. You should then remain upright for 30–60 minutes and avoid lying down. Avoid ingestion of food, beverages (other than water), and other medications for 30–60 minutes after taking this medication.

- Calcitonin nasal spray should be primed prior to use and any unused portion should be discarded after 30 days.

- Teriparatide injection should be refrigerated at all times and should be discarded after 28 days of use.

- Denosumab injection should be refrigerated prior to use and brought to room temperature in its original container prior to injection into the upper arm, thigh, or abdomen. Once at room temperature, the prefilled syringe should be used within 14 days. Injection is typically administered by a health care professional.

- Oral bisphosphonate therapy has been associated with a low potential risk for ONJ. Use of bisphosphonate therapy should be shared with your dental health professional.

GOUT

Definition

Gout is a syndrome of acute or chronic recurrent arthritis characterized by deposits of monosodium urate crystals in synovial fluid and/or tissues and is most often associated with hyperuricemia. Hyperuricemia can result from either an overproduction or under-excretion of uric acid. Overproduction of uric acid is most common in myeloprolifera-tive and lymphoproliferative disorders. A decrease in the renal excretion of uric acid can be the result of renal dysfunction, certain drugs, or a number of predisposing condi-tions, including obesity and hypothyroidism. Acute gouty attacks may be precipitated by a number of conditions including stress, trauma, and alcohol ingestion.

Diagnosis

The diagnosis of gout is based on clinical presentation along with the presence of uric acid crystals detected on joint aspiration of the synovial fluid of affected joints. Eval-uation of a 24-hour urinary uric acid will allow classification of the patient as a uric acid overproducer (urinary uric acid excretion $\geq$600 mg) or a uric acid underexcretor (urinary uric acid >600 mg), which will assist in pharmacotherapeutic decisions.

Signs and Symptoms

Patients presenting with acute gouty arthritis complain of a quick onset of excruciating pain, inflammation, and swelling that most commonly affects the first metatarsopha-langeal (MTP) joint and can also affect the feet, ankles, heels, knees, wrists, fingers, and elbows. Severe cases of gout can result in uric acid nephrolithiasis, nephropathy, or urate deposits (tophi) in affected joints.

Guidelines

Khanna D, Fitzgerald JD, Khanna PP, Bae S, Singh MK, Neogi T, et al; American College of Rheumatology. 2012 American College of Rheumatology Guidelines for Management of Gout. Part 1: Systematic nonpharmacologic and pharmacologic therapeutic approaches to hyperuricemia. *Arthritis Care Res (Hoboken).* 2012;64(10):1431–46.

Treatment of Acute Gouty Arthropathy

- Asymptomatic hyperuricemia does not require therapy.
- First-line treatment for gout includes the use of an NSAID. The majority of acute gout attacks will respond to an NSAID within 72 hours of therapy. Indomethacin is the most common NSAID used in the treatment of gout, but other NSAIDs are also appropriate. Please see the medication chart in the osteoarthritis section of this chapter for more specific NSAID information.

- If patients have a contraindication to the use of an NSAID, evaluation of the time course of symptoms is necessary.

  - If gout symptoms have been present for less than 48 hours, colchicine is recommended for acute treatment.

  - If gout symptoms have been present for more than 48 hours, use of a corticosteroid is recommended.

- If the patient demonstrates an inadequate response to either NSAIDs or colchicine, corticosteroids should be considered.

- The use of oral (preferred) or parenteral corticosteroids is recommended for multijoint involvement, while an intraarticular corticosteroid can be used to target one specific symptomatic joint.

- Allopurinol or febuxostat should never be used in the treatment of acute gout. These agents are reserved for chronic prophylactic therapy in patients with multiple gout exacerbations each year. If these agents are used in the treatment of an acute gout exacerbation, the symptoms may be worsened due to the mobilization of uric acid stores.

Prophylaxis of Gout

- Colchicine maintenance therapy is indicated for prophylaxis in patients with only slightly elevated serum uric acid levels.

- Allopurinol is indicated for prophylaxis of gout exacerbations in patients with a moderately elevated serum uric acid level and a history of nephrolithiasis, tophi, serum creatinine >2.0 mg/dL, or urinary uric acid excretion indicative of overproduction.

- Uricosuric drugs are indicated for prophylaxis of gout exacerbations in patients who are not candidates for allopurinol or febuxostat therapy and have a urinary uric acid excretion indicative of underexcretion.

- When initiating prophylactic therapy in a patient with gout, colchicine should be initiated with allopurinol, febuxostat, or a uricosuric and continued for the first 3–6 months of therapy to avoid causing an exacerbation.

- Pegloticase is indicated for refractory chronic gout in patients that do not respond to or have contraindications to traditional therapy.

Gout Treatment Summary

Drugs for Gout

Generic • Brand • Dose & Max	Contraindications	Primary Side Effects	Key Monitoring Parameters	Pertinent Drug Interactions	Med Pearls
Mechanism of action – colchicine: inhibits lactic acid production, decreases uric acid deposition, reduces phagocytosis, and decreases inflammation					
Colchicine • Colcrys • 1.2 mg then 0.6 mg 1 hr later (max = 1.8 mg)	• Hypersensitivity • Serious GI, renal, hepatic or cardiac disorders	• D/N/V • Rare: bone marrow suppression, aplastic anemia, thrombocyto-penia	• Response to therapy • Serum uric acid • GI symptoms • Periodic CBC	None significant	• Patients may be provided with a prescription to be filled on a PRN basis and used during an exacerbation • Used for treatment and prophylaxis
Mechanism of action – xanthine oxidase inhibitor: by inhibition of xanthine oxidase, impairs the conversion of xanthine to uric acid, thereby decreasing the production of uric acid					
Allopurinol☆ • Zyloprim • 100–800 mg daily (renal dose adjustment necessary)	Hypersensitivity	• Skin rash • Leukopenia • GI upset	• Response to therapy • Serum uric acid • Renal function	• Mercaptopurine • Azathioprine	Adjust dose in renal impairment
Febuxostat • Uloric • 40–80 mg PO daily	Concurrent use with azathioprine, mercaptopurine, or theophylline	• Rash • Liver abnormalities • Arthralgia	• LFTs 2 and 4 months after initiation and periodically thereafter • Serum uric acid levels	• Azathioprine • Mercaptopurine • Theophylline • Didanosine	• No renal dose adjustment necessary • Not to be used during acute gout flares
Mechanism of action – uricosuric agents: increase the renal clearance of uric acid by inhibiting tubular reabsorption					
Sulfinpyrazone • Anturane • 50–800 mg daily (BID)	• Hypersensitivity • CrCl <50 mL/min • History of renal calculi • Overproducers of uric acid • PUD	• GI upset • Rash • Stone formation	• Response to treatment • Serum uric acid • Renal function	• Warfarin (↑ INR) • Salicylates	May precipitate acute gouty attacks; avoid use during acute gouty arthritis
Probenecid • None • 250–2,000 mg daily (BID)	• Hypersensitivity • CrCl <50 mL/min • History of renal calculi • Overproducers of uric acid • PUD	• GI upset • Rash • Stone formation	• Response to treatment • Serum uric acid • Renal function	• Methotrexate (↓ MTX levels) • Salicylates • Penicillins	May precipitate acute gouty attacks; avoid use during acute gouty arthritis

Drugs for Gout *(cont'd)*

Generic • Brand • Dose & Max	Contraindications	Primary Side Effects	Key Monitoring Parameters	Pertinent Drug Interactions	Med Pearls
Mechanism of action – catalyzes oxidation of uric acid to allantoin, thereby decreasing serum uric acid					
Pegloticase • Krystexxa • 8 mg IV infusion (over 2 or more hours) every 2 wk	• Glucose-6-phosphate-dehydrogenase deficiency • Risk of hemolysis • Methemoglobinemia	• Acute gout exacerbation • Infusion reactions • Anaphylaxis	• Response to treatment • Serum uric acid • S/S of anaphylaxis/infusion reactions 1 hr after infusion • Symptoms of congestive heart failure after infusion	None	• Indicated only for refractory cases • Patient should receive pre-treatment with antihistamines and corticosteroids • Gout flare prophylaxis with colchicine or NSAID 1 wk prior to administration is recommended
Mechanism of action – inhibits the transporter proteins involved in renal uric acid reabsorption, uric acid transporter 1 (URAT1), and organic anion transporter 4 (OAT4), which ↓ serum uric acid levels and ↑ renal clearance of uric acid					
Lesinurad • Zurampic • 200 mg daily	• CrCl <45 mL/min • Kidney transplant recipients • Tumor lysis syndrome	• Headache • ↑ serum creatinine • Acute renal failure • Nephrolithiasis • Gastroesophageal reflux disease	• Response to treatment • Serum uric acid • Renal function	• Hormonal contraceptives • Aspirin • Valproic acid	Must be used in combination with xanthine oxidase inhibitor

Storage and Administration Pearls

▪ Medications should be stored in a dry place and protected from light.

Patient Education Pearls

▪ Patient should drink plenty of water (6–8 eight-oz glasses) while taking sulfinpyrazone or probenecid to avoid formation of kidney stones.

LEARNING POINTS

- First-line therapy for mild to moderate osteoarthritis is acetaminophen.

- NSAIDs and other pain medication should be administered with food to minimize stomach upset.

- Biologic therapies for RA suppress immunity and therefore cannot be initiated during infection and may be temporarily withdrawn during active infection.

- Biologic therapy for RA requires parenteral administration.

- First-line therapy for osteoporosis is the bisphosphonate class. Frequency of administration varies greatly from once daily to once annually. Oral formulations require very specific adherence to administration instructions to avoid esophageal side effects.

- Allopurinol and febuxostat are used for gout prophylaxis only and should be avoided during acute attacks because of their ability to exacerbate acute gout arthropathy by mobilizing uric acid stores.

PRACTICE QUESTIONS

1. Which of the following is NOT correctly matched with its trade name?

    (A) Methotrexate – Rheumatrex
    (B) Hydroxychloroquine – Azulfidine
    (C) Leflunomide – Arava
    (D) Etanercept – Enbrel
    (E) Infliximab – Remicade

2. A 60-year-old woman on etanercept 50 mg subcutaneously once weekly is requesting that her immunizations be updated. Which immunization would be contraindicated?

    (A) Varicella zoster
    (B) Seasonal influenza vaccine (intramuscular)
    (C) 23-valent pneumococcal vaccine
    (D) Tetanus, diphtheria, pertussis (Tdap)

3. A 64-year-old asymptomatic man with a medical history significant for hypertension and obesity takes bisoprolol 5 mg daily. His serum uric acid concentration is 7.3 mg/dL on routine laboratory examination. Which is the most appropriate therapeutic strategy?

    (A) Start allopurinol 100 mg/day.
    (B) Start febuxostat 40 mg/day.
    (C) Start probenecid 500 mg twice daily.
    (D) Therapy is not indicated because the patient has not yet experienced a gout attack.

4. A 52-year-old man with a medical history of hypertension, obesity, and gout (one episode, 6 months ago) takes enalapril 40 mg daily, amlodipine 10 mg daily, and aspirin 81 mg daily. He presents with symptoms, starting this morning, of gout in his left first metatarsophalangeal joint and left ankle. The metatarsophalangeal joint is swollen, inflamed, erythematous, and sensitive to light touch. Which is the best approach to therapy?

    (A) Colchicine 1.2 mg by mouth, then 0.6 mg 1 hour later
    (B) Colchicine 1.2 mg by mouth, then 0.6 mg 1 hour later; start allopurinol 300 mg once daily
    (C) Colchicine 1.2 mg by mouth, then 0.6 mg every hour as tolerated
    (D) Colchicine 1.2 mg by mouth, then 0.6 mg every hour as tolerated; start allopurinol 300 mg once daily

5. An 80-year-old woman is diagnosed with osteoarthritis of the right hand. Her medical history is significant for of peptic ulcer disease (PUD), hypertension, and hyperlipidemia. Which is the most appropriate therapy recommendation?

    (A) Glucosamine sulfate 500 mg by mouth three times daily
    (B) Naproxen 500 mg by mouth twice daily
    (C) Diclofenac 1% gel topically four times daily
    (D) Duloxetine 60 mg by mouth once daily

6. A 62-year-old man with hyperlipidemia, allergic rhinitis, and a history of PUD with an upper gastrointestinal bleed 2 years ago is diagnosed with osteoarthritis of the knee. He has tried maximum-dose, scheduled acetaminophen with insufficient pain relief. Current medications include atorvastatin and loratadine. Which is the best recommendation for the management of this patient's osteoarthritis of the knee?

    (A) Naproxen
    (B) Naproxen plus esomeprazole
    (C) Intraarticular corticosteroid
    (D) Diclofenac topical gel

7. A 44-year-old woman is newly diagnosed with rheumatoid arthritis (determined to be moderate–high disease activity) following more than 3 months of bilateral symptoms involving her metacarpophalangeal (MCP) and wrist joints. Laboratory results include AST 33 IU/L, ALT 36 IU/L, SCr 1.0 mg/dL, Hgb 13 g/dL, Hct 39%, (+) RF. Which is the most appropriate therapy selection?

    (A) Hydroxychloroquine
    (B) Methotrexate
    (C) Leflunomide
    (D) Adalimumab

8. A 56-year-old woman with rheumatoid arthritis complains of worsening joint pain in wrists and elbows over the past month. Upon physical exam, new rheumatoid nodules are noted on both elbows. Current medications include adalimumab, methotrexate, and folic acid. Prior medications include hydroxychloroquine (in combination with methotrexate), leflunomide, and etanercept. Which is the most appropriate therapy recommendation?

    (A) Replace adalimumab with abatacept
    (B) Replace methotrexate with sulfasalazine
    (C) Add sulfasalazine
    (D) Add minocycline

9. A 72-year-old woman with osteoporosis and a history of multiple vertebral fractures presents with intolerance to both alendronate and risedronate due to dyspepsia and esophageal irritation. She has followed administration instructions closely but continues to complain of bothersome side effects and indicates that she will no longer consider taking the medications. Her medical history is significant for chronic heart failure and history of venous thromboembolism (×2). Current medications include calcium, vitamin D, lisinopril, digoxin, furosemide, and rivaroxaban. Which of the following is the most appropriate therapy for her osteoporosis?

(A) Ibandronate
(B) Raloxifene
(C) Denosumab
(D) Teriparitide

ANSWERS AND EXPLANATIONS

1. B

Hydroxychloroquine is generic for Plaquenil. Azulfidine is the brand name for sulfasalazine. The other answer choices are correctly matched with their trade names. Methotrexate (A) is generic for Rheumatrex or Trexall.

2. A

Patients with RA receiving biologic DMARDs should not be administered live vaccines such as varicella zoster. Trivalent seasonal influenza vaccine (B) and 23-valent pneumococcal vaccine (C) are acceptable to give to all patients, according to the schedule recommended by the Centers for Disease Control and Prevention (CDC) and Advisory Committee on Immunization Practices (ACIP). The Tdap vaccine (D) may also be safely administered to patients who are considered (non-HIV) immune compromised or receiving immune system–compromising agents.

3. D

Patients should not receive treatment for asymptomatic hyperuricemia until they have experienced their first gouty attack. One to 2 weeks after the first attack, patients may begin uric acid–lowering therapy, and they should be treated to a serum uric acid concentration of <6 mg/dL.

4. A

Because this patient is suffering from an acute gouty attack, the use of allopurinol (B and D) is not appropriate. Allopurinol should be initiated only after the episode of acute gout has resolved. With respect to the colchicine dose, current recommendations support the lower cumulative dose due to equal efficacy and superior tolerability (fewer GI adverse events). The "as-tolerated" instructions for choices (C) and (D) put the patient at risk of overdosing and could potentially cause the patient GI adverse effects and even life-threatening hematologic effects.

5. C

First-line options for osteoarthritis of the hand include topical and oral NSAIDs, topical capsaicin, and tramadol. The ACR 2012 guidelines do not recommend glucosamine (A) for the treatment of OA of the hand. For patients over age 75, topical NSAIDs are preferred over oral NSAIDs, making choice (B) incorrect. Although duloxetine (D) is a second-line option in osteoarthritis of the knee and hip, this agent is not recommended prior to topical NSAIDs and is not preferred in OA of the hand.

6. B

Patients with a history of a GI bleed >1 year ago should receive an NSAID plus a proton pump inhibitor (B) or a COX2 selective NSAID. According to the ACR 2012 guidelines, oral NSAIDs such as naproxen (A) are the first-line option following inadequate response to maximum dose acetaminophen in patients with OA of the knee. Duloxetine, tramadol, and intraarticular injections (C) are reserved for patients with NSAID nonresponse or NSAID contraindications. Diclofenac topical gel (D) is also reserved for patients with NSAID contraindication or over the age of 75.

7. B

According to the 2015 ACR recommendations, treatment-naive patients with moderate–high disease activity should receive combination DMARD therapy with methotrexate unless contraindicated.

8. A

Based upon the 2015 ACR recommendations for rheumatoid arthritis treatment in patients with established disease, health care providers should replace adalimumab in patients with high disease activity (persistently worsening symptoms on escalating therapy); the options include an alternate anti-TNF agent, rituximab, or abatacept. Using an alternate nonbiologic DMARD such as sulfasalazine in place of (B) or in addition to methotrexate (C) would not likely alter the disease progression or symptoms at this stage. Minocycline (D) is reserved for patients with low disease activity and good prognostic features.

9. C

Denosumab is an appropriate agent for the treatment of osteoporosis in postmenopausal female patients at high risk of fracture (prior fractures) that have been intolerant to or failed alternate therapy options. Ibandronate (A) is a bisphosphonate; although this is the first-line class, the patient has not tolerated two agents in this class of medications. Raloxifene (B) is contraindicated due to the patient's history of venous thromboembolism. Teriparatide (D) would be an appropriate selection in a patient with osteoporosis and a history of fracture but would interact with this patient's digoxin, increasing the risk of digoxin toxicity.

Ophthalmologic and Otic Disorders

13

This chapter covers the following disorders:

- **Glaucoma**
- **Impacted cerumen, water-clogged ears, and otitis externa**

 Suggested Study Time: **25 minutes**

GLAUCOMA

Definitions

Glaucoma is a group of eye disorders caused by damage to an area of the optic nerve (optic disk), which results in loss of visual sensitivity and field. The two types of glaucoma include open-angle and closed-angle glaucoma. Open-angle glaucoma is the most common form of this disorder and can be due to either genetic causes (most prevalent is primary open-angle glaucoma [POAG]) or other factors such as trauma, surgery, or medications (secondary open-angle glaucoma). Although it was previously believed that increased intraocular pressure (IOP) was solely responsible for the damage to the optic disk, it appears that factors such as ischemia, changes in blood flow, and autoimmune factors may also play a role.

Given that up to 70% of all cases of glaucoma in the United States are characterized as POAG, the discussion in this chapter focuses only on this form of the ocular disorder.

Diagnosis

The diagnosis of POAG is based on the presence of characteristic changes to the optic disk and visual field loss with or without an increased IOP. An increased IOP does not need to be present to confirm the diagnosis of POAG. In general, an IOP greater than 21 mmHg is considered to be elevated.

Signs and Symptoms

Symptoms of glaucoma usually do not develop until significant damage to the optic disk and significant visual field loss has already occurred. Patients may complain of blind spots, reduced peripheral vision, and changes in color perception.

Guidelines

American Academy of Ophthalmology
http://one.aao.org/CE/PracticeGuidelines/default.aspx

Overview of Treatment

Because the guidelines given here do not specify which drugs should be used as first-line or second-line therapy, this section should not be considered a Guidelines Summary, but rather a general overview of the pharmacologic treatment of glaucoma.

The initial goal is to achieve a 20–30% reduction in the IOP. Additional lowering may be necessary based upon the baseline IOP, the extent of damage to the optic disk, and the extent of visual field loss.

- β-blockers or prostaglandin analogs are considered first-line therapy for POAG. Prostaglandin analogs are often used as initial therapy. These agents can be used as monotherapy or in combination with each other.
  - If a patient does not tolerate or does not respond at all (no reduction in IOP) to an agent, an alternative drug should be used.
  - If a patient partially responds to an agent (some reduction in IOP, but not at goal), addition of another drug should be considered.
- α_2 agonists or topical carbonic anhydrase inhibitors can be considered if the patient does not respond to or tolerate one of the above first-line agents.
- Cholinergic agonist are usually considered as last-line drug therapies because of their increased risk of side effects.
- Laser or surgical procedures may also be considered during the course of therapy.

β-Blockers

Generic • Brand • Dose	Contraindications	Primary Side Effects	Key Monitoring	Pertinent Drug Interactions	Med Pearl
Mechanism of action – ↓ IOP by ↓ production of aqueous humor					
Betaxolol ($β_1$- selective) • Betoptic-S • Solution: 1–2 drops BID • Suspension: 1 drop BID Carteolol (nonselective, ISA properties) • Only available generically • 1 drop BID Levobunolol (nonselective) • Betagan • 1–2 drops 1–2 × daily Metipranolol (nonselective) • OptiPranolol • 1 drop BID Timolol ☆ (nonselective) • Solution: Betimol, Istalol, Timoptic, Timoptic-XE • Solution: 1 drop 1–2 × daily • Gel-forming solution: 1 drop daily	• Sinus bradycardia • ≥2nd-degree heart block (in absence of pacemaker) • Decompensated heart failure • Severe chronic obstructive pulmonary disease/asthma	Local effects • Burning • Stinging • Tearing • Blurred vision • Dry eyes Systemic effects • Bradycardia • Heart block • Hypotension • Heart failure exacerbation • Bronchospasm • Fatigue	IOP every 2–4 wk until target achieved, then every 6 mo	• ↑ risk of systemic side effects with oral β-blockers • ↑ risk of bradycardia or heart block with digoxin, verapamil, diltiazem, ivabradine, or clonidine	• All have similar efficacy in ↓ IOP • Tachyphylaxis may occur with long-term use • Effect on IOP may be ↑ in patients receiving oral β-blockers

Prostaglandin Analogs

Generic • Brand • Dose	Contraindications	Primary Side Effects	Key Monitoring	Pertinent Drug Interactions	Med Pearl
Mechanism of action – ↓ IOP by ↑ outflow of aqueous humor					
Bimatoprost ☆ • Lumigan • 1 drop in evening Latanoprost ☆ • Xalatan • 1 drop in evening Tafluprost • Zioptan • 1 drop in evening Travoprost ☆ • Travatan Z • 1 drop in evening	Hypersensitivity	• Change in iris, eyelash, and eyelid pigmentation (become darker) • Growth of eyelashes • Eyelid edema • Itching, redness, blurred vision, dry eyes	IOP every 2–4 wk until target achieved, then every 6 mo	None	• Do not exceed daily dosing (may worsen IOP) • Iris discoloration is not reversible (highest incidence with latanoprost) • Eyelid discoloration and eyelash changes may be reversible • Travatan Z does not contain benzalkonium chloride • Most effective in ↓ IOP • Bimatoprost also available as Latisse →↑ eyelash growth

α₂-Agonists

Generic • Brand • Dose	Contraindications	Primary Side Effects	Key Monitoring	Pertinent Drug Interactions	Med Pearl
Mechanism of action – ↓ IOP by ↓ production of aqueous humor (brimonidine may also ↑ outflow of aqueous humor)					
Apraclonidine • Iopidine • 1 drop TID Brimonidine ☆ • Alphagan P • 1 drop TID	Concurrent or recent use (within 14 days) of monoamine oxidase inhibitors	Local effects • Eyelid edema • Itching, redness, burning Systemic effects • Dizziness • Fatigue • Dry mouth • Headache • Hypotension • Bradycardia	IOP every 2–4 wk until target achieved, then every 6 mo	↑ risk of systemic side effects with central nervous system depressants (e.g., alcohol, opiates, sedatives, barbiturates)	• Structurally similar to clonidine • Apraclonidine primarily used to control postoperative ↑ IOP

Carbonic Anhydrase Inhibitors

Generic • Brand • Dose	Contraindications	Primary Side Effects	Key Monitoring	Pertinent Drug Interactions	Med Pearl
Mechanism of action – ↓ IOP by ↓ production of aqueous humor					
Brinzolamide • Azopt • 1 drop TID Dorzolamide • Trusopt • 1 drop TID	Sulfa allergy (risk of cross-sensitivity)	• Eyelid reactions • Burning, stinging, tearing, blurred vision • Bitter taste in mouth	IOP every 2–4 wk until target achieved, then every 6 mo	None	• Topical therapy rarely associated with systemic side effects • Oral carbonic anhydrase inhibitor therapy (e.g., acetazolamide) may be used in patients refractory to maximal doses of topical therapy; associated with higher risk of side effects

Cholinergic Agonists (Direct-Acting)

Generic • Brand • Dose	Contraindications	Primary Side Effects	Key Monitoring	Pertinent Drug Interactions	Med Pearl
Mechanism of action – ↓ IOP by ↑ outflow of aqueous humor					
Carbachol • Isopto Carbachol • 1–2 drops 2–3 × daily Pilocarpine • Isopto Carpine • Solution: 1–2 drops 3–4 × daily	Ocular inflammatory condition (may worsen condition)	• Impaired night vision • Headache • Eyelid twitching • Stinging, burning, tearing	IOP every 2–4 wk until target achieved, then every 6 mo	None	• Patients with darker eyes may require higher concentrations of pilocarpine to ↓ IOP • Pilocarpine PO (Salagen) used for Sjögren's syndrome

Combination Drugs

Generic	Brand
Brimonidine/brinzolamide	Simbrinza
Timolol/brimonidine	Combigan
Timolol/dorzolamide	Cosopt

Storage and Administration Pearls

- Most ophthalmic preparations (gels, solutions, suspensions) should be stored at room temperature.
  - Latanoprost should be refrigerated until opened; once opened, the bottle can be stored at room temperature.
- Ophthalmic suspensions should be shaken well prior to using.

Patient Education Pearls

- Patient should be educated on the appropriate administration of ophthalmic preparations:

  - Wash and dry hands.

  - If suspension is being used, shake the bottle well.

  - Contact lenses should be removed prior to administration.

  - Tilt head back and look at the ceiling.

  - Pull down the lower eyelid to form a pocket into which the medication will be instilled.

  - Place the dropper over the eye, look up, and then place a single drop in the eye.

  - To avoid contamination, the tip of the dropper should not touch any part of the eye.

  - Close the eyes for several minutes. Do not rub the eyes.

- If the patient is using more than one ophthalmic drug, administration of these drugs should be separated by at least 10 minutes to prevent loss of the initially administered drug.

- Patient should be educated on use of nasolacrimal occlusion when administering eye drops to minimize the development of systemic side effects and to enhance drug efficacy.

  - Once the eye drop is instilled, instruct patient to close eye and place index finger over nasolacrimal drainage system in the inner corner of the eye for 1–3 minutes.

OTIC DISORDERS

Definitions

Impacted cerumen, water-clogged ears, and swimmer's ear (otitis externa) are three common otic disorders that can be managed with various ear drop products. Cerumen normally helps to protect the ear by lubricating the external auditory canal, trapping foreign particles, and preventing organisms from penetrating into the ear. However, certain individuals, including those who have abnormally shaped external auditory canals, increased hair growth in their ears, or hearing aids, may be at increased risk for the cerumen to become impacted. Water-clogged ears are most likely to occur in patients who have abnormally shaped external auditory canals or excessive cerumen in their ears. Otitis externa occurs when inflammation or infection of the external auditory canal or outer ear develops.

Signs and Symptoms

- Impacted cerumen: Fullness/pressure in ear, hearing impairment, vertigo, tinnitus, otalgia
- Water-clogged ears: Fullness/pressure in ear, hearing impairment
- Otitis externa: Otalgia, otorrhea

Overview of Treatment

Drugs for Treatment of Impacted Cerumen

- Carbamide peroxide (Debrox)

Drugs for Treatment of Water-Clogged Ears

- 95% isopropyl alcohol in 5% anhydrous glycerin (Auro-Dri; Swim Ear)

Drugs for Treatment of Otitis Externa

- Acetic acid otic solution (VoSol) (also available with hydrocortisone [VoSol HC Otic])
- Neomycin with polymyxin B and hydrocortisone (Cortisporin Otic)
- Neomycin with colistin, hydrocortisone, and thonzonium (Coly-Mycin S)
- Ofloxacin (only available generically)
- Ciprofloxacin (Cetraxal)
- Ciprofloxacin with hydrocortisone (Cipro HC)
- Ciprofloxacin with dexamethasone (Ciprodex)
- Finafloxacin (Xtoro)

Storage and Administration Pearls

- Most otic preparations should be stored at room temperature
- Otic solutions/suspensions should be warmed to body temperature by holding containers in hand for a few minutes.
- Otic suspensions should be shaken well before using.

Patient Education Pearls

- Patient should be educated about the appropriate administration of otic preparations:
  - Wash and dry hands.
  - If a suspension is being used, shake the bottle well.
  - Warm the solution/suspension container in the hand for a few minutes.

- Carefully wash and dry outside of the ear (being careful not to get water inside the ear canal).
- Tilt head to the side or lie down with affected ear up.
- Position the dropper tip near, but not inside, the opening of the ear canal. To avoid contamination, the tip of the dropper should not touch any part of the ear.
- Pull the ear backward and upward to open the ear canal. If the patient is younger than 3 years, pull the ear backward and downward.
- Instill the appropriate number of drops into the ear canal.
- Gently press the small skin flap over the ear canal opening to push the ear drops down into the canal.
- Remain in the same position for ≥1 minute to allow penetration of the medication.
- Wash hands.

LEARNING POINTS

- Know examples of ophthalmic β-blockers, prostaglandin analogs, and α_2 agonists.
- β-blocker eye drops can cause systemic adverse effects. Use caution in patients also receiving oral β-blocker therapy.
- Prostaglandin analogs can cause pigmentation changes in the iris, eyelid, and eyelashes.
- Carbonic anhydrase inhibitors should not be used in patients with sulfa allergies.
- Know ophthalmic combination drug products.
- Know which otic products are used for impacted cerumen, water-clogged ears, and otitis externa.

PRACTICE QUESTIONS

1. Which of the following medications is likely to cause a darkening of the iris of the eye?

    (A) Apraclonidine
    (B) Carbachol
    (C) Dorzolamide
    (D) Latanoprost
    (E) Timolol

2. Lumigan belongs to which of the following classes of medications?

    (A) α_2 agonist
    (B) Antihistamine
    (C) β-blocker
    (D) Cholinergic agonist
    (E) Prostaglandin analog

3. Which of the following products contains a carbonic anhydrase inhibitor?

    (A) Alphagan P
    (B) Azopt
    (C) Betoptic-S
    (D) Combigan
    (E) Lumigan

4. A patient with glaucoma has a history of anaphylaxis when taking trimethoprim/sulfamethoxazole. Which of the following medications should be avoided in this patient?

    (A) Alphagan P
    (B) Betoptic S
    (C) Combigan
    (D) Simbrinza
    (E) Travatan Z

5. Which of the following medications can be used to clear impacted cerumen in the ear?

    (A) Cetraxal
    (B) Cortisporin Otic
    (C) Debrox
    (D) Xalatan
    (E) Xeljanz

ANSWERS AND EXPLANATIONS

1. D

Latanoprost, an ophthalmic prostaglandin analog, is likely to cause darkening of the iris, so choice (D) is correct. This class of drugs may also cause increased pigmentation of the eyelid and eyelashes.

2. E

Lumigan, the brand name for bimatoprost, is a prostaglandin analog, so choice (E) is correct.

3. B

Azopt contains brinzolamide, which is a carbonic anhydrase inhibitor. Alphagan-P (A) contains brimonidine, an α_2-agonist. Betoptic-S (C) contains betaxolol, a β-blocker. Combigan (D) is a combination product that contains timolol (β-blocker) and brimonidine (α_2-agonist). Lumigan (E) contains bimatoprost, a prostaglandin analog.

4. D

The ophthalmic carbonic anhydrase inhibitors—brinzolamide and dorzolamide—are sulfa derivatives and should be avoided in patients with a history of anaphylaxis to sulfa products (e.g., trimethoprim/sulfamethoxazole). Simbrinza (D) (brimonidine/brinzolamide) contains a carbonic anhydrase inhibitor. Alphagan P (A) contains brimonidine (α_2-agonist); Betoptic S (B) contains betaxolol (β-blocker); Combigan (C) contains timolol (β-blocker) and brominidine (α_2-agonist); and Travatan Z (E) contains travoprost (prostaglandin analog).

5. C

Debrox (C) (carbamide peroxide) can be used to clear impacted cerumen in the ear. Cetraxal (A) (ciprofloxacin) and Cortisporin Otic (B) (neomycin with polymixin B and hydrocortisone) are used to treat otitis externa. Xalatan (D) (latanoprost) is used to treat glaucoma. Xeljanz (E) (tofactinib) is not used to treat ophthalmologic disorders; it is used to treat rheumatoid arthritis.

Hematologic Disorders

14

This chapter covers the following diseases:

- **Iron deficiency anemia**
- **Anemia of chronic kidney disease and dialysis**
- **Megaloblastic anemias**
- **Sickle cell disease**

 Suggested Study Time: **45 minutes**

IRON DEFICIENCY ANEMIA

Definitions

Iron deficiency anemia (IDA) is a common disorder worldwide. In the United States, most cases are caused by menstrual blood loss, gastrointestinal (GI) blood loss, and increased iron requirements of pregnancy. Low iron absorption or high iron requirements from other conditions may also lead to iron deficiency.

Diagnosis

- Evidence of a source of blood loss should be sought.
- Iron deficiency anemia is classically described as a microcytic (mean corpuscular volume [MCV] <80 fL), hypochromic (mean corpuscular hemoglobin concentration [MCHC] <31 g/dL)
- The differential diagnosis of iron deficiency anemia includes thalassemia, sideroblastic anemias, some types of anemia of chronic disease, and lead poisoning.
- Cells start out normochromic but become more hypochromic as the anemia progresses.

- Serum ferritin is the preferred initial diagnostic test. Total iron-binding capacity (TIBC), transferrin saturation, serum iron, and serum transferrin receptor levels may be helpful if the ferritin level is between 46 and 99 ng/mL; bone marrow biopsy may be necessary in these patients for a definitive diagnosis.
- Laboratory tests:
  - Low serum Fe
  - Low ferritin (main lab indicator)
  - High TIBC
  - Hemoglobin (Hgb) and hematocrit (Hct) low in later stages
  - Low MCV, MCHC
  - Low transferrin saturation

Signs and Symptoms

There are many symptoms of IDA. Different patients will experience different combinations of symptom. If the anemia is mild, it is possible that the symptoms may not be noticeable. Some of the symptoms are: pale skin color, fatigue, irritability, dizziness, weakness, shortness of breath, sore tongue, brittle nails, decreased appetite (especially in children), and frontal headaches.

Guidelines and References

World Health Organization. Iron Deficiency Anaemia; Assessment, Prevention, and Control: A Guide for Programme Managers. Geneva, Switzerland: World Health Organization; 2001.

Goddard AF, James MW, McIntyre AS, Scot BB. British Society of Gastroenterology. Guidelines for the management of iron deficiency anemia. Gut. 2011;60:1309–1316.

Short MW, Domagalski JE. Iron Deficiency Anemia: Evaluation and Management. Am Fam Physician. 2013;87:98–104.

Guidelines Summary

In children, adolescents, and women of reproductive age, a trial of iron is a reasonable approach if the review of symptoms, history, and physical examination are negative; however, the Hgb should be checked at one month. If there is not a 1 g/dL increase in the Hgb level in that time, possibilities include malabsorption of oral iron, lack of compliance, continued bleeding, or presence of an unknown lesion.

- Dose of elemental iron needed to treat IDA is 120 mg per for 3 months in adults and 3 mg/kg/day in children (max of 60mg/day).

- An increase in the Hgb level of 1 g/dL after 1 month of treatment is an indicator of adequate response to iron therapy.

- Therapy should be continued for 3 months after correction of IDA to allow for replenishment of iron stores.

- Iron sulfate in a dose of 325 mg provides 65 mg of elemental iron, whereas 30 mg of iron gluconate provides 38 mg of elemental iron.

- GI absorption of elemental iron is enhanced in the presence of an acidic gastric environment, which can be accomplished through simultaneous intake of ascorbic acid (i.e., vitamin C).

- Patients should be counseled to take iron 2 hours before or 4 hours after antacids to minimize the potential for chelation and decreased absorption.

- Although iron absorption occurs more readily when taken on an empty stomach, this increases the likelihood of iron-induced stomach upset. Increased patient adherence that may result from taking the iron with food should be weighed against the inferior iron absorption that may occur.

- Laxatives, stool softeners, and adequate intake of liquids can alleviate the constipating effects of oral iron therapy.

- Indications for the use of intravenous (IV) iron include:
  - Intestinal malabsorption
  - Intolerance to oral iron, which often results in patient nonadherence

Medications for Iron Deficiency Anemia

Generic • Brand • Dose/Dosage Forms	Contraindications	Primary Side Effects	Key Monitoring	Pertinent Drug Interactions	Med Pearl
Mechanism of action – replaces iron found in hemoglobin, myoglobin; allows the transportation of oxygen via hemoglobin					
Ferrous sulfate, gluconate, fumarate • Sulfate: Feosol, Fer-In-Sol, Fer-Iron, Slow-FE • Gluconate: Ferate • Fumarate: Ferrocite • Sulfate: treatment: 300 mg 2–4 × /day • Gluconate/fumarate: 60 mg 2–4 × /day • ER tabs, solution, tabs	• Hypersensitivity to iron salts • Hemochromatosis (GI tract absorbs excess iron) • Hemolytic anemia	• GI irritation • Epigastric pain • Nausea/vomiting (N/V) • Dark stools • Stomach cramping • Constipation	• Serum iron • TIBC • Serum ferritin • Reticulocyte count • Hgb/Hct	• ↓ absorption of tetracyclines, fluoroquinolones, levodopa, methyldopa, and penicillamine • Proton pump inhibitors (PPIs), H₂ blockers, and antacids can ↓ iron absorption	Administer with vitamin C or orange juice to ↑ absorption

Medications for Iron Deficiency Anemia *(cont'd)*

Generic • Brand • Dose/Dosage Forms	Contraindications	Primary Side Effects	Key Monitoring	Pertinent Drug Interactions	Med Pearl
Mechanism of action – iron complex taken up by reticuloendothelial system and then released for storage or for transport and incorporation into Hgb; eventually replenish depleted iron stores in the bone marrow					
Iron dextran complex • Infed (IM or IV) • Dose (in mL) = 0.0442 (desired Hgb − observed Hgb) × lean body weight (LBW) + (0.26 × LBW) • Max dose = 100 mg/day	Hypersensitivity	• Anaphylaxis • Hypotension • Tightness in the chest • Wheezing • Flushing	• Anaphylactic reaction • Serum iron • TIBC • Serum ferritin • Transferrin saturation • Reticulocyte count • Hgb/Hct • Blood pressure • Heart rate	None	• Test dose is required • Anaphylaxis may still occur despite having an uneventful test dose • If flushing or hypotension occur, ↓ infusion rate
Sodium ferric gluconate • Ferrlecit • 125 mg via IV infusion infused (usually × 8 doses) • Injection	Hypersensitivity	• Anaphylaxis • Tachycardia • Hypotension • Chest pain • Dizziness		May ↓ absorption of oral iron	• A safer form of parenteral iron compared to iron dextran • No test dose required
Ferumoxytol • Feraheme • 510 mg via IV infusion followed by 510 mg via IV infusion 3–8 days later • Injection	• Hypersensitivity • History of allergic reaction to any IV iron product	• Anaphylaxis • Diarrhea • Constipation • Hypotension • Dizziness		May ↓ absorption of oral iron	• Patients with multiple drug allergies at ↑ risk for anaphylactic reaction • May interfere with MRI readings for up to 3 mo after use • No test dose required
Iron sucrose • Venofer • Hemodialysis-dependent: 100 mg IV 1–3 ×/wk during dialysis until cumulative dose of 1,000 mg achieved (10 doses) • Peritoneal dialysis-dependent: 300 mg IV, then 300 mg IV 14 days later, then 400 mg IV 14 days later • No dialysis: 200 mg IV administered on 5 separate occasions during a 14-day time period • Injection	Hypersensitivity	• Anaphylaxis • Hypotension • Headache • Chest pain • Dizziness		May ↓ absorption of oral iron	• Can be administered as a slow IV injection (2–5 min) or as an IV infusion (time is dose dependent) • No test dose required
Ferric carboxymaltose • Injectafer • <50 kg: 15 mg/kg IV, then 15 mg/kg IV ≥7 days later (max = 1500 mg/treatment course) • ≥50 kg: 750 mg IV, then 750 mg IV ≥7 days later • Injection	Hypersensitivity	• Anaphylaxis • Hypertension • Nausea • Flushing • Hypophosphatemia • Dizziness		Unknown	• Can be administered as a slow IV injection (100 mg/min) or as an IV infusion (over ≥15 min) • No test dose required

Storage and Administration Pearls

- Oral iron is a leading cause of fatal poisoning in children. Store out of children's reach and in child-resistant containers.

Patient Education Pearls

- Oral iron products can be taken with vitamin C or orange juice to increase absorption.

ANEMIA OF CHRONIC KIDNEY DISEASE AND DIALYSIS

Definitions

Anemia of chronic kidney disease (CKD) is a hypoproliferative disorder associated with certain infectious or inflammatory processes, tissue injury, or conditions that release proinflammatory cytokines. It is attributed primarily to a decrease in endogenous erythropoietin (EPO) production and may occur as the creatinine clearance declines below approximately 50 mL/min. Eventually, the patient may require dialysis to filtrate metabolic waste. There are several types of dialysis, including:

- Hemodialysis—diffuses small molecular-weight solutes across a semipermeable membrane.
- Peritoneal dialysis—uses the peritoneum as a dialysis membrane.
- Ultrafiltration and hemofiltration—remove large volumes of fluid with minimal removal of metabolic wastes.

Diagnosis

- There is currently no definitive test for anemia of CKD. It is a diagnosis of exclusion.
- May coexist with iron deficiency and folate deficiency
- Low serum iron
- Normal or high ferritin
- Low TIBC
- Normal MCV, MCHC
- Normochromic, normocytic red blood cells on peripheral smear

Signs and Symptoms

There are many symptoms of anemia of CKD. Different patients will experience different combinations of symptoms. If the anemia is mild, it is possible that the symptoms may not be noticeable. Symptoms include pale skin color, fatigue, irritability, dizziness, weakness, shortness of breath, sore tongue, brittle nails, decreased appetite (especially in children), and frontal headaches.

Guidelines

KDIGO Anemia Work Group. KDIGO clinical practice guideline for anemia in chronic kidney disease. *Kidney Int Suppl.* 2012;2:279–335.

Guidelines Summary

- Treatment guidelines are based on Hgb.
- ESAs should be used in caution with patients with malignancy if cure of malignancy is an option.
- The upper limit of Hgb should not exceed 11.5 g/dL in adults.
- In pediatric patients, the range of Hgb should be between 11–12 g/dL.
- Iron therapy may be used if TSAT is < 30% and ferritin is < 500 ng/mL.

Medications for Anemia of Chronic Kidney Disease and Dialysis

Generic • Brand • Dose/Dosage Forms	Contraindications	Primary Side Effects	Key Monitoring	Pertinent Drug Interactions	Med Pearl
Erythropoietin Stimulating Agents					
Mechanism of action – induce erythropoiesis by stimulating the division and differentiation of committed erythroid progenitor cells; induce the release of reticulocytes from the bone marrow into the bloodstream					
Epoetin alfa • Procrit, Epogen • Initial: 50–100 units/kg IV or subcut 3 ×/wk • Injection Darbepoetin alfa • Aranesp • CKD patients on dialysis: 0.45 mcg/kg IV or subcut weekly or 0.75 mcg/kg IV or subcut every 2 wk • CKD patients not on dialysis: 0.45 mcg/kg IV or subcut every 4 wk • Injection	• Hypersensitivity • Uncontrolled hypertension • Pure red cell aplasia	• Hypertension • ↑ mortality, myocardial infarction, stroke, or thromboembolism (if target Hgb >11 g/dL) • Seizures • Peripheral edema • Headache • Nausea • Arthralgia	• Hgb • Ferritin • Transferrin saturation • Iron stores • Blood pressure	None	• IV route preferred for patients on hemodialysis • In patients with CKD on dialysis, initiate treatment if Hgb <10 g/dL • Do not ↑ dose more frequently than every 4 wk • If Hgb ↑ by >1 g/dL in a 2-wk period, ↓ dose by ≥25% • If Hgb has not ↑ by >1 g/dL in 4-wk period, ↑ dose by 25% • For CKD patients on dialysis, if Hgb >11 g/dL, ↓ or interrupt dose • For CKD patients NOT on dialysis, if Hgb >10 g/dL, ↓ or interrupt dose

Medications for Anemia of Chronic Kidney Disease and Dialysis *(cont'd)*

Generic • Brand • Dose/Dosage Forms	Contraindications	Primary Side Effects	Key Monitoring	Pertinent Drug Interactions	Med Pearl
Dialysate Iron Replacement					
Mechanism of action – Binds to transferrin for incorporation into hemoglobin					
Ferric pyrophosphate citrate • Triferic • 1 ampule: 2.5 gal. bicarbonate concentrate; 2 micromolar concentration	Hypersensitivity	• Peripheral edema • Urinary tract infection • Pain • Headache • Fatigue • Fistula thrombosis • Fistula hemor-rhage	Predialysis iron status	None	Only used in dialysis patients

Storage and Administration Pearls

- Refrigerate ESA vial between 36–46°F.
- Do not freeze or shake ESA vials.
- ESA multidose vials, with preservative, are stable for 1 week at room temperature.
- Ferric pyrophosphate should be stored protected from light in the aluminum pouch at room temperature.

Patient Education Pearls

- These medications can be administered only by infusion or injection.
- Frequent blood tests will be needed to determine appropriate dosages.
- Avoid alcohol and do not make significant changes in dietary iron without consulting prescriber.
- Check blood pressure frequently.

MEGALOBLASTIC ANEMIAS

Definitions

Megaloblastic anemias is a decrease in red blood cells that occurs when the body cannot properly absorb vitamin B_{12} (cyanocobalamin) from the GI tract or is deficient in folate. Vitamin B_{12} is necessary for the formation of red blood cells. Megaloblastic anemia is a blood disorder characterized by red blood cells that are larger than normal due to deficiency in folate or cyanocobalamin. Pernicious anemia is another name for vitamin B_{12} deficiency.

Diagnosis

- Detecting antibodies to intrinsic factor is specific for the diagnosis of pernicious anemia.
- A Schilling test may be used to detect antibodies to intrinsic factor.
- Serum vitamin B_{12} and folate concentrations should be measured.
- A serum vitamin B_{12} concentration <200 pg/mL is diagnostic of vitamin B_{12} deficiency.
- A serum folate concentration <2 ng/mL is diagnostic of folate deficiency.
- Serum methylmalonic acid and homocysteine are elevated in pernicious anemia.
- High MCV and MCHC.

Signs and Symptoms

- Symptoms similar to IDA.
- Findings may include glossitis, jaundice, and splenomegaly.
- Neurologic symptoms (e.g., ataxia, paresthesias, confusion, and dementia) may be present with vitamin B_{12} deficiency; folate deficiency does *not* cause neurologic symptoms.

Treatment Summary

- No major guidelines have been recently published on the treatment of pernicious anemia or folate deficiency.
- Treatment is directed toward replacing the deficient factor.
- Blood transfusions are rarely required.
- Treatment is often initiated with intramuscular injections before moving to oral formulations.
- With therapy, reticulocytosis should begin within 1 week, followed by an increased Hgb over 6–8 weeks.
- Coexisting iron deficiency is present in one-third of patients and is a common cause of incomplete response to therapy with vitamin B_{12} or folic acid.

Medications for Megaloblastic Anemias

Generic • Brand • Dose/Dosage Forms	Contraindications	Primary Side Effects	Key Monitoring	Pertinent Drug Interactions	Med Pearl
Mechanism of action – coenzyme for various metabolic functions, cell replication, and hematopoiesis					
Cyanocobalamin (vitamin B_{12}) • Nascobal • IM: Initial: 1,000 mcg daily for 1 wk, then 1,000 mcg monthly for 6 mo • IM: Maintenance: 1,000 mcg monthly • PO: 1 mg daily • Intranasal: 500 mcg in 1 nostril weekly	Hypersensitivity	• Anxiety • Itching • Diarrhea	• Serum vitamin B_{12} • Hgb/Hct • Reticulocyte count • Serum folate • Serum iron	• Metformin and proton pump inhibitors may ↓ vitamin B_{12} absorption	Hydroxocobalamin is a longer-acting form of vitamin B_{12}
Mechanism of action – coenzyme in many metabolic systems, particularly for purine and pyrimidine synthesis					
Folic acid (folate) ☆ • Only available generically • 0.4–1 mg daily • Prevention of neural tube defects: 0.4–0.8 mg daily	Hypersensitivity	• Allergic reaction • Bronchospasm • Flushing • Malaise • Pruritus • Rash	• Serum folate • Hgb/Hct • Reticulocyte count • Serum iron	• May ↓ phenytoin and phenobarbital levels • Phenytoin and sulfasalazine may ↓ folate absorption	Products containing >0.8 mg of folic acid are Rx only

Storage and Administration Pearls

- Cyanocobalamin injection is clear pink-to-red solution; stable at room temperature.
- Cyanocobalamin must be protected from light.
- Intranasal spray must be stored in the refrigerator and not frozen.

Patient Education Pearls

- Pernicious anemia may require treatment for life.
- Report rashes on extremities or acute persistent diarrhea.

SICKLE CELL DISEASE

Definition

Sickle cell disease (SCD) is a collection of hereditary red blood cell disorders. Sickle cell hemoglobin differs from normal hemoglobin in that it is shaped in rods or crescent shapes instead of the normal disc shape. The alteration in shape causes the sickled hemoglobin to lose flexibility, stick to vessel walls, and create blockages. SCD is life long and can only be cured with hematopoietic stem cell transplantation.

Diagnosis

SCD is usually diagnosed based on standard neonatal blood screening. If a screen is positive, a second test is performed at 2 months of age for confirmation.

Signs and symptoms

SCD may involve many organs and manifests differently, depending on the genotype. The predominant features of SCD include hemolytic anemia and occlusion of vessels. Other clinical features include episodes of pain, anemia, and enlargement of the liver, spleen, and heart.

Acute complications of SCD include fever and infections due to functional asplenia. Cognitive deficits may also be seen in the presence of cerebrovascular occlusion. Acute chest syndrome is a common cause of hospitalization in patients with SCD and is characterized by pulmonary infiltrates with cough, dyspnea, tachypnea, chest pain, fever, wheezing, and hypoxia. Pain episodes may be due to occlusion of vessels, but also from bone or muscle infarction. Splenic sequestration of red blood cells leads to an acute enlargement of the spleen.

Chronic complications of SCD may include pulmonary hypertension, osteonecrosis, visual blindess or visual field deficits, gallstones, cardiac enlargement, left ventricular hypertrophy, nephropathy, delayed growth, depression, and anxiety.

Guidelines

Yawn BP, Buchanan GR, Afenyi-Annan AN, et al. Management of sickle cell disease: summary of the 2014 evidence-based report by expert panel members. *JAMA*. 2014;312:1033–48.

Guideline Summary

Medication related considerations for patients with SCD:

- Prevent pneumococcal disease with use of immunizations. May also use penicillin as a prophylactic agent up to age 5.
- Progestin-only hormonal contraceptives, levonorgestrel and intrauterine devices can be used in patients with SCD without concern.
- Rapidly assess and treat pain using nonopioid and opioid analgesics.
- May consider the use of hydroxyurea if an adult patient experiences 3 or more moderate-to-severe pain crises in a 12-month period.

LEARNING POINTS

- Coexisting iron deficiency is present in many forms of anemia and should always be assessed.
- When treating with ESA, Hb should not be greater than 13.0 g/dL due to the all-cause mortality and adverse cardiovascular event in patients with CKD and Hb greater than 13.0 g/dL.
- ESAs may be used for chemotherapy associated anemia if cure is not the goal of chemotherapy.
- Iron absorption is enhanced through simultaneous intake of ascorbic acid (i.e., vitamin C).
- Laxatives, stool softeners, and adequate intake of liquids should be regularly recommended to patients taking iron therapy, to alleviate the medication's constipating effects.
- Long-term metformin therapy can decrease the absorption of vitamin B_{12}.

PRACTICE QUESTIONS

1. Which of the following can be administered with ferrous sulfate to increase absorption?

    (A) Ascorbic acid
    (B) Calcium carbonate
    (C) Famotidine
    (D) Omeprazole

2. Which of the following is an adverse effect associated with epoetin alfa?

    (A) Bradycardia
    (B) Constipation
    (C) Hypertension
    (D) Thrombocytopenia

3. Absorption of which of the following medications may be impaired if given concurrently with oral ferrous sulfate? (Select ALL that apply.)

    (A) Amoxicillin
    (B) Ciprofloxacin
    (C) Tetracycline
    (D) Trimethoprim

4. Which of the following can be used to prevent neural tube defects?

    (A) Cyanocobalamin
    (B) Ferrous gluconate
    (C) Ferumoxytol
    (D) Folic acid

5. Which of the following is a precaution for using darbepoetin?

    (A) BP of 110/72
    (B) CKD
    (C) HgB of 12 g/dL
    (D) Palliative chemotherapy

6. Which of the following statements regarding cyanocobalamin is TRUE?

    (A) Injection solution is red to pink in color.
    (B) It is used for the treatment of folate deficiency.
    (C) It must be initiated with the nasal form.
    (D) Levels may be depleted by sulfonylureas.

ANSWERS AND EXPLANATIONS ON FOLLOWING PAGE

ANSWERS AND EXPLANATIONS

1. **A**

Oral iron products need an acidic environment for absorption. Ascorbic acid (vitamin C) or a glass of orange juice can be administered with oral iron products to increase absorption. Calcium carbonate (B) is an antacid, famotidine (C) is an H_2 agonist, and omeprazole (D) is a proton pump inhibitor; all of these would decrease the acidification needed for iron absorption.

2. **C**

Hypertension is associated with the use of ESAs and should be monitored for while on therapy. If a patient has uncontrolled HTN before starting ESAs, it may preclude the use until the blood pressure is more optimally managed. Bradycardia (A), constipation (B), and thrombocytopenia (D) are not associated with ESAs.

3. **B, C**

Oral iron products can bind to both quinolone and tetracycline antibiotics, leading to a decreased serum concentration for the quinolone or tetracycline antibiotic if given concurrently. If iron needs to be given with either a quinolone or a tetracycline antibiotic, the antibiotic should be given 2–4 hours prior to or 2–8 hours after the oral iron product is administered.

4. **D**

Folic acid can be used to prevent neural tube defects. Cyanocobalamin (A) (vitamin B_{12}) is used to increase B_{12} levels and prevent pernicious anemia. Ferrous gluconate (B) and ferumoxytol (C) are used to increase iron levels.

5. **C**

ESA agents should be used in caution in patients with Hgb levels >11 g/dL, as there is an increased risk of death or adverse cardiovascular events in these patients. ESAs may increase BP (A) but are only contraindicated in patients with uncontrolled HTN. CKD (B) is an indication for use of ESAs, but there is a caution for use in patients with Hgb levels >11 g/dL. ESAs can be used in patients receiving palliative chemotherapy (D), but they should not be used in patients receiving curative chemotherapy.

6. **A**

The injection solution for cyanocobalamin is red to pink and is stable at room temperature. Cyanocobalamin is used to treat B_{12} deficiency, not folate deficiency (B). B_{12} therapy is often initiated with the IM formulation and is then transitioned to oral therapy; the nasal formulation (C) is rarely used. Levels of B_{12} may be depleted with metformin, not sulfonylureas (D).

Dermatologic Disorders 15

This chapter covers the following disease states:

- **Acne**
- **Psoriasis**

 Suggested Study Time: **15 minutes**

ACNE

Definitions

Acne vulgaris is an inflammatory skin disorder that results in comedones, papules, pustules, nodules, or cysts on the face, back, or chest. The disorder occurs most commonly in teenagers at or near puberty but can occur at any age.

Diagnosis

Although no strict diagnostic criteria exist, the presence of five or more lesions (of any type) is generally considered sufficient for diagnosis.

Signs and Symptoms

Acne vulgaris lesions appear most commonly on the face but also on the back and chest. The severity of acne vulgaris varies and is based on the types of lesions present. Type I acne is the mildest form and is associated with a mostly noninflammatory presentation of open and closed comedones. Type II acne is a more moderate form with multiple papules present. Type III acne is associated with a more severe form of acne consisting of an inflammatory condition with multiple pustules. Type IV is the most severe form, consisting of inflammatory nodules and cysts that lead to scarring.

Guidelines

Zaenglein AL, Pathy AL, Schlosser BJ, et al. Guidelines of care for the management of acne vulgaris. *J Am Acad Dermatol.* 2016;74:945–73.

Guideline Summary

- Topical benzoyl peroxide is the first-line therapy recommendation for most mild to moderate forms of acne vulgaris (type I).

- Topical antibiotics and topical retinoids are considered first-line for moderate acne vulgaris (type II) and second-line for mild-moderate acne vulgaris (type I).

- Topical antibiotics are most effective when used in combination with benzoyl peroxide or a retinoid due to risk of antibiotic resistance when used as monotherapy.

- Moderate to severe, inflammatory acne (type III) should be treated with topical therapy (benzoyl peroxide, retinoids, or antibiotics) plus oral antibiotics.

- Severe, inflammatory acne (type IV) can be treated with the combination of oral antibiotics and topical therapy but often requires the use of oral isotretinoin therapy.

- Oral isotretinoin is an effective therapy option for the treatment of severe, inflammatory acne, or more moderate forms that have been refractory to other treatment options.

- All females of child-bearing age who have been prescribed isotretinoin must agree to use two forms of contraception during isotretinoin use. Because of the known teratogenic risk associated with isotretinoin therapy, all patients, pharmacies, physicians, and wholesalers must register with the iPLEDGE program. This is an program sponsored by the Food and Drug Administration that is designed to monitor and ↓ the risk of fetal exposure to isotretinoin.

Medications for Acne

Generic • Brand • Dose/Dosage Forms	Contraindications	Primary Side Effects	Key Monitoring Parameters	Pertinent Drug Interactions	Med Pearls
Topical					
Nonprescription					
Benzoyl peroxide • Many • 2.5–10% cream, lotion, gel, wash	Hypersensitivity	• Excessive drying • Photosensitivity • Peeling • Erythema	• Presence of side effects • ↓ lesions	Concurrent use with retinoids causes significant irritation	Available over-the-counter
Sulfur • SAStid • 3–8% soap				Concurrent use with other topical agents cause additive drying	
Salicylic acid • Many • 0.5–2% wash					
Antimicrobials					
Clindamycin • Cleocin T, Clindagel, Evoclin • Lotion/solution: Apply BID • Foam/gel: Apply daily • 1% foam, gel, lotion, solution	• Hypersensitivity • History of ulcerative colitis • History of antibiotic-associated colitis	• Burning • Itching • Dryness • Irritation	• Presence of side effects • ↓ lesions	May ↑ effects of neuromuscular blocking agents	
Erythromycin • Akne-Mycin, Erygel • Apply 1–2 ×/day • 2% gel, ointment, pads, solution	Hypersensitivity			None	
Retinoids					
Tretinoin • Atralin, Avita, Renova, Retin-A • Apply daily • 0.01–0.1% gel, cream	Hypersensitivity	• Photosensitivity • Burning • Dryness • Erythema • Irritation	• Presence of side effects • ↓ lesions	• Concurrent use with other topical drying agents may cause additive drying • Concurrent use with other photosensitizing medications ↑ risk of photosensitivity	• Tretinoin and tazarotene should be applied after freshly washed face is completely dry
Tazarotene • Avage, Fabior, Tazorac • Apply daily • 0.05–0.1% gel, cream, foam	• Hypersensitivity • Women who are or may become pregnant				
Adapalene • Differin • Apply daily • 0.1% gel, cream, lotion; 0.3% gel	Hypersensitivity				• Adapalene does not require waiting until face is dry for application • Adapalene now available over-the-counter

Medications for Acne *(cont'd)*

Generic • Brand • Dose/Dosage Forms	Contraindications	Primary Side Effects	Key Monitoring Parameters	Pertinent Drug Interactions	Med Pearls
Other					
Azelaic acid • Azelex, Finacea • Apply BID • 15% gel, foam; 20% cream	Hypersensitivity	• Burning • Stinging • Tingling • Pruritus • Photosensitivity	• Presence of side effects • ↓ lesions	None	
Dapsone • Aczone • 5% gel: Apply daily • 7.5% gel: Apply BID • Gel	None	• Oiliness • Peeling • Dryness • Erythema	• Presence of side effects • ↓ lesions	• Trimethoprim/ sulfamethoxazole may ↑ effects and risk of toxicity • Concurrent use with benzoyl per- oxide may cause yellow or orange skin discoloration	• Apply after freshly washed face is completely dry • Reassess need for treat- ment if no improvement after 12 wk
Oral					
Antimicrobials					
Tetracycline • Only available generi- cally • 1,000 mg/day in 2–4 divided doses initially, then 125–500 mg daily once improve- ment observed Doxycycline ☆ • Acticlate, Doryx, Monodox, Oracea, Vibramycin • 50–100 mg BID Minocycline ☆ • Minocin, Solodyn • 100 mg PO q12h	Children ≤8 yr and pregnant/breast- feeding women (may cause permanent teeth discoloration and impaired teeth/bone growth)	• Nausea/vomit- ing/diarrhea (N/V/D) • Photosensitivity • Rash	• Presence of side effects • ↓ lesions	• CYP3A4 substrates and inhibitors • Absorption ↓ with antacids, dairy products, and products contain- ing iron, magne- sium, aluminum, calcium, or zinc (separate by 2 hr) • CYP3A4 inhibitors may ↑ risk of side effects • CYP3A4 inducers may ↓ effects • May ↑ effect/ toxicity of CYP3A4 substrates • May ↑ effects of warfarin • May ↓ effects of oral contraceptive	

Medications for Acne *(cont'd)*

Generic • Brand • Dose/Dosage Forms	Contraindications	Primary Side Effects	Key Monitoring Parameters	Pertinent Drug Interactions	Med Pearls
Antimicrobials (cont'd)					
Erythromycin • E.E.S, EryPed, Ery-Tab, Erythrocin, PCE • 250–500 mg PO q6h	• Hypersensitivity • QT interval prolongation • Concurrent use with other drugs that prolong QT interval	• QT interval prolongation interval • N/V/D	• Presence of side effects • ↓ lesions	• CYP3A4 substrate and inhibitor • CYP3A4 inhibitors may ↑ risk of side effects • CYP3A4 inducers may ↓ effects • May ↑ effect/ toxicity of CYP3A4 substrates • ↑ risk of torsade de pointes with other drugs that prolong QT interval • May ↑ effects of warfarin • May ↑ risk of digoxin toxicity	Significant drug interactions and gastrointestinal side effects limit use
Isotretinoin					
Isotretinoin • Absorica, Amnesteem, Claravis, Myorisan, Zenatane • 0.5–1 mg/kg/day in 2 divided doses	• Hypersensitivity • Pregnancy	• Cheilitis • Dry mouth • Dry skin • Pruritus • Erythema • Gastrointestinal upset • Headache • Hyperlipidemia • Depression • Suicidal thoughts • Aggression • Rash (Stevens-Johnson syndrome possible) • Pancreatitis • Hearing impairment • Hepatotoxicity • Arthralgia • ↓ bone mineral density • Corneal deposits • ↓ night vision • Hyperglycemia	• ↓ lesions • Pregnancy test • Lipid panel • Complete blood count with differential • Fasting plasma glucose • Mental status • Changes in vision • Liver function tests	• Concurrent use with vitamin A may lead to ↑ risk of toxicity • ↑ risk of intracranial hypertension with tetracycline	• Females must have 2 urine or blood pregnancy tests before initiating therapy (interval between 2 tests must be ≥19 days), then single pregnancy test must be performed monthly after initiating therapy • Females must agree to at least 2 forms of contraception for 1 mo before therapy initiated and during therapy • Must register in iPLEDGE program • Highly teratogenic • Take with full glass of water

Available combination products:

- Adapalene/benzoyl peroxide (Epiduo, Epiduo Forte)
- Benzoyl peroxide/hydrocortisone (Vanoxide HC)
- Clindamycin/benzoyl peroxide (Acanya, BenzaClin, Duac, Neuac, Onexton)
- Clindamycin/tretinoin (Veltin, Ziana)
- Erythromycin/benzoyl peroxide (Benzamycin)
- Sulfur/sulfacetamide (Plexion, Prascion, Rosanil, Rosula Wash, Sumadan, Sumaxin TS, Zencia)

Storage and Administration Pearls

- Apply topical acne products only after washing the face and then waiting for the skin to dry completely (approximately 30 minutes).
- Protect tetracycline from light. Tetracycline, doxycycline, and minocycline should be taken 2 hours before or after a meal; they interact with calcium-containing products such as dairy items.

Patient Education Pearls

- Topical agents and antimicrobials increase the risk of excessive burning from the sun. Apply sunscreen prior to sun exposure.

PSORIASIS

Definitions

Psoriasis is a chronic inflammatory skin disease associated with silvery scalelike lesions. There are two primary types of psoriasis identified: Type I is diagnosed early in life in patients with a family history, while type II develops later in life and generally has no family history present.

Diagnosis

Diagnosis is based on thorough history and physical and depends primarily on the observation of lesions.

Signs and Symptoms

Sharp, demarcated, erythematous papules and plaques covered with silvery scales are a sign. Affected areas may include the scalp, trunk, back, arms, legs, palms, soles, face, and/or genitalia. Psoriatic arthritis refers to secondary joint inflammation that occurs in patients with psoriasis. The most commonly affected joints are the elbows, wrists, ankles, and knees.

Guidelines

Menter A, Gottlieb A, Feldman SR,et al. Guidelines of care for the management of psoriasis and psoriatic arthritis: Section 1. Overview of psoriasis and guidelines of care for the treatment of psoriasis with biologics. *J Am Acad Dermatol.* 2008;58:826–50.

Menter A, Korman NJ, Elmets CA,et al. Guidelines of care for the management of psoriasis and psoriatic arthritis. Section 3. Guidelines of care for the management and treatment of psoriasis with topical therapies. *J Am Acad Dermatol.* 2009;60:643–59.

Gottlieb A, Korman NJ, Gordon KB, et al. Guidelines of care for the management of psoriasis and psoriatic arthritis: Section 2. Psoriatic arthritis: overview and guidelines of care for treatment with an emphasis on the biologics. *J Am Acad Dermatol.* 2008;58:851–64.

Menter A, Korman NJ, Elmets CA, et al. Guidelines of care for the management of psoriasis and psoriatic arthritis: section 4. Guidelines of care for the management and treatment of psoriasis with traditional systemic agents. *J Am Acad Dermatol.* 2009;61:451–85.

Summary of Treatment Recommendations

- The goal of therapy is complete resolution of lesions.
- There is significant interpatient variability in response to the available medications. Options for initial treatment include topical agents such as emollients and keratolytics (salicylic acid or sulfur), coal tar, anthralin, calcipotriene, or retinoids.
- Systemic treatment is considered as initial therapy in very severe cases or as second-line therapy in patients that do not respond to topical options. Systemic options include antimetabolite therapy (methotrexate, cyclosporine, tacrolimus), oral corticosteroids, psoralens, immunosuppressants, or retinoids.

Medications for Psoriasis

Generic • Brand • Dose/Dosage Forms	Contra-indications	Primary Side Effects	Key Monitoring Parameters	Pertinent Drug Interactions	Med Pearls
Topical					
Coal tar					
Coal tar • Medotar, Fototar • Apply 1–4 × /day • 1–25% cream, lotion, ointment	Hypersensitivity	Photosensitivity	• Presence of side effects • ↓ lesions	Concurrent use with other photosen-sitizing agents may ↑ risk of photosensitivity	Over-the-counter
Retinoids					
Tretinoin • Atralin, Avita, Renova, Retin-A • Apply daily • 0.01–0.1% gel, cream	See details in Acne section				
Tazarotene • Tazorac • Apply daily • 0.05% gel, cream					
Adapalene • Differin • Apply daily • 0.1% gel, cream, lotion; 0.3% gel					
Anthralin					
Dithranol • Psoriatec, Zithranol • Apply daily • 0.5–1% cream	• Hypersensitivity • Inflamed eruptions	• Discoloration of skin, hair, fabrics, irritation	• Presence of side effects • ↓ lesions	None	Staining of fabric can be permanent
Calcipotriene					
Calcipotriene • Dovonex, Sorilux • Apply BID • 0.005% cream, foam, ointment, solution	• Hypersensitivity • Hypercalcemia • Vitamin D toxicity	• Burning • Itching • Skin irritation • Drying	• Presence of side effects • ↓ lesions	Concurrent use with other topical agents may cause additive drying	Do not apply cream or ointment to face
Combination products: Betamethasone dipropionate/calcipotriene (Enstilar, Taclonex)					

Medications for Psoriasis *(cont'd)*

Generic • Brand • Dose/Dosage Forms	Contra-indications	Primary Side Effects	Key Monitoring Parameters	Pertinent Drug Interactions	Med Pearls
Vitamin D analog					
Calcitriol • Vectical • Apply BID (max = 200 g/wk) • Ointment	None	• Pruritis • Erythema • Blisters • Dermatitis • Hypercalcemia • Photosensitivity	• Presence of side effects • ↓ lesions	Concurrent use with vitamin D or calcium supplements, thiazide diuretics, or calcium or magnesium-containing antacids may ↑ risk of hypercalcemia	• Do not apply to face or eyes • Topical product unlikely to cause drug interactions or serum abnormalities due to limited systemic absorption
Corticosteroids					
Halobetasol • Ultravate • Apply BID for up to 2 wk (max = 50 g/wk) • Lotion	Hypersensitivity	Pruritis	• Presence of side effects • ↓ lesions	None	Not approved for use in children <18 yr
Betamethasone dipropionate • Sernivo • Apply BID for up to 4 wk • Spray	Hypersensitivity	• Tingling • Application site reaction	• Presence of side effects • ↓ lesions	None	Not approved for use in children <18 yr
Combination products: Betamethasone dipropionate/calcipotriene (Enstilar, Taclonex)					
Systemic					
Antimetabolites					
Methotrexate ☆ • Otrexup, Rasuvo, Rheumatrex, Trexall • 10–25 mg PO/subcut/IM weekly • Injection, tabs	• Hypersensitivity • Alcoholism • Liver disease • Immunodeficiency • Significant blood dyscrasias • Pregnancy • Lactation	• Gastrointestinal upset (nausea, diarrhea, abdominal pain) • Stomatitis • Thrombocytopenia • Leukopenia • Anemia • ↑ liver function tests (LFTs) • Interstitial lung disease • Rash (Stevens-Johnson syndrome possible) • Malaise • Fatigue • Fever/chills • Infection	• Pain relief • LFTs • Complete blood count (CBC) with differential • Folate concentrations • S/S of infection	• Nonsteroidal anti-inflammatory drugs and salicylates ↑ risk of toxicity • Penicillins, sulfonamides, and tetracyclines may ↑ risk of toxicity	• May supplement with folic acid to ↓ side effects and prevent folate deficiency • Myelosuppression is biggest concern • Should be taken with food • Necessary to use contraception in female patients

Medications for Psoriasis *(cont'd)*

Generic • Brand • Dose/Dosage Forms	Contra-indications	Primary Side Effects	Key Monitoring Parameters	Pertinent Drug Interactions	Med Pearls
Immunosuppressants					
Etanercept • Enbrel • Plaque psoriasis: 50 mg twice weekly × 3 mo, then 50 mg weekly • Psoriatic arthritis: 50 mg weekly • Injection	Sepsis	• Injection site reactions • Anaphylaxis • Infection (esp. latent tuberculosis [TB] reactivation, fungal infections and hepatitis B virus [HBV] reactivation) • Lymphoma • Leukemia • Skin cancer • Heart failure exacerbation • Bone marrow suppression • Lupus-like syndrome • Demyelinating disorders	• S/S of infection • S/S of heart failure • CBC with differential	Not to be given with live vaccines	• PPD and HBV screening should be done before initiating treatment • Refrigerate prior to use • Discontinue if serious infection occurs • Use with caution in patients with heart failure • Can be self-administered • For psoriatic arthritis, can be used alone or in combination with methotrexate • Pregnancy registry for pregnant females on medication
Infliximab • Inflectra, Remicade • Plaque psoriasis and psoriatic arthritis: 5 mg/kg IV infusion at initiation, wk 2 and wk 6, then every 8 wk • Injection	Hypersensitivity	• Infusion reactions (hypotension, dyspnea, urticaria) • Delayed hypersensitivity reactions (fever, rash, myalgia, headache, sore throat, hand/facial edema, dysphagia, arthralgias) • Infection (esp. latent TB reactivation, fungal infections, or HBV reactivation) • Heart failure exacerbation • Bone marrow suppression • Lymphoma • Leukemia • Skin cancer • Hepatotoxicity	• Blood pressure • LFTs • S/S of infection • S/S of heart failure • CBC with differential	Not to be given with live vaccines	• Delayed hypersensitivity reaction may occur as early as after 2nd dose • Premedicate with H_1 antagonist, H_2 receptor antagonist, acetaminophen, and/or corticosteroid • PPD and HBV screening should be done before initiating treatment • Discontinue if serious infection occurs

Medications for Psoriasis *(cont'd)*

Generic • Brand • Dose/Dosage Forms	Contra-indications	Primary Side Effects	Key Monitoring Parameters	Pertinent Drug Interactions	Med Pearls
Immunosuppressants (cont'd)					
Ustekinumab • Stelara • Plaque psoriasis: ≤100 kg: 45 mg subcut at initiation and wk 4, then every 12 wk; >100 kg: 90 mg subcut at initiation and wk 4, then every 12 wk • Psoriatic arthritis: 45 mg subcut at initiation and wk 4, then every 12 wk • Injection	Hypersensitivity	• Infection (esp. latent TB reactivation or bacterial/viral infections) • Malignancy • Hypersensitivity • Reversible posterior leukoencephalopathy (RPLS) syndrome • Headache • Fatigue	• S/S of infection • S/S RPLS • CBC with differential	Not to be given with live vaccines	• PPD screening should be done before initiating treatment • Refrigerate prior to use • Discontinue if serious infection occurs • Can be self-administered • For psoriatic arthritis, can be used alone or in combination with methotrexate
Golimumab • Simponi • Psoriatic arthritis: 50 mg subcut monthly • Injection	None	• Injection site reactions • Anaphylaxis • Infection (esp. latent TB reactivation, fungal infections and HBV reactivation) • Lymphoma • Leukemia • Skin cancer • Heart failure exacerbation • Bone marrow suppression • Lupus-like syndrome • Demyelinating disorders	• S/S of infection • S/S of heart failure • CBC with differential	Not to be given with live vaccines	• PPD and HBV screening should be done before initiating treatment • Can be used alone or in combination with methotrexate • Use with caution in patients with heart failure • Discontinue if serious infection occurs • Can be self-administered • Refrigerate prior to use

Medications for Psoriasis *(cont'd)*

Generic • Brand • Dose/Dosage Forms	Contra-indications	Primary Side Effects	Key Monitoring Parameters	Pertinent Drug Interactions	Med Pearls
Immunosuppressants (cont'd)					
Adalimumab • Humira • Plaque psoriasis: 80 mg subcut initially, then 40 mg subcut every other wk starting 1 wk after initial dose • Psoriatic arthritis: 40 mg subcut every other wk • Injection	None	[Same as above]	[Same as above]	[Same as above]	• PPD and HBV screening should be done before initiating treatment • Use with caution in patients with heart failure • Discontinue if serious infection occurs • Can be self-administered • Refrigerate prior to use • For psoriatic arthritis, can be used alone or in combination with nonbiological disease-modifying antirheumatic drugs
Certolizumab pegol • Cimzia • Psoriatic arthritis: 400 mg subcut at initiation, wk 2, and wk 4, then 200 mg subcut every other wk • Injection	None				• PPD and HBV screening should be done before initiating treatment • Use with caution in patients with heart failure • Discontinue if serious infection occurs • Can be self-administered • Refrigerate prior to use

Medications for Psoriasis *(cont'd)*

Generic • Brand • Dose/Dosage Forms	Contra-indications	Primary Side Effects	Key Monitoring Parameters	Pertinent Drug Interactions	Med Pearls
Immunosuppressants (cont'd)					
Secukinumab • Cosentyx • Plaque psoriasis: 300 mg subcut at initiation, wk 1, 2, 3, and 4, then 300 mg subcut every 4 wk • Psoriatic arthritis: 150 mg subcut at initiation, wk 1, 2, 3, and 4, then 150 mg subcut every 4 wk; OR 150 mg subcut every 4 wk • Injection	Hypersensitivity	• Infection (esp. latent TB reactivation or bacterial/viral/ fungal infections) • Inflammatory bowel disease • Hypersensitivity • Diarrhea	• S/S of infection • S/S of inflammatory bowel disease	Not to be given with live vaccines	• PPD screening should be done before initiating treatment • Refrigerate prior to use • Discontinue if serious infection occurs • Can be self-administered • For psoriatic arthritis, can be used alone or in combination with methotrexate
Ixekizumab • Taltz • Plaque psoriasis: 160 mg subcut initially, then 80 mg subcut at wk 2, 4, 6, 8, 10, and 12, then 80 mg subcut every 4 wk starting wk 16 • Injection	Hypersensitivity	• Infection (esp. latent TB reactivation or bacterial/viral/ fungal infections) • Inflammatory bowel disease • Hypersensitivity • Injection site reactions • Neutropenia	• S/S of infection • S/S of inflammatory bowel disease	Not to be given with live vaccines	• PPD screening should be done before initiating treatment • Refrigerate prior to use • Discontinue if serious infection occurs • Can be self-administered
Phosphodiesterase-4 inhibitor					
Apremilast • Otezla • Plaque psoriasis or psoriatic arthritis: 10 mg PO on Day 1, then 10 mg PO BID on Day 2, then 10 mg PO in AM, 20 mg PO in PM on Day 3, then 20 mg PO BID on Day 4, then 20 mg PO in AM, 30 mg PO in PM on Day 5, then 30 mg PO BID starting on Day 6 • Tabs	Hypersensitivity	• Depression • ↓ weight • N/D • Headache	• Weight • Renal function • Mood changes, depression, or suicidal thoughts	• CYP3A4 substrate • CYP3A4 inhibitors may ↑ effects/ toxicity • CYP3A4 inducers may ↓ effects	• Adjust dose in renal impairment • Do not crush, chew, or split tabs

Medications for Psoriasis *(cont'd)*

Generic • Brand • Dose/Dosage Forms	Contra-indications	Primary Side Effects	Key Monitoring Parameters	Pertinent Drug Interactions	Med Pearls
Retinoids					
Acitretin • Soriatane • 25–50 mg PO daily • Caps	• Hypersensitivity • Pregnancy • Hypersensitivity • Severe hepatic or renal impairment • Concurrent use with methotrexate or tetracyclines	• Hepatotoxicity • Skeletal abnormalities • Dyslipidemia • Dry eyes • Loss of eyebrows/eyelashes • Capillary leak syndrome • Exfoliative dermatitis/erythroderma • Depression • Suicidal thoughts • Aggression • ↓ night vision	• Pregnancy test • Lipid panel • CBC • Renal function • Mental status • Changes in vision • LFTs	• Concurrent use with vitamin A may lead to ↑ risk of toxicity • ↑ risk of intracranial hypertension with tetracycline • ↑ risk of hepatotoxicity with methotrexate • May ↑ risk of hypoglycemia with glyburide	• Highly teratogenic • Females must have 2 urine or blood pregnancy tests before initiating therapy, then single pregnancy test must be performed monthly after initiating therapy; pregnancy test must also be performed every 3 mo for ≥3 yr after discontinuing therapy • Females must agree to at least 2 forms of contraception for 1 mo before therapy initiated, during therapy, and for ≥3 yr after discontinuing therapy • Patients should not donate blood for ≥ 3 yr after discontinuing therapy • Take with food • Law requires medication guide be given to the patient each time acitretin is dispensed

Storage and Administration Pearls

- Store out of reach of children.
- Avoid application of topical agents near the eyes.
- Ustekinumab should be stored in a refrigerator between 2–8°C (36–46°F), protected from light, and retained in drug/diluent pack until time of use.
- Etanercept solution, golimumab syringes, adalimumab syringes/pens, certolizumab syringes, and secukinumab syringes/pens must be refrigerated at 2–8°C (36–46°F) and should not be frozen.

Patient Education Pearls

- Wash hands thoroughly after application of topical agents.
- Keep topical agents away from eyes.

LEARNING POINTS

- First-line therapy for mild to moderate acne vulgaris is topical benzoyl peroxide.
- Topical retinoids should not be combined with other topical acne agents due to risk of excessive drying and photosensitivity.
- Oral isotretinoin is reserved for refractory or severe cases of acne vulgaris. Patients, pharmacists, and physicians must register with the FDA iPLEDGE program to use this medication.
- Oral isotretinoin is associated with significant teratogenicity. Females on isotretinoin therapy must agree to use two forms of contraception during the course of therapy.
- Significant interpatient variability exists in the response to psoriasis treatments. Initial therapy generally consists of topic agents such as keratolytics, coal tar, or anthralin.
- Antimetabolite and immunosuppressant therapy carries significantly greater adverse effect risk and therefore should be reserved for severe or refractory cases.

PRACTICE QUESTIONS

1. Which of the following is appropriate initial treatment for type III acne?

    (A) Topical antibiotics and topical retinoids
    (B) Topical retinoids and oral antibiotics
    (C) Topical benzoyl peroxide
    (D) Oral antibiotics
    (E) Isotretinoins

2. Which of the following topical products should be applied after the face
    is washed and completely dried to minimize the risk of excessive drying?
    (Select ALL that apply.)

    (A) Clindamycin gel
    (B) Tretinoin cream
    (C) Alitretinoin gel
    (D) Adapalene cream

3. A 22-year-old woman is diagnosed with moderate acne vulgaris (type II). She has
    no significant medical history and takes no medications. Which of the following is
    the best therapy recommendation?

    (A) Benzoyl peroxide wash
    (B) Adapalene gel
    (C) Doxycycline oral
    (D) Isotretinoin oral

4. Live vaccines should be avoided with which of the following medications for
    psoriasis? (Select ALL that apply.)

    (A) Calcipotriene
    (B) Dithranol
    (C) Alefacept
    (D) Efalizumab

ANSWERS AND EXPLANATIONS ON FOLLOWING PAGE.

ANSWERS AND EXPLANATIONS

1. **B**

First-line therapy for type III acne is topical therapy (benzoyl peroxide, retinoids, or anti-biotics) plus oral antibiotics. First-line therapy for type I acne is topical benzoyl peroxide (C). First-line therapy for type II acne is topical antibiotics and topical retinoids (A). Oral antibiotics are not used alone (D) without topical agents. Isotretinoins (E) are usually reserved for type IV or other types that are refractory to other treatment options.

2. **B, C**

Retinoids including tretinoin (B) and alitretinoin (C) should be applied only after the face is washed and completely dried in order to minimize risk of excessive drying. This precaution is not necessary with topical antibiotics such as clindamycin (A) or with adapalene (D), a retinoid.

3. **B**

Preferred treatment for moderate (type II) acne vulgaris is topical retinoid or topical antibiotic therapy. Topical benzoyl peroxide (A) is preferred for mild (type I) acne vulgaris. Oral antibiotics such as doxycycline (C) are recommended in combination with topical retinoids, benzoyl peroxide, or antibiotics for moderate–severe (type III) or type II that is unresponsive to topical monotherapy. Isotretinoin therapy (D) is reserved for severe (type IV) or treatment-resistance/refractory acne vulgaris.

4. **C, D**

Live vaccines should be avoided in combination with immunosuppressants. Alefacept (C) and efalizumab (D) are both immunosuppressants. Calcipotriene (A) and dithranol (B) are topical agents and do not interact with immunizations.

Antidotes

The following chapter addresses drugs that are used as antagonist drugs:

- **Antidotes**
- **General antidotes**

 Suggested Study Time: **15 minutes**

ANTIDOTES

Definitions

The drugs included in this chapter act in a variety of ways to counter the toxic effects of exogenous and endogenous substances in the body. Therefore, they are used in the management of poisoning and overdosage. Many antidotes are used to protect against the toxicity of drugs such as antineoplastics, and in the management of metabolic disorders such as Wilson's disease, where toxic substances accumulate.

Accidental and deliberate drug overdosage is a common problem seen by ambulance staff and emergency workers. The majority of these episodes of poisoning are dealt with along similar lines with general supportive care, but some require more specific action.

Some antagonists, such as the opioid antagonist naloxone, compete with the poison for receptor sites. Other antagonists, such as atropine, block substances that mediate the effects of the toxin. These actions may reduce absorption of the toxin from the gastrointestinal tract, inactivate or reduce the activity of the toxin, or increase the toxin's elimination.

Some antidotes, such as fomepizole in methyl alcohol poisoning, act by reducing the rate of metabolism to a toxic metabolite. Others, such as methionine and glutathione, promote the formation of inactive metabolites. Acetylcysteine also acts by bypassing the effect of the toxin. On the NAPLEX, antidote questions can be an easy way to earn points if you learn the correct antidote for the toxicity.

ACUTE POISONING

In the management of suspected acute poisoning, it is often impossible to determine with any certainty the identity of the poison or the size of the dose received. As a result, a common procedure needs to be in place:

- First, call the poison control center: (800) 222–1222.
- Next, take a history of the event and drug, or substance, involved.
  - What mode of poisoning has occurred (i.e., ingestion or inhalation)? What drug or substance was involved?
  - When did it happen?
  - Has any treatment occurred yet (i.e., induced vomiting)?

Few poisons have specific antidotes or methods of elimination, and the mainstay of treatment for patients with suspected acute poisoning is therefore supportive and symptomatic therapy; in many cases, nothing further is required. Clinicians should assess the ABCDs: airway, breathing, circulation, dextrose, decontamination. Symptoms of acute poisoning are frequently nonspecific, particularly in the early stages. Maintenance of the airway and ventilation is the most important initial measure; other treatment—for example, for cardiovascular or neurological symptoms—may be added as appropriate.

Some centers also recommend the routine administration of dextrose to all unconscious patients since hypoglycemia may be a cause of unconsciousness, although blood glucose measurements should be obtained first where facilities are immediately available.

Specific antidotes are available for a number of poisons and are the primary treatment where there is a severe poisoning with a known toxin. These antidotes may be life-saving in such cases but their use is not without hazard. In many situations, the use of antidotes is not necessary. These agents are discussed in greater detail in the chart that follows.

Measures to reduce or prevent the absorption of the poison are widely advocated. For inhalational poisoning, the victim is removed from the source of poisoning. Some toxins, particularly pesticides, may be absorbed through the skin, and clothing should be removed and the skin thoroughly washed to avoid continued absorption. Caustic substances are removed from the skin or eyes with copious irrigation. However, for orally ingested poisons the best method of gastrointestinal (GI) decontamination remains controversial; this is addressed in the following sections.

GENERAL ANTIDOTES

Activated Charcoal

Activated charcoal absorbs a wide range of toxins and is often given to reduce absorption within the GI tract. A single dose is generally effective, particularly if it is given within

1 hour of ingestion. Delayed use, however, may be beneficial for modified-release preparations or for drugs that slow GI transit time, such as those with antimuscarinic properties. Charcoal is generally well tolerated, although vomiting is common, and there is a risk of aspiration if the airway is not adequately protected. Repeated doses may be useful in eliminating some substances even after systemic absorption has occurred.

Active removal of poisons from the stomach by induction of emesis or gastric lavage has been widely used, but there is little evidence to support its role. Emesis should not be induced if the poison is corrosive or petroleum-based, or if the poison is removable by treatment with activated charcoal.

Gastric Lavage

Gastric lavage may occasionally be indicated for ingestion of noncaustic poisons that are not absorbed by activated charcoal, but only if less than 1 hour has elapsed since ingestion. Gastric lavage should not be attempted if the airway is not adequately protected.

Whole-bowel irrigation using a nonabsorbable osmotic agent such as a macrogol has also been used, particularly for substances that pass beyond the stomach before being absorbed (e.g., iron preparations or enteric-coated or modified-release formulations); however, its role is not established.

Antidotes

Toxic/Overdose Substance	Generic Name for Antidote • Brand Name/Dosage Form • Dose	Contraindications	Primary Side Effects	Key Monitoring	Med Pearl
Mechanism of action – pure opioid antagonist that competes and displaces narcotics at opioid receptor sites					
Opioids	Naloxone • Narcan, Evzio • 0.4–2 mg IV/IM/subcut every 2–3 min PRN; after reversal, repeat dose every 20–60 min PRN • Evzio: 0.4 mg IM/subcut every 2 min until emergency medical assistance is available • Narcan Nasal Spray: 1 spray (4 mg) every 2–3 min in alternating nostrils until emergency medical assistance is available • Injection, nasal spray	Hypersensitivity	• Tachycardia • Anxiety • Diaphoresis • Agitation • ↑ blood pressure (BP)	• Respiratory rate (RR) • Heart rate (HR) • BP	• Adverse affects can occur secondarily to reversal (withdrawal) • IV route is preferred due to quick effect • Nasay spray onset is longest (~8–13 min)

Antidotes *(cont'd)*

Toxic/Overdose Substance	Generic Name for Antidote • Brand Name/Dosage Form • Dose	Contraindications	Primary Side Effects	Key Monitoring	Med Pearl
Mechanism of action – acts as a competitive antagonist at opioid receptor sites					
Opioids	Naltrexone • Revia, Vivitrol • PO: 25 mg initially, then 50 mg daily on weekdays with 100 mg on Saturdays or 150 mg every 3 days • IM: 380 mg every 4 wk • Injection, tabs	• Hypersensitivity • Acute opioid withdrawal • Failure to pass naloxone challenge • Positive urine drug screen for opioids	• Hepatotoxicity • Syncope • Headache • Sedation • Nausea/vomiting (N/V) • Depression • Suicidality • Injection site reactions • Muscle cramps	• Opioid withdrawal • Liver function tests (LFTs) • Mental status	• Do not give until patient is opioid-free for 7–10 days (to minimize risk of withdrawal) • Indicated for treatment of alcohol and opioid dependence • Highest affinity for mu receptors
Mechanism of action – competitively inhibits the activity at the benzodiazepine recognition site on the GABA/benzodiazepine complex					
Benzodiazepines	Flumazenil • Only available generically • 0.2 mg IV over 30 sec; if desired consciousness not achieved 30 sec after dose, repeat with 0.3 mg IV over 30 sec; if desired consciousness not achieved, can then repeat with 0.5 mg IV over 30 sec every minute • Injection	• Hypersensitivity • Receiving benzodiazepine for potentially life-threatening condition • Showing signs of serious cyclic antidepressant overdosage	• Palpitations • Blurred vision • Ataxia • Agitation • Dizziness • Seizures • ↑ sweating • Headache	• BP • HR • RR • Benzodiazepine reversal may result in seizures in some patients • May cause return of residual effects of benzodiazepines	• If patient has not responded 5 min after receiving a cumulative dose of 5 mg, the sedation is likely not due to benzodiazepines • Reversal may affect nonbenzodiazepines (eszopiclone, zaleplon, zolpidem)
Mechanism of action – competitively inhibits alcohol dehydrogenase, an enzyme that catalyzes the metabolism of ethanol, methanol, and ethylene glycol					
• Methanol • Ethylene glycol	Fomepizole • Antizol • 15 mg/kg IV, then 10 mg/kg IV every 12 hr × 4 doses, then 15 mg/kg IV every 12 hr until ethylene glycol levels <20 mg/L and patient asymptomatic (with normal pH) • Injection	Hypersensitivity	• Headache • Nausea • Metallic taste • Drowsiness • Dizziness	• Fomepizole plasma levels • Plasma/urinary ethylene glycol or methanol levels • Plasma/urinary osmolality • Renal function • LFTs • Electrolytes • Arterial blood gas • Anion/osmolar gaps • S/S of methanol or ethylene glycol toxicity	• Therapy should be initiated immediately upon suspicion of methanol or ethylene glycol ingestion • Can be used alone or with hemodialysis

Antidotes (cont'd)

Toxic/Overdose Substance	Generic Name for Antidote • Brand Name/Dosage Form • Dose	Contraindications	Primary Side Effects	Key Monitoring	Med Pearl
Mechanism of action – inhibits destruction of acetylcholine by acetylcholinesterase which prolongs effects of acetylcholine (anticholinergic drug overdose)					
Anticholinergic drugs	Physostigmine • Only available generically • 0.5–2 mg IM/IV to start; repeat every 10–30 min until response • Injection	• GI or genitourinary obstruction • Asthma • Gangrene • Severe cardiovascular disease • Concurrent use of depolarizing neuromuscular blocking agents	• Palpitation • Bradycardia • Restlessness • Seizure	• HR • RR • Electrocardiogram (ECG)	
Mechanism of action – antigen-binding fragments (Fab) are specific for the treatment of digitalis intoxication					
Digoxin	Digoxin Immune Fab • DigiFab • 40 mg will bind to 0.5 mg of digoxin • Injection	Hypersensitivity to sheep products	• Exacerbation of heart failure • Rapid ventricular response • Hypokalemia	• Serum potassium concentrations • BP • ECG • Renal function	Digoxin levels will greatly ↑ with digoxin Fab use and are not an accurate determination of body stores; do not monitor serum digoxin concentrations for several days to >1 wk
Mechanism of action – supplies a free thiol group which binds to and inactivates acrolein, the urotoxic metabolite of ifosfamide and cyclophosphamide					
• Cyclophosphamide • Ifosfamide	Mesna • Mesnex • IV-only regimen: 20% of ifosfamide dose IV at time of ifosfamide dose, and then at 4 and 8 hr after ifosfamide dose • IV and PO regimen: 20% of ifosfamide dose IV at time of ifosfamide dose, then 40% of ifosfamide dose PO at 2 and 6 hr after ifosfamide dose • Injection, tabs	Hypersensitivity	• Anaphylaxis • Rash (including Stevens-Johnson syndrome) • N/V/D • Constipation • Leukopenia • Thrombocytopenia • Anemia • Fatigue • Fever	• Urinalysis • Inputs/outputs	Only indicated for prevention of hemorrhagic cystitis induced by ifosfamide; off-label use for prevention of hemorrhagic cystits induced by cyclophosphamide
Mechanism of action – cardioprotective by converting intracellularly to a ring-opened chelating agent that interferes with iron-mediated oxygen free radical generation					
Doxorubicin	Dexrazoxane • Zinecard • 10:1 ratio of dexrazoxane:doxorubicin IV • Injection	Hypersensitivity	• Myelosuppression (additive to chemotherapy) • Phlebitis	• Complete blood count with differential • LFTs • Renal function • Echocardiogram	• Only used if patients have received cumulative doxorubicin dose of 300 mg/m² and are continuing with doxorubicin therapy • Can also be used to treat anthracycline-induced extravasation (Totect)

Antidotes (cont'd)

Mechanism of action – free thiol metabolite is available to bind to and detoxify reactive metabolites of cisplatin

Toxic/Overdose Substance	Generic Name for Antidote • Brand Name/Dosage Form • Dose	Contraindications	Primary Side Effects	Key Monitoring	Med Pearl
Cisplatin	Amifostine • Ethyol • 910 mg/m^2 IV daily given 30 min prior to chemotherapy • Injection	Hypersensitivity	• Hypotension • N/V • Rash (including Stevens-Johnson syndrome) • Anaphylaxis • Hypocalcemia	• BP (every 5 min during the infusion) • Serum calcium concentrations	• Indicated to ↓ cumulative renal toxicity associated with repeated cisplatin administration (in ovarian cancer) • Antiemetic recommended prior to and in conjunction with amifostine • Hold antihypertensive medications for 24 hr before amifostine therapy

Mechanism of action – combines with strongly acidic heparin to form a stable complex (salt) neutralizing the anticoagulant activity of both drugs

Heparin	Protamine • Only available generically • 1 mg of protamine IV neutralizes ~100 units of heparin (max dose = 50 mg) • Injection	Hypersensitivity	• Hypersensitivity • Hypotension • Flushing • Dyspnea • Thromboembolism	• Activated partial thromboplastin time (aPTT) • BP • S/S of bleeding • S/S of thromboembolic events	Will also partially reverse anticoagulant effects of low-molecular weight heparins

Mechanism of action – promotes liver synthesis of clotting factors (II, VII, IX, X) which counteracts the mechanism of warfarin

Warfarin	Vitamin K (phytonadione) • Mephyton • Depends on international normalized ratio (INR) and bleeding risk factors (i.e., INR >10: hold warfarin and give 2.5–5 mg vitamin K PO) • Injection, tabs	Hypersensitivity	• Anaphylaxis (especially with IV administration) • Thromboembolism	• Prothrombin time (PT) • INR • S/S of bleeding • S/S of thromboembolic events	• IM route should be avoided due to hematoma formation • Subcut is the preferred parenteral route • IV recommended only when major bleeding present at any INR • Expect INR to ↓ within 24–48 hr

Mechanism of action – Monocolonal antibody fragment that binds to dabigatran and its metabolites

Dabigatran	Idarucizumab • Praxbind • 5 g administered as 2 separate doses of 2.5 g IV ≤15 min apart • Injection	None	• Headache • Thromboembolism • Hypersensitivity	• aPTT • S/S of bleeding • S/S of thromboembolic evnts	

Mechanism of action – reduced form of folic acid: supplies the necessary cofactor blocked by methotrexate

Methotrexate	Leucovorin • Only available generically • 15 mg PO/IM/IV every 6 hr × 10 doses, until levels normalize • Injection, tabs	• Pernicious anemia • B$_{12}$-deficient megaloblastic anemias	• Anaphylaxis • Rash	Plasma methotrexate concentrations	Continue leucovorin until plasma methotrexate level <0.05 mmol/L

Antidotes *(cont'd)*

Toxic/Overdose Substance	Generic Name for Antidote • Brand Name/Dosage Form • Dose	Contraindications	Primary Side Effects	Key Monitoring	Med Pearl
Mechanism of action – absorbs toxic substances or irritants, thus inhibiting GI absorption					
Numerous toxic substances	Activated charcoal • Actidose • 25–100 g/dose	• Unprotected airway • Non-intact GI tract • GI perforation • Intestinal obstruction	• Hypernatremia • Hypokalemia	• Constipation • Diarrhea	Sorbitol accelerates bowel evacuation
Mechanism of action – exact mechanism of benefit in countering acetaminophen toxicity is unknown					
Acetaminophen	Acetylcysteine • Acetadote, Cetylev • PO: 140 mg/kg, then 70 mg/kg every 4 hr × 17 doses • IV: 150 mg/kg (max = 15 g) over 60 min, then 50 mg/kg (max = 5 g) over 4 hr, then 100 mg/kg (max = 10 g) over 16 hr • Effervecent tabs, injection	Hypersensitivity	• Anaphylaxis • N/V • Rash	• Serum acetaminophen concentrations • LFTs • Bilirubin • PT/INR • Hemoglobin/hematocrit • Renal function	• Therapy should continue until acetaminophen levels are undetectable and there is no evidence of hepatotoxicity • Treatment should begin within 8 hr of acute ingestion
Mechanism of action – blocks the action of acetylcholine at parasympathetic sites in the smooth muscle, secretory glands, and the central nervous system					
Cholinergics	Atropine • AtroPen • 2 mg IM; may repeat with 2 additional doses every 10 min	None	• Anaphylaxis • N/V • Fatigue • Insomnia • Weakness • Tachycardia	• ECG • Respiratory status • HR • BP	Dose until symptoms subside
Mechanism of action – stimulates adrenergic receptors resulting in relaxation of smooth muscle of the bronchial tree, cardiac stimulation and dilation of skeletal muscle vasculature					
Hypersensitivity reactions	Epinephrine • Adrenalin, EpiPen, EpiPen Jr. • 0.2–0.5 mg IM or subcut every 5–15 min until improvement • EpiPen Jr. 0.15 mg IM/subcut every 5–15 min until improvement	None	• Angina • Arrhythmias • Anxiety • Flushing • Dyspnea	• RR • HR • BP	IM administration in the anterolateral aspect of the middle third of the thigh is preferred
Mechanism of action – stimulates adenylate cyclase to produce increased cyclic AMP, which promotes hepatic glycogenolysis and gluconeogenesis					
Hypoglycemia	Glucagon • GlucaGen • 1 mg IV, IM, or subcut; may repeat in 15 min as needed	• Hypersensitivity • Insulinoma • Pheochromocytoma	• Hypersensitivity • Hypotension • Nausea	• BP • Blood glucose • ECG • HR • Mental status	IV dextrose should be given as soon as available

Storage and Administration Pearls

- Protamine: Refrigerate; stable for 2 weeks at room temperature.
- Fomepizole: If solution becomes solid in the vial, warm carefully by running warm water over the vial.
- Naltrexone: Should be stored in the refrigerator. May be kept at room temperature for <7 days prior to use.
- Digoxin immune Fab: Should be refrigerated.
- Activated charcoal: Absorbs gas from air; store in closed container.
- Idarucizumab: Refrigerate (36–46°F), do not freeze, do nto shake. Vial may be stored in original packaging at room temperature for up to 48 hours (or up to 6 hours, if vial was exposed to light).

Patient Education Pearls

- Patient should stay calm and call the poison control center.
- If patient currently has ipecac in their home, it is better to dispose of it, according to the research.
- Most drugs do not have antidotes; therefore, it is important to take medication as prescribed.

LEARNING POINTS

- It is important to memorize the phone number for the poison control center. The number should also be pasted on every telephone in your pharmacy.
- Few poisons have specific antidotes or methods of elimination; therefore, the mainstay of treatment for patients with suspected acute poisoning is supportive and symptomatic therapy.
- Flumazenil is the antidote for benzodiazepines.
- Do not confuse Fomepizole and flumazenil. At first glance they may seem similar, but they have completely different uses.
- Protamine is the antidote for heparin, and vitamin K is the antidote for warfarin. Protamine and vitamin K are not interchangeable and have different mechanisms of action. These two antidotes are used for both inpatient and outpatient treatment.

PRACTICE QUESTIONS

1. Which drug is used to decrease toxicities associated with cisplatin?

    (A) Amifostine
    (B) Physostigmine
    (C) Nalmefene
    (D) Fomepizole
    (E) Leucovorin

2. How many doses of activated charcoal are typically effective?

    (A) 1
    (B) 2
    (C) 3
    (D) 4
    (E) 5

3. Which of the following should be monitored in a patient receiving acetylcysteine?

    (A) AST
    (B) Glucose
    (C) Methotrexate concentrations
    (D) Potassium

4. Which of the following agents could correct an INR of 11.4?

    (A) Protamine
    (B) Vitamin K
    (C) Atropine
    (D) Glucagon

5. Atropine is used to treat which of the following?

    (A) Opioid toxicity
    (B) Hemorrhagic cystitis
    (C) Hypoglycemia
    (D) Cholinergic toxicity

6. A patient accidentally ingests antifreeze and has been diagnosed with ethylene glycol toxicity. Which of the following may be helpful in treating ethylene glycol poisoning?

    (A) Atropine
    (B) Flumazenil
    (C) Fomepizole
    (D) Nalmefene

7. A patient presents with an anaphylactic reaction secondary to nafcillin therapy that was administered despite a noted penicillin allergy. Which of the following may be used to treat the anaphylactic reaction?

    (A) Acetylcysteine
    (B) Activated charcoal
    (C) Leucovorin
    (D) Epinephrine

8. Which of the following should be monitored when glucagon is administered? (Select ALL that apply.)

    (A) Blood glucose
    (B) Hemoglobin A1c
    (C) ECG
    (D) Mental status

9. Which of the following is a contraindication to using physostigmine in the treatment of anticholinergic poisoning?

    (A) Asthma
    (B) Hyperglycemia
    (C) INR >4
    (D) Opioid withdrawal

10. Before starting naltrexone, which of the following should the patient achieve?

    (A) Normalization of blood pressure
    (B) Resolution of bradycardia
    (C) Negative urine drug screen
    (D) Normalization of platelet count

ANSWERS AND EXPLANATIONS

1. **A**

Amifostine is used to prevent cisplatin toxicities associated with renal toxicity. Physostigmine (B) is used primarily to reverse toxic CNS effects caused by anticholinergic drugs. Nalmefene (C) is used as a partial reversal of opioid drug effects. Fomepizole (D) is used for methanol and ethylene glycol poisoning, and leucovorin (E) is used as an antidote for folic acid antagonist.

2. **A**

Activated charcoal typically requires only a single dose to be effective, particularly if it is given within 1 hour of toxin ingestion.

3. **A**

Acetylcysteine is used in the treatment of acetaminophen overdose, which could produce liver toxicity and/or hepatic failure. AST, ALT, bilirubin, prothrombin time, and serum creatinine should be monitored in the presence of possible liver toxicity and acetylcysteine use.

4. **B**

An elevated INR is a result of an overdosage of warfarin. Vitamin K is the reversal agent and is recommend for use in patients with an INR >10 or significant bleeding. Protamine (A) can be used to reverse heparin; atropine (C) is used to reverse cholinergic toxicity; and glucagon (D) treats hypoglycemia.

5. **D**

Atropine is used to treat cholinergic toxicity. Nalaxone is used to treat opioid overdoses or respiratory depression associated with opioids (A). Hemorrhagic cystitis (B) secondary to ifosfamide is treated with mesna, and glucagon can be used to treat hypoglycemia (C).

6. **C**

Fomepizole is the antidote for ethylene glycol or methanol toxicity; it works by inhibiting alcohol dehydrogenase. Atropine is (A) used as an antidote for cholinergic toxicity. Flumazenil (B) is used to treat benzodiazepine toxicity. Nalmefene (D) is used to reverse opioid toxicity.

7. **D**

IV or subcutaneous epinephrine is used to treat anaphylactic reactions. Epinephrine stimulates adrenergic receptors to relax bronchial smooth muscle. Acetylcysteine (A) is used in the treatment of an acetaminophen overdose. Activated charcoal (B) is used to bind a wide-variety of toxins within in the GI tract. Leucovorin (C) is administered to treat methotrexate toxicity.

8. **A, C, D**

Blood glucose, ECG, and mental status are all correct monitoring parameters for glucagon. Blood glucose is monitored to evaluate the resolution of hypoglycemia. ECG and mental status are monitored to ensure patient stability in the presence of hypoglycemia. A1c levels (B) are not monitored, because A1c is a sign of glucose control over the previous 3 months; it would not be an indication of acute glucose control.

9. **A**

Asthma may be exacerbated by physostigmine and is a contraindication in the presence of anticholinergic toxicity. Hyperglycemia (B), an elevated INR (C), and opioid withdrawal (D) are not contraindications to use of physostigmine.

10. **C**

Before starting naltrexone, a patient should be in an opioid-free state. Naltrexone is used to maintain patients in an opioid-free state and should not be used in a patient who has taken opioids in the last 7–10 days.

Reproductive Health and Urologic Disorders

17

This chapter covers the following topics:

- **Contraception**
- **Hormone replacement therapy**
- **Erectile dysfunction**
- **Benign prostatic hyperplasia**
- **Urinary incontinence**

 Suggested Study Time: **60 minutes**

CONTRACEPTION

Definition

Contraception refers to the prevention of pregnancy and is accomplished pharmacologically through two general mechanisms: (*1*) inhibition of contact between sperm and egg, and (*2*) prevention of implantation of the fertilized egg in the endometrium. Available products most commonly contain estrogen, progestin, or both. The estrogen component suppresses follicle-stimulating hormone (FSH) and prevents the development of a viable follicle. The progestin component contributes to the production of thick cervical mucus and the involution of the endometrium, and blocks ovulation.

Therapy Selection

Available Prescription Therapies

- Combination estrogen and progestin
  - Monophasic
  - Multiphasic
- Progestin only
- Implantable
- Emergency contraception
  - Start within 72 hours of unprotected intercourse
  - Approved over-the-counter (OTC) (regardless of age)
  - Plan B (OTC)
    » 2 tablets 0.75 mg levonorgestrel (taken every 12 hr × 2 doses)
  - Plan B One Step (OTC)
    » 1 tablet by mouth, levonorgestrel 1.5 mg
  - Ella (Rx only)
    » Ulipristal acetate 30 mg by mouth within 120 hr of unprotected intercourse

Advantages and Disadvantages of Contraception

Product Type	Advantages	Disadvantages
Combination products	Long history of superior efficacy; multiple formulations allow opportunity to try multiple-dose combination of estrogen/progestin components in different dosage forms (transdermal patch, oral, multiphasic, continuous); ↓ length of menses; ↓ incidence of cramping; ↓ risk of ectopic pregnancy	Drug interactions present; need for backup contraception with missed pills
Progestin only	Can be used safely in patients who are breastfeeding, are >35 years of age, and/or have systemic lupus erythematosus or intolerable estrogen-related side effects	Slightly less effective; require even stricter compliance than combinations; higher incidence of breakthrough bleeding; need for backup contraception with missed pills
Implantable	Longer-term efficacy	Not readily reversible; requires insertion at medical office

Adverse Effects Associated with Hormonal Imbalance

Estrogen Excess	Estrogen Deficiency	Progestin Excess	Progestin Deficiency
• Breast tenderness • Cyclic weight gain • Edema • Bloating • Hypertension • Melasma • Migraine • Nausea	• Vasomotor symptoms (hot flashes) • Spotting • Breakthrough bleeding (early) • ↓ libido • Dyspareunia	• ↓ libido • Depression • Fatigue • Weight gain • Acne • Hypomenorrhea • Vaginal candidiasis	• Heavy menstruation • Weight loss • Delayed menses • Spotting • Breakthrough bleeding (late)

Pharmacologic Contraceptives

Generic • Brand • Dose & Max	Contraindications	Primary Side Effects	Key Monitoring Parameters	Pertinent Drug Interactions	Med Pearls
Hormonal Contraceptives					
Oral monophasic/high-dose estrogen					
Ethinyl estradiol and norgestrel ☆ • Ovral, Ogestrel • 50 mcg E. estradiol/0.5 mg norgestrel Ethinyl estradiol and ethynodiol diacetate • Demulen 1/50, Zovia 1/50 • 50 mcg E. estradiol/1 mg E. diacetate Mestranol and norethindrone ☆ • Ortho-Novum 1/50, Necon 1/50, Norinyl 1/50 • 50 mcg mestranol/1 mg norethindrone	• Pregnancy • Breast cancer • History of deep vein thrombosis (DVT) or pulmonary embolism (PE) • Lactation (<6 wk postpartum) • Smoker >35 years old	• Breast tenderness • ↑ breast size • Nausea • Edema • Bloating • Cyclic weight gain • DVT/PE • Headaches during active pills • Thrombophlebitis (rare) *Estrogen-excess side effects most common*	• Presence of side effects • Pregnancy	↓ effect of oral contraceptive: • Antibiotics (ampicillin, sulfonamides, tetracycline) • Anticonvulsants (phenytoin, topiramate, barbiturates) • Protease inhibitors • Rifampin Need backup method of contraception during use and for ≥1 wk after; for chronic therapy with above medications use another form of contraception	Take 1 tablet daily at the same time of day for 21 days, followed by 7 days of inactive placebo pills

Pharmacologic Contraceptives *(cont'd)*

Generic • Brand • Dose & Max	Contraindications	Primary Side Effects	Key Monitoring Parameters	Pertinent Drug Interactions	Med Pearls
Oral monophasic/low-dose estrogen					
Ethinyl estradiol and levonorgestrel • Alesse, Aviane, Lessina, Levlite, Lutera, Sronyx • 20 mcg E. estradiol, 0.1 mg levonorgestrel • Levlen, Levora, Nordette, Portia, Seasonale, Lo Ovral, Quasense, Jolessa • 30 mcg E. estradiol, 0.15 mg levonorgestrel	• Pregnancy • Breast cancer • History of DVT or PE • Lactation (<6 wk postpartum) • Smoker >35 years old	• Nausea/vomiting (N/V) • Breakthrough bleeding • Spotting • Melasma • Headache • Weight change • Edema • DVT/PE • Side effects associated with hormonal imbalance (see preceding Adverse Effects table)	• Presence of side effects • Pregnancy	Same as high-dose	Seasonale is taken continuously for 84 days with 7 placebo pills; menses only every 3 mo
Ethinyl estradiol and drospirenone☆ • Yasmin, Yaz, Beyaz (has added folate), Safyral (has added folate), Syeda, Gianvi, Loryna, Ocella, Vestura, Zarah • 20–30 mcg E. estradiol, 3 mg drospirenone			• Serum potassium concentrations • Pregnancy		• ↓ duration of menses • Drospirenone is a structural analog to spironolactone
Ethinyl estradiol and norgestrel☆ • Cryselle, Low-Ogestrel • 30 mcg E. estradiol, 0.3 mg norgestrel			• Presence of side effects • Pregnancy		Take 1 tablet daily at the same time of day for 21 days, followed by 7 days of inactive placebo pills
Ethinyl estradiol and norethindrone acetate☆ • Loestrin 21 1/20, Loestrin Fe 1/20, Microgestin Fe 1/20, Lo Loestrin Fe • 10–20 mcg E. estradiol, 1 mg n. acetate					
Ethinyl estradiol and norethindrone☆ • Ovcon 35, Balziva, Femcon Fe • 35 mcg E. estradiol, 0.4 mg norethindrone • Brevicon☆, Modicon, Neocon 0.5/35, Nortrel 0.5/35 • 35 mcg E. estradiol, 0.5 mg norethindrone • Necon 1/35☆, Norinyl 1/35, Nortrel 1/35, Ortho-Novum 1/35 • 35 mcg E. estradiol, 1 mg norethindrone					
Ethinyl estradiol and desogestrel • Kariva, Azorette, Mircette • 10–20 mcg E. estradiol, 0.15 mg desogestrel • Emoquette, Apri, Desogen, Reclipsen • 30 mcg E. estradiol, 0.15 mg desogestrel					
Ethinyl estradiol and levonorgestrel • Seasonique Lo Seasonique • 10–20 mcg E. estradiol, 0.15 mg levonorgestrel 10–20 mcg E. estradiol, 0.1 mg levonorgestrel					
Ethinyl estradiol and norgestimate☆ • Ortho cyclen, Sprintec, MonoNessa, Previfem • 35 mcg E. estradiol, 0.25 mg norgestimate					

Pharmacologic Contraceptives *(cont'd)*

Generic • Brand • Dose & Max	Contraindications	Primary Side Effects	Key Monitoring Parameters	Pertinent Drug Interactions	Med Pearls
Oral biphasic					
Ethinyl estradiol and norethindrone ☆ • Ortho-Novum 10/11, Necon 10/11 • 35 mcg E. estradiol, 0.5–1 mg norethindrone	• Pregnancy • Breast cancer • History of DVT or PE • Lactation (<6 wk postpartum) • Smoker >35 years old	• N/V • Breakthrough bleeding • Spotting • Melasma • Headache • Weight change • Edema • DVT/PE • Side effects associated with hormonal imbalance (see preceding Adverse Effects table)	• Presence of side effects • Pregnancy	↓ effect of oral contraceptive: • Antibiotics (ampicillin, sulfon-amides, tetracycline) • Anticon-vulsants (phenytoin, topiramate, barbiturates) • Protease inhibitors • Rifampin Need backup method of contraception during use and for ≥1 wk after; for chronic therapy with above medica-tions use another form of contraception	• Created to ↓ overall hormone exposure • High incidence of breakthrough bleeding
Oral triphasic					
Ethinyl estradiol and norethindrone ☆ • Tri-Norinyl, Necon 7/7/7, Ortho-Novum 7/7/7, Estrostep 21, Estrostep Fe • 35 mcg E. estradiol, 0.5–1 mg norethindrone	• Pregnancy • Breast cancer • History of DVT or PE • Lactation (<6 wk postpartum) • Smoker >35 years old	• N/V • Breakthrough bleeding • Spotting • Melasma • Headache • Weight change • Edema • DVT/PE • Side effects associated with hor-monal imbalance (see Table 2)	• Presence of side effects • Pregnancy	Same as biphasic	• Many tripha-sics approved for treatment of acne as well • More difficult to deal with missed pills • ↓ overall hormone exposure
Ethinyl estradiol and desogestrel • Cyclessa • 25 mcg E. estradiol, 0.1–0.15 mg desogestrel					
Ethinyl estradiol and norgestimate ☆ • Trinessa, Ortho-TriCyclen • 35 mcg E. estradiol, 0.18–0.25 mg norges-timate • Orth-TriCyclen Lo • 25 mcg E. estradiol, 0.18–25 mg norgestimate					
Ethinyl estradiol and levonorgestrel • Enpresse, Tri-Levlen, Triphasil, Trivora • 30–40 mcg E. estradiol, 0.075–0.125 mg levonorgestrel					

Pharmacologic Contraceptives *(cont'd)*

Generic • Brand • Dose & Max	Contraindications	Primary Side Effects	Key Monitoring Parameters	Pertinent Drug Interactions	Med Pearls
Oral four-phasic					
Estradiol valerate and dienogest • Natazia • Days 1–2: 3 mg estradiol valerate • Days 3–7: 2 mg estradiol valerate + 2 mg dienogest • Days 8–24: 2 mg estradiol valerate + 3 mg dienogest • Days 25–26: 1 mg estradiol valerate • Days 27–28: inactive	• Pregnancy • Lactation • Breast cancer • History of DVT or PE • Hepatic disease • Abnormal uterine bleeding • Vascular disease • Hypercoagulopathy	• N/V • Break-through bleeding • Spotting • Melasma • Headache • Weight change • Edema • DVT/PE • Side effects associated with hormonal imbalance (see preceding Adverse Effects table)	• Presence of side effects • Pregnancy	Same as triphasic	• Only 4-phasic option available • ↑ efficacy for heavy menstrual bleeding
Transdermal					
Ethinyl estradiol and norelgestromin • Xulane • 35 mcg E. estradiol and 0.15 mg norelgestromin	• Pregnancy • Breast cancer • History of DVT or PE • Lactation (<6 wk postpartum) • Smoker >35 years old	• N/V • Break-through bleeding • Spotting • Melasma • Headache • Weight change • Edema • DVT/PE • Side effects associated with hormonal imbalance (see preceding Adverse Effects table)	• Presence of side effects • Pregnancy	Same as oral contraceptives	• Safe with usual activities • Do not apply lotion to site of application • Improved compliance over oral • Apply weekly for 3 wk • Avoid if >90 kg

Pharmacologic Contraceptives *(cont'd)*

Generic • Brand • Dose & Max	Contraindications	Primary Side Effects	Key Monitoring Parameters	Pertinent Drug Interactions	Med Pearls
Other					
Ethinyl estradiol and etonogestrel☆ • NuvaRing • 0.015 mg E. estradiol and 0.12 mg etonogestrel released daily • Inserted by patient intravaginally every 4 wk (active for 3 wk)	Negative pregnancy test needed for initiation	Same as oral contraceptives (systemic absorption occurs)	Same as oral contraceptives (systemic absorption occurs)	Same as oral contraceptives (systemic absorption occurs)	• May be removed before intercourse • Not to be used >4 mo after being dispensed
Oral progestin-only					
Norethindrone • Ortho Micronor, Errin, Jolivette, Nor-QD, Nora-BE, Camila • 0.35 mg daily	Negative pregnancy test prior to initiation	• ↓ libido depression • Fatigue • Weight gain • Acne • Hypomenorrhea	Presence of side effects	None	Can be used in breastfeeding women, those >35 yr who smoke, and those at risk of coronary heart disease
Norgestrel • Ovrette • 0.075 mg daily					
Parenteral progestin-only					
Medroxyprogesterone☆ • Depo-Provera, Depo-Subq Provera 104 • 150 mg IM every 12 wk; or 104 mg subcut every 12 wk	• Must have negative pregnancy test to start therapy or to continue therapy if >14 wk since last injection • Breast cancer • Liver disease	• Weight gain • ↓ bone mineral density • Acne • Delayed return of fertility after discontinuation	Bone mineral density	None	• Supplement calcium and vitamin D due to potential bone loss • Do not use for >2 yr unless unable to use other forms of contraception

Pharmacologic Contraceptives *(cont'd)*

Generic • Brand • Dose & Max	Contraindications	Primary Side Effects	Key Monitoring Parameters	Pertinent Drug Interactions	Med Pearls
Implantable/intrauterine					
Levonorgestrel ☆ • Mirena • 20 mcg released daily • Intrauterine	• History or high risk of pelvic inflammatory disease (PID) or ectopic pregnancy • Breast cancer • Abnormal uterine bleeding • High risk for sexually transmitted infections (STIs) (multiple sexual partners) • Uterine or cervical cancer	• Spotting • Breakthrough bleeding • Amenorrhea • Mastalgia • Headache • Abdominal pain • PID	• Presence of side effects • Pregnancy	None	Remains in place for up to 5 yr
Levonorgestrel • Skyla • 6 mcg released daily • Intrauterine					Remains for 3 yr
Etonogestrel • Implanon, Nexplanon • 68 mg subdermal implant in upper arm • Replace every 3–5 yr	History or high risk of PID or ectopic pregnancy	• Amenorrhea • Infrequent menses • Weight gain			Not studied in women >130% ideal body weight
Nonhormonal					
Copper–T380 • ParaGard • Intrauterine placement for up to 10 yrs	History or high risk of PID or ectopic pregnancy	• Heavy bleeding • Cramping	None	None	Can remain in place for up to 8–10 yr with efficacy

Storage and Administration Pearls

- Store at controlled room temperature 20–25°C (68–77°F) in a dry area, protected from direct light.
- After use, discard NuvaRing away from children or pets.
- Store NuvaRing in refrigerator prior to use.

Patient Education Pearls

- Hormonal contraceptives do not prevent the transmission of STIs.
- Establish a regular time to take oral contraceptive, preferably as a part of daily routine, such as brushing teeth.
- Plan a backup contraceptive method.

- Contact physician immediately if any of the following occur:
  - Abdominal pain
  - Chest pain (severe), shortness of breath
  - Headache (severe), dizziness, weakness, or numbness
  - Eye problems (vision loss or blurring), speech problems
  - Severe leg pain (calf or thigh)
- Specific instructions for missed doses:

Doses Missed	Instructions for Patient
1	Take missed dose immediately and next dose at regular time
2 (during first 2 wk)	Take two doses daily for the next 2 days, then resume taking; use backup method for 7 days
2 (during third wk)	Sunday start: Take one dose daily until Sunday, dispose of current pack, then begin next pack without placebo pills. Backup method required for 7 days.
≥3	Other: Dispose of current pack and begin new pack. Backup method required for 7 days.

HORMONE REPLACEMENT THERAPY

Definitions

- Menopause is the cessation of menses after the loss of ovarian follicular activity.
- Perimenopause refers to the period of time immediately prior to menopause and the 1 yr following menopause onset.

Diagnosis

Diagnosis is made when amenorrhea occurs for a minimum of 12 consecutive months.

Signs and Symptoms

Symptoms are related primarily to lack of estrogen and include vaginal dryness, vaginal atrophy, hot flashes, and night sweats. Other potential symptoms include arthralgia, depression, migraine, mood swings, myalgia, and insomnia.

Guidelines

North American Menopause Society. The 2012 hormone therapy position statement of: The North American Menopause Society. *Menopause* 2012;19:257–271.

Guideline Summary

- All women should undergo careful evaluation prior to initiation of hormone replacement therapy (HRT), including comprehensive history and physical, mammography, and, potentially, bone densitometry.

- The benefit:risk ratio for HRT is highly individualized and based on a patient's symptoms, impact on quality of life, and degree of risk for adverse effects.

- The primary indication for HRT is vasomotor symptoms of hot flashes and night sweats.

- Local vaginal therapy is recommended when vaginal symptoms are the only complaint.

- Prevention of osteoporosis with HRT should be considered only for women with a very strong risk of osteoporosis and in whom other available therapies are not options.

- In women who are receiving HRT and who have an intact uterus, progestin is indicated as a means of decreasing the risk of endometrial hyperplasia and cancer that exists with unopposed estrogen use in these patients.

- Due to an unclear evidence-based benefit:risk ratio, HRT is not recommended for use for any of the following indications: cardiovascular disease, stroke prevention, hyperlipidemia, or dementia prevention.

- The Women's Health Initiative (WHI) indicated increased risks of venous thromboembolism, stroke, coronary disease, and breast cancer in women who receive HRT for an extended period of time. The risk was greatest in patients on estrogen-progestogen combination therapy and lower in estrogen only therapy.

- Combination therapy should be limited to 3–5 year or less whenever possible. Longer term use of estrogen only therapy may be considered.

- Nonhormonal options are available for the treatment of vasomotor symptoms in patients with contraindications to hormone therapy or preference to avoid hormone therapy. Evidence-based options include venlafaxine, paroxetine, fluoxetine, and gabapentin. (These agents are detailed in drug tables in the Neurological Disorders and Psychiatric Disorders chapters.) Brisdelle is a low-dose paroxetine product that is approved by the Food and Drug Administration solely for the treatment of vasomotor symptoms related to menopause.

Hormone Replacement Therapy

Generic • Brand • Dose/Dosage Form	Contraindications	Primary Side Effects	Key Monitoring Parameters	Med Pearls
Oral Preparations				
Estrogens				
Conjugated equine estrogens ☆ • Premarin • 0.3–2.5 mg daily	• Hypersensitivity • Abnormal bleeding • Breast cancer • History of DVT or PE • Pregnancy • Estrogen-dependent tumor • History of stroke or myocardial infarction (MI) • Hepatic impairment • Protein C, protein S, or antithrombin deficiency	• Nausea • Fluid retention • Bloating • Headaches • Mood changes • Breast tenderness • ↑ risk of DVT/PE, stroke, MI, and breast cancer • ↑ blood pressure (BP)	• Vaginal bleeding • S/S of DVT/PE • S/S of stroke • S/S of MI • BP • Pap smear • Breast exam • Mammogram	• Most studied • No generic equivalent • Should not be abruptly discontinued; taper
Synthetic conjugated estrogen • Enjuva • 0.3–1.25 mg daily				• Long half-life • Most potent hepatic effects • Should not be abruptly discontinued; taper
Micronized estradiol • Estrace • 1–2 mg daily				
Estropipate • Only available generically • 0.75–6 mg daily				
Esterified estrogens • Menest • 0.3–2.5 mg daily				Should not be abruptly discontinued; taper
Progestins				
Medroxyprogesterone ☆ • Provera • 2–10 mg daily	• Hypersensitivity • Abnormal bleeding • Breast cancer • History of DVT or PE • Pregnancy • Estrogen- or progesterone-dependent tumor • History of stroke or MI • Hepatic impairment	• ↓ libido • Cramping • Mood changes • Bloating • Nausea • Depression • Headache • ↑ risk of DVT/PE, stroke, MI, and breast cancer	• Vaginal bleeding • S/S of DVT/PE • S/S of stroke • S/S of MI • Pap smear • Breast exam • Mammogram	
Micronized progestin • Prometrium • 200 mg daily				Primary use in patients with adverse effects associated with synthetic progestin
Selective Estrogen Receptor Modulator/Estrogen Agonist–Antagonist				
Ospemifene • Osphena • 60 mg daily	• Hypersensitivity • Abnormal bleeding • Breast cancer • History of DVT or PE • Pregnancy • Estrogen-dependent tumor • History of stroke or MI	• ↑ risk of DVT/PE, stroke, MI, and breast cancer • Vasomotor symptoms	• Vaginal bleeding • S/S of DVT/PE • S/S of stroke • S/S of MI • Pap smear • Breast exam • Mammogram	

Hormone Replacement Therapy *(cont'd)*

Generic • **Brand** • **Dose/Dosage Form**	**Contraindications**	**Primary Side Effects**	**Key Monitoring Parameters**	**Med Pearls**
Combination Oral Preparations				
Conjugated equine estrogens and medroxyprogesterone ☆ • Prempro • 0.3–0.625 mg estrogen/1.5–2.5 mg progestin • Premphase • 0.625 mg/0 mg × 14 days then 0.625/5 mg × 14 days	• Hypersensitivity • Abnormal bleeding • Breast cancer • History of DVT or PE • Pregnancy • Estrogen-dependent tumor • History of stroke or MI • Hepatic impairment • Protein C, protein S, or antithrombin deficiency	• Nausea • Fluid retention • Bloating • Headaches • Mood changes • Breast tenderness • ↑ risk of DVT/PE, stroke, MI, and breast cancer • ↑ BP	• Vaginal bleeding • S/S of DVT/PE • S/S of stroke • S/S of MI • BP • Pap smear • Breast exam • Mammogram	
Estradiol and drospirenone • Angelique • 0.5-1 mg/0.25–0.5 mg daily				
Ethinyl estradiol and norethindrone acetate • FemHRT • 2.5–5 mcg/0.5–1 mg daily • Activella • 0.5–1 mg/0.1–0.5 mg daily				
Transdermal and Topical Preparations				
17β Estradiol transdermal ☆ • Alora, Climara, Estraderm, Mini-velle, Vivelle, Vivelle-Dot • 25–50 mcg/24 hours • Applied 1–2 × wk	• Hypersensitivity • Abnormal bleeding • Breast cancer • History of DVT or PE • Pregnancy • Estrogen-dependent tumor • History of stroke or MI • Hepatic impairment • Protein C, protein S, or antithrombin deficiency	• Skin irritation • Nausea • Fluid retention • Bloating • Headaches • Mood changes • Breast tenderness • ↑ risk of DVT/PE, stroke, MI, and breast cancer • ↑ BP	• Vaginal bleeding • S/S of DVT/PE • S/S of stroke • S/S of MI • BP • Pap smear • Breast exam • Mammogram	• Limited hepatic effects • Useful in patients with gastrointestinal disturbances • Side effects less common in general
17β Gel • Divigel, Elestrin, Estrogel • 0.25–1.25 g daily				
17β Topical emulsion • Estrasorb • 2 packets (3.48 g) daily				
17β Transdermal spray • Evamist • 1 spray (1.53 mg) daily; may ↑ to 2–3 sprays daily				

Hormone Replacement Therapy *(cont'd)*

Generic • Brand • Dose/Dosage Form	Contraindications	Primary Side Effects	Key Monitoring Parameters	Med Pearls
Vaginal Preparations				
Conjugated estrogen cream • Premarin • 0.5 g 1–2 × /wk to daily (for 21 days, 7 days off)	• Hypersensitivity • Abnormal bleeding • Breast cancer • History of DVT or PE • Pregnancy • Estrogen-dependent tumor • History of stroke or MI • Hepatic impairment • Protein C, protein S, or antithrombin deficiency	Systemic side effects possible but rare	• Presence of adverse effects • Efficacy	• Used in cases of vaginal symptoms only • Effective for stress incontinence
Estradiol ring • Estring • 2 mg intravaginally; should remain in place for 90 days • Femring • 0.05–0.1 mg intravaginally; should remain in place for 90 days				Long-term use associated with endometrial hyperplasia
17β Cream • Estrace cream • 2–4 g intravaginally daily × 1–2 wk, then 1–2 g daily × 1–2 wk, then 1 g/day 1–3 × /wk				• Used in cases of vaginal symptoms only • Effective for stress incontinence
Estradiol tablet • Vagifem • 1 tab (10 mcg) intravaginally daily × 2 wk , then 1 tab (10 mcg) twice weekly				

Drug Interactions

	Interacting Drug(s)	Result
Estrogen	3A4 inducers: barbiturates, carbamazepine, phenytoin rifampin, St. John's wort	↓ effect of estrogen
	Levothyroxine, warfarin	↓ Effect of interacting drug
	3A4 inhibitors: azole antifungals, macrolide antibiotics, ritonavir, grapefruit juice	↑ effect of estrogen
	Corticosteroids	↑ effect of interacting drug
Progestin	3A4 inducers: barbiturates, carbamazepine, phenytoin rifampin, St. John's wort	↓ effect of progestin

Storage and Administration Pearls

- Store at controlled room temperature in a dry location.
- Dispose of patches in a safe place inaccessible to children or pets.

Patient Education Pearls

- Potential risks of HRT should be discussed thoroughly with every patient.
- Side effects may be decreased if a low dose is used for a short period of time.
- Contact physician promptly for any of the following: Abnormal vaginal bleeding, abdominal pain or tenderness, speech or visual disturbance, breast lumps, numbness in extremities, severe headache, vomiting, sharp pain in leg or chest, shortness of breath.

ERECTILE DYSFUNCTION

Definition

Erectile dysfunction (ED) is often referred to as impotence and is defined as the inability to achieve a penile erection suitable for sexual intercourse.

Diagnosis

Diagnostic workup of ED includes an assessment of the severity of the dysfunction, a complete history and physical, a review of medications, a physical examination, and selected laboratory tests (serum glucose, lipid profile, thyroid function). Each component of the evaluation is used to rule out potential reversible causes of the ED.

Signs and Symptoms

The inability to achieve or maintain an adequate erection is the hallmark symptom; however, symptoms such as depression and anxiety are also commonly associated with ED.

Guidelines

Erectile Dysfunction Guideline Update Panel. The management of erectile dysfunction: an update. Linthicum, MD: American Urologic Association Education and Research, Inc.; 2006 May. www.guideline.gov/summary/summary.aspx?doc_id=10018&nbr=0053 32&string=erectile+AND+dysfunction.

Guidelines Summary

- Initial treatment for most patients will consist of therapy with a phosphodiesterase-5 (PDE-5) inhibitor because these agents are known to be efficacious and are minimally invasive.

- PDE-5 inhibitors are contraindicated in patients who are currently taking nitrates, due to a risk of significant, dangerous hypotension when these agents are used concomitantly.

- If a patient does not respond to therapy with a PDE-5 inhibitor, alternate therapy options should be considered, including a different PDE-5 inhibitor, alprostadil intraurethral suppositories, intracavernous injection, vacuum constriction devices, and penile prostheses.

- Lifestyle modification and treatment of underlying cause/secondary cause should also be encouraged (hypertension, diabetes, hyperlipidemia).

Erectile Dysfunction Treatment Summary

Medications for Erectile Dysfunction

Generic • Brand • Dose/Dosage Forms	Contraindications	Primary Side Effects	Key Monitoring Parameters	Pertinent Drug Interactions	Med Pearls
Oral					
Mechanism of action – PDE-5 inhibitors: enhance the activity of nitric oxide by inhibiting an enzyme (PDE-5) responsible for its degradation; enhanced nitric oxide allows relaxed smooth muscles and ↑ vasodilation and blood flow to the penis following stimulation					
Sildenafil☆ • Viagra • 25–100 mg PRN 0.5–4 hr prior to sexual activity (max = 1 dose daily) • Tabs Tadalafil☆ • Cialis • 5–20 mg PRN prior to sexual activity; or 2.5–5 mg daily • Tabs Vardenafil • Levitra, Staxyn • 5–20 mg (max = 10 mg for ODTs) PRN ~1 hr prior to sexual activity • ODTs, tabs Avanafil • Stendra • 50–200 mg PRN 15–30 min prior to sexual activity • Tabs	• Use with nitrates (continuous or intermittent) • Hypersensitivity • Concurrent use with riociguat	• Hypotension • Dizziness • Headache • Flushing • Dyspepsia • Priapism (not common) • Vision changes • Hearing changes	• Efficacy • Presence of side effects • BP	*Nitrates—**Combination results in potentially fatal hypotension. Avoid concomitant use within ≥24 hours; 48 hours with tadalafil.*** • Concurrent use with alpha-blockers may ↑ risk of hypotension; avoid combination or use lowest dose of each agent used with close monitoring • 3A4 substrates • 3A4 inhibitors may ↑ effects/toxicity • 3A4 inducers may ↓ effects	• Dose adjustments when used with strong 3A4 inhibitors: sildenafil (use initial dose of 25 mg); tadalafil (max dose = 10 mg every 72 hr; or 2.5 mg daily); vardenafil (max dose = 2.5–5 mg every 24–72 hr based on drug; do not use with ODTs); avanafil (avoid concurrent use)

Medications for Erectile Dysfunction *(cont'd)*

Generic • Brand • Dose/Dosage Forms	Contraindications	Primary Side Effects	Key Monitoring Parameters	Pertinent Drug Interactions	Med Pearls
Topical					
Testosterone transdermal patch • Androderm • 2.5–6-mg patch daily • Transdermal patch	• Hypersensitivity • Breast or prostate cancer	• ↑ liver enzymes • ↑ risk of DVT/PE, stroke, and MI • Edema • Hyperlipidemia • Depression • Aggression	• Liver function tests (LFTs) • Serum testosterone concentrations • Prostate-specific antigen • Lipid panel	May ↑ effects/toxicity of warfarin	• Only useful in ED due to hypogonadism • Schedule III controlled substance
Testosterone gel ☆ • AndroGel, Fortesta, Testim, Vogelxo, • AndroGel 1%: 50–100 mg daily • AndroGel 1.62%: 40.5–81 mg daily • Fortesta: 40–70 mg daily • Testim: 50 mg daily • Vogelxo: 50 mg daily					
Testosterone intranasal gel • Natesto • 1 pump per nostril (total = 11 mg) TID					
Testosterone buccal • Striant • 30 mg BID (apply to gum, above incisor)					
Intramuscular					
Testosterone • Depo-Testosterone (cypionate), Generic (enanthate), Aveed (undecanoate) • Cypionate or enanthate: 50–400 mg IM every 2–4 wk • Undecanoate: 750 mg IM, then 750 mg IM 4 wk later, then 750 mg IM every 10 wk	• Hypersensitivity • Breast or prostate cancer • Serious cardiac, renal or hepatic disease	• ↑ LFTs • ↑ risk of DVT/PE, stroke, and MI • Edema • Hyperlipidemia • Depression • Aggression	• LFTs • Serum testosterone concentrations • PSA • Lipid panel	May ↑ effects/toxicity of warfarin	• Only useful in ED due to hypogonadism • Schedule III controlled substance

Medications for Erectile Dysfunction *(cont'd)*

Generic • Brand • Dose/Dosage Forms	Contraindications	Primary Side Effects	Key Monitoring Parameters	Pertinent Drug Interactions	Med Pearls
Intraurethral					
Alprostadil • Muse • 125–250 mcg pellets 5–10 min before intercourse	• Hypersensitivity • Urethral stricture • Chronic urethritis	• Urethral pain • Burning • Priapism • Hypotension	• Presence of side effects • Efficacy • BP	None	Duration of effect is 30–60 min
Intracavernosal					
Alprostadil • Caverject, Edex • 1–40 mcg 5–20 min before intercourse injected intracavernosal	• Hypersensitivity • Sickle-cell trait • Multiple myeloma • Leukemia	• Pain at injection site • Erythema • Priapism • Hypotension	• Presence of side effects • Efficacy • BP periodically	None	Self-injection training should be done in physician's office

Storage and Administration Pearls

- Sildenafil should be taken at least 30 minutes prior to sexual activity and can be taken, at earliest, 4 hours prior.

- Vardenafil should be taken approximately 1 hour prior to anticipated activity.

- Tadalafil can either be taken prior to activity or as a scheduled daily dose.

- Alprostadil intraurethral: Store unopened foil pouches in a refrigerator at 2–8°C (36–46°F). Do not expose alprostadil urethral suppository to temperatures above 30°C (86°F). Alprostadil urethral suppository may be kept at room temperature (below 30°C [86°F]) for up to 14 days prior to use.

- Alprostadil intracavernosal: Prepare the solution immediately before use. Do not administer unless solution is clear. Do not add any drugs or other solutions to this solution. Discard any unused solution remaining in the cartridge.

Patient Education Pearls

- Androderm is applied to the arm, back, abdomen, or thigh.

- Testosterone gel is applied to shoulders, arms, abdomen, or thighs (product dependent).

- Males using testosterone products should not allow direct contact between the testosterone product and a pregnant female, as teratogenic effects are possible. They should also avoid direct contact between the testosterone product and children as virilization can occur.

BENIGN PROSTATIC HYPERPLASIA

Definition

Benign prostatic hyperplasia (BPH) is an enlargement of the prostate gland due to the proliferation of smooth muscle and epithelial cells. BPH often leads to lower urinary tract symptoms (LUTS) due to direct bladder outlet obstruction and increase smooth muscle tone/resistance from within the enlarged gland.

Diagnosis

Diagnosis of BPH primarily is made based upon symptoms. The American Urological Association Symptom Index (AUA-SI) and other similar symptom scores are used to determine the degree of impact the LUTS are having on an individual patient's quality of life and to guide therapy decisions.

Questions included in the AUA-SI include quantification of how frequently specific symptoms have occurred over the preceding month. Responses of higher frequency are assigned a higher point value. The overall score on the AUA-SI is a validated measure used to determine symptom severity and initiate patient-specific dialog regarding benefits and risks of treatment. In general, pharmacological therapy is considered for patients with moderate–severe symptoms (AUA-SI scores >8).

Signs and Symptoms

Symptoms of BPH include LUTS such as urinary urgency, leaking, dribbling, hesitancy, frequency (especially nocturia), straining/weak stream, and incomplete bladder emptying.

Signs of BPH may include an enlarged prostate identified during a digital rectal exam (DRE) or an elevated serum PSA.

Guidelines

American Urological Association Guideline: Management of Benign Prostatic Hyperplasia (BPH). Linthicum, MD: American Urologic Association Education and Research, Inc.; 2010. http://www.auanet.org/education/guidelines/benign-prostatic-hyperplasia.cfm

Guidelines Summary

- Watchful waiting (no pharmacologic therapy) is appropriate for patients with mild symptoms (AUA-SI scores <8).

- In general, pharmacologic therapy is considered for patients with moderate–severe symptoms (AUA-SI scores ≥8).

- Alpha-antagonists are the treatment of choice for patients with LUTS and are used as monotherapy or in combination with 5-alpha reductase inhibitors or anticholinergics.

  - Nonselective alpha-antagonists such as terazosin and doxazosin are equally effective as the alpha 1A selective antagonists, tamsulosin, alfuzosin, and silodosin.

  - Nonselective alpha-antagonists require slow dose titration and lower BP; therefore, these agents should be used with caution in patients at risk of hypotension.

  - First-dose syncope and dizziness are common side effects, especially with the nonselective alpha-antagonists. Dosing at bedtime can minimize this side effect, but patients should be educated to stand up slowly to avoid falls.

  - Intraoperative floppy iris syndrome (IFIS) is a potential side effect of the alpha-antagonists that can significantly complicate cataract surgery. Patients with planned cataract surgery should not initiate new alpha-antagonist therapy until cataract surgery is complete.

- 5-alpha reductase inhibitors are appropriate as monotherapy or combination therapy with alpha-antagonists in patients with enlarged prostate glands.

  - Although earlier guidelines suggested use of 5-alpha reductase inhibitors in patients with prostate glands >50 mL (50 g), newer studies have demonstrated benefits in patients with prostate glands >30 mL (30 g).

- Anticholinergic agents such as tolterodine may be considered in patient with LUTS (primarily irritative) and without an elevated postvoid residual (<250 mL). Please see the Urinary Incontinence section of this chapter for specifics related to anticholinergic medications.

PDE-5 inhibitors are now clinically indicated for daily use for the treatment of LUTS/BPH (tadalafil is approved by the Food and Drug Administration for this indication) but are generally reserved for patients who have not responded to more conventional therapies. Because PDE-5 inhibitors exhibit a significant drug interaction with nonselective alpha-antagonists, special care should be taken to monitor for and avoid this combination.

BPH Treatment Summary

Medications for BPH

Generic • Brand • Dose/Dosage Forms	Contraindications	Primary Side Effects	Key Monitoring Parameters	Pertinent Drug Interactions	Med Pearls
Nonselective Alpha-1 Antagonists					
Doxazosin ☆ • Cardura, Cardura XL • IR: 1–8 mg at bedtime • ER: 4–8 mg in AM • ER tabs, tabs	Hypersensitivity	• Orthostatic hypotension • Dizziness • Reflex tachycardia • Peripheral edema • Headache • Drowsiness • Priapism (rare)	• BP • Heart rate • LUTS	↑ risk of hypotension with PDE-5 inhibitors (avoid concurrent use)	• Dosed at bedtime (except for doxazosin ER which is dosed in AM) to prevent dizziness/ falls during the day • ↑ risk of IFIS in patients undergoing cataract surgery
Terazosin ☆ • Only available generically • 1–10 mg at bedtime • Caps					
Selective Alpha 1A Antagonists					
Tamsulosin ☆ • Flomax • 0.4–0.8 mg daily	Hypersensitivity	• Orthostatic hypotension • Dizziness • Headache • Priapism (rare)	• BP • LUTS	• CYP3A4 substrate • CYP3A4 inhibitors may ↑ effects/toxicity; avoid use with strong CYP3A4 inhibitors • CYP3A4 inducers may ↓ effects • ↑ risk of hypotension with PDE-5 inhibitors • Cimetidine may ↑ levels	• Expensive relative to nonselective agents • ↑ risk of IFIS in patients undergoing cataract surgery
Alfuzosin • Uroxatral • 10 mg daily • ER tabs	• Hypersensitivity • Moderate to severe hepatic impairment • Concurrent use with strong 3A4 inhibitors			• CYP3A4 substrate • CYP3A4 inhibitors may ↑ effects/toxicity; concurrent use with strong CYP3A4 inhibitors contraindicated • CYP3A4 inducers may ↓ effects • ↑ risk of hypotension with PDE-5 inhibitors	• Take with food • Do not crush or chew • Expensive relative to nonselective agents • ↑ risk of IFIS in patients undergoing cataract surgery
Silodosin • Rapaflo • 8 mg daily • Caps	• Hypersensitivity • Severe renal or hepatic impairment • Concurrent use with strong 3A4 inhibitors	• Orthostatic hypotension • Dizziness • Headache • Diarrhea • Retrograde ejaculation • Priapism (rare)			• Adjust dose in renal impairment • Take with food • Expensive relative to nonselective agents • ↑ risk of IFIS in patients undergoing cataract surgery

Medications for BPH *(cont'd)*

Generic • Brand • Dose/Dosage Forms	Contraindications	Primary Side Effects	Key Monitoring Parameters	Pertinent Drug Interactions	Med Pearls
5-Alpha Reductase Inhibitors					
Finasteride ☆ • Proscar • 5 mg daily • Tabs	• Hypersensitivity • Pregnant women or women of childbearing potential	• ↓ libido • ED • Gynecomastia	• PSA • LUTS	None	• Cause significant ↓ in PSA; should establish new PSA baseline ≥6 mo after initiation of therapy
Dutasteride ☆ • Avodart • 0.5 mg daily • Caps				• CYP3A4 substrate • CYP3A4 inhibitors may ↑ effects/ toxicity • CYP3A4 inducers may ↓ effects	• Dutasteride caps and crushed/broken finasteride tabs should not be handled by pregnant women or women of childbearing potential (potentially teratogenic for male infants) • Men taking dutasteride should not donate blood for ≥6 mo after discontinuing therapy • Onset of effect can be up to 6 mo

Combination Products: See individual drug components for important points		
Brand	**Components**	**Dosing**
Jalyn	Dutasteride + Tamsulosin	1 cap (0.5 mg dutasteride/0.4 mg tamsulosin) daily (~30 min after a meal)

Storage and Administration Pearls

- Nonselective alpha-antagonists (with exception of ER doxazosin) should be taken at bedtime to avoid side effects of syncope and orthostasis while awake.

- Tamsulosin and silodosin should be taken with food.

- Alfuzosin cannot be crushed, chewed, or broken in half; tablets must be swallowed whole.

- Silodosin caps may be opened and contents sprinkled on a tablespoon of applesauce.

Patient Education Pearls

- Patients taking nonselective alpha-antagonists should be educated to take dose at bedtime and to rise slowly when waking to use toilet at night. ER doxazosin should be taken in A.M. Dizziness may occur and may require some time before patient feels steady on his or her feet. This side effect likely will be most pronounced immediately following dose changes and should subside over time.

- If receiving an alpha-antagonist, rise slowly from seated position to avoid potential dizziness associated with the medication.

- If receiving an 5-alpha reductase inhibitor, know that reaching full benefit of this medication may take up to 6 months. An adequate trial should be allowed.

- For alpha-antagonists, patients should be advised to tell their doctor about any planned cataract surgery.

- Women who may be pregnant or are of childbearing age should not handle 5-alpha reductase crushed or broken finasteride tabs or intact dutasteride caps. These medications can cause birth defects in male infants.

URINARY INCONTINENCE

Definitions

This is a condition associated with the involuntary loss of urine. There are multiple subtypes of urinary incontinence differentiated by etiology. The major classifications are: (*1*) urethral underactivity (stress incontinence), (*2*) bladder overactivity (urge incontinence), and (*3*) urethral overactivity/bladder underactivity (overflow incontinence).

Diagnosis

Diagnosis is based primarily on patient complaints and a thorough history and physical.

Signs and Symptoms

Symptoms of stress incontinence include the loss of small amounts of urine during activities such as sneezing, coughing, laughing, or running. Symptoms of urge incontinence include urinary urgency and frequency that may be associated with the loss of large or small amounts of urine. Overflow incontinence is associated with the loss of a large amount of urine which may be accompanied by symptoms of frequency, nocturia, hesitancy, or weak urinary stream.

Guidelines

Because a nationally recognized guideline for the treatment of urinary incontinence does not currently exist, the following represents general recommendations for treatment of the various subtypes based on multiple primary and tertiary resources.

Summary of Treatment Recommendations

- General
  - Nonpharmacological therapy is important as either monotherapy or an adjunct to pharmacotherapy. Options such as Kegel exercises and scheduled voiding are common.
- Stress incontinence
  - Options for treatment include topical estrogen, alpha agonists, and tricyclic anti-depressants. Alpha agonists carry the risk of ↑ BP and heart rate, and should be used with extreme caution in patients with pre-existing hypertension or heart conditions.
- Urge incontinence
  - Options for treatment include anticholinergic medications and imipramine.
- Overflow incontinence
  - Treatment options are varied based upon the determined etiology. Since many cases of overflow incontinence are secondary to BPH, see the BPH section of this chapter for recommendations.

Medications for Urinary Incontinence

Generic • Brand • Dose/Dosage Forms	Contraindications	Primary Side Effects	Key Monitoring Parameters	Pertinent Drug Interactions	Med Pearls
Topical vaginal estrogen preparations: used in the treatment of stress incontinence (first-line) and urge incontinence (third-line); refer to the Hormone Replacement Therapy section of this chapter for more detailed information					
Tricyclic antidepressants: imipramine and desipramine are most commonly used in incontinence; used primarily in urge incontinence and stress incontinence; refer to the Psychiatric Disorders chapter for more detailed information					
Anticholinergic/Antimuscarinic Agents					
Oxybutynin ☆ • Ditropan XL • IR: 5 mg 2–4 × /day • ER: 5–30 mg daily • ER tabs, tabs • Oxytrol • Apply 1 patch (3.9 mg/day) twice weekly • Transdermal patch • Gelnique • 3%: Apply 3 pumps (84 mg) daily • 10%: Apply contents of 1 sachet (100 mg /g) daily • Transdermal gel	• Hypersensitivity • Urinary retention • Gastric retention • Narrow-angle glaucoma	• Dry mouth • Dry eyes • Constipation • Urinary retention • Dizziness • Somnolence • Hallucinations • Agitation • Confusion • Blurred vision • ↑ intraocular pressure • Angioedema	• S/S of incontinence • Presence of side effects	Additive effects with other anticholinergic medications	• Side effects less common with ER tabs and transdermal formulations • Transdermal patch available over-the-counter
Tolterodine ☆ • Detrol, Detrol LA • IR: 1–2 mg BID • ER: 2–4 mg daily • ER caps, tabs				• CYP2D6 and CYP3A4 substrate • CYP2D6 and CYP3A4 inhibitors may ↑ effects/ toxicity • CYP3A4 inducers may ↓ effects • Additive effects with other anticholinergic medications	• Side effects less common with ER tabs • Adjust dose in renal or hepatic impairment

Medications for Urinary Incontinence *(cont'd)*

Generic • Brand • Dose/Dosage Forms	Contraindications	Primary Side Effects	Key Monitoring Parameters	Pertinent Drug Interactions	Med Pearls
Anticholinergic/Antimuscarinic Agents (cont'd)					
Darifenacin ☆ • Enablex • 7.5–15 mg daily • ER tabs	[Same as above]	[Same as above]	[Same as above]	• CYP3A4 substrate • CYP3A4 inhibitors may ↑ effects/ toxicity • CYP3A4 inducers may ↓ effects • Additive effects with other anticholinergic medications	• Adjust dose in renal or hepatic impairment • Max dose = 7.5 mg daily with potent 3A4 inhibitors
Solifenacin ☆ • Vesicare • 5–10 mg daily • Tabs					• Adjust dose in hepatic impairment • Max dose = 5 mg daily with potent 3A4 inhibitors
Fesoterodine ☆ • Toviaz • 4–8 mg daily • ER tabs					• Adjust dose in renal impair- ment • Max dose = 4 mg daily with potent 3A4 inhibitors
Trospium ☆ • Only available generically • IR: 20 mg BID • ER: 60 mg daily • ER caps, tabs				• Metformin may ↓ levels • Additive effects with other anticholinergic medications	• Take 30 min before meals or on an empty stomach • Adjust dose in renal impairment and in patients ≥75 yr

Medications for Urinary Incontinence *(cont'd)*

Generic • Brand • Dose/Dosage Forms	Contraindications	Primary Side Effects	Key Monitoring Parameters	Pertinent Drug Interactions	Med Pearls
Mechanism of action – beta-3 adrenergic receptor antagonist					
Mirabegron • Myrbetriq • 25–50 mg daily • ER tabs	Hypersensitivity	• Hypertension • Angioedema • Headache	• BP • S/S of in-continence	• CYP2D6 inhibitor • May ↑ effects/toxicity of CYP2D6 substrates • May ↑ serum digoxin concentrations • May ↑ effects of warfarin • Additive effects with other anticholinergic medications	• Adjust dose in renal or hepatic impairment • Newer agent with fewer anticholinergic side effects • Hypertension may limit use • Very expensive
Alpha Agonists					
Pseudoephedrine • Sudafed • 30–60 mg every 4–6 hr PRN (max = 240 mg/24 hrs) Phenylephrine • Many • 10–20 mg every 4 hr PRN	• Hypersensitivity • Concurrent use of monoamine oxidase inhibitors (MAOIs) • Uncontrolled hypertension	• ↑ blood pressure • ↑ heart rate • ↑ blood sugar • Irritability • Insomnia	• BP • Heart rate • Fasting plasma glucose (if diabetes)	Concurrent use MAO inhibitors may ↑ risk of hypertensive crises	Use with caution in HTN or pre-existing cardiac conditions

Storage and Administration Pearls

- Store all medications at room temperature and out of the reach of children.

- Apply oxybutynin transdermal gel to abdomen, thighs, or upper arms/shoulders.

- Apply oxybutynin transdermal patch to abdomen, hip, or buttock.

Patient Education Pearls

- Anticholinergic medications may make patient experience dry mouth, dry eyes, blurred vision, drowsiness, or constipation.

PRACTICE QUESTIONS

1. Which of the following is most accurate regarding the coadministration of sildenafil and nitroglycerin?

    (A) There is no drug interaction between the two medications.
    (B) There is a minor drug interaction between the two medications. The patient should be counseled to monitor for signs and symptoms of the interaction.
    (C) There is a major drug interaction between these two agents, but they can be safely coadministered as long as doses are separated by at least 1 hour.
    (D) There is a major drug interaction between sildenafil and some forms of nitroglycerin. The specific formulation of nitroglycerin should be determined before the medications are taken.
    (E) There is a major, potentially life-threatening drug interaction between the two agents. Coadministration should be strictly avoided.

2. In which of the following clinical scenarios would hormone replacement therapy be contraindicated?

    (A) Breast cancer
    (B) Obesity
    (C) Stage III chronic kidney disease
    (D) Diabetes mellitus
    (E) History of hysterectomy

3. Which of the following is the correct trade name for tadalafil?

    (A) Viagra
    (B) Levitra
    (C) Cialis
    (D) Caverject
    (E) Proscar

4. Which of the following describes drugs most likely to cross the placenta?

    (A) High molecular mass (1,500 Da)
    (B) Highly protein bound
    (C) Highly lipophilic
    (D) Highly ionized

5. A 74-year-old man with benign prostatic hyperplasia (BPH) has taken terazosin for 6 months with some symptom improvement. He still complains of urinary urgency. His prostate size is 20 g and postvoid residual volume is 50 mL. Which medication is most appropriate in combination with his current treatment to address his symptoms?

   (A) Tolterodine
   (B) Dutasteride
   (C) Sildenafil
   (D) Saw palmetto

6. A 32-year-old woman with hypertension, headaches, and seasonal allergies expresses a desire to become pregnant. She is currently taking nifedipine 60 mg PO daily, lisinopril 10 mg daily, acetaminophen 500 mg 1–2 PRN Q 4–6 hours, and loratadine 10 mg daily. Which of the patient's medications is a known teratogen and should be discontinued prior to conception?

   (A) Nifedipine
   (B) Lisinopril
   (C) Acetaminophen
   (D) Loratadine

7. A 24-year-old woman on a monophasic oral contraceptive informs you that she missed the last 2 doses of her contraceptive tablets in the first 2 weeks of the pack. In addition to using a back up form of contraception for at least the next 7 days, which of the following is the most appropriate set of instructions to provide?

   (A) Take 1 extra dose today, the next dose at the regularly scheduled time, and resume 1 tablet daily.
   (B) Take 2 doses daily for next 2 days, then resume 1 tablet daily.
   (C) Take 1 tablet daily until Sunday, start a new pack without taking placebo pills.
   (D) Dispose of the current pack, wait until Sunday and restart a new pack on that day.

8. Which of the following contraceptives could be used safely in a 26-year-old woman who is 12 weeks postpartum and breastfeeding her baby?

   (A) Ortho Micronor
   (B) NuvaRing
   (C) Ovcon 35
   (D) Loestrin Fe

9. A 67-year-old man with BPH has an AUA-SI score of 10, prostate size of 15 g, and postvoid residual of 100 mL. He has a medical history of hypertension and cataracts and is scheduled to have cataract surgery in 2 weeks. Which of the following is the best recommendation?

   (A) Watchful waiting for 6 months.
   (B) Initiate alfuzosin today.
   (C) Initiate alfuzosin in 1 month.
   (D) Initiate dutasteride today.

ANSWERS AND EXPLANATIONS

1. **E**

There is a major, life-threatening drug interaction between these two medications. When coadministered, the two agents can result in a life-threatening drop in blood pressure. All forms of nitroglycerin carry this risk, and coadministration should be avoided for *at least* 24 hours.

2. **A**

Hormone replacement therapy is contraindicated in patients with breast cancer due to the potential to exacerbate tumor growth. Obesity, kidney disease, and diabetes are not contraindications to hormone replacement therapy. Patients with a history of hysterectomy may take unopposed estrogen but do not need progestin.

3. **C**

Cialis is the trade name for tadalafil. Viagra is the trade name for sildenafil, Levitra is the trade name for vardenafil, Caverject is the trade name for alprostadil, and Proscar is the trade name for finasteride.

4. **C**

Greater fat solubility increases the likelihood that a drug will cross the placenta. Small molecular mass (<500 Da) agents are more likely to cross the placenta, as are drugs with lower degree of protein binding and drugs that are un-ionized.

5. **A**

Therapy with an anticholinergic drug such as tolterodine can be used in combination with alpha-blockers to treat symptoms of urinary urgency if the postvoid residual volume is below 250 mL. Dutasteride (B) is beneficial in combination with alpha-blockers in men with elevated prostate size (30–60 g or greater) and this patient's size is 20 g. Sildenafil (C) is appropriate for erectile dysfunction; however, phosphodiesterase inhibitors are reserved for patients that have not responded to conventional therapies, and tadalafil is the only currently FDA approved agent for LUTS associated with BPH. Saw palmetto (D) has limited evidence of benefit and would not be the best recommendation in this case.

6. **B**

ACE inhibitors such as lisinopril are pregnancy category D and are known to cause renal defects and restrict fetal growth patterns. Nifedipine (A) is classified as category C by the FDA but is endorsed and recommended by the ACOG guidelines as a potential first-line antihypertensive during pregnancy. Acetaminophen (C) and loratadine (B) have not demonstrated teratogenicity and are thought to be safe for use during pregnancy.

7. **B**

Taking 2 doses daily for the next 2 days, then resuming 1 tablet daily is appropriate. An extra dose today, then resuming 1 tablet daily (A) would be correct if the patient had missed only 1 dose but it will not provide enough contraceptive medication if she missed 2 doses. Starting a new pack on Sunday (C and D) would be appropriate if the patient had missed 3 or more doses or if she had missed 2 or more doses in the third week of the pack.

8. **A**

Progestin-only contraceptives such as Ortho Micronor are safe options during breastfeeding. NuvaRing (B), Ovcon 35 (C), and LoestrinFe (D) are all estrogen-containing contraceptives and cannot be used during breastfeeding.

9. **B**

The patient's AUA-SI score (≥ 8) warrants pharmacological treatment, thus watchful waiting (A) is incorrect. Alpha antagonists including alfuzosin (C) would be the appropriate first-line therapy; however, it should not be started until after the patient's cataract surgery. Alfuzosin has the potential to cause intraoperative floppy iris syndrome (IFIS) in patients undergoing cataract surgery. And 5 alpha reductase inhibitors such as dutasteride (D) are reserved for patients with prostate glands >30 mL (30 g); this patient's prostate size is 15 g.

Solid Organ Transplant/ Immunosuppression

18

This chapter covers the following procedure:

- **Solid organ transplantation**

 Suggested Study Time: **30 minutes**

SOLID ORGAN TRANSPLANTATION/IMMUNOSUPPRESSION

Definitions

Solid organ transplantation is a common treatment strategy for patients with organ failure. Immunosuppressive therapy is needed to prevent organ rejection and maintain graft function. Organs commonly transplanted include liver, kidney, heart, pancreas, and lung. Most commonly, transplants occur between individuals of the same species who are not genetically identical. These types of grafts are considered allograft transplants.

Hyperacute graft rejection occurs within minutes to hours after the graft has been revascularized. *Acute graft rejection* usually occurs within the first 6 months after the transplant, but it may occur anytime post-transplant. Maintenance immunosuppression is then initiated and maintained for the life of the graft to reduce the risk of *chronic organ rejection,* which can occur months to years after transplant or acute rejection episodes. Chronic graft rejection may occur due to chronic inflammation or fibrotic vascular changes, which diminish the blood supply; over time, ischemia can lead to graft loss.

Induction therapy is used during the initial period post-transplant, when higher levels of overall immunosuppression are required to prevent acute graft rejection. Induction therapy requires selecting different combinations of therapies or using higher dosages of medications. Agents selected may include antibody therapies, IV corticosteroids, and other drugs. Maintenance therapy is used for the lifetime of the graft to reduce the risk of both acute and chronic organ rejection. Combinations of agents are selected and titrated to balance efficacy and toxicity.

Patients taking immunosuppressive therapies must be monitored for risk of infection, especially those who are taking multiple immunosuppressants, because overall immunosuppression is generally increased with the use of multiple immunosuppressive therapies. This encompasses any drug with immunosuppressive properties, including immunosuppressants used for oncologic or rheumatologic conditions.

Diagnosis

Diagnosis of acute organ rejection is dependent upon the specific organ that was transplanted. For acute renal allograft rejection, evidence of histologic changes, donor-specific antibodies, and antibody infiltration of endothelium are needed for diagnosis. Acute hepatic allograft rejection is diagnosed based on elevation of liver function tests (LFTs) and histologic changes.

Signs and Symptoms

Fever, malaise, and pain are nonspecific symptoms that may be seen with organ rejection. Hepatomegaly, abdominal pain, or jaundice may be present for hepatic rejection. Renal allograft rejection may present with rising serum creatinine levels, oliguria, graft pain, and hypertension.

Guidelines

There are no guidelines for immunosuppressive therapy. Regimens vary based on the organ, the patient population, and the transplant center.

Induction Immunosuppression Therapy

Generic • Brand • Dose/Dosage Forms	Contraindications	Primary Side Effects	Key Monitoring Parameters	Pertinent Drug Interactions	Med Pearls
Mechanism of action – antibody that acts on T-cell surface antigens and depletes CD4 lymphocytes					
Antithymocyte globulin • Thymoglobulin (rabbit) • 1.5 mg/kg/day IV × 7–14 days • Injection	• Hypersensitivity to antithymocyte globulin or rabbit proteins • Infection	• Chills • Fever • Headache • Malaise • Pain • Hypertension • Leukopenia • Thrombocytopenia • Dyspnea • Anaphylaxis • Infection	• Complete blood count (CBC) with differential • Heart rate (HR) • Blood pressure (BP) • S/S of graft rejection • S/S of infection	• Not to be given with live vaccines • May ↑ effects/ toxicity of other immuno- suppressants	• Indicated for treatment of acute renal transplant rejection • Premedicate with corticosteroid, acetaminophen, and/or anthistamine

Maintenance Immunosuppression Therapy

Generic • Brand • Dose/Dosage Forms	Contraindications	Primary Side Effects	Key Monitoring Parameters	Pertinent Drug Interactions	Med Pearls
Mechanism of action – limits activity and volume of lymphatic system					
Prednisone ☆ • Only available generically • 5–60 mg daily initially; individualized • Solution, tabs	• Systemic fungal infection • Hypersensitivity	• Hyperglycemia • ↑ BP • ↓ bone mineral density (BMD) • Fluid retention • Impaired wound healing • Infection • Hyperglycemia • ↑ appetite • Irritability • Insomnia • Weight gain	• S/S of graft rejection • S/S of infection • Blood glucose • BP • Electrolytes • BMD	• Not to be given with live vaccines • May ↑ effects/toxicity of other immunosuppressants • May ↑ anticoagulant effect of warfarin	• Take with food • Taper if discontinuing high doses that have been used for long periods

Maintenance Immunosuppression Therapy *(cont'd)*

Generic • Brand • Dose/Dosage Forms	Contraindications	Primary Side Effects	Key Monitoring Parameters	Pertinent Drug Interactions	Med Pearls
Mechanism of action – inhibit inosine monophosphate dehydrogenase which blocks purine synthesis and lymphocyte function					
Mycophenolate mofetil • CellCept • 1–1.5 g PO/IV BID • Caps, injection, suspension, tabs Mycophenolic acid • Myfortic • 720 mg BID • ER tabs	Hypersensitivity	• Diarrhea • Neutropenia • Anemia • ↑ LFTs • ↑ SCr • Hypertension • Hypotension • Edema • Chest pain • Tachycardia • Headache • Insomnia • Rash • Infection • Malignancy	• CBC with differential • LFTs • SCr • BP • S/S of graft rejection • S/S of infection • Pregnancy test	• Not to be given with live vaccines • May ↑ acyclovir levels • Antacids, proton pump inhibitors, cholestyramine, and sevelemer may ↓ its absorption • Cyclosporine may ↑ levels • Telmisartan and rifampin may ↓ levels • May ↑ effects/toxicity of other immunosuppressants	• Teratogenic • Women must use appropriate contraception during therapy and for 6 wk after discontinuing therapy • Take on an empty stomach
Mechanism of action – inhibit calcineurin, which inhibits the activation of T-cells and downregulation of interleukins and tumor necrosis factor-alpha					
Cyclosporine • Gengraf, Neoral, Sand-IMMUNE • 7–10 mg/kg/day PO in 2 divided doses • 3–7.5 mg/kg/day in 1–3 divided doses IV • Caps, injection, solution	Hypersensitivity	• Hypertension • Nephrotoxicity • Hepatotoxicity • Edema • Hypertrichosis • Hirsutism • Infection • Tremor • ↑ triglycerides • Gingival hyperplasia • Malignancy • Seizures • Encephalopathy • Anaphylaxis • Hyperkalemia	• Trough concentrations • BP • LFTs • Renal function • Lipids • Electrolytes • S/S of graft rejection • S/S of infection	• CYP3A4 substrate and inhibitor • CYP3A4 inhibitors may ↑ effects/toxicity • CYP3A4 inducers may ↓ effects • May ↑ effects/toxicity of CYP3A4 substrates • Not to be given with live vaccines • ↑ risk of nephrotoxicity when used with amphotericin B, loop diuretics, nonsteroidal anti-inflammatory drugs, or cisplatin • May ↑ effects/toxicity of other immunosuppressants • Angiotensin-converting enzyme inhibitors (ACEIs), angiotensin receptor blockers (ARBs), aldosterone receptor antagonists (ARAs), potassium-sparing diuretics, and potassium supplements may ↑ risk of hyperkalemia	• Therapeutic range dependent on organ transplanted (general range of 100–400 ng/mL) • Also available as eye drops (Restasis) for dry eye disease

Maintenance Immunosuppression Therapy *(cont'd)*

Generic • Brand • Dose/Dosage Forms	Contraindications	Primary Side Effects	Key Monitoring Parameters	Pertinent Drug Interactions	Med Pearls
Tacrolimus☆ • Astagraf XL, Envarsus XR, Prograf • IR: 0.075–0.2 mg/kg/day PO in 2 divided doses • ER: 0.15–0.2 mg/kg daily • IV: 0.01–0.05 mg/kg/day continuous infusion • Caps, ER caps, ER tabs, injection	Hypersensitivity to tacrolimus or polyoxyl 60 hydrogenated castor oil	• Hypertension • Edema • Chest pain • Headache • Insomnia • Diabetes mellitus • Dyslipidemia • Diarrhea • Nephrotoxicity • Hepatotoxicity • Infection • Malignancy • Anaphylaxis • Encephalopathy • QT interval prolongation	• Renal function • LFTs • Electrolytes • Glucose • Lipids • BP • Whole blood trough concentrations • S/S of graft rejection • S/S of infection • Electrocardiogram	• CYP3A4 substrate • CYP3A4 inhibitors may ↑ effects/toxicity • CYP3A4 inducers may ↓ effects • Not to be given with live vaccines • ↑ risk of nephrotoxicity when used with amphotericin B, loop diuretics, nonsteroidal anti-inflammatory drugs, or cisplatin • May ↑ effects/toxicity of other immunosuppressants • ACEIs, ARBs, ARAs, potassium-sparing diuretics, and potassium supplements may ↑ risk of hyperkalemia • ↑ risk of torsade de pointes with other drugs that prolong QT interval	• Therapeutic range dependent on organ transplanted • IR: Must be consistent with taking medication with or without food • ER: Administer on an empty stomach (1 hr before or 2 hr after a meal) • Also available as ointment (Protopic) for atopic dermatitis

Mechanism of action – inhibits mammalian target of rapamycin which inhibits the transduction of the signal generated by IL-2 binding to the IL-2 receptor which affects cell growth

Sirolimus • Rapamune • 2–40 mg daily • Solution, tabs	Hypersensitivity	• Hypertension • Edema • Headache • Dyslipidemia • Constipation • Anemia • Nephrotoxicity • Infection • Malignancy • Anaphylaxis • Interstitial lung disease	• LFTs • CBC • Lipids • BP • Renal function • Trough concentrations • S/S of graft rejection • S/S of infection	• CYP3A4 substrate • CYP3A4 inhibitors may ↑ effects/toxicity • CYP3A4 inducers may ↓ effects • Not to be given with live vaccines • ↑ risk of nephrotoxicity when used with amphotericin B, cyclosporine, loop diuretics, nonsteroidal anti-inflammatory drugs, or cisplatin • May ↑ effects/toxicity of other immunosuppressants	• Should be taken 4 hr after cyclosporine • Solution should be diluted in water or orange juice • To be used with cyclosporine (renal transplant)
Everolimus • Zortress • 0.75–1 mg BID • Tabs	Hypersensitivity to everolimus or sirolimus	• Hypertension • Edema • Chest pain • Headache • Insomnia • Anemia • Diabetes mellitus • Dyslipidemia • Diarrhea • Nephrotoxicity • Infection • Malignancy • Angioedema • Interstitial lung disease	• Renal function • LFTs • CBC • Electrolytes • Glucose • BP • Whole blood trough concentrations • S/S of graft rejection • S/S of infection		• Also available as Afinitor and Afinitor Disperz for treatment of various malignancies • To be used with cyclosporine (renal transplant) or tacrolimus (liver transplant)

Maintenance Immunosuppression Therapy *(cont'd)*

Generic • Brand • Dose/Dosage Forms	Contraindications	Primary Side Effects	Key Monitoring Parameters	Pertinent Drug Interactions	Med Pearls
Mechanism of action – selective T-cell costimulation inhibitor by binding to CD80 and CD86 receptors on antigen presenting cells					
Belatacept • Nulojix • 10 mg/kg IV on Day 1, Day 5, and at the end of Wk 2, Wk 4, Wk 8, and Wk 12 after transplantation, then 5 mg/kg IV every 4 wk beginning at Wk 16 after transplantation • Injection	• Hypersensitivity • Epstein-Barr virus (EBV) seronegative or unknown EBV status	• Infection • Anemia • Leukopenia • Diarrhea • Constipation • Hypo- or hyperkalemia • Peripheral edema • Hypertension • Hypotension • Post-transplant lymphoproliferative disorder • Malignancy • Progressive multifocal leukoencephalopathy	• S/S of graft rejection • S/S of infection • S/S of malignancy • Epstein-Barr virus status prior to therapy • Cognitive or neurological symptoms	• Not to be given with live vaccines • May ↑ effects/toxicity of other immunosuppressants	

Storage and Administration Pearls

- Refrigerate antithymocyte globulin powder (rabbit); do not freeze, stable for 24 hours if reconstituted at room temperature

Patient Education Pearls

- Avoid live vaccines in immunocompromised patients.
- Assess for signs of infection in immunocompromised patients.

LEARNING POINTS

Induction immunosuppression is administered at the time of transplant to prevent acute graft rejection.

- Maintenance immunosuppression is administered for the life of the graft to prevent chronic graft rejection.
- Immunosuppression increases the risk of infection in transplanted patients.
- Immunosuppressants may be administered as monotherapy or in conjunction with other immunosuppressants for solid-organ transplantation.
- Immunosuppression is increased with multiple immunosuppressive therapies, so pharmacists need to be aware of the risks to patients taking multiple immunosuppressants, even those for nontransplant indications.

PRACTICE QUESTIONS

1. Which of the following is an adverse effect associated with prednisone?

   (A) Hypoglycemia
   (B) Osteoporosis
   (C) Renal dysfunction
   (D) Thyroid dysfunction
   (E) Toxic epidermal necrolysis

2. Which of the following inhibits mammalian target of rapamycin?

   (A) Belatacept
   (B) Cyclosporine
   (C) Everolimus
   (D) Mycophenolate
   (E) Tacrolimus

3. Which of the following should be monitored for tacrolimus? (Select ALL that apply.)

   (A) Blood glucose
   (B) Blood pressure
   (C) Drug levels
   (D) Hepatic function
   (E) Respiratory rate

4. Which of the following should not be administered with cyclosporine?

   (A) Adacel
   (B) Engerix
   (C) Fluzone
   (D) Pneumovax
   (E) Zostavax

5. Which of the following counseling points applies to mycophenolate mofetil?

   (A) ER tablets may be crushed.
   (B) Take on an empty stomach.
   (C) Taper medication upon discontinuation.
   (D) Keep tablets refrigerated.

6. Which of the following is the brand name of tacrolimus?

   (A) Zortress
   (B) Rapamune
   (C) Prograf
   (D) Neoral

7. Which of the following must have Epstein-Barr serology tested before use?

   (A) CellCept
   (B) Nulojix
   (C) Prograf
   (D) SandIMMUNE
   (E) Thymoglobulin

ANSWERS AND EXPLANATIONS

1. B

Long-term treatment with prednisone can result in osteoporosis, which necessitates screening of bone mineral density in those who chronically take prednisone. Prednisone causes hyperglycemia, so hypoglycemia (A) is incorrect. Prednisone is not associated with renal dysfunction (C), thyroid dysfunction (D), or toxic epidermal necrolysis (E).

2. C

Everolimus is an mTOR (mammalian target of rapamycin) inhibitor. Belatacept (A) is a selective T-cell costimulation inhibitor, and mycophenolate (D) inhibits inosine monophosphate dehydrogenase. Cyclosporine (B) and tacrolimus (E) are both calcineurin inhibitors.

3. A, B, C, D

Monitoring for tacrolimus includes blood glucose (A), blood pressure (B), trough concentrations (C), and hepatic function (D), as well as electrolytes, renal function, signs and symptoms of graft rejection, and signs and symptoms of infection.

4. E

Zostavax is a live attenuated vaccine that should not be used in patients taking immunosuppressive therapy due to the risk of disease occurrence caused by the vaccine. Adacel (Tdap) (A), Engerix (HepB) (B), Fluzone (influenza) (C), and Pneumovax (pneumococcal) (D) are inactivated vaccines and can be used in immunosuppressed patients.

5. B

Mycophenolate should be taken on an empty stomach to ensure consistent absorption. ER tablets should not be crushed (A), and the medication does not require tapering upon discontinuation (C). Oral tablets do not need to be refrigerated (D), and can be kept at room temperature.

6. **C**

Prograf is one of the brand names for tacrolimus. Zortress (A) is the brand name for everolimus, and Rapamune (B) is the brand name for sirolimus. Neoral (D) is one of the brand names for cyclosporine.

7. **B**

Nulojix (belatacept) necessitates the patient to have virology test for the Epstein-Barr virus as patients without immunity (EBV seronegative) have an increased risk of post-transplant lymphoproliferative disorder.

Special Populations 19

This chapter covers the following special populations:

- **Pediatrics**
- **Geriatrics**
- **Pregnancy and Lactation**

 Suggested Study Time: **30 minutes**

PEDIATRICS

Physiologic Changes

It is important to understand that the pediatric population should not be considered "little adults." A number of physiologic changes occur as the neonate develops into an infant, child, and then an adolescent that affect body composition and organ function that can ultimately impact drug disposition in the body. The following table reflects that various groups of the pediatric population based on age.

Group	Age
Neonate	Birth to 4 weeks
Infant	1 to <12 months
Child	1 to 12 years
Adolescent	13 to 18 years

Pharmacokinetics

Absorption

- Gastric pH changes
  - Alkaline at birth (pH = 6–8)
    - Result: ↓ absorption of weak acid drugs (e.g., phenobarbital, phenytoin)
  - Becomes more acidic (pH = 1–3) within 24 hours in full-term infants
  - Reaches adult pH by 2 years of age
- Gastric emptying
  - Delayed in neonates
    - Result: ↑ absorption of medications absorbed in stomach; delays absorption of medications absorbed in small intestine
  - Reaches level of adults by 6 months of age
- Surface area
  - Greater in neonates and infants; neonates also have thinner/immature epidermal layer and ↑ skin hydration
    - Result: ↑ absorption of topical medications

Distribution

- Body composition
  - Total body water
    - Neonates have ↑ total body water (75–85%) compared to adults (55–60%)
      - Result: ↑ V_d of hydrophilic drugs (e.g., aminoglycosides)
      - Require ↑ dose of drugs that distribute into total body water
  - Total body fat
    - Neonates and infants have less fat tissue compared to adults
      - Result: ↓ V_d of lipophilic drugs (e.g., diazepam)
- Plasma protein binding
  - Neonates and infants have:
    - Lower concentration of drug-binding proteins
    - Lower protein-binding affinity
    - ↑ competition for binding sites (e.g., from bilirubin)
  - Results
    - ↑ unbound concentration of highly protein-bound drugs (e.g., phenytoin)
    - Sulfonamides may displace bilirubin, causing kernicterus

- Blood brain barrier
  - Incomplete blood brain barrier development in neonates
  - Result: ↑ central nervous system exposure to drugs that cross the blood–brain barrier (e.g., gentamicin, theophylline, phenobarbital, phenytoin)

Metabolism

- Phase I metabolism
  - Level of activity of cytochrome P450 (CYP) enzymes ↓↓ in neonates (level approaches that of adults by ~6 months of age)
    - Enzymes affected: 1A2, 2D6, 2C19, 2C9, 3A4
  - Result: ↑ plasma concentrations of drugs metabolized by affected CYP isoenzymes
- Phase II metabolism
  - Glucuronidation, sulfation, and acetylation ↓ in neonates
  - Result: ↑ plasma concentrations of drugs metabolized by these enzymatic processes

Elimination

- Renal
  - Glomerular filtration rate directly proportional to gestational age and then ↑↑ at birth and then in first 2 weeks of life; reaches adult values by 3–5 months
  - Tubular secretion does not mature as quickly as glomerular filtration (approaches adult levels by 7–8 months)
  - Schwartz equation often used to estimate creatinine clearance in pediatric population:

$$CrCl = \frac{k \times \text{height } (cm)}{SCr}$$

  k = age-specific proportionality constant

Principles of Drug Use

To provide safe and effective drug therapy to the pediatric population, it is essential that pharmacists have an understanding of the drug's pharmacokinetic and pharmacodynamic properties and how these properties will be affected by the various physiologic changes that occur as children mature.

Key References

Taketomo C, Hodding JH, Kraus DM, eds. Pediatric and Neonatal Dosage Handbook. 22nd edition. Hudson, Ohio, Lexi-Comp, Inc.; 2015.

Phelps SJ, Hagemann TM, Lee KR, Thompson AJ, eds. Pediatric Injectable Drugs (The Teddy Bear Book). 10th edition. Bethesda, Maryland, American Society of Health-System Pharmacists; 2013.

GERIATRICS

Physiologic Changes

Many organ systems progressive decline in function with increasing age. Physiologic changes that occur with age often lead to decreased functional capacity and homeostatic reserve leaving older adults more sensitive to the effects of medications.

Pharmacokinetics

Absorption

Most drugs are absorbed via passive diffusion so their absorption is mostly unaffected by age. However, drugs that require active transport for absorption may have reduced bio-availability. First-pass metabolism is decreased, so medications that have a high first-pass effect are noted to have increased bioavailability and increased plasma concentrations.

Distribution

Body composition and protein binding are factors that influence the distribution of medications within the body. Due to a reduction in lean muscle mass and an increase in adipose tissue with aging, the volume of distribution of water-soluble drugs is decreased as opposed to lipophilic drugs that have an increased volume of distribution. For acidic drugs, decreased levels of serum albumin lead to increased free fractions of medication. However, increased levels of α_1-acid glycoprotein lead to decreased free fractions of basic drugs.

Metabolism

Drug metabolism is primarily conducted in the liver. Age-related decline in phase I metabolism (e.g., oxidation) is thought to be due to reduced liver volume and may reduce drug clearance of medications that rely on that pathway. Phase II metabolism (e.g., glucuronidation, acetylation) seems to be relatively unaffected by age.

Elimination

Renal excretion of medications is also affected by age. Glomerular filtration is known to decline with age and results in increased half-lives and serum concentrations of renally eliminated medications.

Pharmacodynamics

Older adults are known to have increased responses to some medications. Medications with an increased pharmacodynamic response include muscarinics, anticoagulants, benzodiazepines, antipsychotics, opioids, and sedatives. In contrast, a decreased pharmacodynamic response has been seen with β-agonists and antagonists.

Principles of Drug Use

Once a thorough medication history that includes both prescription and over-the-counter medications is taken, each medication should be linked to a corresponding diagnosis. As the medical complexity of an older adult grows, this becomes an important step to confirm that older adults actually need all of the medications they are taking and to determine if they have untreated indications. If a medication is needed, the appropriateness with regard to age should be considered. If a safer alternative is available, the possibility of changing medications should be considered. Factors such as life expectancy, time to therapeutic benefit, and goals of care should be considered to determine if a medication should be started or continued. Medications should be started one at a time at low doses and titrated very slowly. If an older adult experiences a new symptom, medication-induced causes should be ruled out to avoid creating a prescribing cascade. Overall, simplifying medication regimens will help prevent medication induced adverse effects and help increase patient adherence.

Key References

The Beers criteria is a reference used to determine the appropriateness of medication use in older adults. The reference is periodically updated by an interprofessional panel of experts that review the literature to alert health care providers to high-risk medications that should be avoided or used with caution in older adults.

American Geriatrics Society 2015 updated Beers criteria for potentially inappropriate medication use in older adults. J Am Geriatr Soc. 2015;63:2227–2246.

PREGNANCY AND LACTATION

Physiologic Changes

Pharmacokinetics

During pregnancy, pharmacokinetic changes impact the action of many pharmacological agents.

Absorption

Gastric motility decreases due to increasing progesterone levels, slowing gastric emptying.

Distribution

Increased plasma volume leads to increased volume of distribution for some drugs. Decreased albumin levels can increase availability of highly albumin-bound drugs.

Metabolism

Altered liver function can interfere with hepatic metabolism. Increased activity of enzymes in the CYP 450 family and others and induction activity may result in clinically significant reductions in active drug levels.

Elimination

Increased plasma volume results in increased renal blood flow and glomerular filtration rate (GFR), thereby increasing the renal excretion of many drugs.

Principles of Drug Use

Although it is ideal for patients to avoid pharmacologic agents during pregnancy, pharmacotherapy is often necessary. Reasons for taking pharmacologic agents during pregnancy include acute illness and chronic illnesses such as diabetes mellitus, hypertension, epilepsy, asthma, depression, anxiety, and bipolar disorder, among others.

One consideration when deciding whether to prescribe a medication to a pregnant patient is the likelihood of that medication crossing the placenta; this helps determine the relative benefit-to-risk ratio of that medication during pregnancy. Crossing the placenta indicates exposure to the fetus and increased risk. Characteristics of pharmacologic agents that are more likely to cross the placenta include:

- Small size: Water-soluble agents with lower molecular mass (<500 Da) more readily cross the placenta, middle range (501–1,000 Da) cross more slowly, and larger (>1,000 Da) will not cross.
- Fat solubility: Agents with greater lipophilicity are more likely to cross the placenta.
- Un-ionization.
- Minimal protein-binding: Lower protein-binding translates to higher percentage of unbound/free drug available to cross the placenta.

Sample Known Teratogens (Commonly Used)

General Class	Drug(s)	Effects
Alcohol	Dose-dependent/cumulative	Fetal alcohol syndrome, abnormal central nervous system (CNS) functioning
Antibiotics	Tetracyclines	Malformations of the teeth and bone
Anticoagulants	Warfarin	CNS and skeletal malformations, hemorrhage
Anticonvulsants	Valproate, carbamazepine	Neural tube defects
	Phenytoin	CNS malformations
Antihypertensives	ACE inhibitors, ARBs	Renal defects, restrict normal growth patterns
Antineoplastic	Any, thalidomide	Multiple, congenital malformations
Antiretrovirals	Efavirenz	Neural tube defects
Nonsteroidal anti-inflammatory medications (NSAIDs)	Ibuprofen, naproxen, ketoprofen, etc.	Premature closure of the ductus arteriosus
Prostaglandin	Misoprostol	CNS and limb malformations
Psychiatric medications	Lithium	Congenital cardiovascular defects
Retinoids	Isotretinoin	Multiple, congenital malformations

The Food and Drug Administration (FDA) removed pregnancy letter categories (A, B, C, D, X) from medication labeling in 2015. The letter categories were believed to oversimplify the assessment of risk and benefits in clinical practice. Pharmacological agent labeling now consists of a pregnancy section that includes a summary of risk, available data, and clinical considerations in addition to a lactation section to address any available data relevant to risks of medication for nursing mothers.

Key References

Individual product package inserts include FDA mandated labeling related to pregnancy and lactation. Additionally, Briggs' *Drugs in Pregnancy and Lactation* is a comprehensive reference guide to fetal and neonatal risks associated with medications.

Briggs G, Freeman R, eds. Drugs in Pregnancy and Lactation. 10th edition. Philadelphia: Wolters Kluwer; 2015.

LEARNING POINTS

- Organ system function generally declines with advancing age.
- Beers criteria are used to determine potentially inappropriate medications for older Americans.
- Simplify medication regimens to avoid polypharmacy and adverse drug events in older adults.

Preventive Medicine

20

This chapter covers the following preventive health care measures:

- **Immunizations**
- **Weight loss**
- **Smoking cessation**

 Suggested Study Time: **45 minutes**

IMMUNIZATIONS

Definitions

Vaccines provide immunization against multiple infectious diseases by stimulating an immune response and subsequent immunologic memory. Vaccines induce active immunity because they are composed of antigens that simulate exposure to an infectious disease caused by a virus or bacteria. Once the body identifies the foreign substance, the immune system creates antibodies to eliminate the pathogen.

Vaccines are categorized as live or inactivated. Live vaccines are made up of attenuated viruses or bacteria. Live vaccine pathogens have the ability to replicate in the body, but because they are weakened, they do not cause clinically significant disease. Immunocompromised patients cannot safely receive live vaccines due to the potential for disease occurrence caused by the vaccine; immunocompromised patients include those with malignant neoplasms of the lymphatic system or bone marrow, patients with human immunodeficiency virus (HIV) or acquired immune deficiency syndrome, and anyone receiving immunosuppressant medications. Live vaccines can be given simultaneously or must be separated by at least 4 weeks to allow the body's immune response to adequately respond to the vaccine.

Inactivated vaccines are composed of inactivated or dead viruses or bacteria. There is no risk of contracting the disease from inactivated vaccines; however, multiple doses may be needed to create or sustain immunity. Inactivated vaccines may be categorized as polysaccharides, polysaccharide conjugates, or toxoids. Polysaccharide vaccinations are not effective in those younger than 2 years of age due to the lack of memory B-cell activity. There is also no additional immune response upon repeated vaccination for polysaccharide vaccines. Polysaccharide conjugated vaccines are polysaccharides linked to specific proteins, which induces a better immune response in those younger than 2 years of age. Toxoid vaccines are produced by the inactivation of a biological toxin.

Immunizations

Vaccine • Brand Name • Route of Administration	Contraindications	Adverse Effects	Target Population	Medication Pearls
Live vaccines				
Herpes zoster (shingles) • Zostavax • Subcut	• History of anaphylaxis to gelatin or neomycin • Immunosuppression or immunodeficiency	• Injection site reactions • Headache • Flu-like symptoms • Fever	All patients ≥60 years of age	
Live attenuated influenza • FluMist Quadrivalent • Intranasal	• Anaphylaxis to previous influenza vaccination • Hypersensitivity to egg protein • Children 2–17 years of age taking aspirin	• Runny nose • Nasal congestion • Fever • Sore throat • Headache • ↓ appetite • Weakness	All patients 2–49 years of age yearly	
Measles, mumps, rubella (MMR) • M-M-R II • Subcut	• Hypersensitivity to any vaccine component • Febrile illness • Immunosuppression or immunodeficiency • Pregnancy	• Injection site reactions • Arthralgia • Myalgia • Rash	Children ≥12 months	
Rotavirus • Rotarix, RotaTeq • Oral	• Hypersensitivity • History of intussusception • Severe combined immunodeficiency disease	• Fever • Diarrhea • Vomiting • Otitis media • Nasopharyngitis	• Infants and children 6–24 weeks (Rotarix) • Infants and children 6–32 weeks (RotaTeq)	
Varicella (chickenpox): • Varivax • Subcut	• Allergic reaction to vaccine, gelatin, or neomycin • Immunodeficiency or immunosuppression • Active, untreated tuberculosis • Pregnancy	• Injection site reactions • Rash • Fever • Malaise • Arthralgia	Children ≥12 months of age	

Immunizations *(cont'd)*

Vaccine • Brand Name • Route of Administration	Contraindications	Adverse Effects	Target Population	Medication Pearls
Inactivated vaccines				
Influenza • Afluria, Fluad, Fluarix Quadrivalent, Flucelvax, Flucelvax Quadrivalent, Flulaval Quadrivalent, Fluvirin, Fluzone High-Dose, Fluzone Intradermal Quadrivalent, Fluzone Quadrivalent • Intradermal (Fluzone Intradermal Quadrivalent) • IM (remainder)	• Allergy to previous influenza vaccination • Allergy to eggs (except for Flucelvax)	• Fever • Malaise • Myalgia • Injection site reactions	All patients ≥6 months of age	Yearly vaccination to account for antigenic drifts and ↓ antibody levels over time
Diphtheria, tetanus, acelluar pertussis • DTaP: Daptacel, Infanrix • IM • Tdap: Adacel, Boostrix • IM • Td: Decavac, Tenivac • IM	**DTaP** • Serious allergic reaction to previous dose of diphtheria toxoid-, tetanus toxoid-, or pertussis-containing vaccine • Encephalopathy within 7 days of previous vaccination • Progressive neurologic disorders **Tdap** • Serious allergic reaction to diphtheria toxoid, tetanus toxoid and pertussis antigen-containing vaccine • Encephalopathy within 7 days of previous vaccination **Td** • Serious allergic reaction to tetanus toxoid or diphtheria toxoid containing vaccine	• Injection site reactions • Arthus reactions • Swelling • Fever	• DTaP: Children 6 week–6 years of age • Tdap: Single dose once >7 years of age or in third trimester of each pregnancy • Td: 1 dose every 10 years once ≥7 years of age	Tdap is needed only once per lifetime (except should be given during each pregnancy)

Immunizations *(cont'd)*

Vaccine • Brand Name • Route of Administration	Contraindications	Adverse Effects	Target Population	Medication Pearls
Inactivated vaccines (cont'd)				
Human papillomavirus (HPV) • Cervarix (HPV2), Gardasil (HPV4), Gardasil 9 (HPV9) • IM	• Hypersensitivity • Allergy to yeast (Gardasil, Gardasil 9)	• Injection site reactions • Headache • Fever • Fatigue • Myalgia	• Cervarix: Females 9–25 years of age • Gardasil: Females and males 9–26 years of age • Gardasil 9: Females and males 9–26 years of age	• Cervarix protects against HPV types 16 and 18 • Gardasil protects against HPV types 6, 11, 16, and 18 • Gardasil 9 protects against HPV types 6, 11, 16, 18, 31, 33, 45, 52, and 58
Streptococcus pneumoniae • Pneumovax 23 (PPSV23) • IM, subcut • Prevnar 13 (PCV13) • IM	• Severe allergic reaction to pneumococcal vaccine • Severe allergic reaction to any diphtheria toxoid-containing vaccine (PCV13)	• Injection site reactions • Fever • Myalgia	• PCV13: children 2–59 months of age; children 60–71 months of age with chronic heart disease, asthma, diabetes, asplenia, or immunosuppressive conditions; children ≥6 years of age, adolescents, and adults with asplenia or immunosuppressive conditions; and all patients ≥65 years of age • PPSV23: All patients ≥65 years of age; children, adolescents, and adults ≥2 years of age at ↑ risk for pneumococcal disease (asplena, sickle cell disease, heart failure, chronic obstructive pulmonary disease, asthma, diabetes, chronic liver disease, cigarette smokers, and immunosuppressed)	• PPSV23 not indicated for children <2 years of age • Second dose of PPSV23 recommended for patients ≥65 years of age with previous dose given ≥5 years ago
Meningococcal • MCV4: Menactra, Menveo • IM • MPSV4: Menomune • Subcut	• Hypersensitivity • Hypersensitivity to diphtheria toxoid (MCV4)	• Injection site reactions • Headache • Fever • Malaise	• MCV4: Adolescents 11–18 years of age with a booster dose after 5 years (if initial dose given before age 16); patients ≥2 months of age at ↑ risk of meningococcal disease (can be used up to age 55) • MPSV4: Unvaccinated adults >56 years of age who are at ↑ risk of meningococcal disease	MPSV4 should not be used in children <2 years of age

Immunizations *(cont'd)*

Vaccine • Brand Name • Route of Administration	Contraindications	Adverse Effects	Target Population	Medication Pearls
Inactivated vaccines (cont'd)				
Hepatitis A • Havrix, VAQTA • IM	• Hypersensitivity • Allergic reaction to vaccine or neomycin	• Injection site reactions • Fever	• All children ≥12 months of age • International travel other than Canada, Europe, Japan, New Zealand, or Australia • Men who have sex with men (MSM) • Illicit drug users • Laboratory workers • Patients with chronic liver disease or clotting disorders	
Hepatitis B • Engerix-B, Recombivax HB • IM	• Hypersensitivity • Allergic reaction to previous hepatitis B vaccination or yeast	• Injection site reactions • Headache • Fatigue • Fever	• Infants at birth • All infants and children • Health care workers • International travel • Patients with multiple sexual partners • MSM • Injection drug users • Adults with diabetes mellitus • HIV • Chronic liver disease • End-stage renal disease	
Haemophilus influenza type B • ActHIB, Hiberix, PedvaxHIB • IM	• Hypersensitivity • Hypersensitivity to tetanus toxoid (ActHIB and Hiberix)	Injection site reactions	All infants and children through age 59 months	
Polio • IPOL • IM, subcut	Hypersensitivity		All infants and children >2 months of age	

Storage and Administration Pearls

- Tetanus, diphtheria, and acellular pertussis: refrigerate; do not freeze; do not administer subcut

- All influenza vaccinations: refrigerate; do not freeze

- Varicella and herpes zoster: must be kept frozen; unreconstituted powder must be used within 72 hours if refrigerated; reconstituted vaccine should be administered within 30 minutes or discarded

- HPV: refrigerate; do not freeze; shake vial before administration

- MMR: may refrigerate or freeze vaccine; do not freeze diluent; reconstituted vaccine should be used within 8 hours or discarded
- PCV13 and PPSV23: refrigerate; do not freeze
- Meningococcal: refrigerate; do not freeze
- Hepatitis A and hepatitis B: refrigerate; do not freeze; shake vial before administration
- Haemophilus influenza type B: refrigerate; do not freeze; shake vial before administration
- Rotavirus: refrigerate; do not freeze
- Polio: refrigerate; do not freeze; shake vial before administration

WEIGHT LOSS

Definitions

Obesity is a chronic problem that increasing numbers of people are battling. Weight loss occurs with a net reduction in total caloric intake and may be accomplished with reduced calorie consumption or increased expenditure of energy.

To classify obesity, body mass index (BMI) is calculated as follows:

$$BMI = weight\ (kg)/[height\ (m)]^2$$

A BMI of <18.5 kg/m^2 is considered underweight, and a BMI of 18.5–24.9 kg/m^2 is considered normal. People are considered overweight with a BMI of 25–29.9 kg/m^2 and obese with a BMI >30 kg/m^2. Obesity is furthered classified as stage I (BMI of 30–34.9 kg/m^2), stage II (BMI of 35–39.9 kg/m^2), and stage III (BMI ≥40 kg/m^2).

Medications may be used to aid weight loss in conjunction with dietary and physical activity modifications. Weight must be monitored to ensure weight loss is occurring, or medication therapy should be modified or discontinued.

Guidelines

Jensen MD, Ryan DH, Apovian CM, et al. 2013 AHA/ACC/TOS guideline for the management of overweight and obesity in adults: a report of the American College of Cardiology/American Heart Association Task Force on Practice Guidelines and The Obesity Society. Circulation. 2014;129(25 Suppl 2):S102–S138.

Guidelines Summary

Health care providers should evaluate a patient's BMI at each visit and create an individualized treatment plan. Weight loss plans need to include moderate caloric reduction, increased physical activity, and behavioral strategies that patients can use to sustain weight loss.

Medications for Weight Loss

Generic • Brand • Dose/Dosage Form	Contraindications	Primary Side Effects	Key Monitoring	Pertinent Drug Interactions	Med Pearls
Mechanism of action – inhibits gastric and pancreatic lipase to inhibit dietary fat					
Orlistat • Xenical, Alli (over-the-counter [OTC]) • Xenical: 120 mg TID with each meal • Alli: 60 mg TID with each meal • Caps	• Hypersensitivity • Chronic malabsorption syndrome • Pregnancy • Cholestasis	• Oily discharge/spotting • Fecal urgency • Hepatotoxicity • Nephrolithiasis • Cholelithiasis • Flatulence	• Weight • BMI • Serum glucose • Thyroid function • Liver function tests (LFTs) • Renal function	• May ↓ absorption of cyclosporine, warfarin, anticonvulsants, amiodarone, levothyroxine, and antiepileptic drugs levels • ↓ absorption of fat-soluble vitamins (A, D, E, K)	• Available OTC • Should supplement with multivitamin
Mechanism of action – stimulates hypothalamus to release norepinephrine (phentermine); suppresses appetite and ↑ satiety through inhibition of neuronal sodium channels and ↑ GABA activity (topiramate)					
Phentermine with topiramate • Qsymia • 3.75 mg/23 mg daily × 14 days, then 7.5 mg/46 mg daily × 12 wk; if 3% of baseline body weight has not been lost, discontinue therapy or ↑ dose to 11.25 mg/69 mg daily × 14 days, then 15 mg/92 mg daily • Caps	• Hypersensitivity to phentermine or sympathomimetics • Pregnancy • Hyperthyroidism • Glaucoma • Use of monoamine oxidase inhibitor (MAOI) within 2 wk	• Tachycardia • Headache • Insomnia • Xerostomia • Constipation • Paresthesia • Difficulty concentrating • Confusion • Memory issues • Speech problems • Depression • Dizziness • Kidney stones • Angle closure glaucoma • Visual field defects • ↓ sweating • Hyperthermia • Metabolic acidosis • ↑ SCr • Hypokalemia	• Weight • BMI • Heart rate (HR) • Blood pressure (BP) • Serum bicarbonate • Serum potassium • Serum glucose • Renal function • Suicidality • Intraocular pressure	• ↑ risk of hypertensive crisis with MAOIs • Other central nervous system (CNS) depressants, including alcohol, may ↑ CNS depressant effects • Concurrent use with loop or thiazide diuretics may ↑ risk of hypokalemia • Phenytoin or carbamazepine may ↓ topiramate levels • Concurrent use with valproic acid may ↑ risk of hyperammonemia or hypothermia • Concurrent use with zonisamide or acetazolamide may ↑ risk of metabolic acidosis or nephrolithiasis	• Schedule IV controlled substance • Adjust dose in renal or hepatic impairment • Teratogenic • Give in AM to minimize risk of insomnia • If patient has not lost 5% of baseline body weight by wk 12 of phentermine 15 mg/topiramate 92 mg daily, discontinue therapy

Medications for Weight Loss *(cont'd)*

Generic • Brand • Dose/Dosage Form	Contraindications	Primary Side Effects	Key Monitoring	Pertinent Drug Interactions	Med Pearls
Mechanism of action – stimulates hypothalamus to release norepinephrine					
Phentermine • Adipex-P • 15–37.5 mg/day in 1–2 divided doses • Caps, tabs	• Hypersensitivity to phentermine or sympathomimetics • History of cardiovascular disease (e.g., coronary artery disease, stroke, arrhythmias, heart failure, uncontrolled hypertension) • Pregnancy • Breast feeding • Hyperthyroidism • Glaucoma • Use of MAOI within 2 wk • Agitation • History of drug abuse	• Hypertension • Tachycardia • Primary pulmonary hypertension • Valvular heart disease • Euphoria • Dizziness • Insomnia • Psychosis • Tremor	• Weight • BMI • BP • HR • S/S of valvular heart disease	↑ risk of hypertensive crisis with MAOIs	• Schedule IV controlled substance • Give before breakfast or 1–2 hr after breakfast
Mechanism of action –activates 5HT2c receptors which stimulates pro-opiomelanocortin neurons that stimulate alpha-melanocortin-4 receptors which lead to ↑ satiety and ↓ appetite					
Lorcaserin • Belviq, Belviq XR • IR: 10 mg BID • ER: 20 mg daily • ER tabs, tabs	• Hypersensitivity • Pregnancy	• Headache • Dizziness • Nausea • Xerostomia • Constipation • Hypoglycemia • Difficulty concentrating • Memory issues • Priapism • Bradycardia • Leukopenia • Hyperprolactinemia • Serotonin syndrome	• Weight • BMI • Complete blood count • Serum glucose • Prolactin levels • S/S of valvular heart disease	• CYP2D6 inhibitor • May ↑ effects/toxicity of CYP2D6 substrates • ↑ risk of serotonin syndrome with MAOIs, selective serotonin reuptake inhibitors, serotonin-norepinephrine reuptake inhibitors, triptans, tricyclic antidepressants, fentanyl, lithium, dextromethorphan, meperidine, buspirone, linezolid, methylene blue, St. John's wort, and tramadol • Thioridazine • Antipsychotics • Ergot derivatives • Bupropion • Metoprolol • Tamoxifen • Serotonin modulators	• Schedule IV controlled substance • If patient has not lost ≥5% of baseline body weight by wk 12, discontinue therapy

Medications for Weight Loss (cont'd)

Generic • Brand • Dose/Dosage Form	Contraindications	Primary Side Effects	Key Monitoring	Pertinent Drug Interactions	Med Pearls
Mechanism of action – not fully understood, weight loss thought to result from regulation of food intake via hypothalmus and mesolimbic influence.					
Naltrexone/ bupropion • Contrave • 8 mg/90 mg daily × 1 wk, then BID × 1 wk, then 2 tabs every AM and 1 tab every PM × 1 wk, then 2 tabs BID (max of 32 mg/360 mg per day) • ER tabs	• Hypersensitivity to naltrexone or bupropion • Concurrent use of other products containing bupropion • Chronic opioid use • Uncontrolled hypertension • Seizure disorders • Bulimia • Anorexia nervosa • Abrupt discontinuation of alcohol, benzodiazepines, barbiturates, or antiepileptic drugs • Use of MAOI within 2 wk • Pregnancy	• Headache • Insomnia • Nausea/vomiting (N/V) • Constipation • Dizziness • Xerostomia • Seizures • Hypertension • Tachycardia • Anaphylaxis • Hepatotoxicity	• Weight • BMI • BP • HR • Renal function • LFTs • Suicidality	• CYP2B6 substrate • CYP2D6 inhibitor • CYP2B6 inhibitors may ↑ effects/toxicity • CYP2B6 inducers may ↓ effects • May ↑ effects/toxicity of CYP2D6 substrates • ↑ risk of hypertensive crisis with MAOIs	• Do not administer with a high-fat meal • Adjust dose in renal or hepatic impairment
Mechanism of action – GLP-1 analog which ↑ glucose-dependent insulin secretion, ↓ inappropriate glucagon secretion, slows gastric emptying, and ↓ food intake					
Liraglutide • Saxenda • 0.6 mg subcut daily × 1 wk, then ↑ by 0.6 mg daily at weekly intervals to target of 3 mg subcut daily • Injection	• Hypersensitivity • History of medullary thyroid carcinoma • Multiple endocrine neoplasia syndrome type 2 • Pregnancy	• Tachycardia • Headache • Hypoglycemia • N/V/D • Constipation • Fatigue • Dyspepsia • Dizziness • ↓ appetite • Anaphylaxis • Cholelithiasis • Pancreatitis • Thyroid tumors	• Weight • BMI • HR • Serum glucose • Renal function • S/S of pancreatitis • S/S hypoglycemia • Thyroid tumors	• May delay absorption of other drugs due to ↑ gastric emptying time (administer other medications 1 hour prior) • Sulfonylureas and insulin ↑ risk of hypoglycemia	If patient has not lost ≥4% of baseline body weight by wk 16, discontinue therapy

SMOKING CESSATION

Definitions

The dependence on tobacco is a chronic disease that often requires repeated intervention and multiple attempts to quit. Tobacco dependence is both physiological and psychological; therefore, treatment interventions must be prepared to target both issues. Informing patients about the dangers of tobacco use is critical, as is educating patients about treatment options available for smoking cessation.

Diagnosis

Patients are not always forthcoming about their use of tobacco, so it is important to assess patients' use status in every interaction possible.

Guidelines

Tobacco Use and Dependence Guideline Panel. Treating Tobacco Use and Dependence: 2008 Update. Rockville (MD): US Department of Health and Human Services; 2008 May.

Guidelines Summary

- The model for treatment and intervention of tobacco use and dependence is summarized by the "5 A's":
  - **ASK.** Identify and document tobacco use status for every patient and every visit.
  - **ADVISE.** Urge every tobacco user to quit in a strong and personalized manner.
  - **ASSESS.** Evaluate if your patient is willing to make a quit attempt.
  - **ASSIST.** For patients willing to make a quit attempt, offer treatment options and additional counseling; for those not willing, use motivational strategies to promote quitting.
  - **ARRANGE.** Schedule follow-ups with those patients willing to make a quit attempt; for those not willing to make an attempt, address willingness to quit at the next visit.
- Tobacco dependence is a chronic disease that often requires repeated intervention and multiple attempts to quit. Effective treatments exist that can significantly increase rates of long-term abstinence.
- It is essential that health care providers consistently identify and document tobacco use status and treat every tobacco user seen in a health care setting.
- Tobacco dependence treatments are effective across a broad range of populations. Clinicians should encourage every patient willing to make a quit attempt to use the counseling treatments and medications recommended.
- Brief tobacco dependence treatment is effective. Clinicians should offer every patient who uses tobacco at least the brief treatments shown to be effective.

Medications for Smoking Cessation

Generic • Brand • Dose/Dosage Forms	Contraindications	Primary Side Effects	Key Monitoring	Pertinent Drug Interactions	Med Pearls
Mechanism of action – partial $\alpha_4\beta_2$ nicotinic receptor agonist; prevents nicotine stimulation of the mesolimbic dopamine system					
Varenicline ☆ • Chantix • 0.5 mg daily × 3 days, then 0.5 mg BID × 4 days, then 1 mg BID × 11 wk • Tabs	Hypersensitivity	• Somnolence • Abnormal dreams • N/V • Constipation • Suicidal/homicidal ideation • Irritability • Depression • Mania • Hostility • Agitation • Anxiety • Panic • Psychotic symptoms • Hallucinations • Paranoia • Delusions • Seizures • Hypersensitivity • Rash (including Stevens-Johnson syndrome)	• Nicotine consumption • Mood changes • Psychotic symptoms • Suicidal/homicidal ideation	• Concurrent use with nicotine replacement products may ↑ risk of N/V • ↑ effects of alcohol	• Start 1 wk prior to target stop day • Take after meal and with full glass of water
Mechanism of action – inhibits neuronal uptake of norepinephrine and dopamine					
Bupropion ☆ • Zyban • 150 mg daily × 3 days, then 150 mg BID × 7–12 wk • ER tabs	• Seizure disorders • Anorexia or bulimia • Abrupt discontinuation of alcohol, benzodiazepines, barbiturates, or antiepileptic drugs • Use of MAOI within 2 wk • Use of MAOI within 14 days • Hypersensitivity • Concurrent use of linezolid or methylene blue	• Insomnia • Xerostomia • Dizziness • Nausea • Constipation • Suicidal/homicidal ideation • Irritability • Depression • Mania • Hostility • Agitation • Anxiety • Panic • Psychotic symptoms • Hallucinations • Paranoia • Delusions • Seizures • Hypertension • Anaphylaxis	• Nicotine consumption • Mood changes • Psychotic symptoms • Suicidal/homicidal ideation • Seizure activity	• CYP2B6 substrate • CYP2D6 inhibitor • CYP2B6 inhibitors may ↑ effects/toxicity • CYP2B6 inducers may ↓ effects • May ↑ effects/toxicity of CYP2D6 substrates • ↑ risk of hypertensive crises with MAOIs	• Start 1 wk prior to target stop day • Can be coadministered with nicotine replacement patches

Medications for Smoking Cessation *(cont'd)*

Generic • Brand • Dose/Dosage Forms	Contraindications	Primary Side Effects	Key Monitoring	Pertinent Drug Interactions	Med Pearls
Mechanism of action – supplements nicotine, which exhibits primary effects via autonomic ganglia stimulation					
Nicotine • Nicoderm CQ, Nicorelief, Nicorette, Nicotrol, Thrive • Gum: 1 piece every 1–2 hr PRN during wk 1–6, then 1 piece every 2–4 hr PRN during wk 7–9, then 1 piece every 4–8 hr PRN during wk 10–12 as needed; max = 24 pieces/day) • Inhaler: 6–16 cartridges/day; duration of treatment = 3 mo • Transdermal patch: >10 cigarettes/day: 21 mg/day × 6 wk, then 14 mg/day × 2 wk, then 7 mg/day × 2 wk; ≤10 cigarettes/day: 14 mg/day × 6 wk, then 7 mg/day × 2 wk • Lozenge: 1 lozenge every 1–2 hr PRN during wk 1–6, then 1 lozenge every 2–4 hr PRN during wk 7–9, then 1 lozenge every 4–8 hr PRN during wk 10–12 as needed; max = 20 lozenges/day) • Nasal spray: 1 spray in each nostril 1–2 × /hr (max = 80 sprays/day); duration of treatment = 3 mo	• Smoking or chewing tobacco • Post- myocardial infarction • Life-threatening arrhythmias • Worsening angina	• Headache • Mouth or throat irritation • Dyspepsia • Cough	• Nicotine consumption • Nicotine toxicity (severe headache, dizziness, confusion)	None	• Can be coadministered with bupropion • Gum or lozenge: use 4-mg dose if smoke first cigarette within 30 min of waking; otherwise, use 2-mg dose • Do not eat or drink within 15 min of using gum or lozenge • Oral inhalation: patient should continuously puff for ~20 min

Storage and Administration Pearl

- Nicotrol inhaler: Protect from light.

Patient Education Pearls

- For improved outcomes, it is important to have consistent and regular interventions with the patient regarding smoking cessation education.
- When working with patient to stop smoking, it is recommended to use the 5 A's: Ask, Advise, Assess, Assist, Arrange.

LEARNING POINTS

- Live vaccines may be administered on the same day or must be separated by at least 4 weeks.
- Live vaccines should not be given to those with immunodeficiency or those who are receiving immunosuppression therapy.
- Caloric reduction and increased physical activity are mainstays for weight loss.
- Medications may be used to aid weight loss but should be used in conjunction with caloric reduction and increased physical activity.
- Smoking cessation counseling is an important consideration for all smokers.

PRACTICE QUESTIONS

1. Which of the following is indicated to prevent HPV infections?

    (A) Gardasil
    (B) Menomune
    (C) Prevnar 13
    (D) Rotarix
    (E) Zostavax

2. Which of the following is a contraindication to using bupropion for smoking cessation?

    (A) Hepatic impairment
    (B) Obesity
    (C) Orthostatic hypotension
    (D) Active seizure disorder

3. Which of the following is contraindicated in a patient taking tacrolimus?

    (A) Hepatitis B vaccine
    (B) Pneumococcal vaccine
    (C) Tdap vaccine
    (D) Varicella vaccine
    (E) All of the above

4. Which of the following formulations are available for nicotine replacement? (Select ALL that apply.)

    (A) Lozenge
    (B) Tablet
    (C) Inhaler
    (D) Gum

5. Which of the following is indicated for weight loss?

    (A) Glargine
    (B) Glimepiride
    (C) Liraglutide
    (D) Pioglitazone

6. A patient needs to receive two live vaccines but is unable to receive both on the same day. How much time must elapse before the second vaccine may be given?

    (A) 1 day
    (B) 1 week
    (C) 2 weeks
    (D) 4 weeks

7. Which of the following should be monitored in a patient taking varenicline?

    (A) Behavioral changes
    (B) Bradycardia
    (C) Pulmonary function
    (D) Weight loss

8. Which of the following vaccines is indicated for all health care workers?

    (A) Haemophilus influenza type B vaccine
    (B) Hepatitis B vaccine
    (C) Human papillomavirus vaccine
    (D) Meningococcal vaccine

9. Which of the following is a counseling point for a patient taking orlistat?

    (A) No dietary modification is needed when taking orlistat.
    (B) Orlistat must be taken on an empty stomach.
    (C) Orlistat works best if taken at bedtime.
    (D) You may experience oily discharge or spotting.

10. Which of the following should be monitored in a patient taking Qsymia? (Select ALL that apply.)

    (A) Weight
    (B) Blood pressure
    (C) LFTs
    (D) Glucose

ANSWERS AND EXPLANATIONS

1. A

Gardasil is the vaccine that targets human papillomavirus types 6, 11, 16, and 18. Menomune (B) is the brand name of meningococcal vaccine. Prevnar (C) is the polysaccharide conjugate vaccine that targets pneumococcal disease. Rotarix (D) is the brand name for the rotavirus vaccine, and Zostavax (E) is the brand name for the herpes zoster vaccine.

2. D

Bupropion is contraindicated in patients with a seizure disorder because the medication causes CNS stimulation. Hepatic impairment (A) is not associated with bupropion, so the medication is not contraindicated in these patients. Weight loss may be seen with the use of bupropion, so the medication can be used in obese individuals (B). Bupropion may also cause blood pressure elevation, so orthostatic hypotension (C) is not a contraindication to use.

3. D

Live vaccines are contraindicated in a patient receiving immunosuppressive therapies. Varicella is a live, attenuated vaccine that, if given to an immunocompromised patient, may cause infection with chickenpox. Vaccines against hepatitis B (A), pneumococcal (B), and Tdap (C) infection are all inactivated vaccines.

4. A, C, D

Nicotine is available as a gum, lozenge, inhaler, patch, and nasal spray for the treatment of smoking cessation. It is not available as a tablet (B).

5. C

Liraglutide, a GLP-1 analog, is indicated to treat obesity under the brand name Saxenda. Liraglutide is also available under the brand name of Victoza, which is used to treat diabetes mellitus. Glargine (A), glimepiride (B), and pioglitazone (D) are not indicated for obesity management.

6. D

A 4-week time period should separate doses of live vaccines if the live vaccines cannot all be given on the same day.

7. A

Behavioral changes such as depression, irritability, suicidal ideation, and agitation should be monitored for in patients taking varenicline for smoking cessation. Bradycardia (B), changes in pulmonary function (C), and weight loss (D) are not associated with the use of varenicline.

8. **B**

Health care workers should receive the hepatitis B vaccine due to potential exposure to blood or to blood-contaminated bodily fluids. OSHA requires the vaccine to be offered to those who have an occupational risk.

9. **D**

Orlistat may cause oily discharge or spotting, especially if dietary fat content is not limited. Patients taking orlistat for weight loss should limit dietary fat consumption and adhere to a low-calorie diet. Orlistat is taken 3 times per day with meals, not on an empty stomach (B) or at bedtime (C).

10. **A, B**

Qsymia is a combination of phentermine and topiramate. Due to the sympathomimetic activity of phentermine, blood pressure should be monitored; weight is also monitored to ensure the effectiveness of the drug. Qysmia is not associated with changes in liver function (C) or blood glucose levels (D), so those parameters do not need to be monitored.

Clinical Lab Tests

21

This chapter covers clinical lab tests for the following:

- **Electrolytes and minerals**
- **Renal**
- **Hepatic**
- **Endocrine**
- **Cardiology**
- **Hematology**
- **Therapeutic drug levels**

 Suggested Study Time: **15 minutes**

Clinical lab tests are very important to pharmacists because they are commonly used to measure the safety and efficacy of medications. It is imperative that a pharmacist have a working knowledge of the most commonly used clinical lab tests in order to be able to recommend testing when necessary, and to interpret the results obtained. Education of the patient regarding clinical lab tests may also be a role of the pharmacist in some instances.

ELECTROLYTES AND MINERALS

Among the most common laboratory tests, electrolyte concentrations are used to detect and assess many medical conditions and are measured most commonly as part of a basic metabolic panel, or Chem 7.

Substance	Normal Reference Range	Most Common Uses/Comments
Sodium	136–145 mEq/L	• May detect hypo- or hypernatremia • Used to monitor serum osmolality to determine total body water balance
Potassium	3.5–5.0 mEq/L	• May detect hypo- or hyperkalemia • Used primarily to monitor safety of medications and renal function
Chloride	96–106 mEq/L	• May detect hypo- or hyperchloremia • Used in evaluation of acid-based balance and to monitor for safety of medications
Magnesium	1.5–2.2 mEq/L	• May detect hypo- or hypermagnesemia and renal function
Calcium	8.5–10.8 mg/dL	• May detect hypo- or hypercalcemia • Used to monitor renal osteodystrophy • Requires correction with serum albumin <4 g/dL
Phosphate	2.6–4.5 mg/dL	• May detect hypo- or hyperphosphatemia • Monitored along with calcium for renal osteodystrophy

RENAL

The kidneys are the body's major filter of toxins. Thus, the renal system plays a large role in the maintenance of physiological homeostasis. The kidneys also serve the role of producing and activating substances that have an impact on red blood cell production, blood pressure regulation, and mineral metabolism.

The following represent the most commonly used lab assays for evaluation of renal function. Urinary sodium, potassium, and chloride as well as hematologic assays and electrolytes may also be used in the assessment.

Substance	Normal Reference Range	Comments
Serum creatinine (SCr)	0.7–1.4 mg/dL	• Excretion of creatinine closely estimates the glomerular filtration rate (GFR) • ↑ serum creatinine is indicative of ↓ GFR • Used to calculate creatinine clearance (CrCl) • May be inaccurate in the very elderly due to ↓ muscle mass
CrCl	90–140 mL/min	• Estimate of GFR • Can be measured over 24 hours or calculated using the Cockgroft-Gault equation (using SCr and ideal body weight)
Blood urea nitrogen (BUN)	8–20 mg/dL	• Used along with other labs to monitor hydration, renal function, protein tolerance, catabolism • Most commonly used in BUN:SCr ratio to determine hydration status
BUN:SCr	1:1–20:1	• >20:1 indicates dehydration in most patients
Urine microalbumin	<30 mg:g creatinine	• Microscopic protein that escapes into the urine when significant glomerular injury is present • Most commonly used to identify nephropathy in patients with diabetes

HEPATIC

The functions of the liver are numerous and varied. Some of the primary functions include the synthesis of bilirubin, coagulation factors, and albumin; amino acid and carbohydrate metabolism; and cholesterol synthesis. Along with these activities, the liver is also the primary site of metabolism for the majority of drugs and hormones. Hepatic assays are important in assessing the overall liver function and also in monitoring the safety of many medications.

The following represent the most commonly used lab assays for the assessment of hepatic function. Viral antigens and antibodies are not reviewed in this chapter.

Substance	Normal Reference Range	Comments
Albumin	3.5–5 g/dL	• Reflects liver's synthetic ability, nutritional status, and hydration • If low, should be factored into serum drug concentrations of highly protein bound drugs such as phenytoin
Total protein	5.5–8.3 g/dL	• Represents estimated sum of albumin and globulin measurements
Prothrombin time (PT)	10–13 seconds	• Represents the time needed for a series of events in coagulation cascade to occur • Helps to determine synthetic ability of liver; if ↑, indicates potential ↓ production of clotting factors
Alkaline phosphatase	Varies with assay used	• Used to detect hepatocellular injury but is not specific; therefore, should be combined with other tests
Aspartate aminotransferase (AST)	8–42 IU/L	• Aminotransferases are the most frequently used assays in monitoring hepatic disease and are sensitive indicators of hepatic injury • If ↑, indicates hepatic injury
Alanine aminotransferase (ALT)	3–30 IU/L	• Used often to monitor potential hepatiotoxicity of medications
Total bilirubin	0.3–1 mg/dL	• If ↑, may indicate hepatocellular injury; however, test is not sensitive
Ammonia	30–70 mcg/dL	• If ↑, may indicate an inability of the liver to remove ammonia from the blood • Used to identify hepatic encephalopathy
Amylase	44–128 IU/L	• Most commonly used to diagnose acute pancreatitis
Lipase	<1.5 U/mL	• Most commonly used in the late diagnosis of acute pancreatitis (3–4 days after onset)

ENDOCRINE

Disorders of the endocrine system most commonly result from the deficiency or excess of a hormone. These hormones act as regulators within the body by stimulating or inhibiting biological responses. The most common endocrine disorder is diabetes mellitus (DM). Thyroid disorders, including hypothyroidism and hyperthyroidism, are also common. Diagnosis of all of these endocrine disorders is discussed further in Chapter 4.

The assays listed in the following table represent the most commonly used measurements to monitor DM and thyroid disorders, and the medications used to treat these disease states.

Substance	Normal Reference Range	Comments
Fasting plasma glucose (FPG)	70–100 mg/dL	• Most commonly used assay for diagnosis of DM; must be repeated on another day to confirm diagnosis • Patients may also self-monitor this value • Used for disease state monitoring and adjustment of medications
2-hour postprandial glucose	100–140 mg/dL	• May be measured as part of an oral glucose tolerance test or by the patient at home • Used for disease state monitoring and adjustment of medications
A1c	4–6%	• Represents blood sugar over an approximate 90-day time frame • Most common lab test to monitor glycemic control in DM • Also used in diagnosis of DM • Although 4–6% is normal range, <6.5–7% is the goal for a patient with DM • May be inaccurate in cases of severe anemia • A1c correlation to plasma glucose: {{TABLE}}
Free thyroxine (T4)	0.8–1.5 ng/dL	• Measures unbound T4 and is the most accurate representation of thyroid activity
Thyroid-stimulating hormone (TSH)	0.25–6.7 mIU/mL	• If ↓, indicates hyperthyroid state; if ↑, indicates hypothyroid state • Used to monitor need for adjustment of thyroid supplementation medications

A1c (%)	Mean Plasma Glucose (mg/dL)
6	126
7	154
8	183
9	212
10	240
11	269
12	298

CARDIOLOGY

Laboratory tests are used both to detect and to monitor cardiac disorders. Because cardiovascular disease is the leading cause of death, it is imperative that pharmacists have a working knowledge of the markers used to evaluate these conditions.

The following measurements represent the most commonly used lab assays to detect acute cardiac conditions and to monitor chronic cardiac risk.

Substance	Normal Reference Range	Comments
Total cholesterol	<200 mg/dL	• Does not require that the patient fast but is most commonly measured as part of a complete fasting lipid panel • Not as useful as low-density lipoprotein cholesterol (LDL-C) and high-density lipoprotein cholesterol (HDL-C) in determining cardiovascular risk
LDL-C	Patient dependent-goals	• Highly atherogenic, known as "bad" cholesterol • Used as the primary marker of cardiovascular risk • Higher values correlate with higher risk • Most often calculated using Friedwald equation rather than measured : LDL = Total cholesterol − (HDL-C + triglycerides [TG]/5) • Calculation inaccurate if TG >400 mg/dL
HDL-C	>40 mg/dL	• Antiatherogenic lipoprotein known as "good" cholesterol • Higher values associated with lower cardiovascular risk
TGs	<150 mg/dL	• Higher values associated with higher cardiovascular risk • Very high levels associated with ↑ risk of pancreatitis
Troponin I (Tn-I)	<1.5 ng/mL	• Elevated levels used to diagnose acute myocardial infarction (MI) • Elevation seen within 3–12 hr and remain elevated for 5–10 days (Tn-I) or 5–14 days (Tn-T)
Troponin T (Tn-T)	<0.1 ng/mL	
Creatine kinase–MB (CK–MB)	<12 IU/L	• Elevated levels used to diagnose acute MI • Specific for cardiac tissue • Elevation seen within 3–12 hr and remains elevated for 1–2 days
B-type natriuretic peptide (BNP)	<100 pg/mL	• Secreted in response to cardiac stretching • Used to diagnose acute decompensated heart failure and to monitor response in chronic heart failure
C-reactive protein (CRP)	≤1 mg/L	• Plasma protein synthesized by the liver • Biomarker of inflammation and cardiovascular risk
International normalized ratio (INR)	1.0	• Measure of coagulability • Goal is patient-dependent • Used to monitor warfarin therapy

HEMATOLOGY

The complete blood count (CBC) is among the most commonly ordered lab tests. The indices described in the following table make up the CBC and are used to detect and monitor anemias and other hematologic disorders.

Indices	Normal Reference Range	Comments
Red blood cells (RBCs)	Males: $4.5–5.9 \times 10^{12}$ cells/L Females: $4.1–5.1 \times 10^{12}$ cells/L	• May be elevated in smokers
Hemoglobin (Hgb)	Males: 14–17.5 g/dL Females: 12.6–15.3 g/dL	• Indicates oxygen-carrying capacity of blood
Hematocrit (Hct)	Males: 42–50% Females: 36–45%	• Percentage of blood made up by erythrocytes; approximately $3 \times$ the Hgb
Mean cell volume (MCV)	80–96 fL	• Hematocrit/RBC • ↓ in iron deficiency • ↑ in vitamin B_{12} and folate deficiency
Mean cell hemoglobin concentration (MCHC)	33.4–35.5 g/dL	• Hgb/Hct • ↓ in iron deficiency
Reticulocyte count	0.5–2.5% of RBCs	• Reticulocytes are immature erythrocytes • ↑ in blood loss (acute) • ↓ in iron, vitamin B_{12}, and folate deficiency
White blood cells (WBCs)	$4.4–11 \times 10^3$ cells/mm^3	• Made up of granulocytes and lymphocytes • ↑ in infection
Platelet count	$150–450 \times 10^3$ cells/mm3	• Important measure of coagulation

THERAPEUTIC DRUG LEVELS

Medications with narrow therapeutic indices and those with established therapeutic and/or toxic serum concentrations often require therapeutic drug monitoring. In general, serum concentrations are best obtained once the medication has reached steady state (in most cases, a minimum of five elimination half-lives), just prior to an administered dose unless otherwise specified.

Drug	Therapeutic Concentration
Aminoglycosides: gentamicin, tobramycin	4–10 mcg/mL (peak) – efficacy, depending on the infection <0.5–2 mcg/mL (trough) – safety, for serious infections <1 mcg/mL (trough) – safety, for hospital-acquired pneumonia (HAP)
Aminoglycosides: amikacin	25–40 mcg/mL (peak) – efficacy, for life-threatening infections 20–25 mcg/mL (peak) – efficacy, for serious infections 15–20 mcg/mL (peak) – efficacy, for urinary tract infections <8 mcg/mL (trough) – safety <4–5 mcg/mL (trough) – safety, for HAP
Carbamazepine	4–12 mcg/mL
Cyclosporine	100–400 ng/mL
Digoxin	0.5–1 ng/mL – for heart failure with reduced ejection fraction 0.8–2.0 ng/mL – for ventricular rate control in atrial fibrillation
Ethosuximide	40–100 mcg/mL
Lidocaine	1.5–5 mcg/mL
Lithium	0.6–1.2 mEq/L
Phenobarbital	10–40 mg/L
Phenytoin	10–20 mg/L Must be corrected for hypoalbuminemia (Corrected phenytoin concentration = measured total concentration/[0.2*albumin] + 0.1)
Primidone	5–12 mcg/mL
Theophylline	10–20 mcg/mL
Valproic acid	50–100 mcg/mL– for seizure disorders 50–125 mcg/mL – for mania
Vancomycin	Peak serum concentrations usually not monitored 15–20 mcg/mL (trough) – efficacy, for bacteremia, endocarditis, osteomyelitis, meningitis, and HAP 10–15 mcg/mL (trough) – efficacy

PRACTICE QUESTIONS

1. Which of the following lab tests is NOT used to monitor hepatic function?

   (A) Total protein
   (B) Ammonia
   (C) Prothrombin time
   (D) Alkaline phosphatase
   (E) Microalbumin

2. Which of the following is used to estimate glomerular filtration rate?

   (A) Ammonia
   (B) Blood urea nitrogen (BUN)
   (C) Serum creatinine
   (D) Urine microalbumin

3. Which enzyme is elevated within 3–12 hours of an acute myocardial infarction and remains elevated for up to 14 days?

   (A) Erythrocyte sedimentation rate (ESR)
   (B) Troponin I
   (C) Troponin T
   (D) Creatine kinase-MB (CKMB)

4. A peak vancomycin level is drawn. What is the best evaluation of the results?

   (A) 30 mcg/mL: Medication dose is safe.
   (B) 50 mcg/mL: Medication dose is safe.
   (C) 10 mcg/mL: Medication dose is effective.
   (D) 30 mcg/mL: Medication dose is effective.

5. A 60-year-old man (6'2", 220 lbs) with diabetes and history of venous thrombo-embolism (VTE) complains of redness and swelling in his left lower extremity. His current medications include warfarin 5 mg daily and metformin 1,000 mg BID. Lab results include serum creatinine 1.2 mg/dL, K 4.5, INR 2.5, WBC 15 cells/mcL, AST 18 IU/L, and ALT 20 IU/L. Based on the lab information available, what is the most likely cause of the patient's complaint?

   (A) VTE
   (B) Infection
   (C) Renal impairment
   (D) Liver impairment

ANSWERS AND EXPLANATIONS ON FOLLOWING PAGE

ANSWERS AND EXPLANATIONS

1. **E**

There are many tests used for the assessment of hepatic function. Total protein (A) represents the estimated sum of albumin and globulin that are produced by the liver. Ammonia (B) is removed from the blood by the liver, and elevations indicate the liver is not able to remove it. The prothrombin time (C) helps determine the liver's ability to make clotting factors under normal circumstances (without anticoagulant therapy). Alkaline phosphatase (D) is used to detect hepatocellular injury and is often combined with AST/ALT. Microalbumin (E) is actually a test of the kidneys and is elevated when glomerular injury is present. Therefore, (E) is correct.

2. **C**

The creatinine clearance is a close estimate to the glomerular filtration rate and is calculated using patient-specific factors including serum creatinine. Ammonia (A) is useful in evaluating liver function but not renal function. BUN (B) and urine microalbumin (D) are used for evaluating renal function but not, specifically, in estimating glomerular filtration rate.

3. **C**

Troponin T is elevated within 3–12 hours of an acute myocardial infarction (MI) and remains elevated for up to 14 days. ESR (A) is a marker of inflammation, but it is not specific to MI and does not rise rapidly in response to myocardial damage. While both Troponin I (B) and CKMB (D) increase within 3–12 hours of an acute MI, Troponin I remains elevated for a maximum of 10 days and CKMB for a maximum of 3 days, not 14 days.

4. **A**

It is appropriate to draw a peak level when assessing vancomycin safety. The safe therapeutic concentration range is 20–40 mcg/mL. Peak level of 50 mcg/mL (B) would be an unsafely high therapeutic concentration, while 10 mcg/mL (C) would be a low peak level and 30 mcg/mL (D) a normal peak level. None of the answer choices would be valuable for assessing efficacy of the medication, because peak levels are not used to assess efficacy. Troughs are used for that purpose. The reference range for troughs is 5–10 mcg/mL.

5. **B**

Elevated WBCs are indicative of infection. Although the patient has a history of venous thromboembolism (A), his INR is within the therapeutic/goal range for a patient with a history of VTE, making that less likely as the cause of his left lower extremity's redness and swelling. Etiology of renal impairment (C) is unlikely because the patient's calculated creatinine clearance is within normal range, and etiology of liver impairment (D) is unlikely because available liver enzymes (AST and ALT) are within the normal reference range.

Over-the-Counter Medications

22

This chapter covers the following drug classes:

- **Vitamins**
- **Common herbals and supplements**
- **Decongestants**
- **Antihistamines**
- **Cough suppressants and expectorants**
- **Antidiarrheals**
- **Laxatives**
- **Antifungals**
- **Pediculocides**
- **Atopic dermatitis medications**
- **Poison ivy medications**
- **Sunscreens**

The text also provides an overview of basic treatment for common ailments treatable by pharmacists. This chapter also makes recommendations as to when self-treatment is not appropriate.

 Suggested Study Time: **75 minutes**

VITAMINS

Definitions

Vitamins are organic substances needed in small quantities for maintenance of health and body systems. Vitamins are often received through dietary intake but can be supplemented if a patient does not obtain adequate quantities through diet alone. Water-soluble vitamins (B vitamins and vitamin C) are excreted via the kidneys and thus do not often reach toxic limits within the body. However, fat-soluble vitamins (vitamins A, D, E, and K) can accumulate and are capable of achieving toxic levels.

Water-Soluble Vitamins

Vitamin	Function	Deficiency Manifestation	Recommended Daily Allowance (RDA)
B_1 (thiamine)	• Energy metabolism and production • Maintenance of nerve function	• Beriberi • Wernicke-Korsakoff syndrome	• Males: 1.2 mg • Females: 1.1 mg
B_2 (riboflavin)	• Energy metabolism and production • Maintenance of vision and skin	• Sore throat • Lesions of the lips and mucosa of the mouth • Glossitis • Normochromic, normocytic anemia	• Males: 1.3 mg • Females: 1.1 mg
B_3 (niacin)	• Energy metabolism and production • Maintenance of nervous and digestive systems and skin	Pellagra	• Males: 16 mg • Females: 14 mg
B_5 (pantothenic acid)	Energy metabolism and production	Paresthesia	5 mg
B_6 (pyridoxine)	• Production of red blood cells • Balance of sodium and potassium	Neuropathy	• Age 19–50 yr: 1.3 mg • Males >50 yr: 1.7 mg • Females >50 yr: 1.5 mg
B_7 (biotin)	• Fatty acid synthesis • Metabolism of amino acids	• Dermatitis • Enteritis • Hair loss	30 mcg
B_9 (folic acid)	• DNA synthesis • Production of red blood cells	• Neural tube defects • Megaloblastic anemia	400 mcg
B_{12} (cobalamins)	• Nerve function • Production of red blood cells • DNA synthesis	Megaloblastic anemia	2.4 mcg
C (ascorbic acid)	• Antioxidant • Enhances immune system	Scurvy	• Males: 90 mg • Females: 75 mg

Fat-Soluble Vitamins

Vitamin	Function	Deficiency Manifestation	RDA
A	Vision	• Night blindness • Xerophthalmia • Hyperkeratosis	• Males: 900 mcg (3,000 units) • Females: 700 mcg (2,330 units)
D	• Calcium and phosphorus regulation • Bone health	Rickets	• Age 19–70 yr: 15 mcg (600 units) • Age >70 yr: 20 mcg (800 units)
E	• Antioxidant • Smooth muscle and nerve function	Hemolytic anemia	15 mg
K	Blood clotting	Bleeding	• Males: 120 mcg • Females: 90 mcg

COMMON HERBALS AND SUPPLEMENTS

Definitions

Assessing herbals and supplements is important for medication therapy management. Data suggest that 1 in every 5 adults in the United States reports having used a natural product at least once in the previous 12 months.

The Dietary Supplement Health and Education Act of 1994 categorizes herbals, vitamins, protein bars, and shakes as dietary supplements. As a result, manufacturers are not required to demonstrate safety, purity, or efficacy of supplements. Labeling must include the following statement: "This statement has not been evaluated by the Food and Drug Administration (FDA). This product is not intended to diagnose, treat, cure, or prevent any disease." Manufacturers cannot make specific claims on labels. The use of phrases such as "helps boost, support, enhance" are acceptable; however, such statements may mislead the public and generate the need for health care assistance. It is important that you recommend only products that have undergone a standardization assurance.

Common Usage

- Saw palmetto
  - Used in men to improve symptoms of benign prostatic hyperplasia (BPH)
- Glucosamine and chondroitin
  - Used widely for treating osteoarthritis and joint structure support
  - Glucosamine: important for maintaining elasticity, strength, and resiliency of the cartilage in articular (movable) joints
  - Chondroitin: promotes flexibility of cartilage

- Fish oils or omega-3 fatty acids
  - Used primarily for hypertriglyceridemia
  - Contain eicosapentaenoic acid (EPA) and docosahexaenoic acid (DHA), and are believed to be efficacious in many people
- St. John's wort
  - Used for mild to moderate depression
  - Used in Europe for centuries for mild to moderate depression and its efficacy is comparable with tricyclic antidepressants; one study suggests it is no more effective than a placebo or sertraline in moderate to severe depression; it should not be used with other selective serotonin reuptake inhibitors (SSRIs) or serotonin norepinephrine reuptake inhibitors (SNRIs)
- Coenzyme Q10
  - Used for cardiovascular diseases, including angina, heart failure, and hypertension, and may help with myalgias due to statin therapy
- Melatonin
  - Used for insomnia, particularly when adjusting to shift-work cycles or jet lag
  - Naturally secreted from the pineal gland and appears to be the sleep-regulating hormone of the body; adults experience about a 37% decrease in daily melatonin output between 20 and 70 years of age
- Echinacea
  - Used as an immune stimulant
  - Has been studied extensively in the area of flu and cold prevention/treatment
- Black cohosh
  - Used for women's health problems, especially postmenopausal symptom relief and painful menses
  - Should be avoided in pregnancy and lactation
- Ginger
  - Used primarily for motion sickness, dyspepsia, and nausea
  - Lacks sedative affects of other antinausea treatments
  - Has been studied in pregnant women at less than 17 weeks' gestation
- Ginkgo biloba
  - Used for vascular dementia, Alzheimer's, and ischemic stroke
  - The ginkgolides are potent platelet-activating factor antagonists
- Ginseng
  - Used to treat diabetes mellitus
  - May also help reduce mental and physical stress

Over-the-Counter Medications

Name • Alternate Name • Dose	Contraindications	Primary Side Effects	Key Monitoring Parameters	Pertinent Drug Interactions	Med Pearls
Mechanism of action – inhibits production of dihydrotestosterone (DHT), inhibits receptor binding, and accelerates the metabolism of DHT					
Serenoa repens • Saw palmetto • BPH: 160 mg BID	• Pregnancy or lactation • Age <12 yr	Nausea/vomiting (N/V)	BPH symptoms	• May ↑ toxicity of estrogens or estrogen-containing contraceptives • May ↑ risk of bleeding with warfarin	Data from meta-analysis do not support use
Mechanism of action – glucosamine is an amino-sugar that is naturally produced and is a key substrate in the synthesis of macromolecules for connective tissues; chondroitin absorbs water; adding to cartilage thickness, and is found in natural physiologic connective tissue; inhibits synovial enzymes that may contribute to cartilage destruction					
Glucosamine/ chondroitin • Glucosamine: 500 mg TID • Chondroitin: 400 mg TID	• Glucosamine: active bleeding • Chondroitin: none	• Flatulence • Abdominal cramps • ↑ blood glucose	Osteoarthritis pain	May ↑ risk of bleeding with antiplatelets or anticoagulants	
Mechanism of action – inhibit diacylglycerol transferase which leads to a ↓ in hepatic synthesis of triglycerides					
Omega-3 fatty acids • Fish oils • Hypertriglyceride-mia: 2–4 g/day	Active bleeding	Gastrointestinal upset	Lipid panel	May ↑ risk of bleeding with antiplatelets or anticoagulants	
Mechanism of action – ↑ concentrations of serotonin in the central nervous system (CNS) and may have some monoamine oxidase inhibitor (MAOI) effects					
Hypericum perforatum • St. John's wort • 300 mg TID	• Pregnancy or lactation • Concurrent use with CYP2C19, CYP3A4, or P-glycoprotein substrates	• Nausea • Xerostomia • Itching • Photosensitivity • Fatigue • Dizziness • Insomnia • Jitteriness • Headache	Depression symptoms	• CYP2C19 and CYP3A4 inducer • May ↓ effects of CYP2C19 or CYP3A4 substrates • ↑ risk of serotonin syndrome with MAOIs, SSRIs, SNRIs, triptans, tricyclic antidepressants (TCAs), fentanyl, lithium, dextromethorphan, meperidine, buspirone, linezolid, methylene blue, and tramadol	Minimum of 4–6 wk of therapy is recommended before results seen
Mechanism of action – involved in adenosine triphosphate generation and serves as a lipid-soluble antioxidant providing protection against free-radical damage within the mitochondria					
Ubiquinone • Coenzyme Q10 • 20–300 mg/day in 2–3 divided doses	None	• Abdominal discomfort • Headache • N/V	Heart failure symptoms	• May ↓ anticoagulant effects of warfarin • May ↑ risk of cardiotoxicity with anthracyclines	

Over-the-Counter Medications *(cont'd)*

Name • Alternate Name • Dose	Contraindications	Primary Side Effects	Key Monitoring Parameters	Pertinent Drug Interactions	Med Pearls
Mechanism of action – supplements the naturally deficient concentrations of melatonin					
N-acetyl-5-methoxytryptamine • Melatonin • 1–5 mg at bedtime	Autoimmune disease	• Morning sedation or drowsiness • Headache • Dizziness • Nausea	Sleep quality/ quantity	• CYP1A2 inhibitor • May ↑ effects/toxicity of CYP1A2 substrates	Drugs that deplete vitamin B_6 may inhibit the ability of the body to synthesize melatonin
Mechanism of action – may stimulate white blood cell function, including cell-mediated immunity					
Echinacea purpurea/ angustifolia/ pallida • Echinacea • 50–1,000 mg TID on day 1, then 250 mg 4 ×/day	• Hypersensitivty to plants in Asteraceae/ Compositae family (including ragweed, chrysanthemums, marigolds, daisies) • Immunosuppressed patients • Rheumatoid arthritis • Systemic lupus erythematosus • Multiple sclerosis • Tuberculosis	• Itching • Rash • N/V	Cold symptoms	• CYP1A2 inhibitor • CYP3A4 inducer • May ↑ effects/toxicity of CYP1A2 substrates • May ↓ effects of CYP3A4 substrates • May ↓ effects of immunosuppressants	Should not use for >10 days in acute infection
Mechanism of action – contains phytoestrogens, which mimic estrogen					
Actaea racemosa or *Cimicifuga racemosa* • Black cohosh • 20–40 mg BID	• History of or at risk for breast cancer • Pregnancy or lactation • Aspirin sensitivity	• N/V • Rash • Hepatotoxicity	Menopausal symptoms	• CYP2D6 inhibitor • May ↑ effects/toxicity of CYP2D6 substrates	Contains salicylates
Mechanism of action – has local affects in the gastrointestinal (GI) tract and in the CNS					
Zingiber officinale • Ginger • 500–2500 mg/ day in 2–4 divided doses	Active bleeding	Generally well tolerated	Degree of nausea	May ↑ risk of bleeding with antiplatelets or anticoagulants	Use during pregnancy for morning sickness remains controversial
Mechanism of action – the flavonoid component protects neurons and retinal tissue from oxidative stress and injury					
Ginkgo biloba • Ginkgo • 120–240 mg/day in 2–3 divided doses	• Pregnancy or lactation • Active bleeding	• Nausea • Constipation • Headache • Dizziness • Palpitations • Allergic skin reactions	Mini mental state exam	May ↑ risk of bleeding with antiplatelets or anticoagulants	

Over-the-Counter Medications *(cont'd)*

Name • Alternate Name • Dose	Contraindications	Primary Side Effects	Key Monitoring Parameters	Pertinent Drug Interactions	Med Pearls
Mechanism of action – ↓ postprandial glucose levels and stimulates the release of insulin					
Panax quinquefolius • Ginseng (American) • Usual: 100–400 mg daily • Diabetes: up to 3 g/day, 2 hr before a meal	Active bleeding	• Insomnia • Headache • Anorexia	Blood glucose	• May ↑ risk of bleeding with antiplatelets or anticoagulants • May ↑ effects of glucose-lowering drugs	Should not use for >3 mo

DECONGESTANTS

Definitions

Vasoconstrictive agents can be used in the treatment of multiple conditions including hemorrhoids, hypotension, ocular procedures and redness, and nasal congestion. Decongestants are the mainstay of therapy for colds and play an important role in the management of allergic rhinitis. Nasal congestion can be treated with topical or oral decongestants that work by stimulating alpha-1 adrenergic receptors. This agonist effect causes vasoconstriction, which reduces the vascular blood supply to the sinuses, relieving intranasal pressure and reducing mucosal edema and mucus production. Decongestants are indicated for temporary relief of nasal congestion and cough associated with postnasal drip. They are no longer approved for sinusitis. The FDA does not recommend over-the-counter (OTC) medications, including decongestants, for children under the age of 2 years because of the increased risk of death.

Signs and Symptoms

- Sinusitis
  - Tenderness over the sinuses; facial pain aggravated by postural changes; fever (temperatute >101.5°F); tooth pain; halitosis; upper respiratory tract symptoms for >7 days with poor response to decongestants
- Common cold
  - Sore throat; nasal congestion; rhinorrhea; sneezing; common, low-grade fever; chills; headache; malaise; myalgia; cough
- Postnasal drip
  - Continued mucus accumulation in the back of the nose and throat leading to or giving the sensation of mucus dripping downward from the back of the nose

Guidelines

American Pharmaceutical Association. *Handbook of Nonprescription Drugs: An Interactive Approach to Self-Care*, 18th ed., 2015.

Adverse Effects

Appropriate FDA-approved doses of decongestants should be used at all times since overdoses can cause excessive central nervous system stimulation and paradoxical depression. The main adverse effects of oral decongestants are cardiovascular stimulation and central nervous system stimulation. Topical nasal decongestants produce fewer systemic adverse effects.

Guidelines Summary

- A pharmacist may appropriately recommend a decongestant once it is determined that the patient does not have any of the following:
  - Fever (temperature >101.5°F)
  - Chest pain
  - Shortness of breath
  - Uncontrolled hypertension
  - Cardiac arrhythmias
  - Insomnia
  - Anxiety
  - Worsening of symptoms or development of additional symptoms during self-treatment
  - Concurrent underlying chronic cardiopulmonary disease
  - Acquired immune deficiency syndrome or chronic immunosuppressant therapy
  - Frail patients of advanced age
  - Children <2 years of age
  - Current use of MAOIs
- Topical decongestants should not be recommended for longer than 3 days due to the risk of rhinitis medicamentosa, a condition of rebound nasal congestion brought on by overuse of intranasal vasoconstrictive medications.

Decongestants

Generic • Brand • Dose	Contraindications	Primary Side Effects	Key Monitoring Parameters	Pertinent Drug Interactions	Med Pearls
Oral Decongestants					
Mechanism of action – alpha-1 adrenergic stimulant					
Phenylephrine • Sudafed PE Maximum Strength • 10 mg every 4 hr PRN	• Uncontrolled hypertension • Ventricular tachycardia • Use of MAOI within 2 wk	• Restlessness • Hypertension • Tremor • Tachycardia • Insomnia	• Blood pressure • Heart rate • Anxiety	↑ risk of hypertensive crisis with MAOIs	Available OTC without restrictions
Pseudoephedrine • Sudafed • IR: 60 mg every 4–6 hr PRN • ER: 120 mg every 12 hr or 240 mg daily					• Available behind the counter • Must provide photo identification and sign log book to purchase • Amount purchased limited to ≤3.6 g/day or 9 g/mo
Topical Decongestants					
Oxymetazoline • Afrin • Intranasal: 2–3 sprays in each nostril BID	Hypersensitivity	• Dryness of nasal mucosa • Stinging • Rebound congestion	Rebound congestion	↑ risk of hypertensive crisis with MAOIs	Not recommended for longer than 3 days
Naphazoline • Clear Eyes • Ophthalmic: 1–2 drops every 6 hr PRN					
Phenylephrine • Neo-Synephrine • 1–2 sprays in each nostril every 4 hr					

ANTIHISTAMINES

Definitions

Antihistamines can be used for multiple roles in patient care, including contact dermatitis, allergic rhinitis, common colds, insomnia, heartburn, and nausea and vomiting.

Stimulation of histamine-1 receptors produces sneezing, pruritus, and mucus production. Stimulation of histamine-2 receptors results in stomach acid production.

Antihistamines that inhibit H_1 receptors are classified as either sedating (first-generation, nonselective) or nonsedating (second-generation, peripherally selective). Second-generation antihistamines are less sedating because they do not cross the blood–brain barrier. These agents are commonly used to treat allergic rhinitis and common cold symptoms. The FDA does not recommend over-the-counter (OTC) medications, including decongestants, for children under the age of 2 years because of the increased risk of death.

Signs and Symptoms

- Contact dermatitis: Papules, vesicles, erythema, crusting, and oozing
- Allergic rhinitis: Nasal stuffiness, rhinorrhea (usually clear), nasal pruritus, sneezing, watery eyes
- Common cold: Nasal stuffiness, sneezing, scratchy throat, cough, hoarseness, headache, fever
- Insomnia: Difficulty initiating sleep at usual time and/or wakefulness during usual sleep cycle, daytime tiredness

Guidelines

American Pharmaceutical Association. *Handbook of Nonprescription Drugs: An Interactive Approach to Self-Care*, 18th edition, 2015.

Guidelines Summary

- Contact dermatitis
  - Identify the cause: chemicals, acids, solvent, fragrances, metals, poison ivy, etc.
  - Clean the area with mild soap and water.
  - Refer patient to physician if the rash causes edema or invades the eyelids, external genitalia, anus, or massive areas of the body.
  - Treatment includes topical treatment with hydrocortisone, bicarbonate pastes, and antihistamines.
- Allergic rhinitis and common cold
  - A pharmacist may appropriately recommend an antihistamine once it is determined that the patient does not have any of the following:
    » Symptoms of otitis media or sinusitis
    » Symptoms of lower respiratory tract infection
    » History of nonallergic rhinitis
- Insomnia
  - Transient or short-term insomnia with no underlying problems are appropriate for self-treatment.
  - Discuss good sleep hygiene practices—no caffeine after 5 P.M., no exercise in the evening.
  - If diphenhydramine is recommended, it should be taken at bedtime only as needed.
  - Patients who complain of continuing insomnia after 14 days of treatment should be referred to a physician.

Antihistamines

Generic • Brand • Dose/Dosage Forms	Contraindications	Primary Side Effects	Key Monitoring Parameters	Pertinent Drug Interactions	Med Pearls
First-Generation Histamine H$_1$ Antagonists					
Mechanism of action – competes with histamine for H$_1$ receptor sites on effector cells in the GI tract, blood vessels, and respiratory tract					
Clemastine • Tavist Allergy • 1.34 mg BID-TID (max = 8.04 mg/day) • Tabs	• Hypersensitivity • Concurrent use with MAOIs • Lactation • Asthma	• Sedation • Dry mouth • Constipation • Blurred vision • Urinary retention	Mental alertness	• Concurrent use with MAOIs may ↑ risk of anticholinergic effects • Additive effects with other anticholinergic medications	• Paradoxic reactions (including stimulatory effects) may be seen • Have more anticholinergic effects than second-generation H$_1$ antagonists • Diphenhydramine also available as injection • NOT for OTC use in children <2 yr
Chlorpheniramine • Chlor-Trimeton • IR: 4 mg every 4–6 hr PRN (max = 24 mg/day) • ER: 12 mg every 12 hr (max = 24 mg/day) • ER tabs, solution, tabs	• Hypersensitivity • Narrow angle glaucoma • BPH • Asthma			• CYP2D6 substrate • CYP2D6 inhibitors may ↑ effects/toxicity • Additive effects with other anticholinergic medications	
Brompheniramine • J-Tan PD • 1–2 mg every 4–6 hr PRN (max = 6 mg/day [2–5 yr]; 12 mg/day [6–11 yr]) • Solution, tabs	None			Additive effects with other anticholinergic medications	
Diphenhydramine • Benadryl, Sominex, Unisom, ZzzQuil • Allergy: 25–50 mg every 4–8 hr PRN (max = 300 mg/day) • Insomnia: 50 mg at bedtime PRN • Caps, chewable tabs, solution, strips, suspension, tabs	• Hypersensitivity • Lactation			Additive effects with other anticholinergic medications	
Doxylamine • Sleep Aid • 25 mg at bedtime PRN • Solution, tabs					

Antihistamines *(cont'd)*

Generic • Brand • Dose/Dosage Forms	Contraindications	Primary Side Effects	Key Monitoring Parameters	Pertinent Drug Interactions	Med Pearls
Second-Generation Histamine H₁ Antagonists					
Mechanism of action – long-acting tricyclic antihistamines with selective peripheral H₁-receptor antagonistic properties; less blood-brain barrier penetration					
Loratadine • Alavert, Claritin • 10 mg daily • Caps, chewable tabs, ODTs, solution, tabs	Hypersensitivity	• Some sedation • Headache • Dizziness • Xerostomia	Relief of symptoms	Additive effects with other anticholinergic medications	• Available in combination with pseudoephedrine • Desloratadine (Clarinex) only available Rx • NOT for OTC use in children <2 yr
Cetirizine • Zyrtec • 5–10 mg daily • Caps, chewable tabs, ODTs, solution, tabs					• Available in combination with pseudoephedrine • Most sedating of the second-generation antihistamines • NOT for OTC use in children <2 yr
Fexofenadine • Allegra, Mucinex Allergy • 60 mg BID or 180 mg daily • ODTs, suspension, tabs		Headache			• Avoid taking with fruit juices • Available in combination with pseudoephedrine • Least sedating of the second-generation antihistamines • NOT for OTC use in children <2 yr

COUGH SUPPRESSANTS AND EXPECTORANTS

Definitions

A cough is caused by irritants or stimuli stimulating receptors located throughout the respiratory tract. The larynx is more sensitive than the trachea and bronchi. When activated, the receptors send signals through the brain-stem reflex pathway, the voluntary cerebral cortex pathway, or both. The signals eventually end up in the "cough center" of the medulla oblongata. The overall objective is to expel the irritant or stimuli.

Diagnosis

- A cough can be classified in the following ways:
  - Acute: duration <3 weeks
    - » Most commonly caused by a virus
  - Subacute: duration of 3–8 weeks
    - » Caused by infection, bacterial sinusitis, asthma
  - Chronic: duration >8 weeks
    - » Smoking, post nasal drip, asthma, and gastroesophageal reflux disease (GERD)
- Angiotensin-converting enzyme inhibitors (ACEIs) cause a dry cough in ≥20% of treated patients.
- Systemic and ophthalmic beta-adrenergic blockers may cause cough in patients with chronic obstructive pulmonary disease (COPD).

Signs and Symptoms

- Productive
  - A wet or "chesty" cough, which expels secretions from the lower respiratory tract.
  - Secretions may be clear, purulent, discolored, or malodorous.
- Nonproductive
  - A dry or "hacking" cough that serves no useful physiologic purpose.
  - Caused by viral respiratory tract infections, atypical bacterial respiratory tract infections, GERD, cardiac disease, and some medications (e.g., ACEIs).

Guidelines

American Pharmaceutical Association. *Handbook of Nonprescription Drugs: An Interactive Approach to Self-Care*, 18th ed., 2015.

Guidelines Summary

- The primary goal of treating a cough is to reduce the number and severity of cough episodes.
- Cough suppressants (antitussives) should only be used to treat nonproductive coughs; should not be used for productive coughs.
- Codeine and dextromethorphan are the cough suppressants of choice for nonproductive cough.

- Antihistamines also have antitussive properties:
  - Diphenhydramine is a better choice for a cough associated with allergies but is highly sedating.
  - A second-generation antihistamine can also be considered since they are associated with less sedation.
- Expectorants include guaifenesin and water. Expectorants can be used to thin out the mucus or phlegm associated with a productive cough; they do NOT act as a cough suppressant.
- Patients should be excluded from self-treatment if they have any of the following:

Cough with thick yellow sputum or green phlegm	Unintended weight loss
Drenching nighttime sweats	History of asthma, COPD, or heart failure
Foreign-object aspiration	Cough duration >7 days
Fever (temperature >101.5°F)	Children <2 yr of age
Hemoptysis	Cough worsens during self-treatment

Cough Suppressants

Generic • Brand • Dose/Dosage Forms	Contraindications	Primary Side Effects	Key Monitoring Parameters	Pertinent Drug Interactions	Med Pearls
Mechanism of action – depresses the medullary cough center					
Dextromethorphan • Robitussin, Delsym • IR: 10–20 mg every 4 hr or 30 mg every 6–8 hr • ER: 60 mg BID • Max = 120 mg/day • Caps, ER suspension, gel, lozenges, solution, strips	Use of MAOI within 2 wk	• Confusion • Irritability	Relief of symptoms	• CYP2D6 substrate • CYP2D6 inhibitors may ↑ effects/ toxicity • ↑ risk of serotonin syndrome with MAOIs, SSRIs, SNRIs, triptans, TCAs, fentanyl, lithium, meperidine, buspirone, linezolid, methylene blue, St. John's wort, and tramadol	• Not for OTC use in children <2 yr • Chemically related to morphine; lacks narcotic properties except in overdose • May require Rx for use in children and adolescents in some states
Codeine • 7.5–15 mg every 4–6 hr (max = 120 mg/day)	• Hypersensitivity • Respiratory depression • Paralytic ileus • Severe or acute asthma • Gastrointestinal obstruction	• N/V • Constipation • Sedation	• CNS depression • Relief of symptoms	• CYP2D6 substrate • CYP2D6 inhibitors may ↑ effects/ toxicity • Other CNS depressants, including alcohol, may ↑ CNS depressant effects	10% of a codeine dose is demethylated in the liver to form morphine

Expectorant

Generic • Brand • Dose/Dosage Forms	Contraindications	Primary Side Effects	Key Monitoring Parameters	Pertinent Drug Interactions	Med Pearls
Mechanism of action – expectorant; irritates the gastric mucosa and stimulates respiratory tract secretions, thereby ↑ fluid volumes and ↓ mucous viscosity					
Guaifenesin • Mucinex • IR: 200–400 mg every 4 hr PRN • ER: 600–1,200 mg BID PRN • Max = 2,400 mg/day • ER tabs, oral packets, solution, tabs	Hypersensitivity	• Dizziness • Kidney stone formation	Relief of symptoms	None	More effective with water intake

ANTIDIARRHEALS

Definitions

Diarrhea is defined as an abnormal increase in stool frequency or liquidity. Each individual has a different frequency, which is affected by many variables. The typical range of stool frequency can be 3 times per day to once every 2 days. More than 3 bowel movements per day is considered to be abnormal.

Diagnosis

- Diarrhea is defined and characterized by more than three bowel movements in 1 day.
- Diarrhea may be acute, persistent, or chronic in nature.
- Acute diarrhea has a duration of <14 days.
- Persistent diarrhea has a duration of 2–4 weeks.
- Chronic diarrhea lasts more than 4 weeks.

Signs and Symptoms

- Symptoms include abdominal pain, cramping, and frequency.

Guidelines

American Pharmaceutical Association. *Handbook of Nonprescription Drugs: An Interactive Approach to Self-Care*, 18th edition, 2015.

Guidelines Summary

- Acute diarrhea can be managed with fluids, electrolyte replacement, dietary interventions, and nonprescription drug treatment.

- Persistent and chronic diarrhea requires medical care, and patients are not candidates for self-treatment if either forms of diarrhea is present.

- Patients should be excluded from self-treatment if any of the following apply:
  - <6 months of age
  - Severe dehydration
  - >6 months of age with persistent high fevers greater than 102.2°F
  - Blood, mucus, or pus in the stool
  - Protracted vomiting or severe abdominal pain
  - Pregnancy
  - Chronic or persistent diarrhea

Antidiarrheals

Generic • Brand • Dose/Dosage Forms	Contraindications	Primary Side Effects	Key Monitoring Parameters	Pertinent Drug Interactions	Med Pearls
Mechanism of action – acts directly on opioid receptors on intestinal muscles to inhibit peristalsis and prolong transit time					
Loperamide • Imodium A–D • 4 mg, followed by 2 mg after each loose stool, (max = 16 mg/day) • Caps, chewable tabs, solution, suspension, tabs	• Hypersensitivity • Abdominal pain without diarrhea • Children <2 yr • Primary tx for acute dysentery, acute ulcerative colitis, bacterial enterocolitis, and pseudomembranous colitis (*C. difficile*)	• Constipation • Abdominal cramping • Abdominal distention	• Bowel movement frequency • CNS depression • Paralytic ileus • S/S of dehydration	None	
Mechanism of action – possesses both antisecretory and antimicrobial effects; may also provides some anti-inflammatory effects					
Bismuth subsalicylate • Pepto-Bismol • 524 mg every 30–60 min PRN for up to 2 days (max = 4,200 mg/day) • Chewable tabs, suspension	• Children or adolescents with influenza or chickenpox (due to risk of Reye's syndrome) • Hx of GI bleed • Pregnancy • Hypersensitivity to salicylates	• Discoloration of tongue and feces (grayish-black) • Hearing loss • Tinnitus	Bowel movement frequency	May ↓ absorption of tetracyclines and fluoroquinolones (separate by 2 hr)	

Antidiarrheals *(cont'd)*

Generic • Brand • Dose/Dosage Forms	Contraindications	Primary Side Effects	Key Monitoring Parameters	Pertinent Drug Interactions	Med Pearls
Mechanism of action – helps reestablish normal intestinal flora; suppresses the growth of potentially pathogenic microorganisms by producing lactic acid, which favors the establishment of an aciduric flora					
Lactobacillus • Culturelle, Lactinex • Culturelle: 1 caplet daily or BID • Lactinex: 4 tabs 3–4 ×/day • Caps. chewable tabs, granules, powder, tabs, wafers	Hypersensitivity to milk protein	• Flatulence • Bloating	Bowel movement frequency	None	Lactinex must be stored in refrigerator
Lactase enzyme • Lactaid • 1–2 capsules taken with milk or meal	None	None	Bowel movement frequency	None	• Used in the treatment of lactose intolerance • Prevents osmotic diarrhea

LAXATIVES

Definitions

Constipation is a symptom-based disorder that is described as a decrease in the frequency of fecal elimination characterized by the passage of hard, dry stools. The Rome III Criteria require a patient to have experienced ≥2 of the following symptoms over the past 3 months: (1) <3 bowel movements per week; (2) straining; (3) lumpy/hard stools; (4) sensation of an obstruction; (5) sensation of incomplete defecation; or (6) manual maneuvering required to defecate. Its occurrence ↑ as the patient ages in both men and women. However, it tends to be more commonly reported in women. Over half of the elderly population is affected by constipation. It is also a main complaint during pregnancy and after childbirth.

Constipation can be caused by various medical conditions, psychological and physiological conditions (e.g., menopause, dehydration), and lifestyle characteristics. There are several medications that can induce constipation, including: antacids, anticholinergics, antidepressants, antidiarrheals, benzodiazepines, calcium channel blockers, iron supplements, MAOIs, opiates, parkinsonism agents, and sucralfate.

Diagnosis

- There are three clinical subgroups of constipation:
  - Normal transit constipation
    - » Most common form (59%)
  - Slow transit constipation
    - » Accounts for 13% of all cases
    - » Due to delayed colonic transit
  - Pelvic floor dysfunction
  - Combination syndrome
- Less frequency of stooling than the "normal" 3–5 times/week
- Harder stool than "normal"
- Smaller stools than "normal"
- Colonoscopy if age >50 years, alarm signs, or additional symptoms present

Signs and Symptoms

- Lack of passing a bowel movement
- Very hard stools and/or lumpy stools
- Need for performing manual maneuvers to pass stools
- Anorexia, dull headache, low back pain, abdominal distention

Guidelines

Bharucha AE, Dorn SD, Lembo A, Pressman A. American Gastroenterological Association medical position statement on Constipation. *Gastroenterology* 2013;144:211–7.

American Pharmaceutical Association. *Handbook of Nonprescription Drugs: An Interactive Approach to Self-Care*, 18th ed., 2015.

Guidelines Summary

- Lifestyle modifications:
  - Educate patient about high fiber and increased hydration in diet.
  - Encourage patients to avoid postponing defecation.
  - Monitor bowel habits with a daily diary.
  - Encourage patients to maintain moderate exercise.

- Patients should be excluded from self-treatment if they have any of the following:
  - Marked abdominal pain or significant distention or cramping
  - Marked or unexplained flatulence
  - Fever
  - N/V
  - Paraplegia or quadriplegia
  - Daily laxative use
  - Unexplained changes in bowel habits and/or weight loss
  - Bowel symptoms that persist for 2 weeks
  - History of irritable bowel disease
- Pharmacologic therapy begins with bulk-forming agents and proceeds to osmotic laxatives.
- If these options are not helpful, stimulant laxatives should be considered.
- Enemas, suppositories, and lubricants are also available as options.

Medications for Constipation

Generic • Brand • Dose/Dosage Forms	Contraindications	Primary Side Effects	Key Monitoring Parameters	Pertinent Drug Interactions	Med Pearls
Mechanism of action – bulk-forming laxatives that work by absorbing water in the intestine to form a viscous liquid that promotes peristalsis					
Psyllium • Metamucil, Konsyl • 2.5–30 g/day in divided doses • Caps, packets, powder	• Fecal impaction • GI obstruction	• Abdominal cramps • Diarrhea	Bowel movement frequency	May ↓ absorption of other medications (space apart by 2 hr)	Take with full glass of water
Calcium polycarbophil • FiberCon • 2 tabs 1–4 ×/day • Tabs					
Methylcellulose • Citrucel • 2 caps up to 6 × /day • 1 tbsp up to 3 ×/day • Powder, tabs					
Mechanism of action – osmotic laxative that causes water retention in the stool					
Polyethylene glycol 3350 • GlycoLax, MiraLax • 17 g daily • Packets, powder	• GI obstruction • Hypersensitivity	• Abdominal cramps • Diarrhea • Bloating	Bowel movement frequency	None	Can reconstitute with 8 oz of water, juice, cola, or tea

Medications for Constipation (cont'd)

Generic • Brand • Dose/Dosage Forms	Contraindications	Primary Side Effects	Key Monitoring Parameters	Pertinent Drug Interactions	Med Pearls
Mechanism of action – stimulant laxatives that stimulates peristalsis by directly irritating the smooth muscle of the intestine					
Senna • Ex-Lax Maximum Strength, Senokot • 17.2 mg daily up to 34.4 mg BID • Chewable tabs, solution, tabs	• Fecal impaction • GI obstruction	• Abdominal cramps • Diarrhea	Bowel movement frequency	None	
Bisacodyl • Dulcolax, Fleet Laxative • 5–15 mg PO daily • Rectal: 10 mg daily • Enema, suppository, tabs				Effect may be ↓ by milk, dairy products, or antacids (separate by 1 hr)	
Mechanism of action – stool softeners that ↓ surface tension of the oil-water interface of the stool, resulting in enhanced incorporation of water and fat which facilitates stool softening					
Docusate sodium • Colace • 100 mg PO BID • Rectal: 1 enema 1–3 ×/day • Caps, enema, solution, tabs Docusate calcium • Kao-Tin • 240 mg daily	• Fecal impaction • GI obstruction	• Diarrhea • Cramping	Bowel movement frequency	None	Take with full glass of water
Mechanism of action – osmotic laxative that promotes bowel evacuation by causing osmotic retention of fluid which distends the colon with ↑ peristaltic activity					
Magnesium hydroxide • Phillips Milk of Magnesia • 1–2 tbsp daily or BID • Chewable tabs, suspension	Hypersensitivity	Diarrhea	Bowel movement frequency	May ↓ absorption of tetracyclines and fluoroquinolones (separate by 2 hr)	• Take with full glass of water • Use with caution in patients with renal impairment
Mechanism of action – lubricant laxative that eases passage of stool by ↓ water absorption and lubricating the intestines					
Mineral oil • Fleet Oil • 1–2 tbsp at bedtime • 1 enema × 1 • Enema, oil	• Children <6 yr • Pregnancy • Elderly • Difficulty swallowing	• Abdominal cramps • Diarrhea • Aspiration pneumonia	Bowel movement frequency	May ↓ absorption of fat-soluble vitamins (A, D, K, E)	Aspiration is possible, especially in elderly population

ANTIFUNGALS

Definitions

Tinea is known to infect the skin, scalp (tinea capitis), and feet (tinea pedis), but may also infect the beard or groin areas (tinea cruris). Ringworm (tinea corporis) is a common skin infection that is characterized by a round, red patch appearance and is found on the body in various areas. Tinea pedis (athlete's foot) is a foot infection that can range from mild itching to a severe inflammatory process characterized by fissuring, crusting, and discoloration of skin.

Tinea pedis can be further broken down into four types.

- Chronic, intertriginous type
  - Most common form
  - Usually found in the lateral toe webs; however, infection is possible by spreading to the sole or instep of the foot
- Chronic, papulosquamous type
  - Found on both feet
  - Characterized by mild inflammation and diffuse, moccasin-like scaling
- Vesicular type
  - Occurs most often in the summer
  - Characterized by small vesicles or vesicopustules near the instep and on the mid-anterior plantar surface
- Acute, ulcerative type
  - Caused from an overgrowth of gram-negative bacteria

Diagnosis

- Ringworm: round, red patch
- Athelete's foot: typically found in the lateral toe webs; may spread to the sole or instep of the foot

Signs and Symptoms

- Round, red patch on skin
- Fissuring and scaling
- Maceration in the interdigital spaces
- Malodorous
- Stinging and burning sensation

Guidelines

American Pharmaceutical Association. *Handbook of Nonprescription Drugs: An Interactive Approach to Self-Care,* 18th edition, 2015.

Guidelines Summary

- Patients should be excluded from self-treatment if they have any of the following:
  - Causative factor unclear
  - Nails or scalp involved
  - Face, mucous membranes, or genitalia involved
  - Signs and symptoms of possible secondary bacterial infection
  - Excessive and continuous exudation, fever, malaise
- Apply a thin layer of medication to affected area for 2–4 weeks (product dependent), even after the signs and symptoms disappear.

Topical Antifungal Medications to Treat Tinea

Generic • Brand • Dose/Dosage Forms	Contraindications	Primary Side Effects	Key Monitoring Parameters	Pertinent Drug Interactions	Med Pearls
Mechanism of action – squalene epoxidase inhibitor results in deficiency of ergosterol within the fungal cell					
Butenafine • Lotrimin Ultra, Mentax • Apply daily × 2 wk (corporis/cruris) or 4 wk (pedis) • Cream	Hypersensitivity	• Burning • Contact dermatitis • Erythema • Irritation • Stinging	Clinical signs of improvement	None	Used to treat tinea pedis, tinea cruris, and tinea corporis
Terbinafine • Lamisil, Lamisil AT • Apply 1–2x/day × ≥1 wk • Cream, gel					
Mechanism of action – binds to phospholipids in the fungal cell membrane, altering cell wall permeability and resulting in loss of intracellular elements					
Clotrimazole • Lotrimin AF • Apply BID	Hypersensitivity	• Burning • Contact dermatitis • Erythema • Itching	Clinical signs of improvement	None	Used to treat tinea pedis, tinea cruris, and tinea corporis
Miconazole • Desenex, Micatin • Apply BID × 2 wk (cruris) or 4 wk (corporis/pedis) • Cream, lotion, ointment, powder, powder spray, solution, spray					

Topical Antifungal Medications to Treat Tinea *(cont'd)*

Generic • Brand • Dose/Dosage Forms	Contraindications	Primary Side Effects	Key Monitoring Parameters	Pertinent Drug Interactions	Med Pearls
Mechanism of action – distorts the hyphae and stunts mycelial growth in susceptible fungi					
Tolnaftate • Tinactin • Apply BID × 2 wk (cruris) or 4 wk (corporis/pedis) • Cream, powder, powder spray, solution, spray	Hypersensitivity	• Burning • Contact dermatitis • Erythema • Itching	Clinical signs of improvement	None	Used to treat tinea pedis, tinea cruris, and tinea corporis
Mechanism of action – inhibits conversion of yeast to the hyphal form (active form) and interferes with fatty-acid biosynthesis					
Undecylenic acid • Fungi-Nail • Apply BID × 4 wk • Solution	Hypersensitivity	High alcohol concentrations may cause burning	Clinical signs of improvement	None	Used to treat tinea pedis and toe fungus

PEDICULOCIDES

Definition

Lice or pediculosis is a parasitic infection that often results in human infestation. Head lice (*Pediculus humanus capitis*) are found in the hair, often on the back of the head and neck. Head lice lay their eggs near the base of the hair shaft. Although lice cannot jump or fly, they are spread from one person to another by close human contact. Pubic lice are most often found in the pubic hair, but may also be found on the body. Body lice are found on the body when feeding, but mostly live in the seams of clothing.

Diagnosis

Diagnosis of lice is made when a live adult louse or nit (lice egg) is found. Head lice are found on the scalp. Use of a fine tooth louse comb may help find the insects as they avoid light and move quickly, making identification difficult. Evidence of nits close to the scalp can suggest the presence of lice but does not provide a confirmation for diagnosis. Pubic lice are diagnosed based on the presence of nits or lice found in the pubic hair. Pubic lice may also be found in other areas of the body (eyebrows, eyelashes, beard, mustache, armpit, groin). A diagnosis of body lice is made with the presence of eggs and live lice found in the seams of clothing.

Signs and Symptoms

Itching is the most common symptoms of a lice infestation and will manifest in the infected area. Inspection of the affected area may show presence of live lice and nits on hair follicles.

Guidelines

American Pharmaceutical Association. *Handbook of Nonprescription Drugs: An Interactive Approach to Self-Care*, 18th ed., 2015.

Guideline Summary

- All members of a household that contain a person with a lice infestation should be screened for lice and treated if they are infected.

- Treatment includes ovicidal agents. Retreatment is only needed for ovicidal agents if lice continue to be seen. Weakly ovicidal agents will require retreatment to make sure all nits have hatched and will be exposed to medication.

- Nonpharmacologic treatment includes washing all items such at hats, towels, and bedding that came into contact with the infected person within 48 hr of treatment in hot water and dried with hot air. If something cannot be washed in a washing machine, other options include dry cleaning or placing the items within a plastic bag for a 2-week period.

- Patients should be excluded from self-treatment if they have any of the following:
  - Children <2 yr
  - Hypersensitivity to chrysanthemums
  - Secondary skin infection in lice-infested areas
  - Pregnancy
  - Lactation

Medications to Treat Pediculosis

Generic • Brand • Dose/Dosage Forms	Contraindications	Primary Side Effects	Key Monitoring Parameters	Med Pearls
Mechanism of action – inhibits respiration of lice by respiratory spiracle obstruction				
Benzyl alcohol • Ulesfia • 4–48 ounces based on length of hair • Lotion	None	• Pruritus • Erythema • Local irritation • Eye irritation	Eradication of lice and nits	• Rx only • Apply to *dry* hair, saturate scalp, leave on for 10 min, rinse, then repeat in 7 days

Medications to Treat Pediculosis *(cont'd)*

Generic • Brand • Dose/Dosage Forms	Contraindications	Primary Side Effects	Key Monitoring Parameters	Med Pearls
Mechanism of action – inhibits sodium influx into nerve cell membranes, causing repolarization and paralysis of the lice				
Permethrin • Elimite, Nix • Cream, lotion	Hypersensitivity	• Pruritus • Erythema • Scalp rash • Burning • Stinging • Scalp discomfort	Eradication of lice and nits	• Elimite is Rx only • Wash hair with conditioner-free shampooo, towel dry, apply sufficient amount of lotion or cream to saturate scalp and hair, leave on for no longer than 10 minutes, rinse with warm water, comb hair with nit comb; may repeat in 7 days, if needed • Do not use near eyes or inside the nose, ear, mouth, or vagina • Elimite can also be used for scabies
Mechanism of action – neurotoxicity caused by stimulation of nerve cells to produce repeated discharges and subsequent paralysis				
Pyrethrins and piperonyl butoxide • A–200, Licide, Pronto Plus, RID • Gel, oil, shampoo, solution	None	• Pruritus • Burning • Stinging • Skin irritation	Eradication of lice and nits	• Apply to *dry* hair, leave on for 10 minutes, wash and rinse, comb hair with nit comb, then repeat in 7–10 days • Do not use near eyes, in eyebrows or eyelashes, or inside nose, mouth, vagina • Solution should only be applied to bedding (not for human use)
Mechanism of action – ↑ permeabilty of cell membranes to chloride, resulting in hyperpolarization and death of lice				
Ivermectin • Sklice • Lotion	None	• Burning • Skin irritation	Eradication of lice and nits	• Rx only • Apply to *dry* scalp and hair, leave on for 10 minutes, rinse with warm water, comb hair with nit comb; do not repeat • Also available as cream (Soolantra) for rosacea
Mechanism of action – inhibits cholinesterase in lice, causing death				
Malathion • Ovide • Lotion	• Hypersensitivity • Neonates or infants	• Chemical burns • Local irritation • Stinging • Conjunctivitis	Eradication of lice and nits	• Rx only • Apply to *dry* hair and scalp, dry hair naturally (do not cover), shampoo off after 8–12 hr, comb hair with nit comb; may repeat in 7–9 days if needed
Mechanism of action – CNS excitation and involuntary muscle contractions produce paralysis and death of lice				
Spinosad • Natroba • Suspension	None	• Erythema • Local irritation • Dry skin	Eradication of lice and nits	• Rx only • Apply to *dry* scalp and hair, leave on for 10 minutes, rinse with warm water, may then shampoo, comb hair with nit comb; may repeat in 7 days if needed

Medications to Treat Pediculosis *(cont'd)*

Generic • Brand • Dose/Dosage Forms	Contraindications	Primary Side Effects	Key Monitoring Parameters	Med Pearls
Mechanism of action – stimulates the nervous system of lice, causing seizures and death				
Lindane • Only available generically • Shampoo	• Hypersensitivity • Premature infants • Uncontrolled seizure disorders • Crusted skin conditions	• Ataxia • Dizziness • Burning • Neurotoxicity • Seizures • Dermatitis	• Eradication of lice and nits • Mental status • Seizures	• Rx only • Apply to *dry* hair and massage in for 4 min, add in water to form a lather, rinse hair thoroughly, comb hair with nit comb; do not repeat • Can also be used for pubic lice or scabies

ATOPIC DERMATITIS MEDICATIONS

Definition

Atopic dermatitis is a condition characterized by itchy, inflamed patches of skin. This condition usually starts during childhood, but can affect people of any age. The most common areas for involvement include the face, hands, feet, the inner elbow, and the back of the knees. The condition is often made worse by irritants or allergy triggers.

Diagnosis

Diagnosis of atopic dermatitis includes the presence of condition at age < 2 years of age, involvement of skin crease areas, history of dry skin, family history, and visual lesions.

Signs and Symptoms

Patches of atopic dermatitis are often itchy, red, and inflamed. Areas may also have scaling, cracking, and blisters.

Guidelines

American Pharmaceutical Association. *Handbook of Nonprescription Drugs: An Interactive Approach to Self-Care*, 18th ed., 2015.

Guideline Summary

- Treatment of atopic dermatitis includes skin hydration, removal of known irritants, and topical steroid creams.
- Patients should be excluded from self-treatment any of the following apply
  - Age < 2 yr
  - Severe dermatitis or pruritus
  - Large body area involvement
  - Skin infection

Medications for Atopic Dermatitis

Generic • Brand • Dose/Dosage Forms	Contraindications	Primary Side Effects	Key Monitoring Parameters	Med Pearls
Mechanism of action – ↓ inflammatory mediators through the induction of phospholipase A2 inhibitory proteins and release of arachidonic acid				
Hydrocortisone • Cortaid • Applied up to 3–4 ×/day • Cream	• Hypersensitivity • Diaper dermatitis	• Acneiform eruptions • Skin irritation • Dry skin • Hypopigmentation	Response to therapy	Avoid use on weeping lesions

POISON IVY MEDICATIONS

Definition

Poison ivy is an allergic condition in which a rash appears due to exposure and contact with urushiol. Urushiol is found in poison ivy, poison oak, and poison sumac, all of which are naturally growing plants. Poison ivy grows as a bush or vine and generally has three leaves. Poison oak has three leaves similar to that of an oak tree and can be found growing as a shrub or vine. Poison sumac generally has 7–13 leaves and can be found growing as a tree or shrub.

Diagnosis

Poison ivy is diagnosed with the appearance of a red, swollen, blistering rash that causes itching after exposure to poison ivy, poison oak, or poison sumac.

Signs and Symptoms

The rash appears in the pattern of the contact with the plant and can be described as red, swollen, blistering, and itchy. The severity of the rash depends on the amount of exposure and develops within 12–24 hours after contact and can last as long as 2–3 weeks. Patients may experience difficulty with breathing if urushiol is inhaled or if the allergic reaction is severe.

Guidelines

American Pharmaceutical Association. *Handbook of Nonprescription Drugs: An Interactive Approach to Self-Care*, 18th ed., 2015.

Guideline Summary

- Remove clothing worn during exposure to urushiol. Wash exposed clothing separately to avoid contaminating other items.
- Wash skin with soap and water to remove urushiol.
- Treatment focuses on the relief of itching and may include the use of topical calamine or hydrocortisone.
- Avoid topical anesthetics, antihistamines, and antibiotics for mild symptoms to prevent sensitization of the skin and a drug-induced dermatitis.
- Nonpharmacologic treatment can include the use of colloidal oatmeal baths, tepid showers, and baking soda compressed.
- Patients should be excluded from self-treatment if they have any of the following:
  - Involvement of rash on the face, eyes, or genitalia
  - Difficulty breathing
  - Exposure to smoke from a burning poison ivy, poison oak, or poison sumac plant
  - Age <2 years
  - Widespread rash involving >25% of body surface area
  - Presence of infection
  - Presence of rash >2 weeks
  - Presence of numerous bullae

Medications for Poison Ivy

Generic • Dose/Dosage Forms	Contraindications	Primary Side Effects	Key Monitoring Parameters	Med Pearls
Mechanism of action – possesses astringent properties to dry weeping lesions; works as a skin protectant				
Calamine • Apply as often as necessary • Lotion	Hypersensitivity	Local irritation	Response to therapy	Do not use on open lesions

SUNSCREENS

Definition

A sunburn is a superficial burn that is characterized by edema and erythema in the affected area. Sunburns arise from exposure to sun without adequate skin protection. Prevention of a sunburn includes avoiding sun exposure, wearing protective clothing, and/or applying sunscreen.

Sunscreen

- The American Academy of Dermatology recommends that everyone wear sunscreen any day they will be outside and exposed to sunlight.
- Application of sunscreen should include agents that are:
  - Broad spectrum to cover exposure to both ultraviolet (UV) A and UVB rays
  - Water-resistant
  - Sun Protection Factor (SPF) of 30 or higher, which will block 97% of UVB rays
- Sunscreen terms:
  - SPF is measure of a suncreen's ability to block UVB rays. SPF is a factor that can estimate how much time one can spend in the sun without getting burned. If a burn would normally start in 10 minutes, using a product with an SPF of 30 will allow an exposure of approximately 300 minutes without a burn (30 times longer).
  - Water-resistant sunscreen is effective for up to 40 minutes in water.
  - Very water-resistant sunscreen is effective for up to 80 minutes in water.
- Guidelines for the application of sunscreen:
  - Sunscreen should not be applied to infants ≤6 mo.
  - Use enough sunscreen to coat the skin; may need ≥1 ounce to cover the body.
  - To protect lips, use a lip balm with at least an SPF of 30.
  - Apply 15 minutes before exposure to sun.
  - Reapply every 2 hours or after swimming.
  - Creams are best for application on dry skin and the face.
  - Sprays may be used, but ensure all areas have been covered.
  - Gels may be used for areas covered in hair.
  - Stick formulations are good for administration around the eyes.

LEARNING POINTS

- Vitamins are categorized as fat soluble or water soluble. Fat-soluble vitamins may accumulate and can lead to toxic levels.

- The Dietary Supplement Health and Education Act of 1994 categorizes herbals, vitamins, protein bars, and shakes as dietary supplements. As a result, manufacturers are not required to demonstrate safety, purity, or efficacy of supplements.

- Decongestants are the mainstay of therapy for colds and play an important role with allergic rhinitis.

- Having more than 3 bowel movements per day is considered to be abnormal.

- Constipation can be caused by medications (anticholinergics, analgesics, benzodiazepines, sucralfate, calcium channel blockers, and more), menopause, dehydration, psychologic conditions, depression, and more.

- A 2-week treatment period is typically required to treat athlete's foot.

- Ringworm is a type of tinea infection and can be treated with topical antifungals.

- Treatment of lice infestations should include all members of the affected household.

- Topical administration of hydrocortisone is the mainstay of therapy for atopic dermatitis.

- Treatment of poison ivy is centered on the relief of pruritus.

- Use of sunscreen with an SPF of 30 or higher is recommended for the prevention of skin cancers.

PRACTICE QUESTIONS

1. Which of the following conditions might St. John's wort be used to treat?

    (A) BPH
    (B) Depression
    (C) Diabetes
    (D) Hypertriglyceridemia
    (E) Lactose intolerance

2. Which of the following vitamins is used to treat Wernicke-Korsakoff syndrome?

    (A) Thiamine
    (B) Folic acid
    (C) Pyridoxine
    (D) Riboflavin

3. Which of the following contain dextromethorphan?

    (A) Astepro
    (B) Delsym
    (C) Mucinex Allergy
    (D) ZzzQuil

4. Which of the following should be used for only 3 days to treat nasal congestion?

    (A) Diphenhydramine
    (B) Doxylamine
    (C) Loratadine
    (D) Naphazoline
    (E) Phenylephrine

5. A patient comes in complaining of bilateral knee pain caused by arthritis. He requests an herbal product. Which of the following herbal medications would help the patient's arthritis?

    (A) Echinancea
    (B) Melatonin
    (C) Osteo Bi-Flex
    (D) Saw palmetto

6. Which of the following is considered a second-generation or less sedating antihistamine?

   (A) Brompheniramine
   (B) Chlorpheniramine
   (C) Doxylamine
   (D) Fexofenadine
   (E) Pseudoephedrine

7. Which condition can terbinafine be used to treat?

   (A) Athlete's foot
   (B) Constipation
   (C) Diarrhea
   (D) Lactose intolerance
   (E) Seasonal allergies

8. Which of the following vitamins is/are fat soluble? (Select ALL that apply.)

   (A) Vitamin A
   (B) Vitamin B_6
   (C) Vitamin C
   (D) Vitamin D

9. Which of the following medications used to treat constipation should be used with caution in a patient with impaired renal function?

   (A) Ducolax
   (B) Konsyl
   (C) Milk of Magnesia
   (D) Miralax

10. Which of the following is a stool softener that can be used to treat constipation?

    (A) Colace
    (B) Fibercon
    (C) Metamucil
    (D) Miralax
    (E) Sennakot

ANSWERS AND EXPLANATIONS

1. B

St. John's wort is used to treat depression, as it increases the level of serotonin in the CNS. BPH (A) may be treated with saw palmetto, although meta-analysis data has not shown it to be useful. Diabetes (C) may be managed with the herbal supplement ginseng. Hypertriglyceridemia (D) may be treated with omega-3 fatty acids, and lactose intolerance (E) is treated with Lactaid.

2. A

Thiamine (vitamin B1) is used to treat Wernicke-Korsakoff syndrome. The syndrome occurs in severe thiamine deficiency.

3. B

Delsym contains dextromethorphan and is used a cough suppressant. Mucinex Allergy (A) is a brand name for fexofenadine. Astepro (C) is a nasal antihistamine that contains azelastine. ZzzQuil (diphenhydramine) (D) is an antihistamine used for the treatment of insomnia.

4. D

Nasal decongestants—oxymetazoline and naphazoline—should be used for only 3 days to prevent rebound nasal congestion. Diphenhydramine (A), doxylamine (B), and loratadine (C) are oral antihistamines that can be used for more than 3 days and treat postnasal drip or allergic reactions. Phenylephrine (E) is an oral decongestant that can be used for more than 3 days.

5. C

Osteo Bi-Flex (glucosamine and chondroitin) may be useful in treating arthritis pain by altering cartilage. Echinacea (A) may be used as an immune stimulant. Melatonin (B) may be useful for sleep disorders, and saw palmetto (D) may be used to treat benign prostatic hypertrophy.

6. **D**

Fexofenadine is a second-generation antihistamine and is less sedation that other first-generation antihistamines, including brompheniramine (A) and chlorpheniramine (B). Doxylamine (C) is a first-generation antihistamine used for the treatment of insomnia. Pseudoephedrine (E) is an oral decongestant.

7. **A**

Terbinafine is a topical antifungal used to treat athlete's foot. It should be applied to the affected area daily for at least 2 weeks, even after the condition appears to have cleared.

8. **A, D**

Vitamins A and D are fat soluble. Other fat-soluble vitamins include vitamin E and vitamin K. Fat-soluble vitamins may accumulate and cause toxicities if ingested in large quantities. B and C vitamins are water soluble and are excreted by the kidneys when the body has achieved adequate levels.

9. **C**

Milk of Magnesia should be used with caution in patients with renal impairment due to the potential of magnesium to accumulate in the body. Ducolax (bisacodyl) (A), Konsyl (psyllium) (B), and Miralax (PEG3350) (D), can all be used in patients with renal impairment.

10. **A**

Colace is a stool softener and is used to prevent and treat constipation. Fibercon (B) and Metamucil (C) are bulk-forming laxatives that should be taken with a full glass of water. Miralax (D) is an osmotic laxative, and Sennakot (E) is a stimulant laxative.

Pharmaceutical Sciences, Calculations, and Biostatistics Clinical Trial Design

Pharmaceutics

23

This chapter covers the following:

- **Physical pharmacy**
- **Pharmaceutical dosage forms**

 Suggested Study Time: **1.5 hours**

Pharmaceutics encompasses a number of disciplines, including dosage form design, biopharmaceutics, and pharmacokinetics. This chapter focuses on dosage form design (drug dosage forms and the physical and chemical properties that allow these products to be manufactured).

A key concept to keep in mind is that patients don't simply take drugs, they take dosage forms. The active ingredient is not the only substance involved.

PHYSICAL PHARMACY

Physical pharmacy is a branch of pharmaceutics that deals principally with the physical and chemical properties of drugs. It is a highly mathematical subject, but the NAPLEX is not concerned with these aspects except as they relate to chemical kinetics. As you study, focus mainly on how specific properties of drugs make particular types of formulations more or less suitable. A simple example would be antibiotic suspensions that arrive at the pharmacy in dry powder form. The reason that they arrive in dry powder form is that many antibiotics are chemically unstable in liquid formulations; if the water is added only at the time of dispensing, the drug will remain effective long enough for the patient to finish the bottle. If the product were manufactured as a liquid, the drug would be degraded by the time the bottle was processed, shipped, and stored in the pharmacy prior to dispensing.

Preformulation

Preformulation allows the company to make the best decisions about how to formulate the drug into a usable dosage form. Preformulation is an important stage of drug development where the pharmaceutical company characterizes the following physicochemical properties of the drug.

Solubility and Lipophilicity

Every drug must be solubilized before it can be absorbed by the body. A drug must possess at least some aqueous solubility in order to be effective; poorly soluble compounds show incomplete and unpredictable absorption. However, at least some lipophilicity must also be present, as drugs must be able to pass through biological membranes in order to reach their sites of action which are often intracellular. Salts or esters of drugs may be formed to ↑ or ↓ the solubility, depending on the characteristics needed in a particular case. For example, the benzathine salt of penicillin G has a very low solubility, which causes the drug to dissolve slowly after injection, which prolongs the duration of action.

Dissolution rate is improved by ↓ particle size, which ↑ the surface area of the drug that comes into contact with the body fluids. A more in-depth treatment of factors that influence dissolution rate and absorption is contained in the Biopharmaceutics and Drug Disposition chapter.

Ionization Behavior

Ionization behavior is one of the most important factors in drug development. Most drugs are administered as a salt and therefore carry a positive or negative charge in solution. That is, when such a drug goes into solution, a fraction of the molecules dissociate into ions (i.e., charged compounds). The proportion of ionized to unionized drug is very important because the two behave very differently in the body:

- Ionized drug: More soluble, but cannot cross body membranes
- Unionized drug: Less soluble, but can cross body membranes

Salts are often preferred over the weak acid or base because they dissolve more quickly, are more stable during storage, and are easier to crystallize and handle during processing. Different salt forms may have very different properties, and pharmaceutical companies may intentionally modify drugs into more useful salts for a given purpose. Calcium salts, for example, show wide variation in absorption and possible efficacy.

Remember: Until the drug is absorbed across the body membranes it cannot get to the site of action, but it needs to go into solution before that can happen. The equilibrium between the more soluble ionized form and the more absorbable unionized form of the drug is crucial.

The Henderson-Hasselbalch equation (below) can be used to calculate exact ratios of ionized to unionized drug; however, the "Ionization Behavior of Weak Acids and Bases" table below will give you a rough estimate of the ionization behavior of weak acids and bases when comparing the pH of the absorption site to the pK$_a$. In most cases, you will be able to obtain a sufficiently accurate answer by using the table instead of the actual equation, saving valuable exam time.

$$pH = pK_a + \log \frac{[Salt]}{[Acid]} \text{ or } pH = pK_a + \log \frac{[ionized]}{[unionized]} \text{ if the drug is an acid}$$

$$pH = pK_a + \log \frac{[Base]}{[Salt]} \text{ or } pH = pK_a + \log \frac{[unionized]}{ionized} \text{ if the drug is a base}$$

Ionization Behavior of Weak Acids and Bases

	Acidic Drug	Basic Drug
pH > pK$_a$	More ionized	More unionized
pH = pK$_a$	Equal	Equal
pH < pK$_a$	More unionized	More ionized
Note that for pH more than 2 units away from pK$_a$, expect almost complete ionization/unionization.		

The acid or base form is the unionized form and salt form is the ionized form of the corresponding acid or base. Accordingly, ionized and unionized can be substituted in the above equations in order to calculate the amount of ionization or unionization at a particular pH value. To identify which equation to use, you must first know if the drug in question is an acid or a base.

It is impossible to tell if a drug is an acid or a base by looking only at the pK$_a$. Some acids have a higher pK$_a$ (phenytoin = 8.3) than do some bases (morphine = 8.0). You can tell if a drug is an acid or base, however, by what type of salt is used in its formulation. Weak acids form sodium, calcium, potassium, or other cationic salts; weak bases form hydrochloride or other anionic salts.

For example, warfarin is formulated as the sodium salt. Therefore, warfarin is an acid. The positively charged sodium ion is used to displace the proton (i.e., hydronium ion or positively charged hydrogen) from the proton-donating acid in its formulation. In solution, warfarin disassociates from sodium into a negatively charged molecule (i.e., ionized form). If the solution is acidic (e.g., gastric fluid), a proton is likely to be donated back to the negatively charged warfarin to produce the uncharged drug (unionized form). Of course, this is a dynamic state in which the drug is going back and forth between the ionized and unionized form based on the pH of the environment. Determining this ratio provides information about the drug's solubility and its ability to cross biological membranes in any given environment. This is the power of the Henderson-Hasselbalch equation and of the table presented.

Stability

Physical, chemical, and microbiological stability are all very important in preformulation studies. While physical instability does not generally result in ↓ drug concentrations, it can lead to problems with dose uniformity and pharmaceutical elegance (eg., the mottled appearance that can develop in tablets over time, or the formation of a nonsuspendable sediment in a liquid dosage form). Polymorphism and anhydrous-to-hydrate conversions can be considered types of physical instability and are discussed in greater detail in the following section.

Chemical instability does result in loss of drug or excipient molecules. This can lead to either undertreatment, when a patient does not receive the full dose intended, or toxicity from toxic degradation products. In some cases, chemical instability can lead to microbiological instability if a preservative degrades and can no longer protect the formulation from bacterial or fungal overgrowth. The main types of degradation that occur in drug products are:

- Hydrolysis: Occurs in presence of water; typically no change in formulation appearance

- Oxidation: Occurs in presence of atmospheric oxygen; often results in the formation of insoluble precipitates or colored compounds

- Photochemical decomposition: Occurs on exposure to light; often results in the formation of colored compounds

Temperature, humidity, and light often hasten the degradation process, and drug companies use this fact to perform accelerated stability testing and to assign product expiration dates. Finished products must retain 90% of the labeled dose during their shelf life. Studies are performed at extreme storage conditions, and mathematical equations are used to extrapolate the degradation rate constants at normal conditions of storage. A good estimate, however, is that every 10°C ↑ in temperature doubles the rate constant.

Most drugs degrade by either zero- or first-order kinetics (see "Rate and Half-Life Equations" table). Drugs following zero-order degradation have a constant degradation rate that is independent of the drug concentration. First-order degradation, however, is concentration-dependent; therefore, the amount of drug degrading per unit of time is not constant. Suspensions degrade by pseudo–zero-order kinetics, because only the drug molecules that are actually in solution are available for degradation. The concentration of drug in solution is in equilibrium with that in suspension, and the concentration of drug in solution is maintained at a constant level; suspended particles go into solution to replace the degraded drug. This continues as long as some solid is still present.

Rate and Half-Life Equations

Order	Rate Equation		Half-Life Equation
Zero	$C = C_0 - K_0 t$		$t_{1/2} = 0.5 \dfrac{C_0}{K_0}$
First	$\log C = \log C_0 - \dfrac{K_0 t}{2.303}$	$C = C_0 e^{-Kt}$	$t_{1/2} = \dfrac{\ln 2}{K_1} = \dfrac{0.693}{K_1}$

Where C is equal to concentration, C_0 is the initial concentration, K_0 is the zero-order degradation constant, t is time, $t_{1/2}$ is half-life, and K_1 is the first-order degradation constant.

With equations it is possible to calculate the concentration (or amount) of drug at any given time if its degradation rate constant is known. It is not, however, useful to memorize the first-order equation for the NAPLEX because the calculator provided does not include the exponential function. Therefore, the only way to calculate the concentration (or amount) of drug at any given time is to estimate the amount by understanding what the degradation constants represent.

The first thing to do is identify if the question is related to a zero-order or first-order process. If a graphical representation is presented for any problem, a zero-order process will be linear with a constant degradation over time. Therefore, the units for zero-order degradation constants are in terms of amount per unit time (e.g., mg/hr). First-order degradation will be a nonlinear decline that is asymptotic to the x-axis on a graph similar to a drug concentration-time curve seen in pharmacokinetics. The units of the first-order degradation constant are in terms of time^{-1} (e.g., yr^{-1}).

After identifying whether the degradation process is zero-order or first-order, the second step is to estimate how much drug is remaining (or degraded) over some amount of time. This is simple for zero-order processes because a constant amount is being lost over time. For example, if the starting amount of drug is 1,000 mg and 10 mg per year is degraded (i.e., $K_0 = 10$ mg/yr), after 10 years it will have lost 100 mg of drug and have 900 mg remaining. Many zero-order degradation problems can be rationalized without memorizing the equations in the table.

The estimation of amount of drug remaining following first-order degradation is not as straightforward and requires an in-depth understanding of the first-order degradation constant. The degradation constant is in terms of time^{-1}, as mentioned. This represents a percentage of drug lost per unit of time that is being presented. For example, a K_1 of 0.2 yr^{-1} indicates that 20% of the drug is lost every year. Thus, if the starting amount of drug is 1,000 mg of drug, 20% will be lost of that in the first year, or 200 mg, leaving 800 mg. The key in these estimations is to remember that in year 2, the starting amount is 800 mg because 200 mg was lost in year 1. To calculate the amount of drug lost after 2 years, subtract 20% of 800 mg (i.e., 160 mg) from 800 mg. Therefore, the amount of drug remaining after 2 years will be 800 mg minus 160 mg, for a total of 640 mg. This process must be repeated for year 3 and so on.

Solid-State Properties

Because most drugs are given as solid-dosage forms, many properties specific to the solid state are important in pharmacy. These properties are discussed in further detail below.

Crystallization

Solids are present in crystalline or amorphous forms, or as a combination of the two. Crystalline forms show fixed geometric patterns, whereas the atoms in amorphous solids are randomly placed (as they would be in a liquid). The most important things to remember about crystalline versus amorphous solids for the purposes of the NAPLEX are as follows:

- Crystalline solids have definite melting points, whereas amorphous solids melt over a range of temperatures.
- Amorphous solids are more soluble than the corresponding crystalline forms.
- Solids tend to revert to the more stable crystalline form on storage.

Solvates are crystalline structures that contain trapped solvent; when the solvent is water, they are called hydrates. Typically, hydrates are less soluble than their anhydrous counterparts, whereas solvates are more soluble.

Polymorphism

Polymorphs are one of several crystalline structures that have the same chemical formula but show different physical properties. The properties they exhibit can vary substantially, however, and this leads to pharmaceutical companies patenting different polymorphic forms based on variations in solubility, bioavailability, solid-state stability, or processing behavior (such as improved powder flow or tablet compaction).

Metastable polymorphs will revert to the most stable form over time; in some instances, however, the metastable form might have more favorable properties than the stable form (e.g., better solubility). In those cases, even though it is not the most stable form, it may be the best one to market, provided the stability is at least acceptable.

The classic example of excipient polymorphism is cocoa butter, which is often used in suppository and troche formulations. Cocoa butter exists in four polymorphs, but only the β-form is stable. When cocoa butter is heated above 34°C, some of the β-form converts to unstable polymorphs. The unstable polymorphs are liquid at room temperature. The cocoa butter is never able to remain solid outside the refrigerator. This explains why chocolate or cocoa butter that has been overheated does not fully solidify when cooled.

Another pharmacy-related example of polymorphism is ritonavir, a protease inhibitor used to treat human immunodeficiency virus. Initially, it was thought to exist in only one polymorphic form, with relatively poor aqueous solubility. It was marketed in a soft gelatin capsule, which contained an ethanol/water cosolvent system. After drug approval, several batches failed quality control tests. It was discovered that a second polymorphic form with even lower solubility had formed, causing the drug to precipitate out of the cosolvent system. The product had to be reformulated to include Kolliphor (polyethoxylated castor oil) as a solubilizing agent.

Rheology

Rheology is the science of flow properties, which is especially important when discussing liquid and semisolid dosage forms. During manufacturing, rheology is an important concept when mixing and packaging materials. Once the products reach the consumer, the rheology governs the removal of the product from its container, whether by pouring, extruding from a tube, or passing through a syringe needle.

Viscosity and fluidity are two common terms associated with rheology. Viscosity refers to the resistance offered when part of the liquid flows past another part; fluidity is essentially the opposite. Viscous liquids are thick and slow-moving; fluid liquids are thin and flow more readily.

Rheological behavior is divided into two main types: Newtonian flow and non-Newtonian flow. Newtonian materials do not change viscosity with changes in stirring speed; they do, however, become less viscous when heated. True solutions and pure liquid compounds such as water and oil are examples of Newtonian materials. Non-Newtonian materials do change viscosity when stirring speed changes. Three types of non-Newtonian behavior exist: dilatant, plastic, and pseudoplastic. Dilatant materials become more viscous when stirred more rapidly, which can cause manufacturing equipment to malfunction. Plastic and pseudoplastic materials become more fluid when stirred. Plastic flow is best illustrated by a nonpharmacy example: tomato ketchup. It doesn't pour until shaken enough for contacts between adjacent particles to be broken but then acts much like a Newtonian material. Concentrated suspensions show similar behavior. Pseudoplastic flow differs in that flow can start immediately on stirring or shaking; the harder the bottle is shaken, the more fluid the material becomes. Polymer solutions often exhibit pseudoplastic flow.

Thixotropic products are a special case and are actually the ideal situation for pharmaceutical suspensions. They are viscous at rest but become fluid when shaken. Because of this, the suspension settles only slowly, but the liquid pours easily when shaken. After shaking stops, thixotropic products gradually become viscous again. Both plastic and pseudoplastic materials can show thixotropic behavior.

Testing

Numerous quality assurance tests exist for dosage forms, though only four will be discussed here. The four tests used for tablets and sometimes capsules are as follows: friability, hardness, disintegration, and dissolution testing.

Friability and hardness testing evaluate the ability of tablets to withstand manufacturing, packaging, and shipping. Hardness testing measures the force required to cause a tablet to break, and friability testing measures what percentage weight of a tablet is lost after it is tumbled for a specified amount of time in a friabilator. Tablets that are too soft or fragile will suffer too much damage during manufacturing and shipping to be useful, even if they have excellent dissolution and absorption behavior. On the other hand, tablets that are too hard may have poor disintegration, dissolution, and drug absorption.

Disintegration testing is performed by placing tablets into mesh-bottomed cylinders that are immersed in a solution and agitated at a specified rate. The tablets are considered to have disintegrated when the particles are small enough to fall through the mesh screen. It is not a good measure of in vivo behavior, but is a frequently used quality-control measure for tablets.

A better measure of *in vivo* behavior is dissolution testing. Here, the tablets or capsules are immersed in appropriate dissolution liquids (typically, simulated gastric fluid) and samples are taken at specific time points to determine how much of the drug has gone into solution. While this test is still not a true predictor of *in vivo* behavior—because it does not demonstrate absorption—it is an improvement over disintegration testing, as the drug must go into solution with body fluids before being absorbed.

PHARMACEUTICAL DOSAGE FORMS

What things need to be considered when a drug company designs a dosage form for a particular drug? Some of the primary considerations are:

- Nature of the illness
- Manner in which the illness is treated
- Age of the patient
- Condition of the patient
- Stability of the drug

Suppose a patient suffers from motion sickness and is getting ready to go on a cruise. Would a tablet be the best dosage form in which their antinausea medication should be formulated? Probably not, as there is a risk that they could vomit and lose the medication before it had a chance to be absorbed by the body. For this reason, scopolamine is formulated into transdermal patches for motion sickness.

Some drugs can be used to treat different conditions based on their formulation and route of administration. An example is the antifungal product, terbinafine. It is given as cream for surface conditions such as athlete's foot, and as tablets for more deep-seated fungal infections of the toenails and fingernails.

Age of the patient plays a large role in development of dosage forms. Young children and the elderly are much more likely than adults and teenagers are to have difficulty swallowing. Therefore, most medications for small children are marketed as easy-to-swallow dosage forms such as liquids and chewable or rapid-dissolve tablets. Other groups of patients may also lack the ability and willingness to swallow. Patients with psychiatric conditions will often refuse to swallow medication, and rapid-dissolve formulations or injections may be required to ensure that they receive treatment. Severely debilitated or comatose patients cannot swallow and may receive medicine through nasogastric tubes or by injection.

Oral Delivery: Solids

Solid dosage forms are the most commonly prescribed—over 80% of dosage forms are tablets or capsules. These products are convenient for the patient and are the preferred route for giving nonemergency medications. Some benefits of solid dosage forms are that they are already divided into accurate doses and are easy to handle. Taste is generally less of an issue than with liquid dosage forms and can be masked by coating the product, as long as the dosage is not designed to be chewed or dissolved in the mouth.

Solid products, however, are not perfect. If a very rapid response is needed, traditional tablets and capsules are not the best option because they take time to dissolve and become absorbed by the body. If formulated improperly, the absorption of the active ingredient(s) may be irregular or incomplete.

Traditional / Immediate Release

The simplest type of solid dosage form is the powder. Powders taken orally have a few advantages: They are absorbed more rapidly than tablets and capsules because they do not have to undergo a disintegration step, they are easier to swallow than large tablets and capsules, and they are more chemically stable than liquids. It is easier to give large doses of drug in a powder than in a tablet. One gram of drug plus excipients is much easier to stir into water and swallow than it would be if formulated into a tablet.

One of the main drawbacks of powder as a dosage form is that it is very difficult to mask the taste or smell of unpleasant drugs when they are given in powder form. They are also highly inconvenient to handle and, if provided in bulk containers (such as Metamucil), may be subject to dose inaccuracy. Therefore, potent drugs should not be given as powders. If a drug is hygroscopic, it also should not be formulated into a powder dosage form as it will pick up too much moisture from the air. Finally, contrary to expectations, powders can be more expensive to produce than other solid dosage forms; there is a fairly substantial risk of explosion when working with large quantities of powder, and special handling equipment may be necessary to offset this risk.

Granules have many of the same advantages and disadvantages as powders. The primary difference between these two dosage forms is that granules are prepared agglomerations of smaller particles. They behave as single particles but are irregularly shaped and have a larger particle size than the associated powders. Granules therefore flow better than the powders and are more easily wetted by fluids, whether in manufacturing, in administration of the drug, or in the body. A simple example of the differences in properties of granulated versus powdered solids is sugar. Granulated (common table) sugar flows much more readily and dissolves easily in coffee or other liquids. Powdered sugar tends to clump, not flow freely, and dissolve slowly.

Granules are used more as a component of tablets and capsules than they are as dosage forms in their own right. They can be made by wet or dry methods. Wet granulation involves forming a dough of powder and liquid, pressing that dough through a mesh screen to form appropriately sized particles, and drying. In dry granulation, dry powders are compacted together, without the presence of liquid, into ribbons or oversized tablets that are then ground to size.

Capsules are a much more frequently dispensed type of solid dosage form and contain drug and excipients enclosed inside a gelatin, starch, or cellulose shell. Like tablets, capsules have many advantages over powders and granules. Since capsules are essentially unit-of-use products, they have excellent dose accuracy and the ability to mask the taste and smell of unpleasant drugs. They are also easy to administer, as the active ingredient does not need to be measured out. It is also easy to formulate products with multiple active ingredients. One advantage that capsules have over tablets is that they can be extemporaneously prepared in the pharmacy in instances where the prescriber requests a nonstandard dose of drug.

Capsules do have some disadvantages. They are permeable to moisture and may not be a suitable dosage form for moisture-sensitive drugs. They are also not suitable for water- or alcohol-based preparations, as those bases would dissolve the capsule shell. Some liquids, however, can be dispensed in capsules. Oil or nonaqueous water-miscible liquids such as polyethylene glycol (PEG) 400 can be used to dissolve or suspend drugs and vitamins that are then placed into soft gelatin capsules. Finally, gelatin may be inappropriate for certain patient populations who wish to avoid animal (particularly pork-based) products. In those cases, vegetarian capsule shells made of starch or cellulose may be substituted. Many dietary supplements and herbal products are manufactured in such capsules for this reason.

Tablets are the most frequently prescribed dosage form and are preferred for many reasons. In addition to the advantages they share with capsules, they are easy to make in a variety of shapes and colors, aiding in product identification. They are also inexpensive and quick to produce, especially when compared to most other dosage forms.

In order to make a drug into a tablet, however, the drug needs to be compressible. In other words, when force is placed on the powders in tableting equipment, they must be able to stick together sufficiently to make a durable tablet. Not all powders possess this property. If only small amounts of noncompressible active ingredient are needed, a compressible diluent can be used. Failing that, some materials can be granulated to improve compressibility. This does not work in all cases; if the material remains noncompressible, it may be best to formulate the product as a capsule instead of a tablet.

The different types of immediate-release tablets are described in the following table.

Types of Immediate-Release Tablets

Type of Tablet	Key Features	Example
Compressed	All ingredients contained in a single layer; designed to be swallowed whole; may or may not be coated	Various
Multi-compressed	Contain separate layers of drug, for various reasons (incompatibility of drugs, immediate- plus extended-release in the same tablet, etc.)	Mucinex (guaifenesin)
Chewable	Disintegrate rapidly when chewed; usually mannitol-based (pleasant mouth feel, sweet taste)	Children's vitamins Dilantin Infatabs (phenytoin)
Buccal	Dissolve in cheek cavity; may be designed to erode slowly or quickly	Fentora (fentanyl)
Sublingual	Dissolve under the tongue; erode quickly and are absorbed rapidly	Nitrostat (nitroglycerin)
Effervescent	Contain drug that dissolves rapidly after adding to water; results in carbonated liquid that masks taste	Alka-Seltzer

Many immediate-release tablets are coated. This process can help mask unpleasant tastes and odors, as well as improve the appearance of the tablet, protect the drug from the atmosphere, and allow it to be swallowed more easily. The two types of coating used for immediate-release products are sugar and film coatings. Sugar coating produces a very attractive tablet that is typically much larger than the uncoated product, due to the several layers of sugar, color, flavor, and waterproofing shellac added. The process is very time consuming, and batch variations are common in the coated tablets. The coatings are applied manually in coating pans, not mechanically, by highly skilled personnel. Film coatings are much thinner, and leave a coat of opaque, colored polymer on the surface of the tablet. Although they are customarily machine-applied, requiring less skill in application, the following coating defects are possible:

- Picking and peeling: Film fragments flake from the tablet surface
- Orange-peel effect: Coating leaves rough surface on the tablet
- Mottling: Coating has uneven color distribution
- Bridging: Score lines or logos present on tablet are filled in by coating
- Erosion: Coating solution is in contact with tablet for too long and disfigures the core

Extended Release

Extended-release oral products maintain more constant blood levels of the drug than do immediate-release products. Therefore, patients can take the drugs less often (once or twice a day instead of up to four times a day), which improves adherence. Additionally, adverse effects are usually fewer and less severe with extended-release oral products, as the concentration of the drug in the blood does not vary as widely from peak and trough as much as with immediate-release products. However, there is a risk of dose-dumping with extended-release oral products, especially if the patient chews the medication instead of swallowing it whole.

Drugs that are best suited for extended-release formulations are usually given in fairly small doses, as the practical limit for the amount of drug to be contained in an individual tablet or capsule is 500 mg. The drug should also not have either a particularly fast or slow rate of absorption. Drugs that absorb too quickly require too large a dose, and drugs that absorb slowly are inherently long-acting and an extended-release formulation is not needed. Because of the risk of dose-dumping, the drug should have a good margin of safety and be uniformly absorbed from the gastrointestinal (GI) tract. The different types of extended-release tablets are described in the following table.

Types of Extended-Release Tablets

Type of Tablet	Key Features	Example
Enteric coating	Coating remains intact until drug reaches small intestine; can protect drug from stomach acid and enzymes, or can protect stomach from irritating drugs	Enteric-coated aspirin
Diffusion-controlled reservoir system	Beads or pellets are coated with polymer that releases drug at varying speeds; may involve several release rates	Progestasert (Progesterone)
Diffusion-controlled matrix system	Drug is mixed into an inert plastic matrix; drug dissolves and leaves matrix	Glucotrol XL (glipizide)
Wax	Remains intact in GI tract and is eliminated in feces (inform patient that this is normal)	Desoxyn (methamphetamine)
Hydrophilic	Water causes matrix to swell; drug diffuses through gel layer, and may also be released as matrix erodes	Slo-Niacin (niacin)
Dissolution-controlled system	Rate of release affected by dissolution and tablet or bead erosion (some hydrophilic matrices fall into this category as well as diffusion-controlled)	Cardizem CD (diltiazem)

Types of Extended-Release Tablets *(cont'd)*

Type of Tablet	Key Features	Example
Ion-exchange resin	pH conditions of GI tract cause drug to be released from resin	Floxin (ofloxacin)
Osmotically controlled system	Tablet pulls water into system, then releases drug at controlled rate by osmotic pressure; tablet shell eliminated in feces (inform patient that this is normal)	Glucotrol XL (glipizide)
Complex formation	Drug is combined with other agents, forming a slowly soluble chemical complex	Rynatan allergy products

Rapid Release

Rapid-release products are becoming more important, particularly in the over-the-counter (OTC) industry. Because they can be taken without water, rapid-release products are convenient for the patient, and have a rapid onset of action. However, some of the products are very soft, and thereby may require expensive protective packaging. The various types of rapid-release solid dosage forms are described in the following table.

Types of Rapid-Release Solid Dosage Forms

Type of Product	Key Features	Example
Tablets	Product can contain large doses of drug	Claritin RediTabs (loratidine)
Strips	Dissolves before children can spit it out; cannot put large doses of drug into product	Zuplenz (ondansetron)
Lollipops	Absorbed through buccal mucosa	Actiq (fentanyl)

Oral Delivery: Liquids

Oral liquid dosage forms have the same advantages as other oral products, with the additional advantage of being easy to swallow for small children and others who cannot easily swallow solid dosage forms. Several disadvantages exist as well. Liquids are less portable and convenient than solids. Incorrect doses are much more likely, as patients or caregivers could measure using an inappropriate measuring device (i.e., not all spoons are standard size), and product may be spilled before being consumed. Also, taste can be a large issue, as more of the drug will reach a patient's taste buds than with the same drug in a tablet or capsule.

Solvents

Water is the most common solvent for pharmaceutical products; purified water prepared by distillation, reverse osmosis, or ion-exchange treatment is acceptable for oral use. Other commonly used solvents include ethyl alcohol, glycerin, sorbitol, propylene glycol, and some edible oils. Typically, solvents other than water are included to improve solubility and, in some cases, add sweetness to the final product (e.g. glycerin, sorbitol, and propylene glycol). Only small amounts of sorbitol and glycerin should be present in a given dose of liquid, as they may act as osmotic laxatives in higher quantities.

Types of Liquids

Single-phase liquid dosage forms are all variants of the solution. One or more soluble substances are dissolved in one or more solvents, including water. Therefore, the drug(s) must be water-soluble and stable in aqueous solution. The presence of other excipients in varying amounts results in the following designations:

Types of Single-Phase Liquid Dosage Forms

Type of Product	Key Features	Examples
Syrups	• Contain sugar or sugar substitutes • Contain little or no alcohol • Thickeners improve mouth feel and physically conceal the drug from taste buds • Taste pleasant; often used with children	Various cough/cold preparations
Elixirs	• By definition alcoholic, but some nonalcoholic commercial products are mislabeled as elixirs • Slightly sweet; artificial sweetener usually used since sucrose is not very soluble in alcohol • Less viscous than syrups	• Diphenhydramine • Phenobarbital • Digoxin
Tinctures	• 15–80% alcohol • Usually consist of drug extracted from plant material • Unpleasant taste; not commonly used today	• Opium tincture (1,000 mg morphine/100 mL) • Paregoric (camphorated opium tincture; 40 mg morphine/100 mL)
Spirits	• Alcoholic solutions of aromatic or volatile substances • High concentration of alcohol • Active ingredient may precipitate out when added to aqueous preparations	Flavoring agents
Aromatic waters	• Aqueous solutions of volatile oils • Very dilute	Flavoring and perfuming agents
Fluid extracts	• Similar to, but more potent than, tinctures • Used as drug source, not as dosage form	Herbal medications

Multiphase liquids, such as suspensions and emulsions, are more complicated than single-phase liquids. They still possess most of the advantages and disadvantages of other liquid dosage forms but have the additional disadvantage of being nonhomogenous. Because of this, suspensions and emulsions should always have "Shake Well" labels attached.

Suspensions are multiphase products that contain finely divided solid particles distributed through the liquid phase. They can be used on the skin, used in the ear or eye, or given by intramuscular (IM) or subcutaneous (subcut) injection, but are most commonly given by mouth. Some advantages exist over single-phase liquids. Drugs that have an unpleasant flavor are preferred as suspensions, since the drug does not interact with the taste buds as much when it is not dissolved. Also, drugs that have poor stability in water do not degrade as readily in suspension as they do in solution.

The primary concern with making suspensions is to have a particle size that is small enough to remain suspended in the dispersion medium of choice while not being so small that the particles start to attract each other and form clumps that will not resuspend. This can be achieved by two techniques, used separately or in combination: 1) Use of structured vehicles; and 2) Controlled flocculation.

- Structured vehicles: ↑ viscosity and slow the sedimentation of suspended particles. These natural and synthetic polymer solutions are often used (cellulose gels, acacia, bentonite).
- Controlled flocculation: Add materials that promote loose aggregation of suspended particles, but keep their surfaces apart by charge or interaction of polymer chains. These particles will settle, but loosely, and resuspend easily.

Emulsions are dispersions that consist of nonmiscible liquids. The dispersed phase is also called the internal phase, and the dispersion medium is called the external phase. These products are very thermodynamically unstable and require an emulsifying agent to keep them combined properly. A good nonpharmacy example is mayonnaise. Lemon juice or vinegar serves as the external phase, and the lecithin from the egg yolk emulsifies the product so that the oil that is added does not separate out.

Only oil-in-water (O/W) emulsions are used for oral dosage forms, as water needs to be in the external phase to be palatable to the patient; otherwise, all the patient would taste would be the oil in the outer portion of the product. Topical products can be either O/W or water in oil (W/O). When prepared in the pharmacy, emulsions are made by rapid stirring in a mortar and pestle, shaking in a bottle (though only with reasonably thin oils), using a hand blender, or by heating the phases separately and then mixing them. Three types of emulsifiers are used, depending on the product being made:

- Surfactants: Contain hydrophilic and hydrophobic portions, which remain at the interface of the oil, and water phases to stabilize the product. Often used in combination.
- Hydrophilic colloids: Water-soluble polymers that form a film around oil droplets in O/W emulsions. Tend to ↑ viscosity of the product.
- Finely divided solids: Form a film of particles around the droplets of the dispersed phase, but allow interaction with the dispersion medium as well.

The exact quantity of surfactant needed can be determined by the hydrophilic-lipophilic balance (HLB) system. The HLB is a measure of the degree to which a given surfactant is hydrophilic or lipophilic. This number runs anywhere from 0 to 20. A value less than 10 indicates that the given surfactant is lipid soluble, and a value greater than 10 indicates that the given surfactant is water soluble. Surfactants and the ingredients to be emulsified have been assigned experimentally determined HLB numbers, and the exact amount of emulsifier needed can be determined algebraically if a formula has not already been determined.

Topical Delivery

Topical products are used for three primary reasons: 1) to protect injured areas of the skin from the environment; 2) to hydrate the skin; and 3) to apply medication to the skin for local effect. In some cases, drug may reach the blood supply and be systemically absorbed which is not desired with topical delivery. Systemic absorption of a drug applied to the skin is known as transdermal drug delivery and is discussed later in this chapter.

Powders and liquids are used as topical delivery systems, though not as frequently as semisolid preparations. Of the types of liquids mentioned in the oral delivery section, solutions, suspensions, and emulsions may all be used topically. Two external-use–only liquid products are:

- Liniments: Alcoholic solutions used to irritate the skin and relieve more deep-seated pain or discomfort (Heet, Absorbine Jr), or oleaginous emulsions used as emollients or protective agents. Liniments are applied by rubbing and are not suitable for application to bruised or broken skin.
- Collodions: Contain pyroxylin in an alcohol/ether base that evaporates, leaving an occlusive film on the skin; used to hold edges of incised wounds together.

Ointment Bases

Five types of ointment bases exist:

- Hydrocarbon/oleaginous: Greasy, petroleum-based products used for emollient effect (Vaseline, petrolatum)
- Anhydrous absorption: Greasy products that form W/O emulsions when aqueous solutions are added; can be used to incorporate solutions into an otherwise lipophilic base (hydrophilic petrolatum, anhydrous lanolin)
- W/O emulsion: Similar to anhydrous absorption bases, but already contain some water (hydrous lanolin, cold cream)
- O/W emulsion (water-removable): Creamy emulsions that are easily washed from the skin; may be diluted with water to form lotions (hydrophilic ointment, Lubriderm)
- Water-soluble: Greaseless, water-washable bases containing no oleaginous compounds; cannot add large amounts of water or will soften too much (PEG ointment)

Particular bases are chosen on the basis of the desired rate of drug release, stability of the drug in the base, the need for an occlusive barrier, and ability to wash the ointment easily from the skin. When preparing ointments in a pharmacy, if a levigating agent is needed, it should be compatible with the type of ointment base used. For instance, mineral oil will mix well with any ointment base containing hydrocarbons (all except water-soluble bases). Water-miscible liquids such as glycerin and PEG will be more appropriate when using bases that contain water, such as water-soluble or emulsion bases. If solutions need to be incorporated into an ointment base, acceptable options are anhydrous absorption base or either type of emulsion base.

Other topical product definitions are:

- **Creams:** Terminology often used to describe emulsion bases; soft, cosmetically acceptable topical products
- **Pastes:** Very thick semisolids containing at least 20% solids by weight
- **Gels:** Jelly-like dispersions that are water-soluble, water-washable, and greaseless

Rectal, Vaginal, and Urethral Delivery

Rectal, vaginal, and urethral dosage forms such as suppositories and enemas are less frequently prescribed than many other types of dosage form, but they do have an important place in certain types of therapy. They can be useful for local therapy in rectal or vaginal conditions, or when protecting susceptible drugs from GI tract degradation or first-pass metabolism.

Rectal conditions amenable to local therapy with suppositories, enemas, or other rectally administered dosage forms include hemorrhoids, rectal itching, ulcerative colitis, and constipation.

Rectal suppositories can also be used to administer drug for systemic absorption. Usually, this is done when the patient cannot or will not take medication by mouth. Infants, small children, and severely debilitated patients cannot easily swallow. Patients with severe nausea (as a symptom of a condition such as gastroenteritis or migraine, or as a side effect of chemotherapy or anesthesia) cannot hold down oral antiemetics long enough for the medication to take effect; prochlorperazine can be given rectally to avoid this problem.

Vaginal dosing, including suppositories, creams, and other dosage forms, is usually used for local effect, either for treatment of local infections (clindamycin and various azole antifungals) or for contraception (nonoxynol-9). Hormone replacement may also be administered via vaginal cream or suppository, and will have local effects on the vaginal mucosa. Systemic absorption may be seen with higher estrogen doses.

Urethral suppositories are seldom seen. Alprostadil was approved in 1997 for use in erectile dysfunction (as Muse urethral suppository) but is not commonly used now that oral medications are available and more readily acceptable to patients.

The most common bases used in suppositories are fatty bases similar to cocoa butter that melt at body temperature, and water-soluble bases such as PEG and glycerinated gelatin bases that dissolve slowly in body fluids. Fatty bases are more soothing but do not mix well with body fluids and have a tendency to leak from body orifices. For this reason, they are not suitable for vaginal or urethral delivery. Water-soluble bases can be irritating to the mucosa because they take up water from the area. They are frequently used for vaginal or urethral delivery, but seldom for rectal. Different bases release drugs differently based on the water/oil partition coefficient of the base and of the drug. Lipophilic drugs are released slowly from oleaginous bases but more quickly from water-soluble bases. Hydrophilic drugs, on the other hand, are released extremely quickly from fatty bases but more slowly from water-soluble bases.

Pulmonary Delivery

The lung is an increasingly popular delivery site and is no longer reserved only for pulmonary conditions. The lungs possess a large surface area for drug absorption and a good blood supply that bypasses first-pass metabolism. Even though the first inhaled insulin (Exubera) was a market failure, it proved that large-molecule drugs could be delivered effectively via the lung for systemic use. Continued improvement in delivery devices should cause the field of pulmonary delivery to grow rapidly.

Metered-Dose Inhalers

Metered-dose inhalers (MDIs) are primarily used to deliver medications, including bronchodilators and corticosteroids, for the treatment of asthma and chronic obstructive pulmonary disease. While MDIs are portable and able to deliver precise quantities of potent drugs, many patients have difficulty using them properly. MDIs have undergone rapid changes in the last few years, due in part to federal legislation restricting the use of chlorofluorocarbon propellants due to their link to ozone depletion. Beginning in 2009, medical device exemptions will no longer be allowed for these propellants, so companies have redesigned their products as either hydrofluoroalkane propellant devices or dry-powder inhalers (DPIs). Significant engineering challenges were involved in converting products to use these new delivery devices.

Dry-Powder Inhalers

DPIs avoid some of the difficulties with MDIs. They are generally easier for patients to use correctly, since the device can be primed before use and the patient does not have to coordinate their breaths with device actuation. Ease of use, however, depends significantly on the particular type of device. One study indicated that 92% of patients learned to use the Diskus device correctly, whereas only 74% were able to learn proper use of the Turbohaler.

The Diskus device is a classic example of the discrete-dose style of DPI. Individual doses are contained in foil packets, protecting them from humidity and allowing for dose consistency if the device is dropped. Some discrete-dose devices are single-dose units, and the drug is added when the device is ready to be actuated (Rotahaler, Aerosilizer, Handihaler); this is often a necessity if a drug is heat-sensitive and must be kept refrigerated until use, such as Spiriva (tiotropium bromide). The Twisthaler, on the other hand, is an example of a reservoir device. All of the doses are contained in a central compartment; and if the device is dropped or exposed to humidity, all doses are affected. Of currently marketed products, only the Twisthaler and Flexhaler are reservoir devices.

Nebulizers

Nebulizers allow the drug to be delivered directly to the lung in high concentration and without the use of propellant. They are particularly useful for uncoordinated or unable patients, including those who are intubated. Two types exist: 1) Jet; and 2) Ultrasonic. Jet nebulizers can be used with either solutions or suspensions, and operate by the Bernoulli principle, whereby compressed air from the machine flows at high speed over the medicated liquid, atomizing it and carrying it to the patient. Ultrasonic nebulizers can only be used with solutions. Ultrasonic nebulizers use the vibrations of high-frequency sound waves to move liquid from the machine through the face mask. Vibrations are timed to coincide with inhalation; therefore, less medication is lost with the ultrasonic than with the jet nebulizers.

Nasal Delivery

Nasal delivery shares many of the advantages of pulmonary delivery. Drugs that are inactivated by the GI tract or that undergo first-pass metabolism are protected, and large-molecule drugs can be absorbed across the nasal mucosa. The nose has a dense vasculature, which aids in absorption. Viscosity enhancers and mucoadhesives are often included in the formulations to ↑ residence time, as nasal drainage can be a problem. In addition to the many drugs available via nasal delivery (e.g., desmopressin, calcitonin, butorphanol, corticosteroids), the route shows promise for vaccine delivery, with FluMist being the first approved example.

The most commonly used nasal products are saline solutions for dry nasal mucosa, nasal decongestants, and intranasal corticosteroids. Nasal decongestants are adrenergic agents that constrict the nasal vasculature, shrinking the nasal mucosa and making breathing easier. Overuse can lead to a phenomenon called rhinitis medicamentosa (rebound congestion); therefore, patients should be cautioned to use the products only as directed and for no longer than 3 days. Intranasal corticosteroids are commonly prescribed for allergic rhinitis; they may be administered in pump spray containers or as metered-dose aerosols.

Parenteral Delivery

Injectable products have many advantages over other dosage forms but also have more potential complications. No drug is lost to first-pass metabolism or acid- or enzyme-mediated degradation in the GI tract, which makes injection a particularly useful route for protein drug delivery. The rate of delivery can be accurately controlled and drug, nutrients, and fluids can be given when other routes cannot be used. However, injectable drugs must be prepared and administered by highly trained personnel and cannot be retrieved once given. Additionally, the products must be sterile (see table below for various sterilization methods used), free from undesired particulate matter, and pyrogen-free.

Sterilization Methods Used in Industry

Method	How Does It Work?	Advantages	Disadvantages	Products Sterilized by This Method
Steam sterilization	Heat coagulates and kills microorganisms	• Method of choice when applicable • Lower heat than dry heat sterilization	• Cannot use with heat- or moisture-sensitive drugs • Autoclave can have cools spots	• Aqueous solutions in closed containers • Surgical instruments • Glassware
Dry heat sterilization	Heat coagulates and kills microorganisms	Useful for moisture-sensitive material	• Cannot use with heat-sensitive drugs • Autoclave can have cool spots	• Glassware • Surgical equipment • Oleaginous materials • Powders • Moisture-sensitive material
Filtration	Bacteria and particulate matter are physically removed by membrane filters	Inexpensive	• Technique failure • Membrane defects • Drug can absorb to membrane	• Small volumes of thin liquid • Heat-sensitive liquid formulations
Ionizing radiation	Gamma radiation mutates and kills bacteria	Effective for most microorgranisms	Expensive setup	Sterilizing plastic medical devices
Gas sterilization	Ethylene and propylene oxide gases alkylate microbial protein	Good for heat- and moisture-sensitive materials	• Possibility of toxic residue • Explosion hazard • Expensive setup • Cannot penetrate glass to sterilize material in sealed containers	• Heat-sensitive material • Moisture-sensitive material • Medical and surgical equipment wrapped in plastic

Multiple-dose injectable products must contain a preservative in order to ensure that the product remains sterile after the initial use. Large-volume, single-use products, however, cannot contain preservative, as the amount required to reach an effective concentration would lead to preservative-related toxicity. In addition to sterilization and preservation intended to ↓ the likelihood of microbial growth in the product, steps must be taken to ensure that pyrogens (lipopolysaccharides from gram-negative bacterial cell walls that cause high fever, hypertension, and chills) are not present.

The main routes of injectable delivery are intravenous (IV), subcut, and IM. IV products must be solutions or O/W emulsions (e.g., Intralipid, a component of total parenteral nutrition), as particulate matter could lead to phlebitis and other complications. Subcut and IM injections may be solutions or emulsions; however, they may also be suspensions, which exhibit slower absorption since the drug must go into solution in the tissue before being absorbed into the bloodstream. In some injectable suspensions, such as the contraceptive Depo-Provera (medroxyprogesterone acetate), release of medication can continue for several months, improving patient convenience. Medications may also be given by other injectable routes: Allergy or tuberculosis testing is handled by intradermal injection; betamethasone can be injected directly into the joint (intra-articular) in patients with osteoarthritis; anesthesia is often injected into the epidural space (around the nerve roots of the spine); and anesthetics and some chemotherapy agents are injected into the intrathecal (subarachnoid) space (into the cerebrospinal fluid) to bypass the blood-brain barrier.

Ocular and Otic Delivery

Drug delivery to the eye is complicated by two factors: 1) Drug loss due to blinking and lacrimal drainage; and 2) Poor drug penetration through the corneal membrane. Polymers are typically used as viscosity enhancers to prolong the retention time and ↓ lacrimal drainage; some polymers, such as hyaluronic acid, have mild adhesive properties that prolong the retention time even further. Drop size reduction can also serve to improve ocular availability; only about 10 mcL of fluid remains in the conjunctival cul-de-sac after blinking; therefore, dose volumes larger than this lead to waste.

Drug penetration into the eye can be improved by creating a prodrug that is more lipophilic than the original compound. It is then converted to the active substance by enzymes in the body.

Most ocular products are solutions; however, suspensions, ointments, and gels may also be used. These dosage forms prolong drug contact with the eye and may be preferable in some situations.

Ocular products must be sterile when dispensed, and all multidose products must contain preservative. This helps prevent serious ocular infections, which can lead to corneal ulcers and blindness.

Otic products are generally solutions or suspensions, which frequently contain glycerin or propylene glycol to ↑ the viscosity and maximize contact between the product and the ear canal. The hygroscopic nature of these solvents also helps them draw moisture out of the tissues, which can ↓ inflammation and the amount of moisture available for any microorganisms to grow. Most otic products fall into one of the following categories:

- Anti-infective and anti-inflammatory products: May contain analgesics and local anesthetics to ↓ pain associated with otitis externa or otitis media

- Ear-wax removal agents: Contain surfactants (which emulsify ear wax) or peroxides (which release oxygen and disrupt the integrity of the ear wax), which facilitate removal of the ear wax

Transdermal Delivery

Transdermal delivery differs from topical delivery in that the drug is intended for systemic use. The drug molecules must therefore be small enough to penetrate the stratum corneum and reach the general circulation. Some transdermal ointments (nitroglycerin ointment) exist, but most products are available as transdermal delivery systems (patches).

Patches

Transdermal patches attach to the skin with adhesive and contain the drug either in a polymer matrix or in a drug reservoir covered by a rate-controlling membrane. An excess amount of drug is typically present to ensure that a concentration gradient exists, causing the drug to exit the patch and enter the skin passively. Patches provide more uniform blood levels than conventional release products and can improve patient compliance since, depending on the drug, they can be worn for 1 to 7 days. GI absorption problems and first-pass metabolism also are avoided with transdermal delivery. A wide range of drugs are now available in patches, including nitroglycerin, nicotine, and hormones (for contraception or hormone replacement therapy).

Ultrasound

Drug can be transported across skin by mixing it with a coupling agent and using ultrasonic energy to disrupt the stratum corneum and increase penetrability. This method of delivery is not common; however, high-dose hydrocortisone can be delivered in this fashion.

Iontophoresis

This method of transdermal delivery is not widely used but is gaining popularity. It involves delivery of charged compounds across the skin by applying an electrical current. Since the skin is disrupted, larger molecules may pass than is possible with transdermal patches. Local anesthesia (Numby Stuff) and fentanyl (IONSYS) are available in small iontophoretic patches, and the method is being investigated to deliver protein drugs.

LEARNING POINTS

- A drug cannot work until it is absorbed. It cannot be absorbed until it is dissolved.
- Ionized, hydrophilic drugs dissolve more readily; unionized, lipophilic drugs are absorbed more easily.
- Focus on why a particular dosage form might work better for a particular condition or with a particular drug.
- Consider nonoral routes for drugs that undergo extensive first-pass metabolism.
- At this time, protein drugs can be given only by injectable or pulmonary routes. There is future potential with nasal delivery.

PRACTICE QUESTIONS

1. Which of the following dosage forms must be sterile?

   (A) Ophthalmic suspension
   (B) Oral suspension
   (C) Topical suspension
   (D) Suspension for rectal administration
   (E) Otic suspension

2. A 15-year old patient with ADHD who had been stable on a dose of 10 mg BID of Focalin is transitioning to Focalin XR 20 mg QD. After 2 weeks, he returns to the doctor complaining of distractedness during school and a jittery feeling in the morning an hour or two after taking his medication. When asked how he is taking his medication, he states that due to difficulty swallowing he has been opening the capsules of Focalin XR and mixing them with chunky applesauce, which he chews before swallowing. How do you explain the patient's current symptoms?

   (A) The new dose of Focalin XR is too high and should be reduced.
   (B) The patient is experiencing dose-dumping because he is opening the capsules.
   (C) The patient is experiencing dose-dumping because he is chewing the capsule contents with the applesauce.
   (D) The severity of the patient's ADHD has increased and he is suffering from a new-onset anxiety disorder.
   (E) The patient is experiencing dose-dumping because the capsule contents are interacting with the applesauce.

3. What environmental advantage do HFA inhalers have over CFC inhalers?

   (A) They contain less packaging.
   (B) They are less likely to lead to ozone depletion.
   (C) They do not contain mercury.
   (D) They are a pump spray instead of an aerosol spray.
   (E) They do not use petroleum-based mineral oil as an emulsifier.

4. An insulin injection decomposes at a rate of 0.15 yr^{-1}. How many units of an initial 100-unit solution remain after 3 years?

   (A) 70 units
   (B) 67 units
   (C) 65 units
   (D) 63 units
   (E) 61 units

5.   Using the graph below, indicate which of the following statements is true.

Figure 1. Effect of lubricant on dissolution rate of salicylic acid contained in the compressed tablets.

(A)   Sodium lauryl sulfate appears to decrease the rate of dissolution.

(B)   At 10 minutes, approximately 10 mg of salicylic acid have dissolved when formulated with sodium lauryl sulfate.

(C)   The rate of dissolution of tablets containing magnesium stearate is greater than the control.

(D)   The dissolution rate for tablets with sodium lauryl sulfate follows zero-order kinetics.

(E)   None of the above statements is true.

6.   What approximate percentage of phenytoin sodium ($pK_a = 8.3$) is unionized at a physiological pH of 7.3 ?

(A)   99%

(B)   90%

(C)   45%

(D)   10%

(E)   1%

ANSWERS AND EXPLANATIONS

1. A

All ophthalmic dosage forms must be sterile, and either packaged in single-dose containers or formulated to contain a preservative. Sterility is not required for any of the other routes, as the drug is being applied either to an epithelial surface (topical, otic) or to the GI mucosa (oral, rectal). These surfaces are not sterile in their natural state, and dosage forms applied to them need not be sterile.

2. C

Focalin XR derives its extended-release properties from a coating on the beads contained within the capsule. It is therefore appropriate to open the capsule and consume the contents with food or in liquid; applesauce is specifically mentioned in the manufacturer instructions as appropriate. However, crushing or chewing the beads destroys the coating, causing dose-dumping. The patient's jitteriness in the morning and inattention later in the day are symptomatic of too high a dose being absorbed in the morning, and too little medication remaining in his system later in the day.

3. B

HFA inhalers were designed to replace CFC inhalers, which are being phased out due to the Montreal Protocol and the effect of CFCs on ozone depletion. HFA inhalers are similar in size to CFC inhalers. Neither type of product contains the other excipients mentioned in the question.

4. E

The first step toward answering this problem is to determine if this is a zero-order or first-order degradation process. The units of the degradation rate constant are in $time^{-1}$, which indicates a nonlinear process and, therefore, a first-order degradation. The rate constant is given as 0.15 yr^{-1}, indicating that 15% of the insulin injection is lost every year. In year 1, 15% of the initial 100 units are lost, leaving 85 units. In year 2, 15% of the remaining 85 units are lost; that is, 12.75 units (85×0.15) are lost, and $85 - 12.75 = 72.25$ units remain after year 2. In year 3, 15% of the 72.25 units are lost, or 10.84 units (72.25×0.15), and $72.25 - 10.84 = 61.41$ units remain after year 3. This result is rounded to the answer 61 units.

5. D

The rate of dissolution follows zero-order kinetics. This can be observed on the graph because there is a linear relationship between the amount dissolved (y-axis) and time (x-axis). Because this graph is on a linear scale (i.e., it is NOT a log or natural log scale) and the relationship is linear, it is a zero-order process. Choice (A) is incorrect because the rate of dissolution (or any rate) is directly related to the slope of a line. A steeper slope indicates a faster rate. Because sodium lauryl sulfate had a steeper slope than control, it indicates that those tablets dissolved faster. The same concept applies to choice (C), which is incorrect. Choice (B) is also incorrect: Drawing a straight line up from 10 minutes on the *x*-axis to the line indicating sodium lauryl sulfate demonstrates that approximately 40 mg of the salicylic acid has dissolved, not 10 mg.

6. **B**

The first step to answer this question is to determine if phenytoin is an acidic or basic drug. Phenytoin is formulated with sodium; this indicates that phenytoin is a weak acid. The sodium ion replaces a proton on the phenytoin molecule in its salt formulation and disassociates in solution. Once phenytoin is identified as an acid, it is clear that the following equation applies:

$$pH = pK_a + \log \frac{[Salt]}{[Acid]}$$

The salt in the numerator is the ionized form of the drug; the denominator indicates the drug itself, which is unionized. The next step is to fill in the pH and pKA given in the equation and change the ratio to be ionized over unionized as follows:

$$7.3 = 8.3 + \log \frac{ionized}{unionized}$$

To solve this equation, first, move all numeric values to one side of the equation:

$$-1 = \log \frac{ionized}{unionized}$$

Second, get rid of the log function by taking each side of the equation to the power of 10:

$$10^{-1} = 10 \,^{\wedge} \log \frac{ionized}{unionized}$$

The 10 to a log power on the right side of the equation cancels out, and converting from scientific notation gives the following:

$$0.1 = \frac{ionized}{unionized}$$

Note that this is a good time to review general principles of using logarithmic functions and scientific notation. These functions will not be available on the NAPLEX calculator; understanding the simple principles is needed to calculate these problems.

Any number on either side of an equation can be divided by 1 without altering the math, thus the 0.1 on the left side of the equation can be divided by 1 to give ratios on both side of the equation:

$$\frac{0.1}{1} = \frac{ionized}{unionized}$$

Add the 0.1 to the 1 (total drug parts = 1.1). This shows that 0.1 of a total of 1.1 is ionized and 1 of 1.1 is unionized. The question asks for the percentage unionized, so divide 1 by 1.1. The result is a value of 90.9%, which is approximately 90%.

Biopharmaceutics and Drug Disposition

24

This chapter covers the following:

- **Drug liberation and absorption**
- **Drug distribution**
- **Drug metabolism**
- **Drug excretion**

 Suggested Study Time: **2–3 hours**

Biopharmaceutics deal with the relationship between the physicochemical properties of a drug; the dosage form in which the drug is available; and its route of administration, with the rate and extent of its absorption and elimination from the body. It is the science that links together traditional pharmaceutics (physical pharmacy and dosage form design) with pharmacokinetics. The acronym LADME (liberation, absorption, distribution, metabolism, and excretion) is often used to describe the main processes addressed by biopharmaceutics.

DRUG LIBERATION AND ABSORPTION

A key concept to remember is that drugs are administered as dosage forms, not individual chemicals. Once taken, they must first be liberated from the dosage form in question and absorbed into the bloodstream before they become available in the systemic circulation. The exception is IV administered drugs, as they are delivered directly into the systemic circulation.

Liberation from a dosage form can be as simple as powder from a capsule being released from the capsule shell after ingestion, or as complicated as the slow release of drug from a tablet or transdermal patch matrix. Oral compressed tablets are the most commonly dispensed dosage form; in this case, liberation of the drug requires disintegration of the tablet into smaller drug particles that then undergo dissolution.

If a drug is not already in solution within the dosage form (as in an oral syrup or elixir), it must first undergo dissolution. Undissolved drug particles cannot cross biological membranes and are therefore trapped at their site of administration. For oral dosage forms, this means the gastrointestinal (GI) tract; any drug that is not absorbed is lost in the feces. In the case of an eye drop given in suspension form, the drug particles remain on the corneal surface until the drug either dissolves and passes through the corneal membrane or is lost via lacrimal drainage. Similarly, topical products remain on the skin surface, and IM and subcut injections remain in the tissues until the drug is dissolved in the body fluids.

The rate and extent to which the drug contained in the dosage forms described above is absorbed into the systemic circulation is the **bioavailability**. This property plays a very important role in the biopharmaceutics and pharmacokinetics of drugs. The liberation and dissolution of a drug can be affected by processing factors and excipients, which can in turn affect bioavailability. Other factors affecting bioavailability are addressed later in this chapter.

One physicochemical property that can affect bioavailability is particle size. ↓ the particle size of a drug formulation ↑ the surface area, which leads to more rapid dissolution. This is an important factor for drugs with low water solubility; finely milling or micronizing drugs such as griseofulvin and nitrofurantoin can dramatically improve their oral bioavailability.

Many excipients can affect product bioavailability. Some examples are listed in the table below.

Excipients That Affect Product Bioavailability

Excipient Category	Examples	Effect on Drug Particles	Effect on Bioavailability
Disintegrants	Starch, microcrystalline cellulose	Breaks tablet into smaller particles, ↑ dissolution	Possible ↑
Surfactants	Tweens, Spans	Low concentration: ↓ surface tension and ↑ dissolution rate	Possible ↑
		High concentration: Form micelles with drug inside, ↓ dissolution	Possible ↓
Lubricants	Magnesium stearate	Has tendency to waterproof particles in large concentration, making them less soluble	Possible ↓

Drug Transport Across Membranes

There are several ways for drugs to cross body membranes that you should be aware of: 1) passive diffusion; 2) carrier-mediated transport; 3) endocytosis; and 4) drug efflux. In passive diffusion, the drug crosses cell membranes based on a concentration gradient, moving from regions of higher concentration to areas of (relatively) lower concentration. For this mechanism to be practical, the drug must be small enough to be absorbed across cells and lipid-soluble enough to interact with the cell membranes. The rate of transport is described by Fick's first law of diffusion:

$$\frac{dC}{dt} = \frac{DA(C_s - C)}{h}$$

While it is unlikely that the NAPLEX will require you to perform calculations based on this equation, you should be familiar with the items that affect it: The concentration gradient (C_S–C), the thickness of the membrane being crossed (h), the surface area of the membrane (A), and the diffusion coefficient of the drug (D).

As would be expected, drugs diffuse more slowly through thicker membranes. Body locations with larger surface area tend to promote faster diffusion, as there is more available membrane through which the drug molecule can diffuse. The small intestine is thus a prime location for drug absorption, as the surface area is very large due to the presence of villi and microvilli.

Another key factor to remember is that the GI membranes are more permeable to the drug in the unionized form. It would therefore be expected that weakly acidic drugs would be better absorbed in the highly acidic environment of the stomach. In an acidic environment, a weakly acidic drug would be primarily in its unionized form. However, solubility of weakly acidic drugs ↑ as the drug moves from the stomach to the intestines. The reason that weakly acidic drugs are commonly better absorbed in a more basic environment such as the duodenum is not the pH of the environment. The aforementioned factors that affect drug absorption play a bigger role, such as a ↓ membrane thickness and ↑ surface area of the small intestine. Furthermore, even though the unionized form of a drug is more permeable to cell membranes, the ionized form of the drug is more soluble. Therefore, basic drugs will be more soluble in the highly acidic environment of the stomach. Because of this, poorly soluble, weakly basic drugs may be poorly absorbed if taken with drugs that ↓ gastric acid secretion. For example, ketoconazole and atazanavir both exhibit ↓ rate and extent of absorption when taken with antacids, H_2 blockers or proton pump inhibitors. This phenomenon of solubility and permeability is governed by the Henderson-Hasselbalch equation, as explained in the Ionization Behavior section of the Pharmaceutics chapter.

Not all drugs are absorbed by passive diffusion; many undergo carrier-mediated transport processes. Active transport, which requires input of energy and occurs against a concentration gradient, is the most common type of carrier-mediated transport process.

Unlike passive diffusion, the process can be saturated or competitively inhibited by chemically similar substrates. Many drugs are transported via transport systems designed to move amino acids and vitamins across cell membranes (see table). Some drugs undergo simultaneous passive diffusion and active transport.

Active Transport Mechanisms for Drugs in the Body

Transporter	Drugs Transported
Peptide	• Penicillins • Cephalosporins • Angiotensin-converting enzyme inhibitors
Nucleoside	• Anticancer/antiviral nucleosides
Amino acid	• Levodopa • Methyldopa

Facilitated diffusion is another carrier-mediated transport process; it differs from active transport in that it occurs only from high to low concentrations. As with active transport, the transporter may bind to structurally similar inhibitors, which will ↓ the transport rate of the drug. If the inhibitor is present in high concentration, the transporter may become saturated. Furosemide, morphine, and dopamine are examples of drugs that undergo facilitated diffusion.

Macromolecules are most likely to cross cell membranes by endocytosis, a process by which substances are transported across cell membranes by formation of vesicles. Most endocytosis is receptor-mediated; nonreceptor-mediated endocytosis is called either phagocytosis (engulfment of solid particles) or pinocytosis (engulfment of liquid), and is often seen in the GI tract and lungs. Protein and peptide drugs such as insulin, erythropoietin, and growth hormone are transported via receptor-mediated endocytosis. Polio and other oral vaccines are absorbed from the GI tract by phagocytosis.

The final method of drug transport with which you should be concerned is drug efflux. In this case, transporters pump drugs and other substances out of cells rather than into them. P-glycoprotein is the key efflux protein, and is linked to multidrug resistance in tumor cells. In this case, resistance occurs because the transporter pumps drug back out of the tumor site before it can accumulate to an effective concentration. P-glycoprotein is also expressed on the intraluminal surface of the GI tract. In this location, it pumps substrates out of the plasma and back into the intestinal lumen, resulting in a ↓ net absorption (and bioavailability) of some drugs. Digoxin, corticosteroids, and immunosuppressants are just a few of the drugs that can be affected in this way. There is significant overlap between drugs that are inhibitors of the cytochrome P450 3A (CYP3A) isoenzyme and inhibitors of P-glycoprotein. Therefore, many drugs that are known inhibitors of the CYP3A4 can ↑ the absorption and plasma concentrations of digoxin despite the fact that digoxin is not a CYP3A4 substrate. The amiodarone–digoxin interaction is a clinically relevant example of an interaction involving P-glycoprotein that results in ↑ plasma digoxin concentrations since amiodarone is an inhibitor of P-glycoprotein.

Barriers to Drug Absorption

Several factors can affect drug absorption (see table below). The drug not only must dissolve initially but also should stay in solution during the absorption process. The pH of the GI tract varies significantly, and a drug that is in solution at the low pH of the stomach may be less soluble in the higher pH of the small intestine. Food intake can affect absorption and bioavailability in a variety of ways, including ↑ the pH in the stomach, which can in turn affect drug dissolution and absorption (↑ dissolution and absorption for weak acids, and ↓ dissolution and absorption for weak bases). Chemical stability may be affected as well, which can in turn ↓ the amount of drug available for absorption.

Food-Related Absorption and Bioavailability Variations

Process	Explanation	Examples
Food-drug complexation	Can bind and make drug insoluble; prevent absorption	Tetracycline complexes with calcium and iron in food and supplements (↓ bioavailability)
Alteration of pH	Food acts as buffer in stomach; ↑ pH	• ↑ dissolution (and subsequent absorption) of weak acids • ↓ dissolution (and subsequent absorption) of weak bases
Gastric emptying	Foods and some drugs can slow gastric emptying and delay drug onset or speed-up gastric emptying and ↓ drug effect	Metoclopramide and erythromycin can ↑ gastric emptying
Gastric acid secretions	• Pepsin may ↑ drug metabolism • Bile salts ↑ dissolution of poorly soluble drugs, but can form complexes with other drugs	Bile acid-drug complexes: neomycin, nystatin
Competition for specialized absorption mechanisms	Competitive inhibition of drugs by nutrients with similar chemical structures	Amino acids can compete with drugs (e.g. cephalexin) transported by the peptide transporter (PEPT1)
↑ volume and viscosity of GI contents	Presence of food can lead to: • Slower drug dissolution • Slower diffusion of dissolved drug from GI tract	This can affect several drugs
Food-induced changes in first-pass metabolism	↑ bioavailability due to inhibition of CYP450 isoenzymes (primarily CYP3A)	Grapefruit juice may ↑ bioavailability of numerous 3A substrates (e.g. cyclosporine, verapamil, saquinavir)
Food-induced changes in blood flow	• Giving some drugs with food ↑ bioavailability due to ↑ blood flow to the GI tract and liver following a meal • A larger fraction of drug escapes first-pass metabolism because the enzyme system becomes overwhelmed	Drugs with metabolism sensitive to rate of presentation to liver: • Propranolol • Hydralazine

DRUG DISTRIBUTION

Once in the bloodstream, some proportion of the drug may be bound to the plasma proteins while the remainder remains unbound. A key point to remember is that only drug that is unbound can pass out of the plasma to reach the site of action. The amount of drug that is bound to plasma protein is in dynamic equilibrium with the amount that is not.

Volume of Distribution

In the average 70-kg (~155-lb) patient, blood volume is approximately 5 L and total body water is about 40 L. After absorption, a drug will distribute into the body fluids; since the total amount of drug placed into the body is known and the concentration of drug in the plasma can be measured, the volume of fluid through which the drug seems to have distributed throughout the body can be determined. This volume is referred to as the *apparent* volume of distribution (V_d), because it is not a physical volume. Rather, it is a calculated number, dependent on physicochemical properties of the drug, which helps compare the behavior of different drugs. Thus, the apparent V_d may be a much larger value than what is physiologically possible (i.e., $\geq$1,000 L). This indicates that the drug either is primarily distributed into extravascular tissue or is highly protein bound. This phenomenon can be visualized by the following equation to determine a drug's apparent V_d:

$$V_d = \frac{\text{dose}}{C_p} \text{ when dose = IV bolus and } C_p \text{ is unbound plasma drug concentration}$$

measured immediately after injection

Plasma Protein Binding

Most drugs exhibit plasma protein binding, and this affects their V_d. Proteins are large molecules that cannot leave the capillaries; therefore, the drug-protein complex remains in the plasma. However, since the concentration of protein-bound drug is not usually measured, protein binding results in lower free plasma concentrations of the drug, $\uparrow$ the apparent V_d. As protein binding is reversible, equilibrium exists between bound and free drug. As free drug distributes out of the bloodstream, bound drug is released from plasma proteins to maintain the equilibrium.

Although plasma proteins are relatively nonspecific in their binding behavior, the different proteins do tend to bind to different types of drug:

- Albumin: Weak acids
- α_1-acid glycoprotein: Weak bases
- Lipoproteins: Basic and neutral drugs
- Globulins: Steroids, vitamins, metal ions

Dosing a highly protein-bound drug based only on physiological volumes (plasma volume, interstitial volume, or total body water) may not produce a high enough concentration at the site of drug action to yield an adequate pharmacological response. Therefore, a higher dose may need to be given. The protein-drug complex can also act as a drug reservoir, prolonging action of the drug in the body. These factors must be considered when determining dose and dosing frequency. Certain disease states can alter the levels of plasma proteins significantly enough to require drug dose adjustments. Additionally, if a patient is receiving several drugs that all bind to the same plasma protein, one drug may displace another, leading to higher-than-expected drug concentrations and possible toxicity. This is most important in drugs that are more than 95% protein bound, particularly if they have a narrow therapeutic index. Warfarin (99% protein bound) is an excellent example of this potential drug interaction. Even a minor displacement of protein-bound warfarin (e.g., 99% to 98% bound) would double the unbound concentration; therefore the effective concentration of warfarin would ↑ from 1% to 2%. However, there are few examples of clinically relevant drug interactions related to displacing plasma protein binding.

Some Disease States and Physiological Conditions That Affect Plasma Protein Concentration

↓ plasma protein concentration	• Liver disease • Trauma (albumin) • Surgery (albumin) • Burns • Renal failure (albumin) • Hyperthyroidism • Age (neonate, elderly) • Pregnancy
↑ plasma protein concentration	• Hypothyroidism • Schizophrenia • Rheumatoid arthritis • Renal failure (α_1-acid glycoprotein) • Trauma (α_1-acid glycoprotein) • Surgery (α_1-acid glycoprotein)

DRUG METABOLISM

Drugs are eliminated from the body by two processes: metabolism and excretion. Metabolism, also referred to as biotransformation, leads to the chemical conversion of drug to active or inactive compounds called metabolites. These metabolites are generally more polar (and hence more water-soluble) than the parent drugs which allows the metabolites to be more efficiently cleared in the urine. Not all drugs undergo metabolism.

Metabolism is most likely to occur in organs that contain high levels of enzymes. Many microsomal enzymes, including the CYP450 mixed-function oxidases, are found in the liver, which is the primary site of biotransformation. Metabolizing enzymes are found in many other locations of the body, and significant biotransformation of some drugs can occur in the intestinal tract, kidney, and brain. Drugs administered via nasal, pulmonary, or dermal routes often also show significant biotransformation in the nasal tissue, lung, or skin.

One concern with oral delivery of certain drugs is presystemic, or first-pass, metabolism. Because the venous outflow of the GI tract travels directly to the liver via the portal vein, drugs administered via the GI tract are susceptible to hepatic metabolism before they reach the systemic circulation. Bioavailability is ↓; therefore, the drug must be given either in a higher dose or by a delivery route that bypasses the GI tract. Nitroglycerin, for example, is almost completely degraded by first-pass metabolism and is therefore usually formulated as sublingual tablets or spray, or transdermal ointment or patches. Oral extended-release nitroglycerin capsules are also available and are believed to work by saturating the hepatic enzymes responsible for metabolism and by producing metabolites that possess some activity.

Metabolism is classified into Phase I and Phase II reactions. In many cases, a drug may undergo metabolism by competing pathways, leading to multiple metabolites. The metabolites may in turn undergo metabolism. Some of these metabolites may possess therapeutic activity. Some medications are deliberately administered as inactive prodrugs, and the therapeutic component results from the metabolism of the prodrug. Formulating a medication as a prodrug can improve its pharmaceutical, pharmacodynamic, or pharmacokinetic properties.

Phase I Reactions

Phase I reactions are so named because they generally occur before Phase II reactions. However, in some instances, drugs are solely metabolized by Phase II reactions. Phase I reactions are nonsynthetic and introduce or expose a functional group. The primary types of Phase I reactions are oxidation, reduction, and hydrolysis. Oxidation is the most common type of metabolism, and many of these reactions are catalyzed by enzymes in the CYP superfamily.

Phase II Reactions

Phase II reactions are synthetic reactions. They are often called conjugation reactions, as a reactive group on the drug is attached to a polar molecule or group originating inside the body. This generally leads to a polar, water-soluble metabolite. While most drugs undergo Phase I metabolism prior to Phase II, this is not required provided the drug already possesses one or more reactive groups.

Examples of Phase II reactions are listed in the table below, with glucuronidation being the most common example. Since these reactions involve enzymes, the reactions may be capacity limited. If the concentration of drug approaches or exceeds the metabolic capacity of the enzyme, nonlinear drug metabolism may be observed.

Two types of conjugation reactions (methylation and acetylation) lead to metabolites that are less polar, and therefore less soluble, than the original compound. Less soluble metabolites will have extended elimination half-lives. This can extend the duration of action in cases where an active metabolite is formed, such as with *N*-acetylprocainamide. Toxicity may also occur from ↑ blood or tissue levels of toxic metabolites. For example, at high concentrations, the acetylated metabolites of sulfonamides can precipitate in the kidney tubules and lead to kidney damage and crystalluria.

Phase II Reactions

Type of Phase II Reaction	Drugs Metabolized by This Route
Glucuronidation	• Chloramphenicol • Meprobamate • Morphine
Sulfation	• Acetaminophen • Estradiol • Methyldopa • Minoxidil
Amino acid conjugation	• Salicylic acid
Acetylation	• Isoniazid • Procainamide • Sulfonamides • Hydralazine
Methylation	• Catecholamines • Niacinamide
Glutathione conjugation	• Chlorambucil

Factors Affecting Biotransformation

Several factors can affect metabolizing enzyme activity in the body. Disease states, age, gender, or chemical and nutritional exposure to a variety of substances can lead to enzyme inhibition or enzyme induction. Genetic variability also plays a role. Drug–drug interactions are a common result of the metabolic process, as most marketed drugs are metabolized by multiple pathways, and drugs that inhibit or induce enzyme activity can affect the metabolism of many other drugs.

Enzyme Inhibition

Enzyme inhibition describes the situation when an enzyme is prevented from binding with its substrate. The substrate is therefore unable to be properly metabolized, and plasma concentrations ↑, possibly to toxic levels. In cases where a prodrug must be activated by metabolism, enzyme inhibition may limit, delay, or prevent drug activity. Enzyme inhibitors can act by competitive or noncompetitive means.

Drugs that are metabolized by the same metabolic pathways frequently act as competitive inhibitors to each other. Drug metabolites, herbal products, and foods can also act as enzyme inhibitors. Compounds containing imidazole, pyridine, or quinolone groups in particular are often found to be enzyme inhibitors. The table below contains a partial list of common enzyme inhibitors.

One of the most widely known drug–food interactions results from enzyme inhibition. Grapefruit juice is an inhibitor of CYP3A, the isozyme responsible for metabolism of a host of drugs, including macrolide antibiotics, benzodiazepines, calcium channel blockers, and protease inhibitors. While a single portion is unlikely to lead to problems, patients receiving drugs metabolized by this isozyme should be cautioned to avoid grapefruit juice.

Drugs Involved in Inhibition of Metabolic Enzymes

CYP1A2	CYP2C9	CYP2C19	CYP2D6	CYP3A
fluvoxamine	fluconazole	cimetidine	bupropion	indinavir
ciprofloxacin	amiodarone	esomeprazole	fluoxetine	nelfinavir
		lansoprazole	paroxetine	ritonavir
		omeprazole	quinidine	clarithromycin
		pantoprazole	duloxetine	itraconazole
		fluoxetine	sertraline	ketoconazole
		fluvoxamine	terbinafine	nefazodone
		indomethacin	amiodarone	saquinavir
		isoniazid	cimetidine	erythromycin
		ketoconazole	chlorpromazine	fluconazole
		oxcarbazepine	clomipramine	grapefruit juice
		probenecid	doxepin	verapamil
		topiramate	haloperidol	diltiazem
		voriconazole	methadone	cimetidine
				amiodarone

Enzyme Induction

Enzyme induction is essentially the opposite of enzyme inhibition. Enzyme inducers stimulate enzyme activity, which leads to ↓ plasma concentrations of the enzyme's targets. In most cases, this means a ↓ in both activity and adverse effects of the drug. If active or toxic metabolites are produced, however, drug activity and toxic effects may be ↑. A number of commonly prescribed drugs induce metabolic enzymes, as do ethanol, tobacco, marijuana, and certain herbal products, most notably St. John's wort which can lead to clinically significant drug interactions. For example, triazolam is extensively metabolized by CYP3A4. St. John's wort, rifampin, and several seizure medications (carbamazepine, phenytoin, and phenobarbital) induce this isozyme. Using any of these agents with triazolam or other drugs metabolized by 3A4 may lead to significantly ↓ plasma concentrations and therapeutic effect of triazolam. The table below lists some of the most common inducers of drug metabolism. Although there are exceptions, the inducers commonly affect all of the inducible CYP enzymes including CYP1A2, CYP2B6, CYP2C9, CYP2C19, and CYP3A. The CYP2D6 isoenzyme is not inducible.

Some drugs undergo a phenomenon called auto-induction, wherein they stimulate their own metabolism. Carbamazepine is a key example of a drug of this type. Due to auto-induction, administration of carbamazepine especially during the initial 3-5 wk of therapy can lead to ↓ blood concentrations and therapeutic activity.

Drugs Involved in Induction of Metabolic Enzymes

Seizure medications	• Carbamazepine • Phenytoin • Phenobarbital
Tuberculosis medications	• Rifampin

Genetic Variability

Pharmacogenomic variability is an important source of drug variability. The Pharmacogenomics chapter is dedicated to describing variability in drug response based on genetics.

DRUG EXCRETION

The other process by which the body eliminates substances is excretion. Unlike metabolism, excretion eliminates the substances without further chemical change. The kidney is the primary organ involved, and most substances are excreted in the urine.

Polar, water-soluble drugs are usually excreted unchanged; lipophilic drugs are generally excreted as metabolites. There are three components to renal excretion:

1. Glomerular filtration:

   - Blood passes through the capillary network (glomerulus) inside Bowman's capsule.

   - Fenestrated endothelium allows paracellular transport of most solutes (other than macromolecules) into Bowman's capsule.

   - Filtrate (including drug) moves from Bowman's capsule into renal tubules.

   - All nonprotein-bound, small-molecule drugs undergo glomerular filtration; the concentration of drug or metabolite in the filtrate will be equal to the concentration of unbound drug in the plasma.

2. Tubular reabsorption:

   - Many nutrients and ions are actively reabsorbed into the bloodstream.

   - Water is reabsorbed, and filtrate becomes more concentrated as it moves along the tubule.

   - No transporters exist for reabsorption of drug; passive diffusion process is dependent on filtrate pH. Acidic (citrus fruits, cranberry juice, aspirin) and basic (milk products, sodium bicarbonate) foods and drugs can alter urine pH enough to affect reabsorption.

     » In alkaline urine: Acidic drugs are ionized → less reabsorbed → more readily excreted in urine

     » In acidic urine: Basic drugs are ionized → less reabsorbed → more readily excreted in urine

     » Pentobarbital (weak acid) overdose: Treated by alkalinizing urine with sodium bicarbonate injection

3. Tubular secretion:

   - This occurs simultaneously with tubular reabsorption.

   - This removes certain substances from the blood and secretes them back into the filtrate.

   - This occurs against the concentration gradient and is an energy-requiring process that uses protein transporters.

   - Only ionized drugs are bound to and secreted by the transporter proteins; drugs that are highly ionized at pH 7.4 will be secreted to a greater extent.

   - Plasma protein binding has little effect on this process; transporters can strip drug off of protein.

     » Competitive process; can lead to drug interactions

       - Saturable process; at high dose, process plateaus → less drug excreted → higher plasma concentration than expected

The rate of renal excretion of drugs is the net result of the above processes. It depends on blood flow in addition to the physicochemical properties of the drugs in question. More rapid blood flow through the nephron generally leads to an $\uparrow$ in all three processes, with an overall higher drug excretion rate. Glomerular filtration rate (GFR) is normally about 120 mL/min, but may vary widely with the patient's age, body weight, and concomitant disease states. The GFR for an individual is determined by calculating the clearance of creatinine, an endogenous substance that is not reabsorbed or secreted. This value gives an indication of kidney function. A common way to estimate a patient's creatinine clearance (CrCl) is using the Cockroft-Gault equation listed below and should be memorized for the NAPLEX.

$$\text{CrCl (mL/min)} = \frac{(140 - \text{age}) \times \text{wt (kg)}}{\text{Serum Creatinine (mg/dL)} \times 72} (\times 0.85 \text{ if female})$$

Renal clearance (Cl_r) is a measure of the efficiency of renal excretion in removing unchanged drug in the urine. It is an indirect measurement expressed by the following equation, where C_U and V_U are concentration of drug in the urine and volume of urine formation per unit time, respectively:

$$\text{CL}_r = \frac{\text{excretion rate in urine}}{\text{plasma concentration}} = \frac{C_U V_U}{C_P}$$

Nonrenal Excretion

Drugs may also be excreted by the liver into the bile; at this point, one of two things can happen:

- Biliary excretion: Bile (including drug) is emptied into the small intestine, where it is eventually excreted from the body in the feces.
- Enterohepatic recycling: The drug is partially reabsorbed from the intestines (based on pKa and partition coefficient) and re-enters the bloodstream. Drugs undergoing this process may show a secondary peak in plasma concentration; with multiple dosing regimens, the blood-concentration curve can be altered significantly.

Some drugs are excreted into other fluids, though this is usually not a significant route:

- Saliva: Swallowed, leading to salivary recycling; routine and noninvasive way of monitoring for concentrations of certain drugs
- Breast milk: Mostly occurs by passive diffusion (primarily of weak bases); can lead to drug transfer to breastfeeding infants
- Sweat: Small volume; therefore, not a significant mode of drug excretion; could become a convenient method for detecting use of illegal or restricted drugs (cocaine, amphetamines, morphine, and ethanol)
- Expired air: Significant route of excretion for volatile drugs (anesthetics, ethanol); drug volatility is more important than polarity for this method of excretion

LEARNING POINTS

- The prime body location for drug absorption is the small intestine, due to the high surface area; the drug must be dissolved in order to be absorbed. Factors affecting dissolution in the small intestine (i.e., pH) may prevent this from being the prime absorption location for a particular drug.

- Only drugs that are unbound to plasma protein can pass from the plasma to reach the site of action.

- Enzyme inhibition can often lead to toxicity; enzyme induction can lead to inadequate blood concentrations of drug.

- Genetic variations in CYP metabolism lead to fast and slow metabolizers of a variety of drugs; dosage adjustments or alternate therapies must be made in some cases.

- Tubular reabsorption decreases drug and metabolite concentration in the urine, while tubular secretion increases the amount. Water-soluble, ionized drugs are more likely to be excreted.

PRACTICE QUESTIONS

1. A single IV dose of a drug is given and the AUC is calculated. After an adequate washout period, a single oral dose of the same drug and in the same salt form is administered. If the doses are the same amount, which of the following results is NOT possible?

    (A) $AUC_{PO} = AUC_{IV}$
    (B) $AUC_{PO} > AUC_{IV}$
    (C) $AUC_{PO} < AUC_{IV}$
    (D) None are possible
    (E) All are possible

2. The quality control test required for tablets that is intended to reflect the release of the drug is the

    (A) weight variation test.
    (B) content uniformity test.
    (C) dissolution test.
    (D) disintegration test.
    (E) friability test.

3. A 15-year-old patient taking Focalin XR for his ADHD is experiencing inattention later in the day. He admits that after having a cold 2 weeks ago, he started taking 2 g of vitamin C per day to "boost his immune system." What do you think is causing his symptoms?

    (A) He is experiencing vitamin C toxicity.
    (B) The vitamin C is acidifying his urine, causing decreased excretion of Focalin XR.
    (C) The vitamin C is acidifying his urine, causing increased excretion of Focalin XR.
    (D) The vitamin C is inducing CYP2D6, causing increased metabolism of Focalin XR.
    (E) The vitamin C is inhibiting CYP2D6, causing increased metabolism of Focalin XR.

4. In cases of overdose of the sodium salt of a chemotherapeutic drug, the rate of excretion of the drug may be increased by which of the following?

    (A) Intravenous administration of ammonium chloride
    (B) Intravenous administration of calcium chloride
    (C) Acidifying the urine
    (D) Intravenous administration of sodium bicarbonate
    (E) Intravenous administration of monosodium phosphate

5. Acidification of the urine in a patient taking aspirin can be expected to do which of the following?

(A) Increase the rate of excretion of the drug
(B) Increase the blood concentrations of the drug
(C) Cause hydrolysis of the drug
(D) Lower the blood concentration of the drug
(E) Have no effect on the concentration of the drug

ANSWERS AND EXPLANATIONS

1. B

Because the bioavailability of a drug administered intravenously is equal to one, the oral bioavailability of a dosage form containing the same drug may be as high as the IV bioavailability (assuming complete absorption and no first-pass metabolism). The oral AUC is commonly lower than the IV dose given the lower bioavailability. Since bioavailability can never be greater than 1, the oral bioavailability never exceeds the IV bioavailability. Therefore, the AUC_{PO} may be less than or equal to the AUC_{IV} but never greater.

2. C

The quality control test intended to reflect the absorption of the drug is the dissolution test. It is only an approximation; going into solution is the last step before absorption. Weight variation and content uniformity tests assess the distribution of the active ingredients across the tablets and ensure that each dose is approximately the same weight. The disintegration test evaluates how quickly or slowly a tablet disintegrates; disintegration is a necessary step prior to dissolution. The friability test determines how well tablets will hold up to handling.

3. C

Focalin (dexmethylphenidate) is a weakly basic drug primarily excreted via the renal route. Acidification of the urine will cause trapping of the ionized form of the drug in the urine, increasing urinary excretion. Although some quantity of Focalin is metabolized by CYP2D6, vitamin C does not induce this enzyme. Symptoms of vitamin C toxicity do not include inattention.

4. D

Because the drug is formulated as a sodium salt, the drug must be a weak acid. The positive charge of the sodium ion replaces the hydronium ion of the acid through an ionic bond. Placing the drug in its ionized form facilitates excretion and limits reabsorption. To ionize a weak acid, the pH of the ultrafiltrate should be raised with a basic solution. Sodium bicarbonate is the only basic solution provided that can be used clinically and that raises the pH of the ultrafiltrate.

5. **B**

Aspirin is a weak acid. As the pH of the environment is lowered, weak acids will be primarily in the unionized form. Remember that acids are proton donors (i.e., hydronium ion donors). In an acidic environment, weak acids are surrounded by other proton donors; thus they are more likely to have the hydronium ion and be without charge. The uncharged drug molecule is more lipophilic and can cross biological membranes. Hence, in its unionized form, the drug will be without charge and can undergo passive reabsorption to increase blood concentrations.

Pharmacogenomics 25

This chapter covers the following:

- **Definitions**
- **Phase I metabolism**
- **Phase II metabolism**
- **Drug targets**

 Suggested Study Time: **1.5 hours**

Variants (i.e., mutations) in the human genome account for a portion of the clinical variability observed between patients receiving the same drug therapy. *Pharmacogenomics* describes the impact of genetics on the pharmacokinetics and pharmacodynamics of drugs. The most clinically relevant variants that alter drug pharmacokinetics and pharmacodynamics are located in genes that encode drug-metabolizing enzymes, target receptors, or the human leukocyte antigen (HLA). These genes and the effects of genetics on drug therapy are the focus of this chapter.

DEFINITIONS

Proteins (including enzymes) that have different expression profiles are considered to be polymorphically expressed. The expression profile is commonly determined by the presence of functional versus nonfunctional alleles. Alleles are a specific form of a gene. Humans have two alleles, one inherited from each parent. Therefore, patients may have:

- Two functional alleles (wild-type or extensive metabolizer)
- One functional and one nonfunctional allele (intermediate metabolizer)
- Two nonfunctional alleles (poor metabolizer)

Genetic polymorphisms result in allele expression that can lead to a number of metabolism-related issues. For the NAPLEX, it is important to understand how the functional classification of enzymes can alter dosage requirements. For example, you will likely be told if a patient fits into one of the three categories listed. It is unlikely that you will be expected to memorize the nomenclature for functional and nonfunctional alleles for even the most common cytochrome P450 (CYP) enzymes. However, it is useful to know that alleles follow a star nomenclature system, with *1 considered the wild-type for most enzymes. Therefore, if a patient is said to express the *1/*1, it is highly likely that this patient would be considered an extensive metabolizer. If only one *1 is present, they are probably an intermediate metabolizer, and if no *1 is present they are probably a poor metabolizer.

Of course, patients cannot always be simply categorized into one of the three groups listed, and individuals can have polymorphisms that may increase or reduce function to varying extents. For example, polymorphisms of the CYP2D6 enzyme can produce an allele with supraenzymatic activity. These patients would be classified as ultrarapid metabolizers. For the NAPLEX, once you identify the expression profile of a patient, you will likely need to make dosage adjustments to avoid subtherapeutic consequences or toxic effects, depending on the category into which a patient falls and whether the metabolite of the drug is active or inactive.

PHASE I METABOLISM

Cytochrome P450

CYP enzymes, in particular, are highly polymorphic and follow the nomenclature outlined. As mentioned, CYP2D6 can be problematic; variants mean that individuals can be classified as poor, intermediate, extensive, and ultrarapid metabolizers. The percentage of poor metabolizers varies somewhat by ancestry. Approximately 5–10% of Caucasians, 1–2% of Asians, and up to 20% in African Americans are poor metabolizers. When making dosage adjustments, it is important to consider whether (1) the parent drug is active and/or (2) the major metabolite via the CYP pathway in question is active. For example, codeine is metabolized by CYP2D6. Poor metabolizers of CYP2D6 receive less benefit from the drug, because codeine must be metabolized into morphine to exert its full analgesic effect. Pharmacists should be aware of this variability, since poor metabolizers may be falsely labeled as drug-seekers when in fact codeine is an ineffective analgesic for them. These patients should instead be placed on analgesics not activated by CYP2D6, such as morphine itself.

The importance of the field of pharmacogenomics has dramatically increased the ability to determine a patient's genotype. In addition to CYP2D6, the enzymes CYP1A, CYP2C9, and CYP2C19 are polymorphically expressed as outlined. Understanding the drugs metabolized by this pathway and their active metabolites is likely enough to master most of the pharmacogenomics drug dosing questions regarding this topic on the NAPLEX. The following table lists selected drugs metabolized by the most common CYP enzymes.

Common Drugs Metabolized by Pathway

CYP1A2	CYP2C9	CYP2C19	CYP2D6	CYP3A
caffeine	warfarin	omeprazole	codeine	clarithromycin
theophylline	phenytoin	esomeprazole	dextromethorphan	erythromycin
	glipizide	lansoprazole	hydrocodone	quinidine
	glyburide	pantoprazole	oxycodone	midazolam
		citalopram	fluoxetine	alprazolam
		voriconazole	haloperidol	diazepam
		clopidogrel	venlafaxine	cyclosporine
			paroxetine	tacrolimus
			duloxetine	amlodipine
			risperidone	diltiazem
			propranolol	nifedipine
			metoprolol	verapamil
			tamoxifen	atorvastatin
				lovastatin
				simvastatin
				estrogens
				carbamazepine

Glucose-6-Phosphate Dehydrogenase

Glucose-6-phosphate dehydrogenase is an enzyme with over 300 reported polymorphic variants, leading to individuals possessing low, normal, or high levels of the enzyme. This enzyme protects red blood cells from oxidative stress. Consequently, levels combined with certain environmental or pharmacological stresses—such as eating fava beans or taking certain drugs—can lead to life-threatening hemolytic anemia. Prevalence of this deficiency is highest among those of African, Asian, and Mediterranean ancestry, with more severe variants occurring in Mediterranean populations. The high gene frequency in certain populations is believed to be related to its protective effect against malaria.

Substances to Be Avoided in Glucose-6-Phosphate Dehydrogenase Deficiency

- Oxidant drugs
  - Primaquine
  - Chloroquine
- Sulfonamides
- Fluoroquinolones
- Aspirin
- Probenecid
- Vitamin K
- Nitrofurantoin
- Fava beans
- Mothballs

PHASE II METABOLISM

Glucuronidation

Phase II reactions are synthetic reactions. They are often called conjugation reactions, because a reactive group on the drug is attached to a polar molecule or group originating inside the body. Like Phase I enzymes, Phase II enzymes can be polymorphically expressed with altered function.

Irinotecan is a cytotoxic agent used in colorectal cancer that has an important pharmacogenomic profile related to its drug toxicity. The active metabolite of irinotecan is SN-38. SN-38 is primarily eliminated by glucuronidation through the UGT1A1 enzyme. By assessing for the presence of UGT1A polymorphisms, tests can predict severe drug toxicities before ironotecan is administered. For example, homozygotes for the UGT1A1*28 allele significantly reduce elimination of SN-38, predisposing patients to life-threatening myelosuppression. Homozygotes for the UGT1A1*28 allele may also have Gilbert's syndrome, which affects bilirubin elimination.

Acetylation

Acetylation is another aspect of drug metabolism that can be affected by genetic variability. Rapid-metabolizing and slow-metabolizing polymorphic variants of N-acetyl-transferase-2 have therapeutic implications for several drugs, most notably isoniazid. Slow acetylators do not metabolize the drug quickly, so they require lower doses to avoid toxic effects. Rapid acetylators require substantially higher doses, whereas in normal or slow acetylators, therapeutic failure rates are more common.

DRUG TARGETS

Somatic Mutations

The pharmacogenomics of drug targets—including ion channels, G protein–coupled receptors, and other proteins—contribute to variable effects on drug efficacy and toxicity. Currently, the greatest clinical application of pharmacogenomics involves identifying somatic mutations within the field of oncology. *Somatic mutations* refer to genetic variants that occur within the tumor itself and are not a part of the patient's germline. Therefore, screening for somatic mutations requires a biopsy of the tumor; saliva will only reveal the germline DNA. For example, somatic mutations within the epidermal growth factor receptor tyrosine kinase family can help guide the treatment of various cancers, such as non–small cell lung carcinoma.

Vitamin K Epoxide Reductase Complex Subunit 1 (VKORC1)

The VKORC1 gene encodes for the vitamin K epoxide reductase complex subunit 1, which converts inactive vitamin K epoxide to active vitamin K. Active vitamin K is required for several coagulation factors. Patients with mutations at position 1639 (1639G>A) in the VKORC1 gene demonstrate diminished VKORC1 expression. Since VKORC1 is the target for warfarin, patients with diminished VKORC1 expression require lower maintenance doses of warfarin. These patients have a correspondingly higher risk of warfarin-related adverse events at normal doses.

Human Leukocyte Antigen

There is also a clinically important role for pharmacogenomics of the HLA genes. The strongest evidence for adverse effects that have been associated with HLA polymorphisms are serious skin hypersensitivity reactions resulting in Stevens-Johnson syndrome (SJS) or toxic epidermal necrolysis (TEN). Carbamazepine and phenytoin have a strong association with the development of SJS/TEN in patients carrying the HLA-B*1502 allele. The highest allele frequency for this mutation is found in Asian populations, so patients of Asian descent are commonly tested for this mutation before receiving carbamazepine or phenytoin therapy. Additionally, abacavir has a strong association with the development of hypersensitivity reactions in patients carrying the HLA-B*5701 allele. Patients should be tested for this mutation before receiving abacavir therapy, and abacavir should be avoided in patients who test positive for this mutation.

LEARNING POINTS

- Genetic variations in CYP metabolism lead to extensive and poor metabolizers of a variety of drugs. In some cases, dosage adjustments must be made or alternate therapies selected.

- The CYP enzymes CYP2D6, CYP1A, CYP2C9, and CYP2C19 are polymorphically expressed with clinically relevant changes in pharmacokinetics.

- There are important genetic differences in Phase II enzymes (e.g., glucuronidation and acetylation) that have clinically relevant consequences.

- The HLA gene has known polymorphisms that increase the risk of hypersensitivity reactions to drugs like carbamazepine.

PRACTICE QUESTIONS

1. A 55 year-old Asian patient presents to your clinic with a new prescription for carbamazepine. Which of the following genes is MOST important to be included in the genotype testing for this patient?

   (A) CYP2D6
   (B) HLA
   (C) EGFR
   (D) VKORC1
   (E) UGT1A1

2. Which of the following statements regarding CYP2D6 poor metabolizers is/are TRUE? (Select ALL that apply.)

   (A) CYP2D6 poor metabolizers commonly are carriers of at least one *1 allele.
   (B) CYP2D6 poor metabolizers demonstrate unusually high morphine concentrations following codeine administration.
   (C) CYP2D6 poor metabolizers have polymorphisms that result in an allele with supra-enzymatic activity.
   (D) CYP2D6 poor metabolizers will form fewer metabolites through the CYP2D6 pathway than extensive metabolizers.
   (E) A CYP2D6 poor metabolizer is a phenotype that can be predicted by a patient's genotype.

3. A 22-year-old woman presents to the ER with nystagmus and excessive sedation. She has been on phenytoin therapy for 18 months for primary generalized epilepsy. Plasma phenytoin concentration is 34.4 µg/mL. Which of the following is the most likely genotype of this patient?

   (A) CYP2C9*2*3
   (B) CYP2C19*1*17
   (C) CYP2D6*1*4
   (D) CYP1A2*1A*1C
   (E) UGT1A1*28

4. Which of the following is the most likely clinical outcome in a CYP2D6 poor metabolizer being treated for pain?

   (A) Hallucinations associated with morphine
   (B) Failed pain management with codeine
   (C) Respiratory depression with hydrocodone
   (D) Failed pain management with hydromorphone
   (E) None of the above would be expected

5. Which of the following comorbidities in the past medical history would be the most concerning in a patient being started on irinotecan?

(A) Non–small cell lung carcinoma (NSCL)
(B) Paget's disease
(C) Parkinson's disease
(D) Gilbert's syndrome
(E) Stevens-Johnson syndrome

6. Which of the following genes has/have known genetic variations that can alter dosing requirements for warfarin? (Select ALL that apply.)

(A) CYP2D6
(B) VKORC1
(C) HLA
(D) CYP2C9
(E) CYP2C19

ANSWERS AND EXPLANATIONS

1. B

Patients receiving carbamazepine are at an increased risk of developing severe skin reactions such as Stevens-Johnson syndrome or toxic epidermal necrolysis. The patients at the greatest risk have polymorphisms in the HLA gene, with the strongest correlation found in patients of Asian descent. The other genes (CYP2D6, EGFR, VKORC1, and UGT1A1) do not have clinically significant polymorphisms related to carbamazepine therapy.

2. D, E

A poor metabolizer (PM) has decreased CYP2D6 function, resulting in fewer metabolites formed through that pathway (D). A PM is a phenotype that can be predicted by a patient's genotype (E); a phenotype is the observable characteristic and is affected by genetic and environmental factors. The *1 alleles refer to the wild-type allele, and homozygotes (i.e., carriers of two *1 alleles) would be considered extensive metabolizers, while carriers of one *1 allele would likely be intermediate metabolizers depending on the other allele, not poor metabolizers (A). Option (B) is incorrect since morphine is a metabolite formed via CYP2D6 following codeine administration. Supraenzymatic activity (C) describes an ultra-rapid metabolizer phenotype, not a PM.

3. A

Phenytoin is metabolized by CYP2C9, and both the *2 and *3 alleles are decreased-function alleles. Patients with these mutations would have decreased CYP2C9 activity, resulting in higher phenytoin concentrations and potentially the adverse effects listed in this case. The other enzymes (CYP2C19, CYP2D6, CYP1A2, and UGT1A1) do not have polymorphisms that are known to alter phenytoin to any great extent.

4. B

The parent drug codeine has minimal analgesic effectiveness. It primarily exerts its analgesic effect through activation to morphine by cytochrome P450 2D6 (CYP2D6). Therefore, a poor metabolizer of CYP2D6 would have negligible morphine concentrations and would likely lack a clinically effective analgesic effect from codeine.

5. **D**

Patients with Gilbert's syndrome are homozygous for the UGT1A1*28 allele, which is a decreased-function allele. Since the active metabolite (SN-38) of irinotecan is eliminated through glucuronidation, patients with Gilbert's syndrome would be at an increased risk of severe toxic effects such as myelosuppression. The other diseases listed would be unlikely to influence the administration of irinotecan.

6. **B, D**

Warfarin targets the VKORC1 gene product, which is necessary for the proper function of the vitamin K–dependent coagulation factors. There are known VKORC1 mutations that decrease the function of the enzyme and increase sensitivity to warfarin. The most active enantiomer of warfarin is metabolized by CYP2C9; decreased function of this enzyme will also increase sensitivity to warfarin. By contrast, CYP2D6 (A) and CYP2C19 (E) do not have polymorphisms that are known to have significant clinical effects on warfarin. Polymorphisms in the HLA gene (C) likewise have not been associated with warfarin hypersensitivity.

Pharmacokinetics 26

This chapter covers the following:

- **Plasma drug concentration profiles**
- **Theoretical compartments**
- **Basic pharmacokinetic parameters**
- **Oral dosing**
- **Multiple drug dosing**
- **Multiple dosing factor and accumulation factor**
- **Nonlinear pharmacokinetics**

 Suggested Study Time: **3 hours**

Pharmacokinetics is the mathematical study of drug concentration in the body. It is dependent on the absorption, distribution, metabolism, and excretion (ADME) discussed in the Biopharmaceutics chapter and is the quantitative description of what happens to the drug in the body. Clinical pharmacokinetics applies the concepts directly to individual patients, making individualized drug therapy and therapeutic drug monitoring possible.

Many equations are employed in pharmacokinetics. The more complicated of these equations are unlikely to be used in calculations on the NAPLEX due to time constraints, but you should be familiar with their concepts because they could form the basis for theoretical questions. Studying for this section of the exam should focus primarily on being able to perform calculations related to the basic pharmacokinetic parameters discussed and being able to properly interpret graphs of plasma concentration data. Calculations involving drugs most likely to be monitored clinically (e.g., digoxin, phenytoin, aminoglycosides, vancomycin) are the most important to focus on.

PLASMA DRUG CONCENTRATION PROFILES

Plasma drug concentration versus time curve charts are used extensively in pharmacokinetics. A known dose of drug is given to a patient, and blood samples are taken at various time intervals following drug administration. The concentration of drug in plasma following IV and oral administration is measured and plotted in the following figure. The shape of the curve depends on the relative rates of absorption, distribution, and elimination of the drug.

Plasma Concentration versus Time Curves for Intravenous and Oral Drug Administration

The preceding graphs represent drug plasma concentration (Cp) versus time profiles following an IV bolus and oral administration of a mock drug. Following IV administration, the drug will reach its maximum plasma concentration (C_{max}) at time 0 (leftmost point on the X-axis). Therefore, the time to maximum plasma concentration (T_{max}) is at time 0 following an IV bolus. The only route of administration that can be deciphered from the concentration-time curve alone is an IV bolus due to the C_{max} occurring at time 0.

The time 0 on the oral concentration-time profile does not display measurable plasma concentrations. This is true for any route of administration for which absorption into the systemic circulation is required (e.g., sublingual, inhalation, subcutaneous, etc). Following the lag time for absorption, a rise in drug plasma concentration is seen until it reaches a plateau, which represents the C_{max} on the oral curve. The time of this plateau (i.e., C_{max}) is the T_{max}. At the T_{max}, there is a brief time period where this is no net change in drug plasma concentration. This represents the time when the rate of drug absorption is equal to that of elimination. Beyond the C_{max}, elimination will be greater than absorption and is represented by a decline in the drug plasma concentration.

THEORETICAL COMPARTMENTS

From a pharmacokinetic perspective, the body is considered to consist of compartments, inside each of which the drug can be considered evenly distributed. These compartments are interconnected, and the drug moves between them at defined rates. Although compartments are completely theoretical (consisting of groups of tissues with similar blood flow and drug affinity, not actual body regions), they serve a useful purpose in simplifying calculations. Several models exist, but only two are likely to be considered on the NAPLEX:

- One-compartment model:
  - Body consists of one homogenous central compartment.
  - Drug distributes rapidly and uniformly to this compartment.
- Two-compartment model:
  - Central compartment is still present, and includes highly perfused organs (e.g., liver, kidneys).
  - There is a slow distribution of drug into a peripheral compartment that consists of poorly perfused tissue (e.g., muscles, connective tissue).

One-Compartment Model

The basic structure of a one-compartment drug is displayed on the left, with a corresponding drug log concentration-time curve on the right. At time 0, the drug is administered into the central compartment. This can be observed on the concentration-time curve by the C_{max} at time 0. The central compartment represents plasma and tissue to which the drug rapidly distributes. The slope of the concentration time curve on a log or natural log scale is directly proportional to the first-order elimination rate constant and therefore the drug half-life. The elimination rate constant can be calculated by taking the difference of the natural log of two concentrations and dividing by the difference of the two corresponding times.

Two-Compartment Model

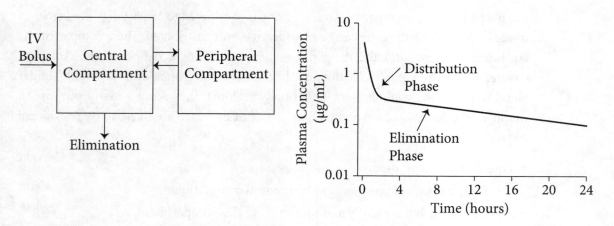

The general structure of a two-compartment model is displayed on the left of the figure. The right side of the figure represents the log concentration-time profile following an IV bolus of a two-compartment drug. As displayed on the concentration-time curve, there are two distinct slopes labeled as the distribution phase and the elimination phase. The C_{max} following an IV bolus in a two-compartment model is still at time 0. However, the slope of the line at time 0 is representative of both the elimination from the central compartment and slow distribution into peripheral tissue. This phase, commonly called the *distribution phase* of the drug, is not directly representative of elimination. Therefore, it is inappropriate to calculate an elimination rate constant or half-life while a drug is in the distribution phase. Once drug accumulates in the peripheral tissue to a point of equilibrium (i.e., drug diffuses from peripheral tissue back into the central compartment), the change in the concentration-time curve is solely due to the elimination of the drug. The half-life of the drug can be calculated only in the elimination phase.

BASIC PHARMACOKINETIC PARAMETERS

Most calculations you are likely to see on the NAPLEX involve the parameters listed here.

Bioavailable Fraction

The bioavailable fraction (F) is the portion of dose administered that reaches the systemic circulation. For IV administration, $F = 1$. A drug given by any other route can have an F ranging from 0 to 1; the F will never be >1. Two factors can ↓ the F of a drug:

- Incomplete absorption
- First-pass metabolism

The equation governing F is given below. fa represents the fraction of administered dose absorbed into the bloodstream, and ffp represents the fraction of absorbed drug escaping first-pass metabolism. It should be noted that first-pass metabolism is generally in the liver but can also occur through gut-wall metabolism or enzymatic degradation.

$$F = ffp \cdot fa$$

Hepatic Extraction Ratio

The hepatic extraction ratio (E) is the fraction of drug in the blood that is metabolized during each pass of blood through the liver.

$$(1 - E) = ffp$$

High-E drugs are extensively metabolized by the liver enzymes. Low-E drugs are metabolized by enzymes with relatively low affinity for the drug. Knowing a drug's E value is useful in predicting the effects of first-pass metabolism, disease states, and drug–drug interactions on the metabolism of the drug.

Plasma Concentrations

The plasma concentration of the drug (Cp) can be determined by a number of equations. The most basic version, for a drug following a one-compartment model for a first-order process, is given here in three formats.

$$Cp = C_0 e^{-kt}$$
$$\ln Cp = \ln C_0 - kt$$
$$\log Cp = \log C_0 - \frac{kt}{2.3}$$

In this equation, C_0 is the initial concentration, k is the first order elimination rate constant and t is time. Note that the calculator available to you during the NAPLEX does not have an exponential or log function. However, you may be asked to estimate drug concentration at any given time or estimate a half-life ($t_{1/2}$). These estimations will be provided later in this chapter, and you can check your answers by using the equations shown here.

Elimination Rate Constant

The first-order elimination rate constant, k, represents the fraction of drug eliminated per unit time, and thus has units of reciprocal time (i.e., hr^{-1}). It can be obtained graphically (see the figure that follows) or from the drug $t_{1/2}$:

$$k = \frac{\ln 2}{t_{1/2}} = \frac{0.693}{t_{1/2}}$$

Graphical Calculation of Elimination Rate Constant

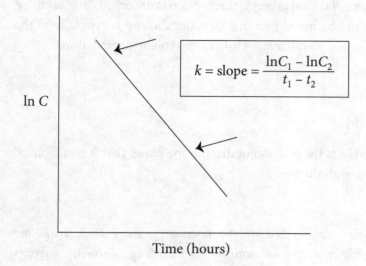

$$k = \text{slope} = \frac{\ln C_1 - \ln C_2}{t_1 - t_2}$$

Half-Life

The elimination $t_{1/2}$ of a drug is the time required for its serum concentration to ↓ by half. It can be obtained mathematically or graphically:

$$t_{1/2} = \frac{\ln 2}{k} = \frac{0.693}{k}$$

The $t_{1/2}$ can also be calculated from clearance (CL) and volume of distribution (V_d). While these parameters do not influence or depend on one another, half-life depends on both of them:

$$t_{1/2} = 0.693 \cdot \frac{Vd}{CL}$$

Clearance

CL refers to the efficiency of the body in removing drug from the blood. The liver and kidney are the primary organs involved, and body CL refers to the sum of the hepatic (CL_h) and renal clearances (CL_r), plus any CL from other organs, usually negligible:

$$CL = CL_h + CL_r$$

Some drugs are cleared primarily by one organ (propranolol has a CL_h of 840 mL/min and a total clearance of only 848 mL/min), while others have a more mixed CL (procainamide has a CL_h of 268 mL/min and a CL_r of 303 mL/min). Knowledge of drug CL can help determine when dosage adjustments are needed in patients with hepatic or renal impairment. Using the previous examples, patients with renal impairment would need dose adjustments for procainamide but not for propranolol. Patients with hepatic impairment would need dose adjustments for both drugs.

If $CL\uparrow$, the drug is more efficiently removed from the body and the drug $t_{1/2}\downarrow$.

Population CL values are typically based on body weight; CL corresponds to ideal body weight (IBW):

- Tall, lean individuals have larger eliminating organs resulting in a higher CL than a shorter lean person.

- Adipose tissue does not affect the size of eliminating organs; thus actual body weight should not be used to determine CL in obese patients. In many instances these patients will need to be dosed on an adjusted body weight, which is derived from their IBW.

$$\text{IBW (males)} = 50 \text{ kg} + [2.3 \cdot (\# \text{ of inches of height} > 60")]$$

$$\text{IBW (females)} = 45 \text{ kg} + [2.3 \cdot (\# \text{ of inches of height} > 60")]$$

Volume of Distribution

Apparent V_d describes the volume of body fluids required to account for all drugs in the body. As mentioned in the Biopharmaceutics chapter, it is not a real volume but a calculated number that helps to compare the behavior of different drugs. Several equations can be used to calculate apparent V_d, depending on the information you have available:

$$V_d = \frac{\text{dose}}{C_{peak}} = \frac{F \cdot \text{Dose}}{AUC \cdot k} = \frac{CL \cdot t_{1/2}}{0.693}$$

V_d has the following effect on $t_{1/2}$:

- Small V_d:
  - Drug mostly located in blood
  - Liver and kidneys only clear drug in blood
  - Fewer passes needed to rid body of drug
  - Shorter $t_{1/2}$
- Large V_d:
  - Drug is extensively distributed into extravascular tissues
  - Liver and kidneys only clear drug in blood
  - More passes are required to clear drug from body
  - Longer $t_{1/2}$

Area under the Curve

Area under the curve (AUC) is a measure of the extent of drug exposure. It is defined as the area under the drug plasma level – time curve from $t = 0$ to infinity. It can be calculated by the trapezoidal rule (unlikely to appear on the NAPLEX, due to time constraints), or by the other listed equations, and has units of concentration/time. S is the salt factor for a given drug formulation and refers to the percentage of administered product that is the active moiety (the acid or base, not the salt). A commonly used example of a drug with a salt factor is aminophylline ($S = 0.8$), as compared to theophylline ($S = 1$).

Trapezoidal rule:

$$AUC = \frac{C_{n-1} + C_n}{2}(tn - t_{n-1})$$

where n refers to the concentration and time associated with it and $n-1$ is the previous concentration and associated times.

Other equations:

$$AUC = \frac{F \cdot S \cdot D_0}{CL} = \frac{F \cdot D_0}{k \cdot V_D}$$

AUC is often directly proportional to dose, such that $\uparrow$ the dose of a drug from 500 mg to 1,000 mg will lead to a twofold $\uparrow$ in AUC. This is not always the case, however. If a pathway for drug elimination becomes saturated, as can happen with the enzyme-dependent metabolism of certain drugs (e.g., phenytoin, salicylates), $\uparrow$ the dose can lead to a disproportionately large $\uparrow$ in AUC.

ORAL DOSING

Most immediate-release oral dosage forms follow a first-order absorption model, as do some non-oral dosage forms such as suppositories and intramuscular (IM) injections. When plotting log C versus time (see figure that follows), the following equation of the "$y = mx + b$" format applies:

First-Order Drug Plasma-Level-versus-Time Curve

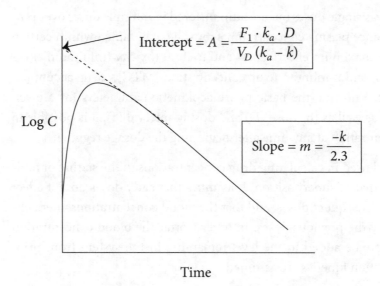

The absorption rate constant, k_a, cannot be measured directly. It can be calculated by several methods, which are fairly lengthy mathematical processes and are unlikely to be tested on the NAPLEX. General questions about the methods could be asked, however.

- Method of residuals (feathering, peeling)
  - The difference between the extrapolated line (shown in a dashed line) in the graph and the point directly below it on the absorption portion of the curve (the residual) is plotted versus time.
  - k_a can be derived by the substraction of the extrapolated line from elimination phase above (dashed line) and the concentrations in the absorption phase.
- Wagner-Nelson method
  - Plots fraction of drug unabsorbed versus time
  - Can use blood level and/or urinary excretion data
- Loo-Riegelman method
  - Plots percent of drug unabsorbed versus time
  - Used for two-compartment model drugs
  - Must give drug IV and orally to obtain all necessary information

MULTIPLE DRUG DOSING

Most drugs are not given as single doses but are administered in multiple doses over prolonged periods of time. Since plasma concentrations must be maintained within certain levels in order to achieve maximum effectiveness and to limit toxicity (minimum effective concentration [MEC] and minimum toxic concentration [MTC]), drug accumulation must be considered. Knowing the basic pharmacokinetic parameters for a given drug (k, V_d, and/or CL), as well as the dose (D) and dosing interval (τ), it is possible to predict the plasma concentration at any time after beginning the dosage regimen.

The most common model used in calculating drug concentrations in the setting of multiple-dosage regimens is that of superposition. It assumes that early doses do not affect the pharmacokinetics of subsequent doses, and that the blood concentrations after subsequent doses will overlay the previous doses. In other words, the blood concentration after each dose can simply be added to the level remaining in the system from prior doses. First-order elimination kinetics are assumed.

If the same dose of drug is given at a fixed-dose frequency, eventually the plasma concentration curve reaches a plateau and a steady-state plasma concentration (C_{SS}) is reached. At this point, the rate of the drug entering the body equals the rate of drug leaving the body. Blood concentrations are constant from interval to interval, provided the patient's pharmacokinetic parameters do not change and the dose and dosing interval stay the same. Ninety percent of the C_{SS} is attained after three half-lives; after five half-lives, 97% is attained. These numbers are very important to remember as they will allow you to estimate some answers on the NAPLEX.

MULTIPLE DOSING FACTOR AND ACCUMULATION FACTOR

The extent of accumulation can be predicted by using the multiple dosing factor (MDF), where $N =$ the number of doses:

$$MDF = \frac{1 \cdot e^{-N \cdot k \cdot \tau}}{1 - e^{-k \cdot \tau}}$$

Single-dose equations can be converted to multiple-dose equations simply by multiplying each exponential term that contains time as a variable by the MDF.

At steady state, the MDF simplifies to the following accumulation factor (AF):

$$AF = \frac{1}{1 - e^{-k \cdot \tau}}$$

As the equation for *AF* shows, two things affect how much drug accumulates between the first dose and a dose at steady state:

- Elimination constant or half-life
- Dosing interval

We cannot control the half-life; it is dependent on the drug in question. However, the dosing interval can be adjusted to increase or decrease the drug accumulation factor. A simple estimation of this can be described by:

- Dosing interval < drug half-life → C_{SS} will be much higher than the concentration after the first dose.
- Dosing interval = drug half-life → C_{SS} will be twice as high as the concentration after the first dose.
- Dosing interval > drug half-life → C_{SS} will be similar to the concentration after the first dose (because the drug is almost completely washing out before the next dose is given).

Peak-to-Trough Ratio

Multiple intermittent dosing results in peak and trough drug concentrations. As will be discussed, a dose and dosing interval (τ) are calculated to achieve a desired steady-state plasma concentration average ($C_{SS, avg}$). The $C_{SS, avg}$ represents the average concentration between the peak and trough. Shorter dosing intervals for a particular dose will lead to a decreased *P:T* ratio, meaning that less fluctuation in peak-to-trough is occurring.

The peak-to-trough ratio can be especially useful when predicting the effect of switching a patient from a regular to a sustained-release formulation. T_{max} represents time to peak concentration within the dosing interval; it is smaller for immediate-release formulations than for sustained-release, as the drug is liberated and absorbed more quickly, and so the peak concentration occurs sooner.

Loading Doses

Loading doses are often used to achieve target plasma drug concentrations as quickly as possible. These large initial doses (which may be given as either a single dose or divided doses over a specified period of time) are especially important in life-threatening conditions such as myocardial infarction, status asthmaticus, and status epilepticus. Loading doses should not be used when there is not an urgent need to achieve target blood concentrations immediately or the patient cannot be supervised for possible toxicity. Loading doses for narrow-therapeutic-index drugs should ideally occur within a clinical setting.

Loading doses that are given slowly can be calculated by the equation given here. If given rapidly (by bolus injection, for example), the volume of the central compartment (V_c) should be used instead of V_d. Lidocaine is an example of a drug that would require a fast loading dose, due to its use in the treatment of life-threatening arrhythmias.

$$F \cdot Loading\ dose = C_{ss(target)} \cdot V_d$$

Loading doses are commonly given by the IV route, so the F will be equal to 1 in these cases. If an oral loading dose is being administered, the bioavailability of the drug MUST be taken into consideration. The target concentration will be given along with the drug's V_d. Therefore, this is a simple and important equation to know for the NAPLEX exam.

If the patient already has drug in his or her system, this needs to be taken into consideration. Simply take the desired concentration ($C_{ss(target)}$) and subtract out the concentration already in the system. Just be sure the units are identical when performing this calculation.

When patients are within 20% of their IBW, total body weight (TBW) should be used when calculating loading dose. For obese patients, the decision to use IBW versus TBW depends on the drug and its ability to partition into adipose tissue.

- Drug fully partitions into fat: V_d will increase with weight gain; use TBW
  - Example: Lidocaine
- Drug does not partition into fat: V_d does not change with weight gain; use IBW
  - Example: Digoxin
- Drug that partially partitions into fat: an intermediate value should be used
  - Example: Theophylline

Constant IV Infusion

Constant-rate infusions do not generate fluctuations in plasma concentrations. Determining the rate for such infusions is relatively simple:

1. Determine the target steady-state plasma concentration (C_{SS}).
2. Find the appropriate population CL.
3. Look up S (if drug is a salt).
4. Calculate infusion rate (R). (The infusion rate is in the units of amount per time [e.g., mg/min].)

$$R = \frac{C_{SS} \cdot CL}{S}$$

In most instances, S will be equal to 1 and can be ignored. Clearance adjustment factors may be available for some drugs. Some conditions that may have corresponding clearance adjustments include patient age, smoking status, and concurrent use of certain drugs. If available, these factors should be used to better predict blood concentrations in the individual patient.

If a drug is infused at a faster rate, a higher steady-state concentration will result. However, the time to steady-state is based on half-life and will remain the same. To achieve and maintain immediate steady-state concentrations:

- Give IV loading dose.
- Begin IV infusion.

Intermittent IV Infusion

Short IV infusions separated by the time required for drug elimination are often given to prevent high drug concentration and associated adverse effects. The drug may not reach steady-state in such cases.

These equations are not important to memorize for the NAPLEX exam because they contain an exponential function. However, the principles should be noted.

$$C = \frac{R}{V_d \cdot k}(1 - e^{-kt})$$

The rate of infusion is equal to the dose/infusion period. After the infusion has stopped, drug concentration at a particular time can be determined by the following equation, given the concentration at the time the infusion was stopped.

$$C = C_{stop}(1 - e^{-kt})$$

Intermittent Oral Dosing

Dose rate in intermittent oral dosing is calculated in a similar fashion to IV infusions. Remember to take F into account with oral dosing, however, since bioavailability may not be equal to IV products. The equation to calculate a dosing rate (dose divided by dosing interval, τ) for an intermittent infusion or oral dosing to a desired steady-state plasma concentration is displayed:

$$\frac{F \cdot Dose}{\tau} = C_{SS}, avg \cdot CL$$

where F is the bioavailability (equal to 1 for IV infusion), dose is the amount administered, τ is the dosing interval, Css, avg is the average steady-state plasma concentration, and CL is the clearance. This is an important equation that can be used to calculate maintenance dosing of drugs to desired steady-state concentrations.

NONLINEAR PHARMACOKINETICS

So far, this chapter has referred to general pharmacokinetic principles. These principles are applicable to most drugs without significant modification, and they result in linear mathematical models. Several assumptions are made when different or multiple doses are given:

- Drug clearance remains constant.
- Doubling the dose results in a doubling of the concentration and AUC.

These assumptions are not always accurate. With some drugs, giving a single low dose of the drug leads to the expected linear pharmacokinetics. However, when higher doses are given, or when the medication is taken chronically, the drug no longer fits the linear pharmacokinetic profile.

Pharmacokinetic Relationships: Linear versus Nonlinear

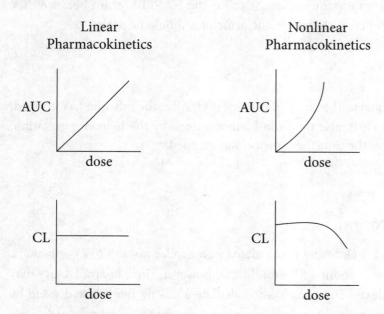

Nonlinear pharmacokinetics generally occur when one or more enzyme- or carrier-mediated systems are saturated. These systems are often referred to as capacity-limited.

- Active drug absorption: Absorption of riboflavin involves saturable gut wall transport
- Drug distribution: Saturable protein binding of salicylates
- Drug metabolism: Saturable metabolism of phenytoin
- Drug excretion: Active secretion of penicillin G

Most elimination processes can be saturated if enough drug is given. Certain drugs (phenytoin in particular) show nonlinear behavior even at normal drug doses.

For drugs exhibiting nonlinear behavior, dose increases lead to half-life increases, and AUC is not proportional to the amount of bioavailable drug. The behavior is described by the Michaelis-Menten equation:

$$\frac{dC}{dt} = \frac{V_{max} - C_{SS}}{K_M + C_{SS}}$$

V_{max} (the maximum elimination rate) and K_M (the Michaelis constant, equal to one-half the concentration at V_{max}) are dependent on both the drug and the enzyme system. Two general situations can apply:

- $C >> K_m$; rate of change simplifies to V_{max}, a constant → zero-order kinetics
- $C << K_m$; rate of change is concentration dependent → first-order kinetics

To determine K_m and V_{max}, steady-state concentrations are measured as the result of two different doses given at different times. Recall that at steady-state, the rate of drug metabolism is assumed to be the same as the rate of drug input. In other words, the change in concentration over time is equal to the dosing rate (*DR*). As most nonlinear calculations that you will encounter involve phenytoin, remember that the salt factor (*S*) for phenytoin sodium is 0.92, and the dose must be multiplied by this number when the salt form (capsules and injection) is used.

$$DR = \frac{V_{max} - C_{SS}}{K_M \cdot C_{SS}}$$

K_m may be obtained in two ways:

1. Graph the data and obtain K_m from the slope.
2. Solve simultaneous equations using two dosing rates and respective C_{SS} (algebraic determination).

$$DR_1 = V_{max} - Km \cdot \frac{DR_1}{C_{ss1}}$$

$$-(DR_2 = V_{max} - Km \cdot \frac{DR_2}{C_{ss2}})$$

Subtracting the second equation from the first, V_{max} will drop out and the equation can be solved for K_m.

V_{max} may be obtained in two ways as well:

1. Graph the data, and determine the *y*-intercept from the graph.
2. Use the dosing rate, C_{ss}, and the newly calculated K_m to solve mathematically.

Graphical data, if available, is the faster way to obtain K_m and V_{max}.

Graphical Determination of K_m and V_{max}

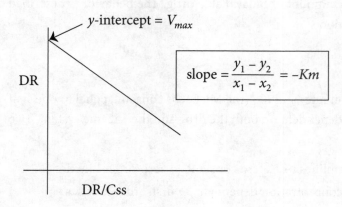

$$\text{slope} = \frac{y_1 - y_2}{x_1 - x_2} = -Km$$

LEARNING POINTS

- Ninety percent of steady-state blood concentrations are achieved after three half-lives; 97% after five half-lives.

- Increasing the infusion rate will lead to higher steady-state concentrations, but the drug will not reach steady state more quickly.

- The main parameters you should be able to calculate are half-life, k, CL, V_d, plasma concentration (simple cases), and R.

- When calculating loading doses, the tendency of drug to partition into fat must be considered when determining whether to use TBW or IBW for obese patients (use TBW for drugs that partition heavily into fat).

- Increasing the dose for nonlinear drugs such as phenytoin increases the half-life and can increase AUC above what would be expected for drugs exhibiting linear behavior. Pharmacokinetic monitoring is especially important in such cases.

PRACTICE QUESTIONS

1. A patient is being started on IV digoxin. What plasma concentration of digoxin would you expect after a loading dose of 0.75 mg? Patient weight $= 65$ kg $\cdot V_d = 6$ L/kg

    (A) 167 mcg/L
    (B) 2.6 mcg/L
    (C) 125 mcg/L
    (D) 1.95 mcg/L
    (E) 11.5 mcg/L

2. What is the half-life of procainamide in a patient whose total clearance is estimated to be 18 L/h and the volume of distribution is 140 L?

    (A) 10.8 hours
    (B) 7.4 hours
    (C) 5.4 hours
    (D) 4.6 hours
    (E) 2.7 hours

3. An investigational drug was intravenously injected into a patient, and serum samples were obtained at specific time intervals, displayed in the table below. What is the half-life of this drug?

Time Following IV Administration (min)	Serum Drug Concentrations (mg/dL)
10	8.6
20	7.5
30	6.5
60	4.2
80	3.2
100	2.4
120	1.8

    (A) 58 minutes
    (B) 48 minutes
    (C) 38 minutes
    (D) 28 minutes
    (E) 18 minutes

4. Which of the following statements is true regarding the administration of theophylline depicted in the following graph?

This graph illustrates the time course of the mean plasma theophylline (administered as the ethylenediamine salt) concentrations when 0.5 g is administered (X) intravenously, (Y) as a retention enema, and (Z) as an oral tablet.

(A) The elimination half-life of theophylline is 3.5 hours.
(B) Theophylline is eliminated from the body by zero-order kinetics.
(C) The bioavailability of theophylline is not affected the route of administration.
(D) The retention enema and oral tablet are bioequivalent to each other.
(E) None of the above statements is true.

5. A patient taking 40 mg of propranolol PO enters the hospital and is switched to propranolol IV. What would be an appropriate dose in milligrams, considering the drug undergoes approximately 90% first-pass effect?

(A)   4
(B)   20
(C)   40
(D)   80
(E)   120

6. The apparent V_d of gentamicin in a patient is 8 L. What dose of the antibiotic should be given to a patient with a current plasma concentration of 2 mg/L when a 6 mg/L concentration is desired?

   (A) 48 mg
   (B) 40 mg
   (C) 32 mg
   (D) 12 mg
   (E) 6 mg

7. 250 mg of an antibiotic with a half-life of 9 hours is given every 6 hours to a patient with a clearance rate of 1.54 L/hr. What is the steady-state concentration of this drug assuming 80% is absorbed?

   (A) 64.2 mg/L
   (B) 51.3 mg/L
   (C) 33.3 mg/L
   (D) 21.6 mg/L
   (E) 3.7 mg/L

ANSWERS AND EXPLANATIONS

1. **D**

$$\text{Use } C = \frac{\text{dose}}{V_d} = \frac{0.75\,\text{mg}}{\dfrac{6L}{kg} \cdot 65\,\text{kg}} = \frac{1,000\,\text{mcg}}{1\,\text{mg}} = \frac{1.95\,\text{mcg}}{L}$$

2. **C**

$$t_{1/2} = 0.693 \cdot \frac{V_d}{CL}$$

$$t_{1/2} = 0.693 \cdot \frac{140}{18} = 5.4 \text{ hours}$$

3. **B**

The elimination rate constant can be directly calculated by first calculating the slope of the line on a natural log scale. The slope is equal to the negative value of the elimination rate constant. Theoretically any two time points and concentrations in the table can be used, but in practice it is important that you avoid choosing points in a distribution phase. It advisable to choose the later time points, as shown here.

$$-k = \text{slope} = \frac{\ln C_1 - \ln C_2}{t_1 - t_2}$$

$$-k = \text{slope} = \frac{\ln 3.2 - \ln 1.8}{80 - 120}$$

$$k = 0.0144$$

$$t_{1/2} = \frac{0.693}{k} \approx 48 \text{ minutes}$$

This answer can also be estimated by simply looking at the time it takes for any given concentration to decrease by half. For example, it took 40 minutes (difference between 120 and 80) for the concentration to go from 3.2 to 1.8. This is just a little less than half, so you know that the half-life of the drug must be slightly >40 minutes. Indeed, the calculated half-life was 48 minutes. This is a good method to check your calculations.

4. **A**

The half-life can be estimated from any of the three administration routes because the elimination phases are parallel to each other and have similar slopes. This indicates that they have identical elimination rate constants and half-lives. The key is to identify two concentrations (one that is half the value of the other) in the elimination phase of any of the routes. The half-life of theophylline can be estimated from the IV curve (X in the graph) because concentration 4 mg/mL and 2 mg/mL are in the elimination phase in the curve. To estimate the half-life, use a straight edge to extrapolate from 4 mg/mL on the y-axis to the IV curve (X on the graph) and then down from that point to the time (x-axis value) that theophylline was at 4 mg/mL. This time is approximately 2 hours following IV administration. Do the same extrapolation for the 2 mg/mL concentration. The time of the 2 mg/mL concentration is approximately 5.5 hours. Therefore, between 2 and 5.5 hours (or 3.5 hours) after IV administration, the concentration of theophylline decreased by half its value from 4 mg/mL to 2 mg/mL. Therefore, choice (A) is a true statement. Choice (B) is false because the elimination of theophylline is linear on the log-axis, indicating a first-order process. Choice (C) is false because the bioavailability is clearly altered by the route of administration. This can be seen by the vastly different AUCs given the same total dosages of each route. Choice (D) is false because the C_{max} and AUCs are different between the retention enema and the oral dose. These, along with T_{max}, must be similar to demonstrate bioequivalence.

5. **A**

If 90% of the oral drug is lost to a first-pass effect, then the bioavailability (F) cannot be greater than 10%. Therefore, one would administer 10% of the oral dose by the IV route; 10% of 40 mg is 4 mg.

6. **C**

$$F \cdot \text{Loading dose} = C_{SS \ (target)} \cdot V_d$$

In this case, an IV drug is being administered, so F is equal to 1. Additionally, there is drug onboard at 2 mg/L with a target of 6 mg/L. These concentrations can be subtracted from each other to get the concentration for the $C_{SS(target)}$ value.

6 mg/L (desired C_{SS}) − 2 mg/L (onboard C) = 4 mg/L

$F \cdot \text{Loading dose} = 4 \cdot 8 = 32$ mg

7. **D**

$$\frac{F \cdot \text{Dose}}{\tau} = C_{SS,avg} \cdot CL$$

$$\frac{0.8 \cdot 250 \, \text{mg}}{6 \, \text{hours}} = C_{SS,avg} \cdot 1.54 \, \text{L/hr}$$

$$C_{SS,avg} = 21.6 \, \text{mg/L}$$

Calculations 27

This chapter covers the following:

- **Problem-solving techniques**
- **Fundamentals of units and measurement**
- **Density, specific gravity, and specific volume**
- **Reducing and enlarging formulas**
- **Percentage, ratio strengths, and parts per million**
- **Dosage calculations**
- **Dilution, concentration, and alligation**
- **Electrolyte solutions**
- **Compounding calculations**

 Suggested Study Time: **4 hours**

This section contains a quick review of the types of calculation questions likely to be covered on the NAPLEX. Practice is the key to this section. Keep in mind that you will be restricted to using a basic calculator (provided by testing centers).

If you would like additional review, older editions of pharmacy calculation text books will be helpful—the techniques involved have not changed. Two suggestions are *Pharmaceutical Calculations* by Ansel and Stockton, and *Pharmaceutical Calculations* by Zatz and Teixeira.

PROBLEM-SOLVING TECHNIQUES

Ratio-Proportion and Dimensional Analysis

There are two techniques that can be used to solve most pharmaceutical calculations: ratio-proportion and dimensional analysis. Either of these techniques is acceptable, and you should use whichever one you find most comfortable.

Ratio-proportion is a one-step calculation technique that is probably the easiest to use for simple (one- or two-step) calculations. In this process, you set up a likeness between a fraction involving known quantities and one that includes your unknown, and solve the equation by cross-multiplying. An example is given here, illustrating how to convert 3 fluid ounces to milliliters:

$$\frac{30\,\text{mL}}{1\,\text{fl oz}} = \frac{x\,\text{mL}}{3\,\text{fl oz}}$$

$$(30\,\text{mL})(3\,\text{fl oz}) = (x\,\text{mL})(1\,\text{fl oz})$$

$$\frac{(30\,\text{mL})(3\,\text{fl oz})}{(1\,\text{fl oz})} = x\,\text{mL}$$

$$x = 90\,\text{mL}$$

While ratio-proportion is often the most intuitive method, and is something with which you have been familiar since early grades of school, it has no inherent error-checking and it is not ideal for multistep calculations. When using ratio-proportion for multi-step problems, you will have to write down intermediate steps; rounding intermediate answers reduces your accuracy, and writing them down takes time. Both of these can be problems when taking exams, so dimensional analysis might be preferred for these reasons.

To avoid rounding errors, keep as many decimal points as possible until the last step in the calculation. If the question is fill-in-the-blank style, it will instruct you regarding how many decimals points to include in the final answer. An advantage of the ratio-proportion method is that it is more logical than using a dimensional analysis, which is primarily set up based on units alone.

Dimensional analysis is a technique, often used in chemistry and other sciences, which allows you to set up long calculations in a single step. Using the short example given earlier, the problem would be solved:

$$3\,\text{fl oz} \cdot \frac{(30\,\text{mL})}{(1\,\text{fl oz})} = 90\,\text{mL}$$

As you can see, the fluid ounces cancel out and leave you with the correct units of milliliters. This serves as an internal error-check and is especially helpful in longer, more complex problems. Also, it saves you from having to write down intermediate steps, and helps prevent "kitchen-sink" syndrome (using every bit of information given, whether it will help solve the problem or not). This method also helps you to avoid the problem of rounding too early; you round once, when the problem is finished.

When you have completed a calculation, regardless of the method you choose, always ask yourself if the answer makes sense. You won't always be able to determine this, but in many cases you can tell if something has gone wrong in your calculation just by looking at the final answer. For example, it would be impractical to have an IV drip rate of 1,000 mL/min, or a dose rate of 52 tablets per day. If your answer doesn't make sense, check your calculation to find out where you went wrong.

Estimation

Estimation is not always appropriate; when working in pharmacy, you want the most accurate answer possible, especially when working with drugs with narrow therapeutic indices, or for dosing of infants and children. However, for exam purposes you will often be able to eliminate several, if not all, incorrect options by using estimates, particularly of some of the conversion factors listed in the upcoming section. This could allow you more time to focus on other portions of the exam.

FUNDAMENTALS OF UNITS AND MEASUREMENT

The metric system is the standard system used for science worldwide. It is not, however, the only system used in pharmacy. The avoirdupois, or "common," system is the customary measure in the United States, and most patients will communicate with you in this system. Because of this, you will have to convert between systems of measurement on the NAPLEX. Unfortunately, cross-system conversions are inherently inexact. Therefore on the NAPLEX, convert from one system of measurement to another only once in a problem, not multiple times, and use the most direct conversion possible. Otherwise, the measurement error will be compounded.

The following conversions need to memorized for the NAPLEX:

- Avoirdupois refers to solid measures only (pounds and ounces).
  - 1 pound = 16 ounces
- Common or household liquid measurements start with the teaspoon:
  - 1 teaspoon (tsp) = 5 mL
  - 3 tsp = 1 tablespoon (T) = 15 mL
  - 2 T = 1 fluid ounce (fl oz) = 30 mL = 1/8 cup
  - 1 cup = 8 fl oz

- 1 pint = 16 fl oz (or 2 cups)
- 1 quart = 32 fl oz (or 4 cups)
- 1 gallon = 128 fl oz (or 16 cups)

- Apothecary measures, the measures pharmacists originally used (drams, grains, and scruples), are no longer used.

  - Some medications (aspirin is one) were traditionally measured in grains, and you may still see strength listed this way; Roman numerals are used instead of Arabic (65 mg = 1 grain [gr]; a gr V aspirin tablet = 325 mg).

  - The apothecary system adopted the common or household liquid measurements of pint, quart, and gallon.

  - Note that the apothecary system has pounds and ounces. These are not the same size as avoirdupois pounds and ounces, and are seldom—if ever—used. The grain, however, is the same size in the avoirdupois and apothecary systems.

Some of the more common conversion factors are given here:

Avoirdupois System	Metric System
1 lb	454 g
2.2 lb	1 kg
1 oz	28.4 g (30 g is an acceptable estimate)
1 grain	64.8 mg (65 g is an acceptable estimate)

Apothecary System	Metric System
1 tsp	5 mL
1 T	15 mL
1 fl oz	29.6 mL (30 mL is an acceptable estimate)
1 cup	240 mL
1 pint	473 mL
1 quart	946 mL
1 gallon	3,785 mL

In addition to converting the avoirdupois or apothecary system to the metric system, it is important to convert units within the metric system itself. Important conversions within the metric system follow:

Prefix	Conversion Factor	Example
Kilo (k)	1,000 or 10^3	1 kilograms (kg) = 1,000 grams (g)
Deci (d)	0.1 or 10^{-1}	1 deciliter (dL) = 0.1 liters (L)
Centi (c)	0.01 or 10^{-2}	1 centimeter (cm) = 0.01 meters (m)
Milli (m)	0.001 or 10^{-3}	1 milligram (mg) = 0.001 grams (g)
Micro (μ)	0.000001 or 10^{-6}	1 microliter (μL) = 0.000001 liters (L)
Nano (n)	0.000000001 or 10^{-9}	1 nanogram (ng) = 0.000000001 grams (g)

DENSITY AND SPECIFIC GRAVITY

Density describes the relationship between the mass of a substance and the volume it occupies. This is a helpful concept in pharmacy, as it allows you to convert between measures of mass and measures of volume. This is most useful with liquid ingredients used in compounded formulations. In compounded recipes, you may see liquid amounts expressed as either weight or volume and, depending on the recipe and the equipment you have available, it might be easier to measure in one form over the other. For instance, viscous liquids might be hard to get out of a graduated cylinder and, if you don't have a dosing syringe in which to measure the liquid, it might be better to weigh the product in a weigh boat.

Density should be treated like a conversion factor, since you are converting between mass and volume.

Example: 450 mL of phenol weighs 482.56 g. What is its density? Express your answer in g/mL.

$$\frac{482.56 \text{ g phenol}}{450 \text{ mL}} = 1.07 \text{ g/mL}$$

Specific gravity (SG) is a related concept, one that many pharmacy students find confusing. SG is simply the density of a substance relative to a reference substance (usually water). It is a unitless number, because it is equal to density divided by density—the units cancel out. Since water has a density of 1 g/mL, the SG will be numerically identical to the density of the substance expressed in g/mL. However, the SG of a substance is the same regardless of what units it was calculated from, so it allows you to compare the relative masses of equal volumes of substances. Also, some sources will list SG instead of density, so you need to be familiar with it to understand these sources.

Example: 150 mL of formaldehyde weighs 121.82 g. What is its specific gravity?

$$\frac{\dfrac{121.82 \text{ g formaldehyde}}{150 \text{ ml}}}{\dfrac{1 \text{ g water}}{1 \text{ mL}}} = 0.81$$

Thus, formaldehyde has a SG of 0.81, which is the same as the density if presented in g/mL. It is recommended to convert SG problems into g and mL as a first step in most calculations.

REDUCING AND ENLARGING FORMULAS

Most compounding formulas are for stock quantities, and how much the formula makes is rarely the amount you are actually wishing to prepare. However, it is simple to reduce or enlarge the formula to make the amount you need, provided you keep the ingredients in the same proportion with one another. In many ways, this is similar to doubling a recipe when you are cooking for a crowd. Compounding recipes come in two formats:

1. The amount of product produced is specified (formula makes 1,000 mL, for instance).

2. The quantity of each ingredient is specified, either in measured units or in parts. You figure out how much product will be made.

Example: Say you wish to make 50 capsules from the following recipe:

Rx   *Ketoprofen 2.5 g*
        Phenyltoloxamine citrate 6 g
        Caffeine 6 g
        Lactose 70.5 g

        M et div caps 200

First of all, how many doses is this recipe for? "M et div" means "mix and divide," so the recipe is for the entire amount of capsules (200), not for a single capsule. What do you do now? You can either reduce each ingredient by the same proportion (which is easy to figure out but involves lots of writing) or create a single conversion factor and apply it to each ingredient. Since you want 50 capsules and your recipes makes 200, your conversion factor would be 50 capsules/200 capsules = 0.25. Multiplying each ingredient by 0.25 yields:

2.5 g ketoprofen × 0.25	=	0.625 g
6 g phenyltoloxamine citrate × 0.25	=	1.5 g
6 g caffeine × 0.25	=	1.5 g
70.5 g lactose × 0.25	=	17.625 g

This method also works well if you do not have enough of a particular ingredient in stock. Say you have only 4 g of caffeine and want to use the recipe given here, which calls for 6 g. You can reduce the recipe to fit the amount of your limiting ingredient. Simply multiply each ingredient by the conversion factor of 4 g/6 g = 0.667.

If you have a recipe that does not have a total amount calculated, you will need to add up the amounts represented by each ingredient to find your total. Remember that you must add like to like, using density if needed to make sure that all amounts are specified in the same units (usually either g or mL).

Finally, some recipes are given in parts rather than measurements. If total parts are given (total is listed on the recipe, or one or more ingredients is listed as "qs" or "ad"):

- Set total parts to the amount you want to make
- Solve for the value of one part
- Multiply the size of one part by the number of parts for each ingredient

If total parts are not given:

- Add the number of parts for each ingredient to obtain the total number of parts in the recipe
- Proceed as previously noted

Example:

Rx	Bacitracin	105 parts
	Neomycin	35 parts
	Polymyxin B	5 parts
	Petrolatum	qs 10,000 parts

Calculate the quantities of all ingredients to make 30 grams

In this case, 30 g/10,000 parts = 0.003 g/part

Multiplying this factor times the other ingredients gives:

105 parts bacitracin × 0.003 = 0.315 g = 315 mg
35 parts neomycin × 0.003 = 0.105 g = 105 mg
5 parts polymyxin B × 0.003 = 0.015 g = 15 mg

The petrolatum needed may be found by subtracting the masses of the other ingredients from the 30 total grams desired:

30 g total − 0.315 g bacitracin − 0.105 g neomycin − 0.015 g polymyxin B = 29.565 g petrolatum

PERCENTAGE, RATIO STRENGTHS, AND PARTS PER MILLION

Since drugs are administered as dosage forms that contain more than just the active ingredient, the amount of the active ingredient needs to be expressed. There are several ways to do this:

- Amount per individual dosage form (capsule, tablet, suppository)
- Concentration per dosing volume (oral liquids, certain topical products)
- Percent
- Ratio strength
- Parts per million or billion

Percent describes the number of parts of active drug relative to 100 parts of the total. In pharmacy, simply stating % is incomplete; you must attach the appropriate descriptor from the following list:

- % w/w: g of active drug per 100 g of product
- % w/v: g of active drug per 100 mL of product
- % v/v: mL of active drug per 100 mL of product

Examples:

(1) 10% w/v = 10 g of drug in every 100 mL of the total

(2) 10% w/w = 10 g of drug in every 100 g of the total

Ratio strength is another way of expressing concentration, in terms of parts of active drug related to any number of parts of the whole. Ratio strength is usually expressed in terms of 1 part of active drug relative to the total number of parts of the product, as opposed to percent, which is any number of parts of active drug relative to 100 parts of product. For example, 5% means 5 parts per 100, or 5:100, or 1:20. Ratio strength is used for low-concentration solutions, and triturations of high-potency powders (e.g., 1:75 trituration of estradiol).

Example: Express 1 g of epinephrine in 1 L of solution as a percent strength and as a ratio strength.

First convert the units to g and mL:

$$1\,L = 1{,}000\,mL$$

To convert to **percentage strength**, set the denominator on the right side of the ratio-proportion equation to 100 and calculate for the numerator.

$$\frac{1\,g\,epinephrine}{1{,}000\,mL} = \frac{g\,active}{100\,mL\,product} = 0.1\%\,w/v$$

To convert to **ratio strength**, set the numerator on the right side of the ratio-proportion equation to 1 and calculate for the denominator.

$$\frac{1\,g\,epinephrine}{1{,}000\,mL} = \frac{1\,active}{X\,mL\,product} = 1{:}1{,}000\,w/v$$

Example: How much sodium benzoate do you need to preserve 10 L of a solution at a concentration of 1:10,000?

$$\frac{1\,g\,sodium\,benzoate}{10{,}000\,mL} \times \frac{1{,}000\,mL}{1\,L} \times 10\,L = 1\,g$$

Parts per million (ppm) is a special case of ratio strength. Instead of fixing the numerator as 1, in this case you fix the denominator constant as 1,000,000. Parts per billion (ppb) and trillion (ppt) are handled in an analogous fashion. These are used to express very small concentrations; for example, the EPA action level for lead in drinking water is 15 ppb (or 0.015 mg/L).

DOSAGE CALCULATIONS

Pharmacists frequently need to calculate the size of a dose or total amount of medication to dispense, even for noncompounded prescriptions. The following general equation applies:

Number of doses × size of dose = total amount

Example:

How many milliliters of a liquid medicine would provide a patient with 2 teaspoons three times a day for 7 days?

$$\frac{2\,\text{tsp}}{\text{dose}} \times \frac{3\,\text{doses}}{\text{day}} \times 7\,\text{days} \times \frac{5\,\text{mL}}{\text{tsp}} = 210\,\text{mL}$$

DILUTION, CONCENTRATION, AND ALLIGATION

In some cases, you may receive a prescription in which you need to either dilute a product you have on hand or make a product more concentrated. These problems can generally be solved by:

1. Using the equation: (quantity) × (concentration) = (quantity) × (concentration)
2. Determining the quantity of active ingredient needed and then calculating the quantity of the available solution (usually a concentrated stock solution) that will provide the needed amount of active ingredient

When some ingredients are given as ratio strength, you can convert them to percentage strength before setting up the proportion. Whenever proportional parts enter the calculation, you should reduce them to their lowest terms before beginning (i.e., reduce 75 parts:25 parts to 3 parts:1 part). In both cases, this will simplify your calculations.

Example:

If 250 mL of a 15% v/v solution of methyl salicylate in alcohol are diluted to 1,500 mL, what will be the percentage strength of this diluted solution?

250 mL × 15% = 1,500 mL × X%

X = 2.5% v/v

Stock Solutions

Stock solutions are strong solutions of known concentration that allow the pharmacist to conveniently prepare weaker solutions. They are generally prepared on a w/v basis and their concentration is expressed as a ratio strength.

Example:

How many milliliters of a 1% stock solution of certified red dye should be used in preparing 2,000 mL of an antiseptic that is to contain 1:5,000 of the certified red dye as a coloring agent?

First, how many grams of red dye are needed in the 2,000 mL of antiseptic solution?

$$\frac{1\,g\,red\,dye}{5,000\,mL} = \frac{x\,g\,red\,dye}{2,000\,mL}$$

$$x\,g\,red\,dye = 0.4\,g$$

Next, how much of the 1% stock solution of red dye contains this amount of dye?

$$\frac{1\,g\,red\,dye}{100\,mL} = \frac{0.4\,g\,red\,dye}{x\,mL}$$

$$x = 40\,mL$$

Alligation

Alligation is a method of solving problems that involves mixing multiple products that have different percentage strengths. Two types of alligation exist: Alligation medial and alligation alternate.

Alligation Medial

This method allows the calculation of the weighted average percentage strength of a mixture of two or more substances of known quantity and strength.

Example:

What is the percentage strength (v/v) of alcohol in a mixture of 3,000 mL of 40% (v/v) alcohol, 1,000 mL of 60% (v/v) alcohol, and 1,000 mL of 70% (v/v) alcohol?

$$40 \times 3,000 = 120,000$$
$$60 \times 1,000 = 60,000$$
$$70 \times 1,000 = 70,000$$

$$\text{Totals:}\,5,000 = 250,000$$
$$250,000 / 5,000 = 50\%\,(v/v)$$

Alligation Alternate

This method allows calculation of the number of parts of two or more components of a given strength when they are mixed to prepare a mixture of a desired strength. Crosswise subtraction is used to determine the amounts needed of each component. This method can be used regardless of how concentration is expressed (mg/mL, ratio, parts, %).

Example:

> In what proportion should a 20% benzocaine ointment be mixed with an ointment base to produce a 2.5% w/w benzocaine ointment?

Since there is no active drug in the ointment base, its strength can be expressed as 0%. To complete this problem, set up a table with the high concentration (i.e., 20%) in the upper left corner and the low concentration (i.e., 0%) in the lower left corner. The desired concentration (i.e., 2.5%) is placed in the center column between the low and high concentrations. Note that the desired concentration must always be a value between the high and low concentrations. Subtract diagonally to calculate the parts of the low and high concentration solutions to be mixed. Always subtract in a manner that will get you a positive value in the right column. In this example, 20% − 2.5% = 17.5 parts. Because this value is in the lower row of the table, it indicates that this is the number of parts of the low concentration to add to the mixture. In a similar fashion, you will need 2.5 parts of the high concentration (20% ointment). See the following table for the appropriate setup of this problem.

Strengths to Be Mixed	Desired	Difference in Strength Mixed (crosswise subtraction of absolute values)
20%		2.5 parts (2.5−0) of 20% ointment
	2.5%	
0%		17.5 parts (20 − 2.5) of ointment base

Therefore, 2.5 parts of the 20% w/w ointment should be added to 17.5 parts of the ointment base. Remember that the values are subtracted diagonally, but the identities of the substances are read across the row.

The standard alligation problem on the NAPLEX may provide you with not only the concentrations of both starting amounts and the desired concentration to be made, as described above, but also the total amount that is to be dispensed. Thus, the final step is to take the total amount to be dispensed and calculate the amounts of each ingredient based on the parts that were calculated above. For example, if 12 g were to be dispensed in the problem above, you would use the parts as shown below.

Parts of high concentration: 2.5 parts

Parts of low concentration: 17.5 parts

Total parts (i.e., high plus low concentration): 20 parts

To calculate the amount of the *high* concentration to be mixed:

$$\frac{2.5 \, \text{parts}}{20 \, \text{parts}} = \frac{x \, \text{g}}{12 \, \text{g}}$$
$$x = 1.5 \, \text{g}$$

To calculate the amount of the *low* concentration to be mixed:

$$\frac{17.5 \, \text{parts}}{20 \, \text{parts}} = \frac{x \, \text{g}}{12 \, \text{g}}$$
$$x = 10.5 \, \text{g}$$

Another method is to simply take the total amount to be dispensed (i.e., 12 g) and subtract out the amount of the high concentration to be mixed (i.e., 1.5 g), which was calculated in the first step. That is, 12 g − 1.5 g = 10.5 g, which is the amount of the low concentration to add. This is a good method for checking calculations, because there are two ways to calculate the last amount to be added.

Therefore, to get 12 g of a 2.5% w/w benzocaine ointment, mix 1.5 g of a 20% concentration with 10.5 g of the ointment base (0% concentration).

ELECTROLYTE SOLUTIONS

Electrolyte solutions are frequently prescribed for patients who have lost an essential ion through disease, as they play a critical role in maintaining normal body function. Sometimes the necessary amount of the appropriate salt will be stated on the prescription, but often the prescription will ask for a quantity of the needed ion in chemical units, and the pharmacist will need to calculate how much of the salt will contain the desired amount. Milliequivalents are the most common unit used.

Millimoles and Milliequivalents

A review of several chemistry concepts will be useful before beginning milliequivalent calculations.

- Moles (mol): Measurement of the amount of a substance; Avogadro's number of particles (6.023×10^{23})
- Atomic weight: Found on the periodic table; 1 mol of that atom weighs that many grams (also, 1 mmol of that atom weighs that many mg)

- Molecular weight (MW): The sum of all the atomic weights for all of the atoms in the molecule. 1 **mole** of the molecule will weigh the value of the molecular weight in **grams**. However, in electrolyte solutions and osmolarity calculations, it is necessary to convert to millimoles. This can be done easily by taking the amount of the substance in milligrams and dividing by the molecular weight to get the answer in millimoles. This can be visualized in the following important equations:

$$moles = \frac{Amount\,(grams)}{Molecular\ weight}$$

$$millimoles = \frac{Amount\,(milligrams)}{Molecular\ weight}$$

- Molar solution: The molarity of a solution is the moles of solute in every 1 L of solution. This is an important concept on the NAPLEX, as questions can ask for the answer in terms of molarity; therefore, on the last step of the problem, you would then need to calculate how many moles there are in 1 L for the solutes in the problem.
  - Stock solutions often expressed this way
  - 0.1 M = 0.1 mol of solute/1 L solution

Example:

What is the molar concentration of a 5% w/v $MgCl_2$ solution? MW $MgCl_2$ = 95.

The 5% concentration indicates that there are 5 g of $MgCl_2$ per every 100 mL. The question is asking for the molar concentration, so directly calculate the moles per every 100 mL solution by the following:

$$\frac{5\,g\,MgCl_2}{95} = 0.053\,moles\,per\,100\,mL$$

It is recommended to indicate the volume of solution in each step of the problem, as indicated earlier. Because the answer needs to be in molar concentration, the moles per liter can be calculated as follows:

$$\frac{0.053\,moles}{100\,mL} = \frac{x\,moles}{1{,}000\,mL} = 0.53\,mol/L = 0.53\,M$$

or using dimensional analysis:

$$\frac{1\,mol\,MgCl_2}{95\,g\,MgCl_2} \times \frac{5\,g\,MgCl_2}{100\,mL} \times \frac{1{,}000\,mL}{1\,L} = 0.53\,mol/L = 0.53\,M$$

What if you are interested in moles of atoms instead of moles of molecules? In this case, you need to look at the molecular formula. If there is more than one of an atom in a molecule (such as the chloride in the example), you need to adjust your formula. In that example, you have 1 mol of $MgCl_2$, which contains 1 mol of Mg^{+2} and 2 mol of Cl^-. If you don't have a molecular formula, you can figure one out by balancing charges, provided you know the valencies of the ions involved. The following table displays the valence of the most common ions. This information will likely not be provided on the NAPLEX.

Valence	Ions
+1	Sodium, potassium, lithium
+2	Barium, calcium, magnesium, zinc
+3	Aluminum
+1 or +2	Copper
+2 or +3	Iron, manganese
−1	Acetate, chloride, bicarbonate
−2	Sulfate, carbonate
−1, −2, or −3	Phosphate, citrate

In the magnesium chloride example, Mg^{+2} is divalent; it takes two Cl^- to make as much negative charge as one Mg^{+2}. Therefore, the correct formula is $MgCl_2$, not $MgCl$. $NaCl$, however, is made up of two monovalent ions, so the charges are equal.

Electrolytes are commonly prescribed in terms of equivalents rather than mass. This means 1 mol of hydrogen has 1 mol of positive charge. One equivalent of an ion is the amount required to replace (in positively charged ions) or react with (in negatively charged ions) 1 mol of hydrogen. Monovalent ions (Cl^-, Na^+, K^+, NH_4^+, OH^-) therefore have 1 Eq/mol. Divalent ions like Ca^{+2} are 2 Eq/mol, as it takes 2 mol of hydrogen to replace the charge carried by 1 mol of calcium.

The concept of equivalents is important in pharmacy when dispensing electrolytes or small drug molecules as salts. For example, a prescription that is written for 40 mg of potassium chloride does not contain the same amount of elemental potassium as a prescription written for 40 mg potassium acetate. The reason is that the 40 mg in each prescription is the total weight of potassium and the salt form (i.e., chloride or acetate). Since acetate has a larger molecular weight than chloride, it contributes more to the 40 mg, and therefore, the patient will receive less potassium in this prescription compared with 40 mg of potassium chloride. This concept is also true for drugs for which the amount of drug dispensed is the weight of the drug itself and also the salt that is formulated. However, drugs are much larger molecules than electrolytes. Thus the percentage of salt is so small that switching salt formations of drugs has limited clinical applicability. The only clinical relevance would be for drugs with a narrow therapeutic index or a small molecular weight.

To overcome this problem for electrolytes, the prescriptions will be written in terms of milliequivalents (mEq). For example, a prescription that calls for 40 mEq of potassium chloride will contain the same amount of elemental potassium as a prescription that calls for 40 mEq of potassium acetate.

To calculate mEq, simply calculate the millimoles of the substance and multiply by the valence of either the positive or negative charge of the molecular formula. For example, if $MgCl_2$ is the compound of interest, you would multiply the millimoles by a factor of 2. The factor of 2 is due to the fact that Mg has 2 positive charges and Cl has a negative charge with two of them giving a total negative charge of 2. Remember that the charges of the positive side and the negative side must equal zero.

Use the following equation to calculate mEq:

$$\text{milliequivalents (mEq)} = \frac{\text{Amount (milligrams)}}{\text{Molecular weight}} \times \text{valence}$$

Example:

How many milligrams of potassium citrate powder (MW = 324.41) should be weighed to compound 1 dose of the following prescription?

Rx   *Potassium citrate 20 mEq PO TID*

Recall that potassium has a valence of +1 and citrate has a −3, so the formula must have 3 potassium ions for every citrate or $K_3(C_6H_5O_7)$.

$$20\,\text{mEq} = \frac{x\,\text{mg}}{324.1} \times 3$$
$$x = 2{,}160\,\text{mg}$$

Therefore, 20 mEq of potassium citrate provides 20 mEq of potassium and 20 mEq of citrate. This means that a quantity of 2,160 mg of potassium citrate would provide 20 mEq of potassium and 20 mEq of citrate. The important thing to keep track of with this method is the amount and molecular weight being used. Since we used the molecular weight of potassium citrate (and not just potassium or citrate alone), the amount calculated in milligrams is the weight of both potassium and citrate together. One could calculate the actual amount of potassium in a dose by replacing the molecular weight of potassium citrate with the atomic weight of potassium (i.e., 39.1). NAPLEX questions may provide either the full molecular weight or an atomic weight of one of the components. Remember: Using an atomic weight of one of the components of the prescription means committing to use that atomic weight. However, the milliequivalents will be the same value for the total compound and each of the components.

Osmolarity and Isotonicity

Osmotic pressure is the pressure that exists across a semipermeable membrane due to the free movement of solvent but not solute. Because cell membranes are semipermeable, this concept is important in patients. When administering parenteral drugs, you must balance the osmolarity of your medication with the osmolarity of the body. If not, tissue damage, pain, and possibly death can result due to cells swelling or shrinking with the movement of solvent.

Solutions are considered isotonic when each one has the same osmotic pressure; in pharmacy and medicine, the reference solution is the plasma (280–300 mOsm/L). Hypertonic solutions have higher osmotic pressure than this; hypotonic solutions have lower osmotic pressure. Some other facts you should remember about osmotic pressure are:

- It is a colligative property, based on the number of particles in solution.
- It can be calculated directly, using dissociation constants.
    - NaCl dissociates into sodium and chloride 80% in aqueous solution.
    - For every 100 particles, 80 will have dissociated (making 160 particles) and 20 will not → 180 particles (20 + 160).

$$\frac{180 \text{ particles after dissociation}}{100 \text{ particles before dissociation}} = 1.8 = i$$

- It can be calculated by its effect on other colligative properties, including freezing point, boiling point, and vapor pressure.
    - All colligative properties vary together.
    - A solution with the same freezing point as a reference solution will have the same osmolarity as that reference solution.

- To calculate the milliosmoles (mOsm) in a given solution, multiply the millimoles by the theoretical number of particles that the compound would dissociate into in solution. For example, to calculate the mOsm in an $MgCl_2$ solution, the millimoles would be multiplied by a factor of 3. Theoretically, $MgCl_2$ would dissociate into 1 magnesium and 2 chloride ions in solution. If the dissociation constant is provided in the problem, it would provide a more accurate calculation and should be used as displayed in the equation.

$$\text{mOsm} = \frac{\text{Amount (mg)}}{\text{Molecular weight}} \times \text{Theoretical number of particles}$$
$$\text{(or disassociation constant)}$$

- The NAPLEX may ask for answers to be written in terms of milliosmolarity. Remember: When the suffix "-arity" is at the end of a word in chemistry, it indicates the need to calculate an amount in 1 L of solution. In other words, to calculate milliosmolarity you need to calculate the amount of milliosmoles in the quantity of solution in the problem and convert to 1 L at the end.

Example:

A solute dissociates 50% in aqueous solution. Assuming each molecule of the solute dissociates into two parts, give the dissociation constant (i).

$$\frac{100\,\text{dissociated particles} + 50\,\text{undissociated particles}}{100\,\text{particles before dissociation}} = 1.5 = (i)$$

You can use the ratio form of the dissociation constant as a conversion factor. If $i = 1.5$, 1 mol = 1.5 Osm, and 1 mmol = 1.5 mOsm.

Example:

Calculate the osmolarity of NS in mOsm/L. MW NS = 58.5 and $i = 1.8$.

NS = normal saline = 0.9% w/v NaCl in water

$$\frac{0.9\,\text{g}}{100\,\text{mL}} = \frac{x\,\text{g}}{1{,}000\,\text{mL}}$$

$x = 9$ g or 9,000 mg of NaCl per liter

$$x\,\text{mOsm} = \frac{9{,}000\,\text{mg}}{58.5} \times 1.8$$

$x = 276.9\,\text{mOsm/L}$

Because NS is nearly isotonic with plasma, it is useful for comparison. If we know that a product is isotonic to NS, it will be isotonic to body fluids as well. Sodium chloride equivalents are therefore useful, and are for expression of the amount of NaCl it would take to exert the tonic effect of a particular active ingredient. Some baseline assumptions are:

- The tonic effects of solutes are additive and independent.
- The total tonic effect in the solution is the sum of the effect of each solute.

The following steps can be followed when adjusting tonicity:

1. Determine how much NaCl it would take to exert the tonic effect already seen in the solution.
2. Calculate how much NaCl is required to make the solution isotonic if NaCl is the sole tonicity agent. Compare this to the amount already present (step 1). Proceed only if the total amount of NaCl equivalent already present is less than the amount needed (i.e., solution is currently hypotonic).
3. *Amount needed = Goal amount – Amount you already have*
   a. If adjusting tonicity with NaCl, use amount in step 3.
   b. If adjusting tonicity with another substance, figure out how much of your substance is needed to deliver the required tonic effect, using the E value (1 g of substance has the same tonic effect as E g of NaCl).

If one of your ingredients is already isotonic, you can disregard that volume as you calculate your values.

Example:

How many grams of boric acid (E = 0.52) should be added to make 15 mL of a 3% w/v pilocarpine HCl (E = 0.24) eye drop solution isotonic?

Following the steps:

1. $\dfrac{3\,\text{g pilocarpine}}{100\,\text{mL}} \times 15\,\text{mL} = 0.45\,\text{g pilocarpine}$

   $0.45\,\text{g pilocarpine} \times \dfrac{0.24\,\text{g NaCl(eq)}}{1\,\text{g pilocarpine}} = 0.108\,\text{g NaCl(eq)}$

2. $\dfrac{0.9\,\text{g NaCl}}{100\,\text{mL}} \times 15\,\text{mL} = 0.135\,\text{g NaCl}$

3. $0.135\,\text{g} - 0.108\,\text{g} = 0.027\,\text{g NaCl}$

   $0.027\,\text{g NaCl} \times \dfrac{1\,\text{g boric acid}}{0.52\,\text{g NaCl(eq)}} = 0.05192\,\text{g} = 0.052\,\text{g boric acid}$

Another way to describe and calculate osmolarity and isotonicity is freezing-point depression. As mentioned above, this is a colligative property that varies along with other colligative properties of a solution. Some things to remember:

- Plasma freezes at −0.52°C.
- Solutions isotonic to plasma (such as NS) will also freeze at −0.52°C.
- Pure water freezes at 0°C. Therefore, an amount of solute that will make the solution isotonic depresses the freezing point by 0.52°C.

Example:

Given the following prescription, how many grams of NaCl must be added to make the solution isotonic? The freezing point of a 1% w/v solution of procaine HCl is −0.122°C.

Rx	Procaine HCl	2% w/v
	NaCl	qs
	Sterile water	qs 30 mL

First, what would be the effect of a 2% w/v solution?

$\dfrac{1.22°C}{1\%} \times 2\% = 0.244°C$

The desired freezing point − The depression from the ingredients already in the formulation = The additional depression needed:

$$-0.52°C - (-0.244°C) = -0.276°C$$

So, the required concentration of sodium chloride is:

$$-0.276°C \frac{0.9\% \, NaCl}{-0.52°C} = 0.48\% \, NaCl \text{ or}$$

$$30 \, mL \frac{0.48 \, g \, NaCl}{100 \, g \, NaCl} = 0.144 \, g \, NaCl$$

COMPOUNDING CALCULATIONS

Use of Prefabricated Dosage Forms in Compounding

When compounding, the source of active ingredient will often be prefabricated dosage forms (tablets, capsules, ointments). When performing such calculations, it is important to remember that if your calculation determines that you need 1.3 tablets as your source drug, you must actually crush 2 tablets and then weigh out a proportional amount of the resultant powder. Remember, a tablet contains far more ingredients than just the drug, so take that into account in your calculations.

Example:

Rx	Aspirin	300 *mg*
	Lactose	qs
	M.ft. cap DTD #60	

Using 325-mg aspirin tablets (weighing 430 mg each) as the source drug, how many tablets are needed to compound this prescription? How many grams of the crushed powder should be weighed out?

$$\frac{300 \, mg \, ASA}{capsule} \times 60 \, capsules \times \frac{tablet}{325 \, mg \, ASA} = 55.38 \, tablets \rightarrow 56 \, tablets$$

$$55.38 \, tablets \times 430 \, mg \, total \, tablet \, weight = 23,813 \, mg = 23.813 \, g$$

Suppository Calculations

The density factor method is often used when preparing suppositories. The density factor expresses the relationship between the mass of an ingredient and the volume of suppository base it displaces. Therefore, a drug will have a different density factor in each suppository base.

$$\text{density factor} = \frac{\text{weight of drug}}{\text{weight of base displaced}}$$

Example:

> If a pharmacist needs to prepare six 30-mg phenobarbital suppositories in cocoa butter, how many grams each of cocoa butter and phenobarbital should be weighed? Density factor of phenobarbital in cocoa butter is 1.2. Blank suppositories (base only) weigh 2 g.

If one suppository contains 30 mg drug (0.03 g), it will replace:

> $$\frac{0.03\,\text{g drug}}{1.2\,\text{g}} = 0.025\,\text{g cocoa butter}$$
>
> $2\,\text{g} - 0.025\,\text{g} = 1.975\,\text{g cocoa butter / suppository} \times 6\,\text{suppositories} =$ 11.85 g cocoa butter
>
> $0.03\,\text{g} \times 6\,\text{suppositories} = 0.18\,\text{g phenobarbital}$

Reconstitution Calculations

Some medications, particularly antibiotics for oral suspension or parenteral use, come as powders for reconstitution. While the container or package will include instructions for reconstitution, including what and how much diluent to use, occasionally the prescriber will need to manipulate the final concentration of the drug. Some simple calculations can help you make these adjustments to provide a more dilute or concentrated product.

Example:

> Cefadroxil powder for oral suspension comes in a strength of 250 mg/5 mL. The reconstitution instructions are to add 70 mL of purified water to yield a final solution volume of 100 mL. How many grams of cefadroxil powder are in the bottle?
>
> $$\frac{250\,\text{mg cefadroxil}}{5\,\text{mL suspension}} \times 100\,\text{mL} = 5,000\,\text{mg} = 5\,\text{g}$$

There are a few interesting things to pay attention to here. First, this is an easy example of a question that gives more information than you need to solve the problem (while the 70 mL is necessary for reconstitution, it is not needed to answer this particular question). Be sure to pay attention and use the correct numbers when extra information is given.

Second, if you add only 70 mL of water, how do you get 100 mL of total suspension? The powder takes up space in the final product. This volume is called the powder volume: It is a calculated quantity, not corresponding to the physical volume. The powder volume may be greater than, equal to, or less than zero, depending on the drug and the way it was prepared.

When preparing a final concentration that is different from the package directions, you must first calculate the powder volume. The powder volume is equal to the difference between the diluent volume and the final solution volume.

Example:

Biaxin is available as a powder for reconstitution with instructions to prepare a final concentration of 125 mg/5 mL by adding 55 mL of diluent to make a final volume of 100 mL. How many milliliters of diluent would need to be added to this preparation to make the concentration designated in the prescription given?

Rx   *Biaxin 100 mg/5 mL suspension*
       Sig: 1 tsp PO q 12 hr × 10 days

Given a final volume of 100 mL and a final concentration of 125 mg/5 mL, the amount of active ingredient in the bottle is 2,500 mg. The powder volume = total volume − diluent, so 100 mL − 55 mL = 45 mL.

$$2{,}500 \, \text{mg Biaxin} \times \frac{5 \, \text{mL}}{100 \, \text{mg Biaxin}} = 125 \, \text{mL total}$$

$$125 \, \text{mL total} - \text{PV} = 125 \, \text{mL} - 45 \, \text{mL} = 80 \, \text{mL}$$

Adding 80 mL of diluent will produce 125 mL of solution with a concentration of 100 mg/5 mL.

Drip Rate Calculations

IV medications are regulated by one of the following methods:

- Drip chambers
  - Deliver drops of defined volume
  - Flow is adjusted by the nurse to a set number of *whole* drops per minute
  - Standard sets are 10 gtt/mL or 15 gtt/mL
  - Pediatric and critical care drugs may use microdrop infusion sets: 60 gtt/mL
- Infusion pumps
  - Deliver a rate of mL/hr
  - Round to the nearest 0.1 mL

To calculate the drip rate on the NAPLEX, the question will commonly ask how many gtts/min should be set on the drip chamber. You will be provided with how many drops constitute 1 mL of liquid. Therefore, the first step will be to calculate the infusion rate in mL/min and then convert mL's to gtt's based on the conversion provided in the problem. The following example demonstrates first how to calculate an infusion rate and then extends the answer to a drip rate calculation.

Example:

17 mL of concentrated vancomycin solution is added to a 100-mL piggyback bag of NS. This solution is to be infused over 1 hour. What is the infusion rate?

$$\frac{17 \text{ mL vancomycin} + 100 \text{ mL NS}}{60 \text{ min}} = 117 \text{ mL/60 min} = 117 \text{ mL/hr}$$

What is the infusion rate in drops/min if the drug is administered using an infusion set that delivers 10 gtt/mL?

$$\frac{117 \text{ mL}}{60 \text{ min}} \times \frac{10 \text{ gtt}}{\text{mL}} = 19.5 \text{ gtt/min} = 20 \text{ gtt/min}$$

Enteral Nutrition

Some or all of the patient's nutritional needs are provided by use of orally or enterally administered nutritional products, usually through feeding tubes. Enteral nutrition (EN) products are commercially available, and limited calculations are needed since they are premixed by the manufacturer for different populations. If the patient can tolerate it, EN is usually recommended over parenteral nutrition (PN).

Parenteral Nutrition

Most of the calculations on the NAPLEX exam regarding nutrition will be related to the parenteral route. The cost of TPN therapy is usually 10 times more expensive than EN, with greater possibilities of metabolic and/or infectious complications. Common abbreviations follow:

- **TPN = total parenteral nutrition:** Provides fluid, macronutrients (i.e., dextrose, amino acids, and fatty acids), electrolytes, and micronutrients (i.e., vitamins and trace elements).
- **TNA = total admixture:** Contains all of the macro and micronutrients in a single bag. The terms TNA and TPN are often used synonymously in clinical practice, although there are technical differences.

Calculations Involving Calories

The usual term is Calorie (with a capital C), which is equal to 1 kilocalorie. Therefore, Calories and kilocalories are synonymous. However, many texts do not use a capital C when referring to Calories. Therefore, whenever Calorie is written (with or without the capital C), do not do any metric conversions.

To calculate the caloric requirements for a hospitalized patient, first calculate that patient's basal energy requirement. There are equations to calculate basal energy expenditure based on several patient demographics. The stressed adult in a hospital likely will require additional energy depending on several factors. The calculated basal energy expenditure is then multiplied by a stress factor (usually between 1 and 2) to obtain a total energy expenditure (TEE).

The normal adult requires 25–35 Cal/kg/day. Once the TEE is calculated, the Calories are provided to the patient through dextrose and fatty acids. Amino acids also provide Calories, but those Calories generally are used to meet the TEE in a TPN. The Calories provided by a TPN can be estimated as follows:

Dextrose in the hydrated form (D_5W, $D_{70}W$, etc.)	3.4 Cal/g
Carbohydrates	4 Cal/g
Fats	9 Cal/g
Protein	4 Cal/g

Dextrose in water is the hydrated form and is used in TPN. Although dextrose is a carbohydrate, water molecules are attached to the dextrose to make it more soluble. The water molecules add weight without adding calories, and they dilute the Calorie per gram ratio from 4 to 3.4. Therefore, when calculating caloric content of a TPN, 3.4 Cal/g should be used for the dextrose content.

Dextrose cannot be used alone to meet TEE because there are essential fatty acids that cannot be synthesized by the body. To prevent essential fatty acid deficiency, particularly a deficiency of linoleic acid, fats are incorporated into TPNs usually two to three times weekly. Fats are provided through infusion of oil emulsions. Fatty oil emulsions are approximately isotonic, have a milky appearance, and can be infused into peripheral blood vessels. Every milliliter of 10% fat emulsion has 1.1 Calories, whereas every milliliter of 20% fat emulsion has 2 calories. The emulsions contain glycerol, which provides Calories in addition to the fats. Therefore, there is no easy way to calculate the caloric content of the emulsions and require the memorization of the caloric content per milliliter described.

Calculations Involving Amino Acids

The average adult requires approximately 1 g/kg/day of amino acids. Amino acids are included in TPN primarily to provide protein and nitrogen supplementation. Nitrogen is an important element in the diet that is a precursor to DNA synthesis and other important metabolic functions. On average, 16% of an amino acid solution is nitrogen content.

Example:

How many milliliters of an 8.5% amino acid solution are required to provide 20 g of nitrogen?

$$\frac{16\,g\,nitrogen}{100\,g\,amino\,acids} = \frac{20\,g\,nitrogen}{x\,g\,amino\,acids}$$

$$x = 125\,g\,amino\,acids$$

$$\frac{8.5\,g\,amino\,acids}{100\,mL} = \frac{125\,g\,amino\,acids}{x\,mL}$$

$$x = 1,470\,mL$$

Of importance is the Cal/g nitrogen ratio. The desired ratio is 125/1 up to 150/1. That is, a formula should provide at least 125 Calories for each gram of nitrogen being infused. This amount is needed to provide for normal energy expenditure and calories to aid in the anabolic conversion of nitrogen sources into lean body mass.

Calculations Involving Electrolytes and Micronutrients

There are not many sources of calculations regarding TPN on the NAPLEX outside of the macronutrients described previously. Electrolyte calculations have been described in this chapter related to milliequivalents. For TPN, the most important concept regarding electrolytes is clinical considerations. This includes limiting potassium and sodium in patients with renal, hepatic, or cardiac dysfunction. Similarly, there are not calculations involving vitamins or trace elements as these are added to TPNs via commercially available products.

Compounding Considerations for TPNs

Both calcium and phosphate are essential components of TPN formulas. Sources of calcium include the chloride and gluconate salts. Phosphorus is supplied as combinations of mono- and disodium phosphates or mono- and dipotassium phosphates. The exact ratio depends on the pH of the solution.

Depending upon the relative concentrations of the soluble calcium salts and the phosphate salts, a chemical reaction may occur forming the very **insoluble dibasic calcium phosphate** ($CaPO_4$). This fine, white precipitate may form slowly and be difficult to visualize, especially if a milky fatty oil emulsion is also included in the TPN.

Methods for lessening the incompatibility problem:

1. Keep Ca and PO_4 concentrations below certain limits (solubility curves are available for various mixtures).

2. Agitate the mixture after each ingredient addition.

3. Add Na or K phosphates first and calcium salt last.

4. Add the Na or K phosphates to the amino acid solution, and the calcium salt to the dextrose solution; then, mix by shaking.

5. Use a 0.2 micron filter for nonfat emulsion formulas; a 1.2 micron filter is needed for fatty oil emulsions.

LEARNING POINTS

- Always perform a "sanity" check on your answer. Does it make practical sense? If not, recheck your numbers.

- Remember crucial conversion factors (or at least approximations of these): 1 fluid oz = 30 mL, 2.2 lb/kg (*not* the reverse; remember, your weight is always a smaller number when measured in kilograms; if you get an answer to the contrary, you flipped your conversion).

- Valence of a molecule is equal to the total number of negative charges *or* the total number of positive charges, not the two numbers added together.

- When using prefabricated dosage forms as a drug source, fractions of a dosage form must always be rounded up to the next nearest whole.

- Drops must be rounded to the nearest whole drop. You cannot measure partials.

PRACTICE QUESTIONS

1. How many milliliters of water should be mixed with 240 mL of syrup containing 85% w/v sucrose to make a syrup containing 60% w/v sucrose?

   (A) 80 mL
   (B) 100 mL
   (C) 160 mL
   (D) 240 mL
   (E) 340 mL

2. If 10 mL of a solution are to contain 3 mEq of sodium ion, how many 1-g sodium chloride (MW 58.5) tablets would be required to compound 250 mL of solution?

   (A) 2
   (B) 3
   (C) 4
   (D) 5
   (E) 6

3. You have been asked to prepare 500 mL of a benzalkonium chloride solution. The concentration of the solution you prepare must be such that if 20 mL of your solution are diluted to a liter, a 1:1,470 solution is formed. How many milliliters of a 17% w/v benzalkonium chloride solution will you need to compound the solution?

   (A) 17 mL
   (B) 20 mL
   (C) 100 mL
   (D) 147 mL
   (E) 500 mL

4. A pharmacist has 75 grams of 3% w/w zinc oxide paste in stock, to which she adds 5 g of pure zinc oxide. What is the percent concentration of zinc oxide in the final product?

   (A) 2.4% w/w
   (B) 3% w/w
   (C) 7.25% w/w
   (D) 9.06% w/w
   (E) 9.67% w/w

5. How many milligrams of boric acid are needed to compound the following prescription? (The E values are as follows: zinc chloride 0.62, phenacaine HCl 0.17, and boric acid 0.52.)

Rx Zinc chloride   0.2% w/v

Phenacaine HCl   1% w/v

Boric acid   qs

Purified water qs   60 mL

(A) 92 mg
(B) 189 mg
(C) 339 mg
(D) 364 mg
(E) 699 mg

6. How many milligrams of sodium chloride are needed to compound the following prescription? (The E value of phenylephrine HCl is 0.32.)

Rx Phenylephrine HCl   0.5% w/v

Sodium chloride   qs

Purified water qs   30 mL

(A) 48 mg
(B) 86 mg
(C) 150 mg
(D) 222 mg
(E) 270 mg

7. How many milliliters of a 1% (w/v) stock solution of epinephrine HCl are needed for the following prescription?

Rx Epinephrine HCl sol. 1:500 w/v   60 mL

(A) 0.012 mL
(B) 0.12 mL
(C) 1.2 mL
(D) 12 mL
(E) 120 mL

8. Calculate the percentage (v/v) of witch hazel in the following prescription.

   Rx   *Sulfur ppt*   *15 g*

                   Witch hazel   *45 mL*

                   Alcohol

                   Calamine lotion qs   *120 mL*

   (A) 12.5%
   (B) 25%
   (C) 27.3%
   (D) 37.5%
   (E) 45%

9. The following prescription is written for penicillin suspension to be administered: 1.5 teaspoonfuls PO TID for 12 days. How many milliliters of the suspension should be dispensed?

   (A) 23 mL
   (B) 54 mL
   (C) 90 mL
   (D) 270 mL
   (E) 810 mL

10. A 40-pound child is to receive Dilantin 2.5 mg/kg PO BID. How many milliliters of Dilantin suspension (125 mg/5 mL) should be dispensed for a 30-day supply?

    (A) 55 mL
    (B) 109 mL
    (C) 240 mL
    (D) 265 mL
    (E) 528 mL

11. A patient who weighs 167 pounds is receiving phenylephrine at a dose of 2 mcg/kg/min. How many milligrams of phenylephrine does the patient receive over 2 hours?

    (A) 0.30 mg
    (B) 9.1 mg
    (C) 18.2 mg
    (D) 40 mg
    (E) 5,060 mg

12. A formula for 2,000 levothyroxine tablets contains 274 mg of levothyroxine. How many micrograms of levothyroxine are in each tablet?

    (A) 0.137 mcg
    (B) 1.37 mcg
    (C) 13.7 mcg
    (D) 137 mcg
    (E) 1,370 mcg

13. The formula for an analgesic ointment is 10 g menthol, 95 g benzocaine, 5 g camphor, 40 g mineral oil, and 850 g petrolatum. How many grams of benzocaine are needed to prepare 5 lbs. of this product?

    (A) 0.22 g
    (B) 215.7 g
    (C) 238.3 g
    (D) 253.7 g
    (E) 1,045 g

14. A solution of iodine in chloroform has a strength of 1.4% (w/v). How many milliliters of chloroform must be evaporated from the original 180 mL to adjust the iodine concentration to 2.4% (w/v)?

    (A) 50 mL
    (B) 75 mL
    (C) 105 mL
    (D) 125 mL
    (E) 155 mL

15. How many grams of zinc oxide should be mixed with 8% (w/w) zinc oxide ointment to make 250 g of a 12% (w/w) zinc oxide ointment? Round your answer to one decimal place.

    (A) 10.9 g
    (B) 18.5 g
    (C) 37.9 g
    (D) 100 g
    (E) 239.1 g

16. A patient is to receive 2 mEq of sodium chloride per kilogram of body weight. If the patient weighs 186 lbs., how many milliliters of a 0.9% solution of sodium chloride (MW = 58.5) should be administered?

    (A) 11 mL
    (B) 321 mL
    (C) 550 mL
    (D) 1,099 mL
    (E) 5,320 mL

17. How many milliosmoles of calcium chloride (MW = 147) are represented in 200 mL of a 10% (w/v) calcium chloride solution?

   (F) 8.8 mOsm
   (A) 136 mOsm
   (B) 272 mOsm
   (C) 408 mOsm
   (D) 816 mOsm

18. If an ointment contains 60% (w/w) of polyethylene glycol 400 (specific gravity = 1.13), how many milliliters of polyethylene glycol are needed to prepare 1 kg of ointment?

   (A) 53 mL
   (B) 68 mL
   (C) 354 mL
   (D) 531 mL
   (E) 678 mL

19. How many milliliters of water should be added to 50 mL of zephiran chloride 1:750 solution to obtain a 1:10,000 strength solution?

   (A) 100 mL
   (B) 200 mL
   (C) 250 mL
   (D) 617 mL
   (E) 667 mL

20. You receive a prescription for fluticasone HFA 440 mcg BID with instructions to dispense a 90-day supply. Fluticasone HFA is available commercially as 220 mcg/metered dose with 120 doses per inhaler. How many inhalers should be dispensed for a 90-day supply?

   (A) 1 inhaler
   (B) 2 inhalers
   (C) 3 inhalers
   (D) 4 inhalers
   (E) 6 inhalers

21. You receive a prescription for insulin glargine 65 units subcut once daily with instructions to dispense a 30-day supply. Insulin glargine is available commercially as 100 units/mL in 10-mL vials. How many vials should be dispensed for a 30-day supply?

   (A) 1 vial
   (B) 2 vials
   (C) 3 vials
   (D) 4 vials
   (E) 5 vials

22. You receive a prescription for oxycodone/acetaminophen 5/500 mg 1–2 tablets every 4–6 hours PRN pain. Based upon a maximum daily acetaminophen dose of 4 grams, how many tablets should be dispensed for a 30-day supply?

    (A) 60 tablets
    (B) 120 tablets
    (C) 240 tablets
    (D) 360 tablets
    (E) 480 tablets

23. An elixir contains 250 mg of active ingredient per 5 mL. You receive a prescription for 500 mg PO twice daily with instructions to dispense 120 mL of the elixir. How many days would the elixir last if taken as prescribed?

    (A) 4 days
    (B) 6 days
    (C) 8 days
    (D) 10 days
    (E) 12 days

24. A pediatric ferrous sulfate suspension contains 75 mg/1.5 mL (20% elemental). How many milliliters would provide the patient with 30 mg of elemental iron?

    (A) 0.3 mL
    (B) 0.6 mL
    (C) 1.5 mL
    (D) 3 mL
    (E) 6 mL

25. You are asked to compound a prescription for 120 mL of the following lotion:

Rx	Calamine	80 g
	Zinc oxide	80 g
	Glycerin	20 g
	Bentonite magma	250 mL
	Calcium hydroxide topical solution to make	1,000 mL

    How many grams of calamine should be used to prepare the quantity specified?

    (A) 0.96 g
    (B) 8 g
    (C) 9.6 g
    (D) 80 g
    (E) 96 g

26. You receive a prescription for 60 g of zinc oxide ointment. The following formula is available:

Rx	Zinc oxide	1 part
	Starch	1 part
	Petrolatum	2 parts

    How many grams of zinc oxide should be used to prepare the quantity specified?

    (A) 1 g
    (B) 10 g
    (C) 15 g
    (D) 30 g
    (E) 45 g

27. Approximately how many liters of a 0.9% (w/v) aqueous solution can be made from 30 grams of sodium chloride?

    (A) 1 L
    (B) 2 L
    (C) 3 L
    (D) 4 L
    (E) 5 L

28. You receive a prescription for 500 mL of a 0.5% w/v solution of drug A. You have on hand 10% w/v solution of drug A. How many milliliters of your available solution should be diluted with water to make the 500 mL prescription?

    (A) 5 mL
    (B) 10 mL
    (C) 15 mL
    (D) 20 mL
    (E) 25 mL

29. A prescription is written for a total quantity of 100 mEq of NaCl. You have normal saline solution on hand. How many milliliters of normal saline solution should be dispensed? (MW NaCl = 58.5)

    (A) 58.5 mL
    (B) 65 mL
    (C) 527 mL
    (D) 585 mL
    (E) 650 mL

30. A medication order calls for 75 mL of a 0.8 mEq potassium/mL solution. How many grams of potassium chloride should be used to prepare the quantity specified? (MW KCl = 74.5)

    (A) 4.5 g
    (B) 7.5 g
    (C) 45 g
    (D) 75 g
    (E) 450 g

31. A medication order calls for 10 mL of a 1% (w/v) tobramycin (E = 0.07) ophthalmic solution. You have on hand tobramycin 40 mg/mL solution. How many milligrams of NaCl should be added to make the solution isotonic with tears?

    (A) 7 mg
    (B) 33 mg
    (C) 83 mg
    (D) 100 mg
    (E) 400 mg

32. You receive a prescription for amoxicillin 100 mg/5 mL. You have on hand amoxicillin 125 mg/5 mL powder for reconstitution. The label calls for the addition of 63 mL of water to make 80 mL of the 125 mg/5 mL suspension. How many milliliters of water should be added to prepare the concentration specified?

    (A) 68 mL
    (B) 70 mL
    (C) 83 mL
    (D) 88 mL
    (E) 100 mL

33. How many milliliters of a 10% w/v stock solution should be diluted with water to make 500 mL of a 0.25% w/v solution?

    (A) 12.5 mL
    (B) 25 mL
    (C) 50 mL
    (D) 125 mL
    (E) 200 mL

34. A prescription for lansoprazole suspension is written as follows:

Rx	Lansoprazole	3 mg/mL
	Sodium bicarbonate 8.4% w/v qs	150 mL
	Sig. 5 mL BID	

How many lansoprazole 30-mg capsules are needed to compound the prescription?

(A) 10 capsules
(B) 15 capsules
(C) 30 capsules
(D) 45 capsules
(E) 60 capsules

35. What is the caloric requirement for a 52-year-old female with a calculated basal energy expenditure of 1,200 Calories and a stress factor of 1.5 due to a fever?

(A) 1,200 Calories
(B) 1,400 Calories
(C) 1,600 Calories
(D) 1,800 Calories
(E) 2,000 Calories

36. The daily caloric requirement for a 62-year-old male is 1,950 Calories. If 250 mL of a 10% IV fat emulsion product were to be used daily, how many milliliters of $D_{70}W$ would need to be administered to meet his caloric requirements?

(A) 493 mL
(B) 704 mL
(C) 855 mL
(D) 1,220 mL
(E) 1,675 mL

ANSWERS AND EXPLANATIONS

1. **B**

In this problem, the solution of sucrose in water is being diluted. The $Q_1C_1 = Q_2C_2$ method can be used to solve the problem. The volume that is solved for x is the amount of the 2.4% solution that would be made.

$$8.5\% \,(240\ mL) = 60\% \,(x)$$
$$x = 340\ mL$$

However, the question asks how much water *should be mixed with* the original 240 mL to dilute the concentration of the syrup to 60%. Therefore, this amount (240 mL) must be subtracted from the amount of syrup to be made (340 mL) to determine how much water to add.

$$340\ mL - 240\ mL = \textbf{100 mL of water to be added}$$

2. **D**

$$250\,\text{mL} \times \frac{3\,\text{mEq Na}^+}{10\,\text{mL}} \times \frac{1\,\text{mmol Na}^+}{1\,\text{mEq Na}^+} \times \frac{1\,\text{mmol NaCl}}{1\,\text{mmol Na}^+} \times \frac{58.5\,\text{mg NaCl}}{1\,\text{mmol NaCl}} \times$$

$$\frac{1\,g}{1{,}000\,\text{mg}} \times \frac{1\,\text{tablet}}{1\,g} = 4.4\,\text{tabs} = \textbf{5 tabs}$$

If you are using a partial tablet, you must always round up. If you use 4.4 tablets, you will actually expend 5 tablets from inventory, use 4.4 for your product, and discard the remainder of the fifth tablet.

3. **C**

Final solution: 1 L of 1:1,470 benzalkonium chloride (BC) solution

$$1{,}000\,\text{mL} \times \frac{1\,\text{g BC}}{1{,}470\,\text{mL}} = 0.68\,\text{g BC}$$

This solution was produced by diluting 20 mL of the solution you made. Therefore, the solution you made has 0.68 g of BC in every 20 mL.

$$500\,\text{mL} \times \frac{0.68\,\text{g BC}}{20\,\text{mL}} = 17\,\text{g of BC}$$

You need 17 g of benzalkonium chloride. How many milliliters of a 17% w/v stock solution will be required to deliver 17 g?

$$17\,g \times \frac{100\,\text{mL}}{17\,g} = \textbf{100 mL stock solution}$$

4. **D**

$$75 \text{ g paste} \times \frac{3 \text{ g ZnO}}{100 \text{ g paste}} = 2.25 \text{ g ZnO}$$

$$\frac{(2.25 + 5) \text{ g ZnO}}{(75 + 5) \text{ g paste}} = \frac{7.25 \text{ g ZnO}}{80 \text{ g paste}} = \frac{9.06 \text{ g ZnO}}{100 \text{ g paste}} = \mathbf{9.06\% \ w/w}$$

5. **E**

Step 1: Determine the weight of all chemicals present in this prescription.

$$\text{Zinc chloride}: \frac{0.2 \text{ g}}{100 \text{ mL}} = \frac{x}{60 \text{ mL}}$$

$$x = 0.12 \text{ g}$$

$$\text{Phenacaine}: \frac{1 \text{ g}}{100 \text{ mL}} = \frac{y}{60 \text{ mL}}$$

$$y = 0.6 \text{ g}$$

Step 2: Multiply each weight by the listed E value of the chemical.

Zinc chloride: $0.12 \text{ g} \times 0.62 = 0.0744 \text{ g}$

Phenacaine: $0.6 \text{ g} \times 0.17 = 0.102 \text{ g}$

Step 3: Add the weights from step 2. The sum is the amount of NaCl currently present in this prescription.

$$0.0744 \text{ g} + 0.102 \text{ g} = 0.1764 \text{ g}$$

Step 4: Determine the theoretical amount of NaCl that would be necessary to make this prescription isotonic if no other chemical were present.

$$\frac{0.9 \text{ g}}{100 \text{ mL}} = \frac{p}{60 \text{ mL}}$$

$$p = 0.54 \text{ g}$$

Step 5: Subtract the value in step 3 from the value in step 4 to determine the amount of NaCl that needs to be added to make this prescription isotonic.

$$0.54 \text{ g} - 0.1764 \text{ g} = 0.3636 \text{ g}$$

Step 6: Determine the amount of boric acid that would be used instead of NaCl to make this prescription isotonic.

$$\frac{0.3636 \text{ g NaCl}}{q} = \frac{0.52 \text{ g NaCl}}{1 \text{ g boric acid}}$$

$$q = 0.699 \text{ g} \times 1,000 = \mathbf{699 \text{ mg}}$$

6. **D**

Step 1: Determine the weight of all chemicals present in this prescription.

$$\text{Phenylephrine: } \frac{0.5\,\text{g}}{100\,\text{mL}} = \frac{x}{30\,\text{mL}}$$

$$x = 0.15\,\text{g}$$

Step 2: Multiply each weight by the listed E value of the chemical. The product is the amount of NaCl currently present in this prescription.

Phenylephrine: $0.15\,\text{g} \times 0.32 = 0.048\,\text{g}$

Step 3: Determine the theoretical amount of NaCl that would be necessary to make this prescription isotonic if no other chemical were present.

$$\frac{0.9\,\text{g}}{100\,\text{mL}} = \frac{y}{30\,\text{mL}}$$

$$y = 0.27\,\text{g}$$

Step 4: Subtract the value in step 2 from the value in step 3 to determine the amount of NaCl that needs to be added to make this prescription isotonic.

$0.27\,\text{g} - 0.048\,\text{g} = 0.222\,\text{g} \times 1{,}000 = \textbf{222 mg}$

7. **D**

The concentration of the epinephrine solution is presented as a ratio strength. A concentration of 1:500 translates into 1 g/500 mL. The first step in solving this problem is to determine the amount of epinephrine (in grams) that would be contained in 60 mL of the solution.

$$\frac{1\,\text{g}}{500\,\text{mL}} = \frac{x}{60\,\text{mL}}$$

$$x = 0.12\,\text{g epinephrine}$$

Next, set up a ratio-proportion to determine the volume of the 1% epinephrine stock solution needed to obtain the 0.12 grams of epinephrine.

1% stock solution:

$$\frac{1\,\text{g}}{100\,\text{mL}} = \frac{0.12\,\text{g}}{y}$$

$$y = \textbf{12 mL}$$

8. **D**

To determine the percentage of witch hazel, you must calculate the amount of witch hazel in 100 mL of the compound. According to the problem, there are 45 mL of witch hazel in 120 mL of calamine lotion in this prescription. To solve this problem, set up a ratio-proportion.

$$\frac{45\,\text{mL}}{120\,\text{mL}} = \frac{x}{100\,\text{mL}}$$

$$x = \mathbf{37.5\%}$$

9. **D**

First, calculate the number of teaspoons to be administered on a daily basis.

1.5 tsp/dose × 3 doses/day = 4.5 tsp/day

Next, set up a ratio-proportion to determine the total volume (in mL) of penicillin suspension to be administered (assuming 1 teaspoon = 5 mL).

$$\frac{4.5\,\text{tsp}}{x} = \frac{1\,\text{tsp}}{5\,\text{mL}}$$

$$x = 22.5\,\text{mL}$$

Finally, multiply this daily volume by 12 days to determine the total volume of suspension (in mL) that should be dispensed.

22.5 mL/day × 12 days = **270 mL**

10. **B**

Using dimensional analysis, multiply the weight-based dose by the weight of the child (being sure to convert the weight into kilograms), then by 2 (since the weight-based dose is being given twice daily), and then by 30 (to account for the 30-day supply). You can see here that all the units cancel out except for mg. The answer in this first step is the total number of milligrams of Dilantin that will be dispensed for this child for a 30-day supply.

$$\frac{2.5\,\text{mg}}{\text{kg dose}} \times 40\,\text{lb} \times \frac{1\,\text{kg}}{2.2\,\text{lb}} \times \frac{2\,\text{doses}}{\text{day}} \times 30\,\text{days} = 2{,}727.27\,\text{mg}$$

Next, using the concentration of Dilantin suspension of 125 mg/5 mL given in the problem, set up a ratio-proportion to determine the volume of this suspension to be dispensed that will contain 2,727.27 mg.

$$\frac{125\,\text{mg}}{5\,\text{mL}} = \frac{2{,}727.27\,\text{mg}}{x}$$

$$x = \mathbf{109\,mL}$$

11. **C**

Set up the problem using dimensional analysis: Multiply the weight-based dose by the weight of the patient, being sure to convert into kilograms; convert the units of time to hours; and convert the dose from micrograms to milligrams, since that is what the question is asking. You can see that all the units cancel out except for mg.

$$\frac{2\,\text{mcg}}{\text{kg}/\text{min}} \times 167\,\text{lb} \times \frac{1\,\text{kg}}{2.2\,\text{lb}} \times \frac{60\,\text{min}}{1\,\text{hr}} \times 2\,\text{hr} \times \frac{1\,\text{mg}}{1{,}000\,\text{mcg}} = \textbf{18.2 mg}$$

12. **D**

Given that there are 274 mg of levothyroxine in 2,000 tablets, set up a ratio-proportion to determine how many milligrams are in 1 tablet. Then multiply this answer (in milligrams) by 1,000 to arrive at the answer in micrograms.

$$\frac{274\,\text{mg}}{2{,}000\,\text{tablets}} = \frac{x}{1\,\text{tablet}}$$

$$x = 0.137\,\text{mg} \times 1{,}000\,\text{mcg/mg} = \textbf{137 mcg}$$

13. **B**

The first step is to determine the total amount of the analgesic ointment that will be made given the formula provided.

$$10\,\text{g} + 95\,\text{g} + 5\,\text{g} + 40\,\text{g} + 850\,\text{g} = 1{,}000\,\text{g ointment}$$

Next, convert the total amount of ointment to be prepared, 5 pounds, into grams.

$$5\,\text{lb} \times \frac{454\,\text{g}}{1\,\text{lb}} = 2{,}270\,\text{g}$$

Finally, set up a ratio-proportion to determine how much benzocaine is needed to prepare 2,270 g of ointment, given that 95 g of benzocaine is used to prepare 1,000 g of the same ointment.

$$\frac{95\,\text{g benzocaine}}{1{,}000\,\text{g ointment}} = \frac{x}{2{,}270\,\text{g ointment}}$$

$$x = \textbf{215.7 g}$$

14. **B**

In this problem, the solution of iodine in chloroform is being concentrated (rather than diluted). The $Q_1C_1 = Q_2C_2$ method can be used to solve the problem. The volume that is solved for x is the amount of the 2.4% solution that would be made.

$$(1.4\%)(180\,mL) = (2.4\%)x$$

$$x = 105\,\text{mL (this is the amount of 2.4\% solution)}$$

However, the question asks how much chloroform *must be evaporated from* the original 180 mL to adjust the iodine concentration to 2.4%. Therefore, this amount (105 mL) must be subtracted from the original amount (180 mL) to determine how much solution must be evaporated.

180 mL − 105 mL = **75 mL must be evaporated**

15. **A**

Alligation:

High Concentration [A]		Parts of High Concentration Ingredient [D]
	Desired Concentration [C]	
Low Concentration [B]		Parts of Low Concentration Ingredient [E]

Parts of high-concentration ingredient [D] = [C] − [B]

Parts of low-concentration ingredient [E] = [A] − [C]

Zinc Oxide Ointment:

Assume pure zinc oxide = 100%

100%		12 − 8 = 4 parts
	12%	
8%		100 − 12 = 88 parts
		Total = 92 parts

Quantity of 100% zinc oxide ointment needed:

$$\frac{4\,\text{parts}}{92\,\text{parts}} = \frac{x}{250\,\text{g}}$$

$$x = \textbf{10.9\,g}$$

16. **D**

The first step is to multiply the weight-based dose by the weight of the patient using dimensional analysis, being sure to convert the weight into kilograms.

$$\frac{186\,\cancel{\text{lb}}}{1} \times \frac{1\,\cancel{\text{kg}}}{2.2\,\cancel{\text{lb}}} \times \frac{2\,\text{mEq}}{\cancel{\text{kg}}} = 169.1\,\text{mEq}$$

At this point, the milliequivalent formula below can be used to determine the weight of sodium chloride (in mg) present in 169.1 mEq. Remember that the valence of sodium chloride (NaCl) is 1. The molecular weight of sodium chloride was given to you in the problem (58.5).

$$mEq = \frac{amount\,(mg)}{molecular\,weight} \times Valence$$

$$169.1 = \frac{x}{58.5} \times 1$$

$$x = 9,891.8\,mg\,/\,1,000 = 9.89\,g$$

Once the weight of sodium chloride is known, a ratio-proportion can be used to determine the volume of 0.9% sodium chloride solution to be administered. Remember that a 0.9% solution of sodium chloride contains 0.9 g of sodium chloride in 100 mL of solution.

Volume of 0.9% NaCl needed:

$$\frac{0.9\,g}{100\,mL} = \frac{9.89\,g}{x}$$

$$x = \mathbf{1,099\,mL}$$

17. **D**

The first step is to determine how much calcium chloride (in grams) is contained in 200 mL of a 10% (w/v) solution. Set up a ratio-proportion to solve this step.

$$\frac{10\,g}{100\,mL} = \frac{x}{200\,mL}$$

$$x = 20\,g\,CaCl_2$$

At this point, the milliosmole formula can be used to determine how many milliosmoles are represented by 20 grams of calcium chloride. Remember that calcium chloride dissociates into 3 species. The molecular weight of calcium chloride was given to you in the problem (147).

$$mOsm = \frac{amount\,(mg)}{molecular\,weight} \times \begin{array}{l} Theoretical\,number\,of\,particles \\ (or\,dissociation\,constant) \end{array}$$

$$mOsm = \frac{20,000\,mg}{147} \times 3$$

$$mOsm = \mathbf{408\,mOsm}$$

18. **D**

The first step is to determine how much of the polyethylene glycol 400 would be needed to prepare 1 kg (or 1,000 g) of ointment, starting with a 60% (w/w) polyethylene glycol 400 ointment. A ratio-proportion can be set up to solve this problem.

$$\frac{60\,g}{100\,g} = \frac{x}{1,000\,g}$$

$$x = 600\,g\,of\,polyethylene\,glycol\,400\,needed$$

Next, set up a ratio-proportion with this information to determine the volume of polyethylene glycol solution needed to prepare this compound. Remember that the specific gravity of a substance represents weight/volume in grams per milliliters.

Specific gravity (SG) = wt/vol

$$\frac{1.13\,g}{1\,mL} = \frac{600\,g}{y}$$

$$y = \mathbf{531\,mL}$$

19. **D**

This is a dilution problem that involves ratio strengths. The first step is to determine how much zephiran chloride (in grams) is contained in 50 mL of a 1:750 solution. This can be determined by setting up a ratio-proportion.

$$\frac{1\,g}{750\,mL} = \frac{x}{50\,mL}$$

$$x = 0.067\,g$$

Since the solution will be diluted to a 1:10,000 solution, the next step is to determine what volume of this solution would contain 0.067 g of zephiran chloride. Again, this can be determined by setting up a ratio-proportion.

$$\frac{1\,g}{10,000\,mL} = \frac{0.067\,g}{y}$$

$$y = 666.67\,mL$$

This dilution process involved going from 50 mL of a 1:750 solution to 666.67 mL of a 1:10,000 solution. However, 666.67 mL is not the final answer, as the question asked how many milliliters of water *should be added* to arrive at this amount. Thus, the final step of the problem is to subtract the initial volume from the total volume to arrive at the answer.

666.67 mL − 50 mL = 616.67 mL = **617 mL of water needs to be added**

20. **C**

Solve this problem using dimensional analysis: Multiply the number of doses per day (2) by the strength of each prescribed dose (440 mcg); by the strength per metered dose (220 mcg/dose) and the number of doses per inhaler (120) to factor in the available dosage form; and by the number of days needed (90). Each fraction should be set up such that all the units cancel out except for inhalers.

$$2 \times \frac{440 \text{ mcg}}{1 \text{ day}} \times \frac{1 \text{ dose}}{220 \text{ mcg}} \times \frac{1 \text{ inhaler}}{120 \text{ doses}} \times 90 \text{ days} = \textbf{3 inhalers}$$

21. **B**

Solve this problem using dimensional analysis: Multiply the number of units the patient will need each day (65) by the number of units in each milliliter of insulin (100); by the number of milliliters per vial (10); and by the number of days needed (30). Each fraction should be set up such that all the units cancel out except for vials.

$$\frac{65 \text{ units}}{1 \text{ day}} \times \frac{1 \text{ mL}}{100 \text{ units}} \times \frac{1 \text{ vial}}{10 \text{ mL}} \times 30 \text{ days} = \textbf{1.95 vials}$$

Therefore, **2 vials** should be dispensed.

22. **C**

Solve this problem using dimensional analysis: Convert the maximum daily dose (4 g/day) to milligrams, and multiply by the strength of each tablet (500 mg) and the number of days needed (30). Each fraction should be set up such that all the units cancel out except for tablets.

$$\frac{4 \text{ g}}{1 \text{ day}} \times \frac{1,000 \text{ mg}}{1 \text{ g}} \times \frac{1 \text{ tablet}}{500 \text{ mg}} \times 30 \text{ days} = \textbf{240 tablets}$$

23. **B**

Solve this problem using dimensional analysis: Multiply the strength of the elixir (250 mg/5 mL) by the desired dose (500 mg); by the number of doses per day (2); and by the quantity dispensed (120 mL). Each fraction should be set up such that all units cancel out except for days.

$$\frac{250 \text{ mg}}{5 \text{ mL}} \times \frac{1 \text{ dose}}{500 \text{ mg}} \times \frac{1 \text{ day}}{2 \text{ doses}} \times 120 \text{ mL} = \textbf{6 days}$$

24. **D**

First, use dimensional analysis to determine the amount of elemental iron per milliliter. Multiply the strength of the available suspension (75 mg/1.5 mL) by the percent of elemental iron (20%).

$$\frac{75 \text{ mg ferrous sulfate}}{1.5 \text{ mL suspension}} \times \frac{20 \text{ mg elemental iron}}{100 \text{ mg ferrous sulfate}} = 10 \text{ mg elemental iron/mL}$$

Then, set up a ratio-proportion to calculate the volume of the suspension needed to obtain the 30 mg of elemental iron, and cross-multiply to solve the problem.

$$\frac{10 \text{ mg elemental iron}}{1 \text{ mL}} = \frac{30 \text{ mg elemental iron}}{x}$$

$$10x = 30 \text{ mL}$$

$$x = 30 / 10 = \textbf{3 mL}$$

25. **C**

One approach to solving this problem is to identify the factor that represents the relationship between the desired quantity (120 mL) and the quantity specified in the compounding recipe (1,000 mL), then multiply by this factor to determine the appropriate amount of each ingredient. In this case, the relationship can be expressed by dividing 120 mL by 1,000 mL, yielding a factor of 0.12.

$$\frac{120 \text{ mL}}{1,000 \text{ mL}} = 0.12 \text{ (factor)}$$

Next, multiply the relevant ingredient—in this case, 80 g of calamine—by this factor to calculate the appropriate amount.

$$80 \text{ g calamine} \times 0.12 = \textbf{9.6 g}$$

26. **C**

First, determine the ratio of zinc oxide to the total recipe by finding the sum of the parts: 1 part + 1 part + 2 parts = 4 parts. So the ratio of parts zinc oxide to total parts is 1:4. Next, set up a ratio-proportion to calculate how much zinc oxide is contained in a total weight of 60 grams, and cross-multiply to solve.

$$\frac{1 \text{ part zinc oxide}}{4 \text{ parts total}} = \frac{x \text{ g zinc oxide}}{60 \text{ g total}}$$

$$4x = 60$$

$$x = 60 / 4 = \textbf{15 g}$$

27. **C**

The first step in solving this problem is to set up a ratio-proportion representing the relationship between the desired % w/v (0.9%) and the available weight of the product (30 g).

$$\frac{0.9\,\text{g}}{100\,\text{mL}} = \frac{30\,\text{g}}{x}$$

$$x = 3{,}333\,\text{mL}$$

The problem asks for liters, so convert from milliliters to liters to solve the problem.

$$3{,}333\,\text{mL} \times \frac{1\,\text{L}}{1{,}000\,\text{mL}} = \textbf{3.33\,L}$$

28. **E**

In this problem, the 10% solution is being diluted to a 0.5% solution. The $Q_1 C_1 = Q_2 C_2$ method can be used to solve the problem. The volume that is solved for x is the amount of the 10% solution that you would need to start with.

$$10\%\,(x\,\text{mL}) = 0.5\%\,(500\,\text{mL})$$

$$x = \textbf{25\,mL}$$

29. **E**

Sodium and chloride are monovalent ions, so 1 mol = 1 equivalent. The first step in solving this problem is to determine the number of grams of NaCl per mEq. Because there is 1 mol per equivalent, this is a simple calculation: Divide the molecular weight (which is equal to the EqW) by 1,000 to determine g/mEq.

$$\text{MW NaCl} = 58.5$$

$$\text{EqW} = \frac{58.5\,\text{g}}{1}$$

$$1\,\text{mEq} = \frac{58.5}{1{,}000} = 0.0585\,\text{g}$$

Next, multiply the weight by the desired number of mEq (100) to determine the total weight needed.

$$100\,\text{mEq} = 0.0585\,\text{g} \times 100 = 5.85\,\text{g NaCl needed}$$

Finally, set up a ratio-proportion indicating the relationship between the available concentration (0.9% for normal saline) and the desired weight of NaCl (5.85 g), and cross-multiply to solve the problem.

$$\frac{0.9\,\text{g}}{100\,\text{mL}} = \frac{5.85\,\text{g}}{x}$$

$$0.9x = 585$$

$$x = 585\,/\,0.9 = \textbf{650\,mL}$$

30. **A**

Because KCl is made up of monovalent ions, the molecular weight is equal to the EqW. Divide the number by 1,000 to determine the weight/mEq.

$$\text{MW KCl} = 74.5$$

$$\text{EqW} = \frac{74.5\,\text{g}}{1}$$

$$1\,\text{mEq} = \frac{74.5}{1,000} = 0.0745\,\text{g}$$

From here, the problem can be solved using dimensional analysis: Multiply the desired concentration (0.8 mEq/mL) by the weight/mEq (74.5 g/mEq) and by the total quantity desired (75 mL). Each fraction should be set up such that units cancel out except for grams.

$$\frac{0.8\,\cancel{\text{mEq}}}{1\,\cancel{\text{mL}}} \times \frac{0.0745\,\text{g}}{1\,\cancel{\text{mEq}}} \times 75\,\cancel{\text{mL}} = \textbf{4.5g}$$

31. **C**

First, calculate the total amount of tobramycin in the desired product by multiplying the % w/v by the given volume.

$$\frac{1\,\text{g tobramycin}}{100\,\text{mL}} \times 10\,\text{mL} = 0.1\,\text{g tobramycin}$$

Then, multiply the weight of the active ingredient by the E value of the active ingredient (0.07) to determine the weight of NaCl required to exert the tonic effect represented in the solution.

$$0.1\,\text{g tobramycin} \times \frac{0.07\,\text{g NaCl(eq)}}{1\,\text{g tobramycin}} = 0.007\,\text{g NaCl(eq)}$$

Next, use the % w/v of normal saline (0.9%) to calculate the total amount of NaCl needed to make the solution isotonic if this were the sole tonicity agent.

$$\frac{0.9\,\text{g NaCl}}{100\,\text{mL}} \times 10\,\text{mL} = 0.09\,\text{g NaCl}$$

Finally, subtract the amount of NaCl already present in the tobramycin (0.007 g) from this total amount (0.09 g) to determine how much should be added.

$$0.09\,\text{g} - 0.007\,\text{g} = 0.083\,\text{g NaCl} \times \frac{1,000\,\text{mg}}{1\,\text{g}} = \textbf{83 mg}$$

32. **C**

First, set up a ratio-proportion to calculate the total weight of medication in the bottle.

$$\frac{125\,mg}{5\,mL} = \frac{x}{80\,mL}$$

$$x = 2{,}000\,mg\,amoxicillin$$

Then, set up another ratio-proportion to determine the total volume needed to provide the desired concentration.

$$\frac{100\,mg}{5\,mL} = \frac{2{,}000\,mg}{y}$$

$$y = 100\,mL$$

Next, calculate the volume of the dry powder to be used in this prescription by subtracting the amount of water added from the total end volume.

volume of dry powder = 80 mL − 63 mL = 17 mL

Finally, determine the amount of water to add for reconstitution by subtracting the volume of dry powder calculated in the previous step from the total volume needed.

100 mL − volume of dry powder (17 mL) = water to add = **83 mL**

33. **A**

In this problem, the 10% solution is being diluted to a 0.25% solution. The $Q_1C_1 = Q_2C_2$ method can be used to solve the problem. The volume that is solved for x is the amount of the 10% solution that you would need to start with.

$$10\%\,(x\,mL) = 0.25\%\,(500\,mL)$$

$$x = \textbf{12.5 mL}$$

34. **B**

First, determine the total weight of drug needed by multiplying the concentration (3 mg/mL) by the given volume (150 mL).

$$\frac{3\,mg}{1\,mL} \times 150\,mL = 450\,mg\,lansoprazole\,needed$$

Next, divide the total weight needed by the available capsule strength (30 mg) to determine the number of capsules needed.

450 mg / 30 mg capsules = total number of capsules needed = **15 capsules**

35. **D**

The patient's total caloric requirement can be calculated by multiplying the patient's estimated basal energy expenditure by the stress factor. The patient has an estimated basal energy expenditure of 1,200 and a stress factor of 1.5.

$$1,200 \times 1.5 = \textbf{1,800 Calories}$$

36. **B**

The fat emulsion and dextrose are used in the TPN to meet the patient's caloric requirement. To calculate the amount of dextrose that is needed to meet the caloric requirement, first calculate the calories obtained from the fat emulsion. The fatty acid emulsion contains 1.1 Cal/mL.

Therefore,

$$\frac{1.1 \, \text{Calorie}}{1 \, \text{mL}} = \frac{x \, \text{Calorie}}{250 \, \text{mL}}$$

$$x = 275 \, \text{Calories from the fat emulsion}$$

Next, calculate the calories needed from the dextrose solution by subtracting the fat emulsion calories from the total caloric need. The number of calories required from dextrose would be:

$$1,950 - 275 = 1,675 \, \text{Calories}$$

Then, calculate the amount of dextrose needed to meet the requirements.

$$\frac{3.4 \, \text{Calories}}{1 \, \text{g}} = \frac{1,675 \, \text{Calories}}{x \, \text{g}}$$

$$x = 493 \, \text{g of dextrose}$$

Finally, convert the amount of dextrose into milliliters of solution.

$$\frac{70 \, \text{g dextrose}}{100 \, \text{mL}} = \frac{493 \, \text{g}}{x \, \text{mL}}$$

$$x = \textbf{704 mL of } \mathbf{D_{70}W}$$

Biostatistics

28

This chapter contains the following:

- **Descriptive statistics: Summarizing the data**
- **Inferential statistics: Predicting outcomes**
- **Statistical test selection**

 Suggested Study Time: **2.0 hours**

Statistics play an important role in the development and interpretation of clinical trials. Biostatistics is defined as the application of statistics to biological data. The NAPLEX tests fundamental statistical knowledge. Many times the questions are not math-based problems but are conceptual in nature. This chapter covers the most important definitions in biostatistics and proper uses of the most common statistical tests.

Statistics can be broken into two fundamental parts: descriptive and inferential.

Descriptive statistics are used to organize, summarize, categorize, and display data. If an entire population were to be studied, one would need only to summarize the data. However, in almost all cases, an entire population cannot be studied, and inferential statistics is needed from a sample of the population. **Inferential statistics** are used to make predictions (i.e., infer) about a large amount of information (population) based on a sample. Ultimately, inferential statistics are used in decision making in many fields, including regulatory drug approval and clinical drug usage.

DESCRIPTIVE STATISTICS: SUMMARIZING THE DATA

Central Tendency

A population or sample from that population can generate a lot of data that need to be simplified. One of the most basic forms of descriptive statistics is to take a large amount of information and simplify that into one or two values that can provide information regarding the tendency of the data. **Central tendency** is a general term used to describe the distribution of a set of values or measurements and the simplification to a single value near a point in the dataset that represents where the largest portion of data are located. The following are the most commonly used central tendency measures.

Median (m): The median is the value directly in the middle of the ranked values in a dataset; that is, 50% of all ranked values are smaller than the median and the other 50% of ranked values are larger. The median is **not** influenced by extreme values (outliers). The median is useful in situations in which there are unusually low or high values that would render the mean unrepresentative of the data.

Mean ($\overline{X}$ or μ): The mean is the average of all observations in a dataset. The mean is the most commonly used measure of central tendency because it has properties that make it useful for statistical analyses. It is influenced by extreme values (outliers) and is most useful when the data are symmetrically distributed without outliers (i.e., normal distribution).

Mode: The mode is the value with the greatest frequency of occurrence. It is not generally used because it is often not representative of the data, particularly when the dataset is small.

Variability

The central tendency (e.g., median, mean) does not provide any information about the variability in a given dataset. An additional measure that describes the variability in a dataset is, therefore, generally provided with a central tendency measure to better describe the dataset. The following are the most commonly used measures of variability.

Standard Deviation (SD or σ): The standard deviation is the most common measure of the variability around the mean. It is used with a mean because it is most informative when the dataset is normally distributed, as described below. The mean and standard deviation are commonly used together as the most informative measures of central tendency and variability of a dataset, respectively.

Standard Error of the Mean (SEM): The standard error of the mean is defined as the variability of the sample means. It is calculated as the SD divided by the square root of the sample size. This will always be smaller than the sample SD. It is sometimes reported in the scientific and medical literature and is an intermediary step in calculating confidence intervals.

Absolute Range: The absolute range is simply the difference between the largest and smallest observation in a dataset. A disadvantage is that the range is based solely on two observations and is likely not representative of the whole dataset. Absolute range is particularly susceptible to outliers.

Interquartile Range (IQR): Quartiles are calculated in a way similar to the median, which splits a dataset into two equally sized groups. Quartiles split the data into four approximately equal sized groups. The interquartile range is the range between the lower and upper quartiles. Like the median, the interquartile range is not influenced by unusually high or low values and is particularly useful when data are not symmetrically distributed.

- The lower Quartile (Q_L or Q_1) is the 25th percentile; that is, 25% of the data are below the value of Q_1.
- The upper Quartile (Q_U or Q_3) is the 75th percentile; that is, 75% of the data are below the value of Q_3.

A dataset with a large number of outliers is best described by a median and IQR as opposed to a mean and SD. These datasets are often displayed graphically with boxplots. **Boxplots** are one-dimensional graphs that can be drawn from the range, IQR, and median, as displayed here.

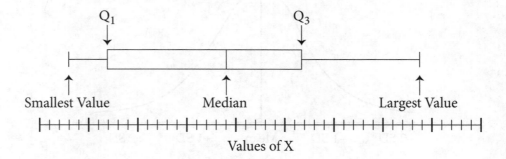

Distributions

Statistical test selection relies heavily on the distribution of data. These distributions can be summarized by a central tendency and variation around that center. The most important distribution is the normal or Gaussian curve. This "bell-shaped" curve is symmetric, with one side the mirror image of the other.

The distribution of any dataset can be assessed visually using a **histogram**. The *x*-axis represents the actual values in the dataset which, for pharmacy, are usually measures made of patients enrolled in a clinical trial (e.g., systolic blood pressure, creatinine clearance, low-density lipoprotein cholesterol concentrations). The *y*-axis represents the frequency of the value or the number of patients who had a value within a defined range. An example of a histogram is displayed here.

As the sample size (*n*) displayed in the histogram here approaches the population size (*N*), the lines on the graph become smooth and look more like following graph for normally distributed data:

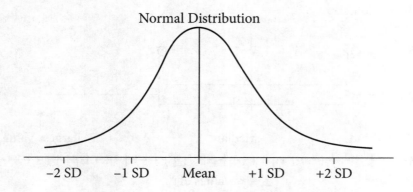

There are important attributes of the Normal Distribution shown in the preceding graph that can be useful in a number of problems on the NAPLEX. Importantly, the data is symmetric about the mean, as shown by the vertical line in the graph. This means that 50% of the values will be greater than the mean and 50% of the values will be less than the mean. Because this is the definition of a median, the mean and median are equal values in a normal distribution. The informative power of the normal distribution comes from the value of the standard deviation:

- The mean ± 1 SD contains 68% of the values in the dataset (or population)
- The mean ± 2 SD contains 95% of the values in the dataset (or population)
- The mean ± 3 SD contains 99.7% of the values in the dataset (or population)

The following graph displays two normal curves with the same means but different standard deviations:

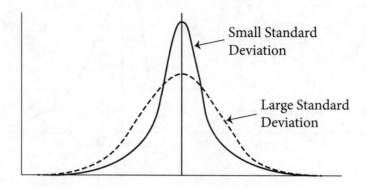

Example:

Patients ($n = 100$) enrolled in a clinical trial have a mean ± SD creatinine clearance of 110 ± 20 mL/min. Approximately how many patients have creatinine clearance values between:

- 90 and 130 mL/min?

  Answer: The value of 90 mL/min is 1 SD away from the mean in the negative direction, and the value of 130 mL/min is 1 SD away from the mean in the positive direction. Approximately 68% of the values will be ± 1 SD away from the mean; therefore, 68% of the sample size of $n = 100$ gives an answer of 68 patients.

- 70 and 110 mL/min?

  Answer: The value of 70 mL/min is 2 SD away from the mean in the negative direction, and the value of 110 mL/min is the value of the mean. Approximately 95% of the values will be ± 2 SD away from the mean. Because the question is asking for only 2 SD in the negative direction and the normal distribution is symmetrical, it will be half the value of 95%. Half of 95% is 47.5%. Therefore, approximately 47.5% of the sample size of $n = 100$ patients will have values in this range. The answer would be approximately 48 patients have creatinine clearance values in this range.

Not all curves are normally distributed. Sometimes the curve is skewed either positively or negatively. As shown in the following graph, a positive skew has the tail to the right with mean greater than the median. A negative skew has the tail to the left and the median greater than the mean.

For skewed distributions, the median is a better representation of central tendency than is the mean, and the IQR is a better measure of the variability than is the SD.

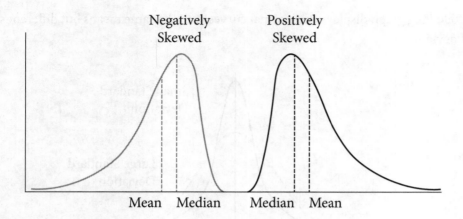

INFERENTIAL STATISTICS: PREDICTING OUTCOMES

The main goal of several studies in the pharmacy literature is to compare measurements from two groups of study patients: a group that receives a standard drug (e.g., control) and a group that receives an investigational drug. Even if both groups are administered placebo, it is highly unlikely that an identical mean and standard deviation of any value will be obtained for both groups. This is due to inherent variability in humans, among other sources, and is termed sampling error. The purpose of inferential statistics is to determine if the observed differences in the measures between the two groups of patients is due to chance (i.e., sampling error) or if one drug is really better than the other.

The following table summarizes important definitions regarding statistical inference.

General Statistical Definitions

Hypotheses	Hypothesis	Theoretical statement that the study is intended to test
	Null hypothesis	States that there is no difference between the study and control groups
	Alternative hypothesis	States that the null hypothesis is incorrect; there is a difference between the study and control groups
Variables	Independent variable	Known variable(s)
	Dependent variable	Variable with a value dependent upon the value of an independent variable
Error	Type I error	Rejecting a true null hypothesis: Finding a difference between the study and control groups that does not exist
	Type II error	Accepting a false null hypothesis: Failing to detect a difference between the study and control groups when a difference truly exists

General Statistical Definitions *(cont'd)*

Tests	Parametric	Requires prior knowledge of the nature of the data under examination; data must fall under a normal (Gaussian) distribution and be measured on an interval or a ratio scale
	Nonparametric	Does not require prior knowledge of the distribution of the observations; data need not follow a normal or Gaussian distribution
Miscellaneous definitions	Accuracy	Measure of how close a measured value is to the expected value
	Precision	Measure of how close a particular measured value is to the other values in a set of measurements; does not imply proximity between measured values and the expected value
	Sample	Data set taken under homogenous conditions; a subset of a population
	Population	Entire group from which a sample is taken
	Gaussian (or normal) distribution	A bell-shaped distribution Given a large enough sample size, the Central Limit Theorem states that the distribution of means will follow this type of distribution even if the population is not Gaussian. • 68% of values fall within ± 1 SD of the mean • 95% of values fall within ± 2 SD of the mean • 99.7% of values fall within ± 3 SD of the mean

Several additional statistical concepts are included below, in slightly greater detail. Many of these concepts apply regardless of the statistical test chosen.

Confidence Intervals

Statistical decisions are made based on sampling from a larger population. The true values for the population may be above or below the sample values. For example, the sample mean is unlikely to be the same value as the actual mean of the entire population. Therefore, confidence intervals are calculated from the sample to provide a range of values that is likely to contain the actual population value. The most common confidence interval used is the 95% confidence interval. This interval implies that you are 95% confident that the actual mean value of the population lies within this range of values. The 5% of uncertainty is the same concept as described with the p-value discussed later in this chapter. Therefore, 95% confidence intervals can be used to determine statistical significance with a Type I error rate of 5%, as demonstrated next.

Example:

The following graph displays the 95% confidence intervals for blood pressure measurements following the administration of three drugs. The closed circle represents the sample mean estimate in each group, and the error bars encompass the values of the 95% confidence interval. Which drugs are statistically different from each other?

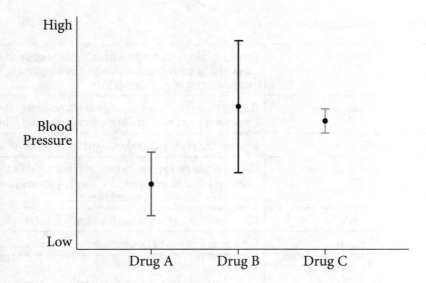

Answer:

When comparing two groups, any overlap of confidence intervals indicates that the groups would have a p-value > 0.05 and are not significantly different. Therefore, if the graph represents 95% confidence intervals and each drug is compared with the others, Drugs B and C are no different in their effects, and Drug B is no different from Drug A. Drug A lowers blood pressure to a greater statistically significant extent than Drug C. Of note, comparing these drugs individually to one another as in this example would increase the Type I error rate >5%, as will be discussed (see ANOVA).

Relative Risk and Odds Ratios

A relative risk (RR) is the ratio of the probability of an event occurring in a treatment (i.e., exposed) group to the probability of the event occurring in a control (i.e., nonexposed) group, as displayed in the following equation:

$$RR = \frac{p(\text{exposure group})}{p(\text{nonexposed group})}$$

Example:

In a local hospital over the last year, the frequency of patients with heart failure developing myopathy among those taking statins was 5 out of 100, and among patients not taking statins, it was 2 out of 100 patients. Calculate the relative risk.

Answer:

$$RR = \frac{5/100}{2/100} = 2.5$$

This implies that patients with heart failure who are taking statins were 2.5 times more likely to develop myopathy than patients who were not taking statins. Clearly, there are many variables in a study that could affect the relative risk beyond that of the statin use. Multivariate regression is commonly used in these types of analyses to account for variables beyond the exposure itself.

Similar to the relative risk, an **odds ratio** (OR) is also a measure of association between an exposure and an outcome. An odds ratio will provide a similar estimate to that of a relative risk, but the calculation is not as intuitive. However, the odds ratio has a mathematical advantage and is commonly reported because it is used in logistic regression to account for study variables beyond the exposure.

It is important to be able to make statistical determinations when provided with confidence intervals for relative risks and odds ratios. Simply put, if the 95% confidence interval contains 1, there is no statistically significant effect of the treatment (i.e., exposure). This is demonstrated in the following table for three hypothetical measures:

Relative Risk or Odds Ratio	Confidence Interval	Interpretation
1.98	(1.45–2.53)	Statistically significant (increased risk)
1.25	(0.78–1.53)	No statistical difference (risk the same)
0.45	(0.22–0.68)	Statistically significant (decreased risk)

Understanding Statistical Inference

The table at the beginning of this chapter introduced the definitions of hypothesis testing that are used after a research question has been identified. The null and alternative hypotheses are tested after the study has been conducted and the data have been collected. The process of running these statistical tests will not be covered on the NAPLEX. However, it is important to be able to interpret the results of the statistical tests. Interpreting statistics is quite simple because most statistical tests convert the output to a single p-value, which always has the same meaning. Therefore, to interpret the output of statistical tests, understanding the p-value is critical. Beyond the p-value, it is important to know what types of statistical error can be made and the power of a given test to determine significance. Finally, for the NAPLEX you will need to know the most commonly used statistical tests and their appropriate uses. All these important topics will be described in detail here.

p-Value and Statistical Significance

The p-value is the probability that the difference measured between your study group and the control group is the result of random chance rather than a true difference. The p-value is expressed as a value between 0 and 1; therefore, the higher the p-value, the more likely it is that a difference in sample means was due to chance and that a drug had no effect. When the p-value is low (e.g., <5%), it indicates that it was unlikely that the difference was due to chance; therefore, the drug had a statistically significant effect.

The null hypothesis may be rejected if there is a sufficiently small probability that it is true. A significance level (or α) of 0.05 is most commonly chosen, although it should be chosen based on the relative consequences of making a Type I or Type II error in the particular study setting. When a 0.05 significance level is chosen, if $p \leq 0.05$, a statistically significant difference in treatment effect exists between the control and treatment groups. If $p > 0.05$, the results of the study are considered to be not statistically significant, meaning no difference exists between the treatment and control groups. Choosing a larger significance level, like $p = 0.1$, gives a higher probability of rejecting a true null hypothesis (Type I error, or false positive test).

Types of Statistical Error

As defined in the table at the beginning of this chapter, there are two types of error that can be made at the end of a statistical test. The significance level (i.e. alpha, α) is commonly set to 0.05. This means that there is a 5% chance that a **Type I error (α error)** will be made during hypothesis testing. A Type I error is the conclusion that there is a statistical difference when in reality there is not one. Of course, you cannot know from a given experiment if you made a Type I error or not. You can only know the rate at which they occur (i.e., 5%).

The other type of error is **Type II error (β error)**, which is the conclusion that there is not a difference between groups when, in reality, there is a difference. A Type II error can only be made when the p-value is > 0.05 and the conclusion is made that there is no statistical difference between groups. As in a Type I error, one cannot know from a single experiment if a Type II error has been made, but can only calculate the frequency of the error. The Type I error rate is set at 5%, but the Type II error rate varies depending on the variable being measured and the study itself (see "Power and Sample Size"). Type II error rates are commonly designed to be <10% or 20%. The factors that affect Type II error are the same that affect study power.

Power and Sample Size

The power of a study is the ability to detect a difference between study groups if one actually exists. Study power is indirectly related to the likelihood of making a Type II (β) error. Therefore, as study power increases, the likelihood of concluding that there is not a difference when one actually does exist decreases. Therefore, as power increases, Type II error rate decreases. The following factors affect the power of a study:

- **Sample size (n):** The closer the sample size is to the actual population size, the easier it is to detect a difference.

- **Difference between the actual population means:** It will be easier to detect a difference between drugs with large effects versus the control or comparator. For example, it is much easier to show that a β-blocker will lower blood pressure compared to a placebo than it would be compared to an angiotensin-converting enzyme (ACE) inhibitor.

- **Variability around the population means (and sample means):** The more variable effect there is, the harder it is to show a difference. For example, if a drug only works in a small percentage of the population, it will be difficult to show statistical significance in a sample from the entire population.

- **Significance level, α:** The Type I error rate directly alters the Type II error rate. This is one reason why the significance level is traditionally set at 5%. If one wanted to decrease the Type I error rate and set it at 1%, it would increase the Type II error rate and, thereby, decrease the power of the study.

Of the factors just listed, the only way to decrease Type II error (increase power) without increasing Type I error is to increase the sample size. The researcher does not have control over the other factors (except the Type I error rate, which should not be changed). Therefore, increasing sample size increases one's power to detect a difference without altering the Type I error rate. Sample size calculations are commonly made before initiating a study. They are made by calculations including the four factors listed. The Type I error rate is set at 5%, and the Type II error rate is determined by the researcher, usually 10% or 20% (to give 90% to 80% power, respectively). The difference in the means is commonly chosen based on clinical significance. For example, if a 45% reduction in blood pressure is considered to be clinically significance, then it would be appropriate to base the sample size on a 45% difference in the means. Finally, the variability is often estimated based on previous research with the same drug or animal studies if human studies have not been conducted.

At the conclusion of a study, if the p-value is > 0.05, the actual study power can be calculated. This is done by simply using the actual values of the factors listed about the study (e.g., the sample size, variability, and mean difference). Of course, it would only make sense to calculate the power of a study if the p-value was > 0.05. If the p-value is < 0.05, it is impossible to make a Type II error. Only a Type I error could have been made with a p-value < 0.05, and the power of the study would be irrelevant.

Correlation

Correlation measures the degree of a linear relationship between two variables. Correlation is often represented by the correlation coefficient (r), which can range in value from −1 to +1. A correlation coefficient of 0 indicates no linear relationship between variables. A coefficient of −1 reflects a perfect inverse relationship between variables, while a value of +1 reflects a perfect direct relationship.

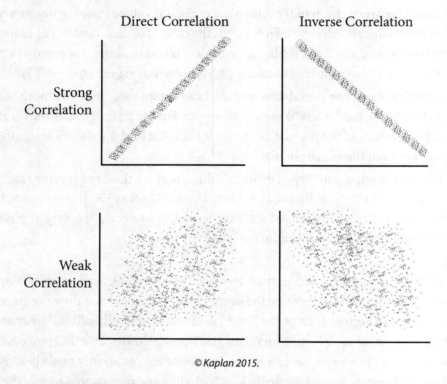

© Kaplan 2015.

A key point to remember is that an observed correlation between two variables does not imply that there is a causal link between the two variables. For example, warm weather causes an increase in both the crime rate and the incidence of sunburn. Crime rate and sunburn incidence will therefore be positively correlated; however, crime does not cause sunburn and sunburn does not cause crime.

Another important point to consider is that correlation coefficient assumes a normal distribution of measured values; if this assumption is incorrect, the coefficient is not relevant.

STATISTICAL TEST SELECTION

The first thing that must be done when determining what statistical test should be employed is to identify the dependent variable and the scale of measurement that will be used for this variable. The scale of measurement may be numeric, ordinal, or nominal.

Tests Appropriate for Numerical Scales of Measurement

Numeric scales (also called interval or ratio scales) of measurement are used when the measured values are numbers. Examples include height, weight, or blood pressure level. When the data follows a Gaussian distribution, parametric statistical tests should be used.

- Two independent groups: *t-test*
- Two dependent groups: *Paired t-test*
- Three or more independent groups: *ANOVA*
- Three or more dependent groups: *Repeated measures ANOVA*

t-Test

The *t*-test is one of the most commonly used statistical tests. It compares means obtained from the numeric data of two groups that are independent of each other. This statistical test is commonly used in the pharmacy literature to compare the outcomes of numeric data (e.g., clinical measures, drug concentrations). in a sample of patients who received an experimental drug versus a different (i.e., independent) sample of patients who received a control drug.

Paired *t*-Test

A paired *t*-test is used when the same sample is being used to compare the experimental and the control drug; that is, this test is appropriate when numeric data is being compared between two dependent groups. This is commonly referred to as a crossover design. A paired *t*-test is the appropriate statistical test for numeric or interval data.

ANOVA

When a third group (or more) is added to a study design for comparison, it is not appropriate to perform multiple *t*-tests. For example, an experimental drug to lower blood pressure is being compared to a group of patients taking β-blockers and another group of patients taking ACE inhibitors. In this study design, one cannot perform a *t*-test to compare the experimental drug to the β-blocker group and then perform another *t*-test to compare the ACE inhibitor group. Each time a *t*-test is performed there is a 5% chance of a Type I error; thus, multiple comparisons increase this rate of Type I error greater than 5%. Therefore, if three or more groups are being compared, it is appropriate to use an analysis of variance (ANOVA). An ANOVA will generate one p-value from the three groups. If the p-value is < 0.05, it states that at least one drug was different than another at lowering blood pressure. Importantly, the Type I error rate is maintained at 5% for an ANOVA.

To determine which drug has a statistically significant effect, additional tests are needed. These statistical tests are referred to as *post-hoc tests*. The most commonly used post-hoc test is Tukey's test. The Bonferroni and Scheffe's tests are also post-hoc tests that can be used to determine which groups were statistically different if an overall p-value from the ANOVA was less than 0.05. If a p-value is > 0.05 following an ANOVA, no further tests are needed.

Repeated Measures ANOVA

The repeated measures ANOVA is the equivalent of using a paired *t*-test instead of a *t*-test. It, therefore, can be used in crossover studies when there are three or more study periods following appropriate wash-out of the drug between each period. This test is referred to as *repeated measures* because it is commonly used when the same measures are being made in patients throughout a study. For example, in many statin clinical trials, the low-density lipoprotein cholesterol (LDL-C) lowering ability of the statins is not determined at only one point but at several points (e.g., 1, 3, 6, 12, 18, and 24 months). To determine if significant LDL-C lowering occurred in patients during these time intervals, a repeated measures ANOVA must be used. The Dunnett's test is the post-hoc test that should be used if an overall p-value < 0.05 is obtained.

When the data does not follow a Gaussian distribution, the same tests used for ordinal data should be employed.

Tests Appropriate for Ordinal Scales of Measurement

Ordinal scales of measurement are used when characteristics have an underlying order to their values but the numbers used are arbitrary (e.g., Likert scales). Various non-parametric tests (e.g., Mann-Whitney U and Wilcoxon Signed-Rank) are used for analyzing such data. Ordinal scales also are used for numeric data that are not distributed normally and that have a small sample size. The following are situations in which a nonparametric test should be considered:

- The outcome is ordinal and the sample is clearly not normally distributed.
- There are values that are too high or too low to obtain accurate measures. It is impossible to analyze such data with a parametric test because the exact value is not determined.

KAPLAN) MEDICAL

- The sample size is small and the sample is not approximately normally distributed. Data transformation can be done by taking the logarithm of the values. This is common for biological data, which often has outliers in the positive direction (i.e., skewed to the right).

The following table lists parametric tests for normally distributed data and the corresponding nonparametric test for ordinal or non-normally distributed data.

Parametric Versus Nonparametric Statistics

Parametric Tests	Nonparametric Equivalent
t-Test $\longrightarrow$	Wilcoxon-Rank Sum (Mann Whitney U)
Paired t-test $\longrightarrow$	Wilcoxon Sign Rank (Sign Test)
ANOVA $\longrightarrow$	Kruskal-Wallis Test
Repeated measures ANOVA $\longrightarrow$	Friedman Test
Note: The Wilcoxon-Rank Sum is the post-hoc test for the Kruskal-Wallis Test	

Tests Appropriate for Nominal Scales of Measurement

Nominal scales are used for characteristics that do not have numerical value (such as gender or race). The Chi-square test and its variants are used to test the null hypothesis that proportions are equal, or that factors or characteristics are not associated with each other.

LEARNING POINTS

- Smaller p-values associated with a statement reflect a greater likelihood that the statement accurately reflects a difference between groups. Larger p-values mean that the difference detected between groups is more likely to have been due to random chance.

- Power is the ability of a study to detect an actual effect. Power can be increased by increasing the number of patients enrolled in a study. Inadequate power may result in a study failing to detect a difference that actually exists between groups.

- The mean is the numerical average of the entire range of data; the median is the central point in the data distribution. In a pure Gaussian distribution, the median will be equal or very close to the mean; large differences between the median and mean value may reflect non-Gaussian distribution or significant outlying data.

- ANOVA and t-tests are appropriate only for numeric data in a Gaussian distribution. Nonparametric tests are appropriate for numeric data in a non-Gaussian distribution, as well as for ordinal data. Chi-square tests should be used for nominal data.

PRACTICE QUESTIONS

1. The median value of a data set is the

   (A) mathematical average of all the values in the data set.
   (B) value equidistant from the extremes of a distribution.
   (C) average of the difference between each value in the set and the mean.
   (D) most commonly occurring value in the data set.
   (E) distance between the smallest and largest values in the data set.

Questions 2–3 refer to the following graph.

Total serum cholesterol concentrations were measured in 175 patients with coronary artery disease. The measured serum cholesterol concentrations are displayed in the grouped frequency distribution histogram using 10 equal intervals, shown below.

2. The class interval as indicated by "B" in the above histogram most likely contains which of the following measures for this dataset?

   (A) Median
   (B) Mean
   (C) Mode
   (D) Standard deviation
   (E) Range

3. Which of the following is the best description of the distribution of this sample dataset?

   (A) Normal
   (B) Positively skewed
   (C) Negatively skewed
   (D) Gaussian
   (E) None of the above

4. A study reports that the mean ± SD peak plasma concentration of a drug is 1.0 ± 0.1 mg/dL in a study consisting of 1,000 patients. Approximately how many patients had values >1.1 mg/dL?

    (A) 840
    (B) 680
    (C) 320
    (D) 160
    (E) 16

5. A clinical study was performed and serum glucose concentrations were measured in 14 diabetic patients following 1 week of an investigational treatment to directly compare it to the decrease following glipizide treatment in a crossover trial. Statistics were performed and a p-value of 0.45 was obtained. Which of the following is (are) the most likely form of statistical error that the researchers could have made?

    (A) Type I error
    (B) Type II error
    (C) Type I or Type II error
    (D) Neither Type I or II error could be made because the results were NOT significant
    (E) Neither Type I or II error could be made because the results were significant

6. In most clinical studies, the Type I error rate is set to 0.05 before the study is performed. This indicates that the research group has a 5.0% chance of making a Type I error. If a research group were to set α at 0.01, corresponding to a Type 1 error rate of only 1.0%, which of the following statements would be true?

    (A) A smaller sample size could be used.
    (B) The study power would increase.
    (C) There would be an increased α error rate.
    (D) There would be an increased β error rate.
    (E) None of the above statements are true.

Questions 7–8 refer to the following table.

A clinical study enrolled 70 patients who were randomized to receive either lisinopril or ramipril (n = 35 per drug). The table shows measures obtained at the end of the study period in patients who received lisinopril and ramipril.

After Drug Treatment (End of Study Period)	Lisinopril n = 35	Ramipril n = 35
Disease states	—	—
Diabetes alone	29%	20%
Atherosclerosis alone	23%	31%
Diabetes and atherosclerosis	43%	34%
Neither disease	5%	15%
Mean serum cholesterol concentrations (mg/dL)	118 ± 4.0	116 ± 4.0
Sex (% male)	62%	46%

Data are presented as percentage of mean ± SD.

7. Which of the following statistical tests would be most appropriate to use to compare the serum cholesterol concentrations in the ramipril versus the lisinopril group?

   (A) *t*-Test
   (B) Paired *t*-test
   (C) Chi-square test
   (D) Wilcoxon sign rank test
   (E) ANOVA

8. Which of the following statistical tests would be most appropriate to use to compare the percentage of males in the ramipril versus the lisinopril group?

   (A) *t*-Test
   (B) Paired *t*-test
   (C) Chi-square test
   (D) Wilcoxon sign rank test
   (E) ANOVA

ANSWERS AND EXPLANATIONS

1. B

The median value is the value equidistant from the extremes of the data set. The mathematical average of the values in the data set (A) is the mean. The average of the difference between each value and the mean (C) is the standard deviation. The most commonly occurring value in the data set (D) is the mode. The distance between the smallest and largest values in the data set (E) is the range.

2. B

The mean is the most likely measure listed in the position marked by "B" on the graph. The mean is susceptible to outliers, and this dataset is skewed to the right, which means that there are outliers in the positive direction. The mean is pulled from the real central tendency of the data marked by "A" on the graph. The "A," most likely, is represented by the median, which is not susceptible to outliers and is the best measure of central tendency for skewed data.

3. B

The dataset is positively skewed because there are outliers on the graph in the positive direction. This pulls the mean to the right of the central tendency as described in the answer to question number 2.

4. D

1.1 mg/dL is 1 SD away from the mean, and the question is asking for values greater than that. With 68% of the dataset ± 1 SD away from the mean, the remaining 32% is outside of this range. Because normally distributed data is symmetrical, there is 16% of the dataset on the two sides that encompass data greater or less than 1 SD away from the mean. Thus, 16% of 1,000 patients equals 160, which is the answer.

5. B

The p-value is > 0.05; therefore, the authors would conclude that the differences observed between the investigational drug and glipizide are due to chance and that the investigational drug was not different than glipizide. Because the authors conclude that there is no difference, the only possible type of error is Type II (β) error. A Type II error is a conclusion that there is no difference when one actually exists. Given the small sample size of this study, the likelihood of a Type II error is likely very high. A Type I error cannot be made because there is no conclusion that a difference exists between the investigational drug and glipizide.

6. **D**

Setting the Type I (α) error rate to 0.01 instead of the traditional 0.05 would increase the Type II (β) error rate. The Type II error is inversely related to power; therefore, the study's power to detect a difference would be smaller. This would mean that a larger sample size would be needed to detect a difference if one actually exists.

7. **A**

The ramipril and lisinopril groups are independent of each other because this study is not a crossover design. Cholesterol concentrations are interval data, thus considered numeric; therefore, the most appropriate test for two independent groups with numeric data is a *t*-test. The sample size is >30, so the data does not have to be normally distributed. If the sample size were small and not normally distributed, the nonparametric Mann–Whitney U test should be used.

8. **C**

The sex of the patients is considered a nominal variable, which is often referred to as *categorical* because the patients can be placed into categories. Each patient is either a male or a female and cannot be classified as both. The fact that the percentages are provided instead of the actual number of males in each group does not change the fact that the data is categorical. The most appropriate statistical test for this type of categorical data is the chi-square test.

Clinical Trial Design 29

This chapter contains the following:

- **Case report/case series**
- **Cross-sectional design**
- **Case-control design**
- **Cohort study design**
- **Randomized controlled trial clinical trials**
- **Meta-analyses**
- **Pharmacoeconomic analyses**

 Suggested Study Time: **1.5 hours**

Clinical trials can be executed using several types of designs. These designs can be retrospective or prospective in time and may be observational or experimental. This section discusses the merits and weaknesses of the most common designs for clinical trials.

ASSESSING CLINICAL TRIAL DESIGN

The optimal study design depends on the type of research question that is being addressed. Some research questions are descriptive in nature; that is, the simple question gets at what currently exists in the world, such as how many patients have diabetes. Research questions can also be relational or causal. Depending on the specific question to be answered, several types of designs can be utilized.

When assessing the strength of a trial design, it is important to know the research question or hypothesis. This should help identify the population of interest, the intervention that is to be studied, and the measure that will be used to determine its efficacy. The following section provides the basics of the most common types of study designs along with a comparison of weaknesses and strengths.

CASE REPORT/CASE SERIES

A **case report** is the simplest form of an observational design, and it describes a unique or unexpected treatment effect or disease. The primary goal of a case report is to describe the experience of a single patient. A **case series** describes the experience of a group of patients that have a common disease, treatment effect, or the like. These types of reports are commonly published in medical journals to disseminate rare or unusual diseases or adverse effects. They are simple observations and form the basis for hypothesis generation. They are not designed or powered to show cause and effect, but they can be important for the design of future experiments to assess unique or uncommon drug effects that are not identified during drug development.

CROSS-SECTIONAL DESIGN

A **cross-sectional study** is a snapshot in time that can describe a pool of existing cases in a population. Each person in this type of study would fall into one of two categories: diseased or disease-free. The common purpose of a cross-sectional study is often to determine the prevalence of a condition. **Prevalence** can be defined as a proportion of the population that is affected by the disease or condition. The prevalence is simply calculated as the proportion of study subjects that is in the diseased state at any given time versus the entire population.

Cross-sectional study designs can also be used to test hypotheses. Although they cannot determine causality, these designs can be used to test associations. However, cross-sectional study designs are not optimal for studying an association between a rare exposure with a disease or between an exposure with a rare disease. The case-control study design would be a better approach for rare occurrences of the exposure or disease.

CASE-CONTROL DESIGN

A **case-control study** is designed to identify a group of subjects with a disease of interest (case) and another group of subjects without the disease (control). The purpose of a case-control study design is to look back in time to find differences in either risk factors or exposures that may have caused the disease. Since these studies look back in time, they employ a retrospective design. These designs promote hypothesis generation by identifying risk factors (such as drug exposure) in the group of subjects that got the disease versus a control group.

The biggest strength of a case-control study is that it is an efficient design to assess rare diseases. This allows the investigator to assess multiple risk factors for the rare disease. For example, torsade de pointes is a rare ventricular arrhythmia that can be triggered by certain medications. Many of the additional risk factors for torsade de pointes were identified through case-control studies. Since the arrhythmia is so rare, it is not feasible to prospectively follow a group of patients until the disease is observed. By pooling several cases of torsade de pointes that have already occurred, an investigator can look back to determine the risk factors versus a matched control group.

The case-control study design also has the advantage of identifying risk factors when long periods exist between the exposure and the disease. The longer the latent period between the exposure and disease, the less feasible it is to prospectively follow patients from the time of exposure to the time of disease. For example, it would be difficult and expensive to assess a group of young healthy subjects who consume high-salt diets and then follow them until the development of hypertension. It is much easier to identify cases of hypertension and then track the history back to assess high-salt diets.

The weaknesses of case-control studies largely concern the observational nature of the design. In addition, even though they are efficient for rare diseases, they are inefficient when there is a rare exposure.

COHORT STUDY DESIGN

In a **cohort study design**, subjects are followed over the defined length of the study. This approach differs from a cross-sectional study, which simply looks at a snapshot in time. The subjects in a cohort study are generally categorized into those that were exposed and those that were not exposed. The subjects are then followed over time prospectively or retrospectively to see if they develop the outcome or disease of interest. This is the opposite of a case-control study, which identifies patients with a disease and then works backward to the exposure. In pharmacy, the exposed cohort is usually the group that received a drug in question, and the nonexposed cohort serves as the control or comparative group. Because the cohorts generally include a control group, these types of study designs can be conducted to test a hypothesis.

A cohort study design can be prospective or retrospective in time. For example, one could place all patients that were prescribed a a drug of interest into the experimental cohort and those that were prescribed an alternative into the control cohort. If the study design is *prospective*, the subjects will be placed into cohorts and followed in real time to obtain outcome measures for the study as they occur for a predetermined length of time. A prospective study could define the exposed and nonexposed cohorts and follow those groups over time. However, at the start of a prospective study, the exposure may or may not have occurred. That is, the study could be implemented at the start of a drug exposure, or a group of subjects could be followed over time and then placed into cohorts as they receive the drug or an alternative exposure. If the study design is *retrospective*, the exposure and outcome has already occurred in the past. The subjects would be identified through medical and prescription records, since the drugs would have been prescribed at an earlier date. The medical record would be mined for the outcomes of interest for the predetermined length of the study design.

A cohort design is useful in tracking a rare exposure or treatment. Given the fact that patients are followed over time, cohort studies also have the advantage of identifying temporal relationships between treatment and disease; this temporal assessment allows for a direct measurement of the incidence of disease. The **incidence** is the rate of occurrence of disease in a given population over a defined period of time.

A weakness of cohort design studies is that they are not useful for rare diseases, because a very large sample size would be needed. They also do not control well for variables, and their outcomes may have been due to some other factor that influenced the drug exposure.

RANDOMIZED CONTROLLED CLINICAL TRIALS

Randomized controlled clinical trials (RCTs) are experimental, whereas cohort studies are **observational**. The experimental nature of RCTs permits the use of a **placebo** in a control group if there is no gold-standard therapy available. Placebo drugs can be used as a control and, in theory, should have no therapeutic effect. They have the advantage of providing a comparative group that will minimize the overall psychological effects of the experimental drug.

Another major difference between RCTs and cohort studies is the process of **randomization**. In an RCT, subjects are randomly assigned to either the treatment group or the control group at the outset of the study. Randomization helps decrease variability between groups and controls for factors that may be correlated to the outcome. This feature overcomes one of the major weaknesses of a cohort design, which is observational and, therefore, can be influenced by variables that are not accounted for.

In addition to placebo control and randomization, RCTs have the distinct advantage of **blinding**. The purpose of blinding in RCTs is to mask the treatment assignment to the patients and investigators. Blinding reduces bias of patients in reporting of adverse effects and other important measures. In a single-blind study, only the patients are unaware of the treatment assignment. In a double-blind study, both the patients and investigators (e.g., the treating physician) are unaware of the treatment assignment.

RCTs are the gold standard for studying interventions (e.g., drug treatment). Due to their randomization and blinding procedures, they have the distinct advantage over the other study designs of minimizing study bias. Nonetheless, RTCs have their weaknesses. The most notable weakness is the lack of generalizability of the results to clinical practice. These studies are highly controlled to minimize bias and, therefore, often include a long list of inclusion and exclusion criteria for subject enrollment. The incorporation of specific criteria for patients results in outcomes that may not be replicable in actual clinical practice.

The best way to show the generalizability of RCTs is to replicate the study. Cohort studies, on the other hand, may have greater generalizability than RCTs, but it is less clear if the outcomes of cohort studies are due to the drug itself or other factors in the study. Whether known and measured or unknown and unmeasured, these confounding factors still affect the outcome of a cohort study. By contrast, they are not usually relevant in an RCT: Given the process of randomization, both the known and unknown confounding factors should be evenly distributed between the groups.

META-ANALYSES

A **meta-analysis** is used to assess a group of studies. In many cases, a meta-analysis will combine the results of several trials and then use specific statistical methods to identify patterns in the outcome of interest. The analysis will put weight on the level of evidence provided from the clinical trials. For example, results of trials that were randomized or had a large sample size could be given heavier weight than those that did not meet these criteria. The goal of the analysis is to gain a more favorable statistical power than the individual trials included in the analysis.

The primary weakness of meta-analysis is that the methods chosen by the investigator can influence the results. These include the criteria for study inclusion, assessment of missing data, and publication bias. A **publication bias** is likely, because investigators are less likely to publish the results of negative trials; consequently, those negative trials would not be available for later analysis. Therefore, if only published trials are incorporated in the meta-analysis, it means that a large amount of important negative trials would be missing and confound the analysis.

PHARMACOECONOMIC ANALYSES

Introduction

The field of pharmacoeconomics falls under the umbrella of health outcomes research. **Health outcomes research** involves the analysis and assessment of outcomes that occur following a patient interaction within the health-care system. The outcomes measured can be those associated with the clinical outcomes or the cost of part or the entire experience to the health-care system. **Pharmacoeconomics** is the assessment of costs to the health-care system that are associated with drug therapy. These analyses can be performed in a comparative manner to assess the cost-effectiveness of more than one drug treatment option. These assessments are crucial to making decisions on drugs to be included on an institutional formulary or developing treatment protocols.

Health outcomes research and pharmacoeconomic-based studies differ from RCTs in that the external validity is prioritized. That is, it is important that the real-world outcomes and costs are accurately measured in the study versus the stringent environment of a RCT. However, the external validity of pharmacoeconomic analyses may have geographical constraints. For example, it is usually not accurate to apply the cost of an intervention from one country to another.

Categorization of Costs

An important measure in pharmacoeconomic analyses is associated with the cost of drug therapy. There are several types of cost that can be collected or predicted in these analyses. It is important to assess how cost is measured in pharmacoeconomic studies before making assessments. The direct costs are the most apparent measured economic outcome. **Direct costs** are the costs associated with the entire course of drug therapy itself. This includes all medical costs associated with administering the drug including the preparation, monitoring, and ancillary support by the entire medical staff. When evaluating the direct costs of drug therapy, it is imperative that the preparation and administration costs are considered along with any necessary monitoring including the cost of technician, pharmacist, nursing, or physician time, etc.

In pharmacoeconomic studies it can be important to assess how drug therapy may improve the morbidity that is associated with disease. **Indirect costs** are commonly associated with morbidity due to an illness that results in loss of income or increased costs due to adverse events. These indirect costs in pharmacoeconomic studies can be more difficult to measure than direct costs. However, in many pharmacoeconomic analyses indirect costs are important to gain an overall understanding of the true costs associated with drug therapy intervention.

In addition to direct and indirect costs, it may be important to consider how the drug therapy intervention is affecting the patient's quality of life. Although it is difficult to assign dollar values to a patient's quality of life issues, these can be important when making decisions based on pharmacoeconomic analyses.

Models of Pharmoeconomic Analyses

Pharmacoeconomic studies can be categorized into four types of analyses. Although, all four types of the assessment measure the cost in dollars, there are distinct differences in the ways that the outcomes or assessed.

The simplest pharmacoeconomic analysis is a **cost-minimization analysis (CMA)**. The underlying principle of this analysis is that the outcomes between the drug therapies being compared are equivalent. This outcome equivalent is referring to the patient outcomes including the potential for adverse effects. The comparison of costs are limited to direct costs being estimated and compared. Therefore, an institution may wish to consider the potential cost-minimization of switching from a twice-a-day regimen to a higher dose once-a-day regimen. If the outcomes are assumed to be similar between the two treatments, the cost-minimization analyses can be used to compare the direct costs of the drugs at each dose, the preparation costs, administration time, etc. The lower cost will give the hospital important economic information to facilitate formulary decisions.

A **cost-benefit analysis (CBA)** is an extension of a CMA but adds an assessment of the savings that may be associated with one of the comparator drugs. Therefore, the outcomes are converted to a monetary value in dollars for the comparison. The advantage of a CBA is that the outcomes do not need to be considered equivalent as in a CMA. Therefore, the addition of a pharmacist to an internal medicine service could be compared to the addition of a pharmacist to a critical care service by an institution. The costs of adding each would be measured as in a CMA but the outcomes achieved by adding a pharmacist would be converted to dollar values for each service and incorporated into this type of analyses. The information gained from this example would help the institution decide if a clinical pharmacist would be more cost effective to be added to an internal medicine service or a critical care service.

A **cost-effectiveness analysis (CEA)** is different from a CBA because the outcomes are measured in units of clinical effectiveness such as hospital length of stay, reduction in weight-loss, emergency room visits, etc. This is different from the CBA since it does not convert the measured outcomes to dollar values. All of the treatments for comparison must have outcomes that can be placed in identical units. For example, a goal of a CEA may be to compare two loop diuretics for effectiveness at symptom relief during exacerbations of heart failure in an emergency department. The cost of each loop diuretic (including preparation and administration time) would be measured in dollars and the outcome could be measured in units of length of hospital stay, etc. Therefore, as an example, the results of a CEA analysis could conclude the following; using Diuretic A over Diuretic B for heart failure symptom relief will cost $1,000 more but decrease the length of stay by 1 hospital day. The CBA analysis would differ from this because it would convert the 1 decreased day in the hospital to a dollar amount saved and could take the difference between the cost of the drug and savings in dollars. Thus, the CEA is usually easier to interpret for most clinicians and is commonly performed.

The fourth type of pharmacoeconomic model is the **cost-utility analysis (CUA)**. A CUA takes into account patient preferences which are referred to as utilities in this type of analyses. The important distinction in this type of analysis versus a CEA can be illustrated using an example of a patient with terminal cancer. A second or third regimen of chemotherapy may be predicted to prolong the patient's life by weeks or months. However, the quality of life could be so poor during those weeks of life that the drugs may not be desired by the patient. To account for this, the length of life from a given chemotherapy regimen can be transformed into **quality-adjusted life years (QALY)**. The QALY unit is a common outcome for a CUA, and it is what distinguishes a CUA from both a CEA (which would just report the outcomes in survival years) and a CBA (which would report the outcome in dollars saved).

Decision Analysis

A decision analysis is an approach to a problem that can be assessed by a pharmacoeconomic analysis. It is similar to the scientific approach utilized to assess several problems as outlined:

- Identify the problem and define in specific terms how a decision will be made. These are considerations that would be needed for most clinical assessments, such as the period of time that the analysis will occur, the primary stakeholder in the analysis (e.g. cost-savings to an institution or individual patient costs).

- Identify the comparator drug. Usually the comparison will be made between the two most effective treatment options for a disease or will compare a newer drug to a gold standard.

- Choose the pharmacoeconomic model that will be used. Since the costs are always computed in dollars, this step eventually comes to deciding how the outcomes will be measured. If the outcomes are considered equivalent, it is a CMA; if the outcomes are measure in dollars, it is a CBA; if the outcomes are measured in clinical outcomes, it is a CEA; or if the clinical outcomes are adjusted for patient preference. it is a CUA. Again, since most of the analyses are performed using the CEA, the clinical outcome just needs to be defined in this step. However, clinical outcomes or adverse events do not occur on an absolute basis and the probability of the event occurring needs to be taken into consideration. For example, the probability of an adverse event may be 40 percent for Drug A and 60 percent for the comparator Drug B in a CEA.

- Construct a decision tree based on the probabilities of treatment success and failures. This is a diagram of all possible options such as the probability of Drug A having treatment success or failure, with and without adverse events. The probabilities and the costs associated with each outcome or adverse event can now be assigned within the decision tree.

- Perform the calculations using the probabilities and costs associated with each possible event.

- Perform a sensitivity analysis by adjusting the probabilities and costs. This is an important step since these inputs were estimates. To do the sensitivity analysis the highest and lowest costs can be used in the calculations to get a range of possible costs associated with each treatment.

LEARNING POINTS

- A case-control study design has the advantage to assess rare diseases, whereas, a cohort design is useful in tracking a rare exposure or treatment.

- Prevalence can be defined as a proportion that describes the fraction of the population that is affected by the disease or condition, whereas, the incidence is the rate of occurrence of disease in a given population over a defined period of time.

- Randomized controlled clinical trials (RCTs) have the distinct advantage over the other study designs of minimizing study bias due to their randomization and blinding procedures.

- Pharmacoeconomics is the assessment of costs to the health-care system that are associated with drug therapy.

- Pharmacoeconomic studies can be categorized into four types of analyses: (1) cost-minimization analysis, CMA; (2) cost-benefit analysis, CBA; (3) cost-effectiveness analysis, CEA; (4) cost-utility analysis, CUA.

PRACTICE QUESTIONS

1. Which of the following is the simplest form of an observational study design to describe a unique event or treatment effect?

    (A) Case report
    (B) Cross-sectional design
    (C) Case-control design
    (D) Cohort study
    (E) Randomized controlled clinical trial

2. Which of the following statements regarding a cohort study design is/are TRUE? (Select ALL that apply.)

    (A) The study design can be retrospective or prospective.
    (B) The primary goal is to look at a snapshot in time.
    (C) The results can identify the incidence of a disease.
    (D) Patients are selected with a disease and then tracked backwards to identify exposure.
    (E) Cohort studies are useful to study rare diseases.

3. A meta-analysis can be best described by which of the following statements?

    (A) A statistical analysis to determine the prevalence of a disease.
    (B) A statistical analysis that is used to test causality.
    (C) An analysis that requires the use of a placebo comparison.
    (D) A large-scale analysis that requires 10,000 or more subjects.
    (E) A statistical analysis of compiled studies to identify patterns in an outcome.

4. Which of the following is a weakness of a randomized clinical trial design? (Select ALL that apply.)

    (A) Lacks internal validity
    (B) Can be used only for hypothesis generation
    (C) Does not allow for appropriate comparator
    (D) Limited generalizability
    (E) Baseline differences between groups frequently confound interpretation

5. Which of the following pharmacoeconomic models measures units in clinical outcomes, and not just monetary outcomes? (Select ALL that apply.)

    (A) Cost-minimization analysis
    (B) Cost-benefit analysis
    (C) Cost-effectiveness analysis
    (D) Cost-utility analysis
    (E) Cost-sharing analysis

6. Which of the following is **NOT** commonly performed when implementing a decision analysis in a pharmacoeconomic study? (Select ALL that apply.)

   (A) The null hypothesis is stated.
   (B) A decision tree is constructed.
   (C) A comparator is identified.
   (D) A cost-sharing analysis is performed.
   (E) The probabilities for the events of interest are estimated.

ANSWERS AND EXPLANATIONS

1. **A**

A case report is the simplest form of an observational design whose goal is to describe a unique or unexpected treatment effect or disease. The remaining trial designs listed have a goal that expands beyond the simple description of an event.

2. **A, C**

Cohort studies can be retrospective or prospective (A), and the results can identify the incidence of a disease (C). Cohort studies follow patients over time and are not a snapshot in time like a cross-sectional design (B). Cohort designs do not select patients with diseases (D), but instead design the cohorts based on the exposure of interest. A case-control design would categorize subjects based on disease and is a useful method to study rare diseases whereas a cohort study (E) would not be useful.

3. **E**

The goal of a meta-analysis is to formally compile and assess outcomes from multiple sources, usually publications. They are not used to determine prevalence of diseases (A) or to test causality (B). A meta-analysis may include data from placebo-controlled trials (C) but it is not a requirement, and there are no set limits to the sample sizes that need to be included (D).

4. **D**

Randomized controlled trials lack generalizability due to the stringent inclusion and exclusion criteria. This characteristic enhances the internal validity over other designs (A) and can be used for hypothesis testing and not just hypothesis generation (B). The baseline differences (E) between groups in a randomized controlled clinical trial are generally minimal, which is a direct result of appropriate randomization.

5. **C, D**

A cost-effectiveness analysis measures clinical outcomes in terms of clinical effectiveness; these can be outcomes such as blood pressure control, event-free days, etc. A cost-utility analysis (D) also measures clinical outcomes beyond cost by also incorporating a measure of a patient's quality of life. Both cost-minimization analysis (A) and cost-benefit analysis (B) report outcomes based on cost savings. A cost-sharing analysis (E) is not a standard pharmacoeconomic model.

6. **A, D**

The null hypothesis is not needed and does not need to be explicitly stated in a decision analysis for a pharmacoeconomic study (A), and a cost-sharing analysis (D) is not one of the four pharmacoeconomic models to be employed. The appropriate steps would include a decision tree (B), a comparator (C), and the estimated probabilities of interest (E).

Part Four

Resources and Policy

Drug Information

30

This chapter provides an overview of common tertiary literature resources that can be used as drug information resources for pharmacists:

- **General drug information resources**
- **Pharmacotherapy resources**
- **Internal medicine resources**
- **Drug interaction resources**
- **Adverse drug reaction resources**
- **Parenteral drug compatibility/stability resources**
- **Pharmacology resources**
- **Compounding and pharmaceutics resources**
- **Drug identification resources**
- **Foreign drug information resources**
- **Pediatric drug information resources**
- **Pregnancy and lactation resources**
- **OTC drug resources**
- **Natural products resources**

 Suggested Study Time: **30 minutes**

GENERAL DRUG INFORMATION RESOURCES

American Hospital Formulary Service (AHFS) Drug Information (published by the American Society of Health-System Pharmacists [ASHP])

- Provides Food and Drug Administration (FDA)-approved and off-label uses
- Each monograph contains general drug information (e.g., pharmacology, pharmacokinetics, side effects, toxicology, drug interactions, dosing, administration, available preparations)

Drug Facts and Comparisons

- Provides information on:
  - Prescription/over-the-counter (OTC) drugs
  - Investigational/orphan drugs
- Each monograph contains general drug information
- Also provides helpful comparison tables

United States Pharmacopeia Drug Information (USP DI)

- Volume I: Drug Information for the Healthcare Professional
  - Provides general drug information
  - Various appendices (poison control centers, drug-induced side effects, selected therapeutic guidelines, drug identification color inserts)
- Volume II: Advice for the Patient: Drug Information in Lay Language
  - Provides supplemental information for patient counseling
- Volume III: Approved Drug Products and Legal Requirements
  - Provides information on therapeutic equivalence (contains FDA Orange Book), labeling/storage/packaging requirements, and pharmacy law

Physicians' Desk Reference (PDR)

- Contains FDA-approved package insert information
  - Does not provide unlabeled drug uses
- Also contains a color insert (for drug identification) and manufacturer information

Drug Information Handbook (published by Lexi-Comp)

- Provides general drug information
- Contains useful charts, tables, and treatment algorithms
- Also available in specialty versions (pediatrics, geriatrics, psychiatric, oncology)

Red Book

- Provides the following information on prescription and OTC drugs:
  - Cost data (average wholesale price [AWP])
  - National Drug Code (NDC) numbers
  - Formulations available (dosage forms, sugar-free/alcohol-free preparations)
  - Drug identification (color inserts)
  - Manufacturer

PHARMACOTHERAPY RESOURCES

Pharmacotherapy: A Pathophysiologic Approach (DiPiro)

- Provides the following information regarding various disease states: pathophysiology, etiology, clinical presentation, diagnosis, treatment

Applied Therapeutics: The Clinical Use of Drugs (Koda-Kimble)

- Focuses on treatment of disease states
- Case-based format

INTERNAL MEDICINE RESOURCES

Harrison's Principles of Internal Medicine

- Focuses on pathophysiology, etiology, clinical presentation, and diagnosis
- Provides an overview of treatment; does not provide detailed information on drugs or dosing recommendations

Cecil Textbook of Medicine

- Not as comprehensive as *Harrison's*

Washington Manual of Medical Therapeutics

- Provides a general overview of disease states and treatment

Merck Manual of Diagnosis and Therapy

- Provides a quick summary of disease-state information (etiology, pathophysiology, clinical presentation, diagnosis, prognosis, treatment)

DRUG INTERACTION RESOURCES

Hansten and Horn's Drug Interaction Analysis and Management

- Provides the following information on drug interactions: Summary of interaction, proposed mechanism, significance, risk factors, treatment options

Drug Interaction Facts (published by Facts and Comparisons)

- Provides similar information as *Hansten and Horn's*

ADVERSE DRUG REACTION RESOURCES

Meyler's Side Effects of Drugs

- Provides critical review of literature regarding drugs' side effects: Effects on organ systems, interference with lab/diagnostic tests, withdrawal, and overdose
- Provides two indexes for ease of reference:
  - Drugs
  - Side effects

PARENTERAL DRUG COMPATIBILITY/STABILITY RESOURCES

Handbook on Injectable Drugs (published by ASHP)

- Previously known as Trissel's
- Provides information regarding compatibility/stability of parenteral drugs
- Also provides information on commercially available dosages, volumes, and sizes

King Guide to Parenteral Admixtures

- Provides similar information as *Handbook on Injectable Drugs*

PHARMACOLOGY RESOURCES

Goodman & Gilman's: The Pharmacological Basis of Therapeutics

- "Gold standard" pharmacology reference
- Provides very thorough discussion of the pharmacology of drugs; also provides information on the drugs' pharmacokinetics, pharmacodynamics, and toxicology

COMPOUNDING AND PHARMACEUTICS RESOURCES

Merck Index

- Different from the *Merck Manual*
- Provides chemical and pharmacologic information on drugs (e.g., chemical name, molecular formula, structure, molecular weight, solubility, drug class, toxicity, data, manufacturer)

Remington: The Science and Practice of Pharmacy

- Provides information on numerous issues concerning pharmacy practice (e.g., pharmaceutical calculations, chemistry, radioisotopes, compounding techniques/ingredients)

DRUG IDENTIFICATION RESOURCES

American Drug Index

- Cross-referenced by brand, generic, and chemical names
- Also provides available dosage forms/strengths and manufacturer information

IDENTIDEX (available through MICROMEDEX)

- Identifies drug after entering in imprint on tablet/capsule

Other useful resources are the color inserts in the following guides:

- *USP DI Volume I*
- *PDR*
- *Red Book*

FOREIGN DRUG INFORMATION RESOURCES

Martindale: The Complete Drug Reference

- Provides information on drugs used throughout the world

Index Nominum: International Drug Directory

- Provides similar information as *Martindale*

PEDIATRIC DRUG INFORMATION RESOURCES

The Harriet Lane Handbook

- Pocket guide that provides brief overview (especially diagnosis and treatment) of common disease states in children

Pediatric Dosage Handbook (published by Lexi-Comp)

- Provides drug information specific to the pediatric population

General drug information resources (e.g., MICROMEDEX, AHFS) also provide general pediatric dosing information.

PREGNANCY AND LACTATION RESOURCES

Drugs in Pregnancy and Lactation (Briggs)

- "Gold standard"
- Focuses on safety of drugs in pregnancy and lactation

La Leche League (www.llli.org)

- Provides practitioners and patients with clinical and practical information on all aspects of breastfeeding

OTC DRUG RESOURCES

Handbook of Nonprescription Drugs: An Interactive Approach to Self-Care (published by the American Pharmacists Association)

- Provides etiology, pathophysiology, clinical presentation, and treatment of disease states that may be amenable to self-care
- Provides comprehensive information on OTC products (e.g., side effects, drug interactions, dosing, dosage forms, patient counseling)

PDR for Nonprescription Drugs

NATURAL PRODUCTS RESOURCES

Natural Standard

- "Gold standard"
- Comprehensive database

PDR for Herbal Medicines

Complete German Commission E Monographs

PDR for Nonprescription Drugs, Dietary Supplements, and Herbs

Comparison of Tertiary Drug Information Resources

Reference	Monograph: Basic Info	Approved Uses	Unapproved Uses	Drug Interactions	Language for Patients	Manufacturer Contact Information	Product ID	Cost	Dosage Form Availability	Pathophysiology	Disease State Management	Treatment of Drug Overdoses	Foreign Drug Identification	IV Drug Compatibility	Chemical Properties	Generic Availability	Compounding Information	Lactation Information	Mechanism of Action
American Hospital Formulary Service Drug Information (AHFS)	X	X	X	X					X			X			X	X		X	X
Physicians' Desk Reference (PDR)	X	X		X		X	X		X			X			X			X	X
Drug Information Handbook (Lexi-Comp)	X	X	X	X					X			X				X		X	X
Facts and Comparisons	X	X	X	X					X			X				X		X	X
Martindale: The Complete Drug Reference													X						
USP DI Drug Information for the Healthcare Provider (Vol I)	X	X	X	X			X		X			X						X	X
USP DI Advice for the Patient: Drug Information in Lay Language (Vol II)					X														
USP DI Approved Drug Products and Legal Requirements (Vol III)		X																	
Pharmacotherapy: A Pathophysiologic Approach (DiPiro's)										X	X	X							X
Remington: The Science and Practice of Pharmacy															X		X		

Comparison of Tertiary Drug Information Resources (cont'd)

Reference	Monograph: Basic Info	Approved Uses	Unapproved Uses	Drug Interactions	Language for Patients	Manufacturer Contact Information	Product ID	Cost	Dosage Form Availability	Pathophysiology	Disease State Management	Treatment of Drug Overdoses	Foreign Drug Identification	IV Drug Compatibility	Chemical Properties	Generic Availability	Compounding Information	Lactation Information	Mechanism of Action
Handbook on Injectable Drugs (Trissel's)									X					X					
King Guide to Parenteral Admixtures														X					
Goodman and Gilman's: The Pharmacological Basis of Therapeutics																			X
Harrison's Principles of Internal Medicine										X	X	X							
Drug Interactions Analysis and Management (Hansten and Horn's)				X															
Drug Interaction Facts				X															
Harriet Lane Handbook	X	X		X							X							X	
Drugs in Pregnancy and Lactation (Briggs)																		X	
Red Book						X	X	X	X										

LEARNING POINTS

- Learn drug information resources by various categories. Once you know the kind of information that you need, you can select the most appropriate reference.

- Do not memorize the table; use it to assess your general knowledge of tertiary literature sources.

- Remember the differences between primary, secondary, and tertiary literature:
  - Primary literature: Original journal articles (research reports, case reports, editorials); serves as information for development of secondary and tertiary literature resources
  - Secondary literature: Indexing and abstracting services (e.g., MEDLINE, IPA, EMBASE, Cochrane)
  - Tertiary literature: Textbooks and review articles; summarize and interpret primary literature

PRACTICE QUESTIONS

1. A physician calls to ask the pharmacist about the mechanism of action of a new drug that has been approved for hypercholesterolemia. Which of the following references is/are most appropriate for obtaining this information? (Select ALL that apply.)

   (A) *AHFS Drug Information*
   (B) *Facts and Comparisons*
   (C) *USPDI Volume III*
   (D) *Red Book*
   (E) *Drug Interaction Facts*

2. A patient comes to your pharmacy and gives you a prescription for an ointment that needs to be compounded. Which of the following references would be most appropriate to obtain information regarding the preparation of this ointment?

   (A) *Martindale: The Complete Drug Reference*
   (B) *Pharmacotherapy: A Pathophysiologic Approach*
   (C) *Physicians' Desk Reference*
   (D) *Remington: The Science and Practice of Pharmacy*
   (E) *Harriet Lane Handbook*

ANSWERS AND EXPLANATIONS

1. **A, B**

AHFS Drug Information (A) and Facts and Comparisons (B) both contain general drug information in monograph format. USP DI Volume III (C) contains information on approved drug products (generic availability) and legal requirements. *Red Book* (D) provides information on drug cost, formulation, and manufacturer. *Drug Information Facts* (E) provides detailed information on specific interactions between medications.

2. **D**

Remington would be the most appropriate reference to obtain information regarding compounding of an ointment, so choice (D) is correct. *Martindale* (A) provides information on foreign drugs. *Pharmacotherapy: A Pathophysiologic Approach* (B) is a general pharmacotherapy resource. *Physicians' Desk Reference* (C) is a general drug information resource. *Harriet Lane Handbook* (E) is a pediatric drug information resource.

Health Policy

31

This chapter covers the following areas of health policy:

- **HIPAA**
- **FDA regulatory process**
- **The Joint Commission accreditation process**
- **Medication therapy management**

 Suggested Study Time: **30 minutes**

HIPAA

The Health Insurance Portability and Accountability Act (HIPAA) of 1996 was established to guarantee patients' access to health care after leaving a job and to regulate the electronic transmission of medical information. Given the risk of disclosure of patient health information, the HIPAA privacy rule provides regulations regarding how covered entities can use and exchange protected health information (PHI). Covered entities include health care plans, health care providers, and health care clearinghouses.

PHI consists of any type of identifiable health information that pertains to the following:

- Past, present, or future medical or mental health conditions
- Provision of health care
- Payment of health care services

The Office for Civil Rights (OCR) enforces the HIPAA privacy rule. The OCR is responsible for investigating any complaints, conducting compliance reviews of covered entities, and providing education about the regulations. Once a complaint is generated, the OCR gathers facts pertaining to the case to determine whether a violation occurred. If the investigation determines that a violation has occurred, the OCR notifies the covered entity named in the complaint. If a compliance issue on the part of the covered entity is found to be valid, the OCR will work with the entity to resolve the complaint. If the covered entity does not fulfill its responsibility in rectifying the complaint, the OCR may impose civil monetary penalties, which are collected and deposited into the U.S. Treasury.

All pharmacies are considered covered entities and must comply with HIPAA regulations. Regulations mandate covered entities to inform patients how their PHI may be used; this includes information about both treatment and payment of services. All pharmacies are also required to provide a paper notice to the public of measures taken to ensure patient privacy. The privacy notice must be:

- Available to everyone, regardless of whether they are patients of the pharmacy.
- Provided to the patient no later than the date of first service, including services conducted electronically. In the event of an emergency, the notice may be provided as soon as possible. Pharmacies can elect to send the notice to all patients at once or give it to each patient as he or she comes in for services.
- Available at the pharmacy for anyone who requests a copy.
- Displayed in a noticeable location in the store for patients to read.

FOOD AND DRUG ADMINISTRATION REGULATORY PROCESS

In the United States, the regulation and approval of new drugs is founded on the New Drug Application (NDA) process. Before any drug may be made commercially available, it is subject to the NDA process to ensure its safety and efficacy. The NDA is a standardized process that documents research from animal and human studies about each new drug.

When a new compound is in development, the sponsor's main goal is to determine whether the drug is safe for human use and whether it has pharmacologic activity for clinical use. Once the sponsor decides to test the compound in humans, the compound changes legal status and becomes a drug under the Federal Food, Drug, and Cosmetic Act, and the sponsor must file an Investigational New Drug (IND) application with the Food and Drug Administration (FDA).

The IND application contains the following information:

- Pharmacology and toxicology data from animal studies to demonstrate that the drug is safe to test in humans.
- Manufacturing information to ensure the stability, safety, and consistency of the drug throughout the manufacturing process.
- Clinical protocols and investigator information to detail trial design and safety precautions for study patients.
- Agreement to adhere to clinical protocols and IND regulations to ensure adherence to regulations.

There are three types of IND applications:

- An **investigator IND application** is submitted by the investigator who initiates and conducts the clinical trials and also oversees the administration and use of the investigational drug. An IND can be used to request approval of either an unapproved drug or a new indication for an existing drug.

- An **emergency-use IND** allows the FDA to authorize the use of an investigational drug for emergency use when time is too short to allow the full NDA process. It also permits individuals to use the drug who would not have been included in clinical trials because they do not meet the study criteria.

- A **treatment IND** is submitted to request authorization to distribute an investigational drug that has shown clinical promise for a serious condition while the remaining clinical trials and FDA review are conducted.

After gathering the data from the IND studies, the sponsoring entity can submit an NDA to the FDA for review. The FDA review evaluates the drug's safety and efficacy for the proposed indication in order to confirm that the benefits outweigh the risks of the medication. The FDA also reviews the medication labeling to ensure that it includes the proper information. Finally, the FDA reviews manufacturing protocols to confirm that adequate quality controls are in place for safe drug preparation.

Types of Clinical Trials

Four types of clinical trials are used in the IND and NDA application process:

- **Phase I** trials are the first studies of investigational new drugs in humans and are focused on drug safety. These trials generally are conducted in small numbers of healthy subjects to determine pharmacologic, pharmacokinetic, and adverse drug reaction information. Dose-ranging data also may be obtained during this phase.

- **Phase II** trials are controlled studies conducted in large numbers of patients to evaluate clinical efficacy. These trials often enroll hundreds of patients to test the effectiveness of the drug in patients with certain health conditions and support clinical indications.

- **Phase III** trials are controlled studies conducted in larger numbers of patients (potentially hundreds or thousands) to evaluate clinical efficacy that can be extrapolated to the general population. Information from Phase III trials contributes to drug labeling and provides guidance for use in clinical practice. The trials may compare the investigational drug to a placebo or to another standard of care.

- **Phase IV** trials are conducted after a drug has been approved for clinical use. These trials conduct post-marketing surveillance to collect information about the use of the medication in various populations and the prevalence of long-term use or rare side effects.

Orphan Drug Products

Orphan drug products are medications that aid in the diagnosis or treatment of rare diseases or conditions. The Office of Orphan Product Development promotes and provides incentives to encourage companies to develop new products for conditions that affect an extremely small number of people.

THE JOINT COMMISSION ACCREDITATION PROCESS

The Joint Commission (TJC) is a private, nonprofit organization that sets the standards by which health care quality is measured. Accreditation by TJC means that health care facilities have demonstrated compliance with the standards of performance in meeting the needs of their patients. To maintain accreditation, health care facilities periodically undergo an extensive on-site review by a team of professionals from TJC. The review evaluates the facility's performance in all areas that affect patient care; accreditation is awarded based on how well the facility met the standards.

National Patient Safety Goals

The following National Patient Safety Goals (NPSG) have been identified for the safe provision of medications.

- NPSG 01.01.01: Use at least two patient identifiers when providing care, treatment, and services
  - Use at least two patient identifiers when administering medications, blood or blood components; when collecting blood samples and other specimens for clinical testing; and when providing treatments or procedures. The patient's room number or physical location is not used as an identifier.
- NPSG 03.04.01: Label all medications, medication containers, and other solutions on and off the sterile field in perioperative and other procedural settings.
  - In perioperative and other procedural settings both on and off the sterile field, label medications and solutions that are not immediately administered. This applies even if there is only one medication being used.
  - In perioperative and other procedural settings both on and off the sterile field, labeling occurs when any medication or solution is transferred from the original packaging to another container.
  - In perioperative and other procedural settings both on and off the sterile field, medication or solution labels include the following: medication or solution name, strength, amount of medication or solution containing medication, diluent name and volume, expiration date when not used within 24 hours, expiration time when expiration occurs in less than 24 hours.

- Verify all medication or solution labels both verbally and visually. Verification is done by two individuals qualified to participate in the procedure whenever the person preparing the medication or solution is not the person who will be administering it.

- Label each medication or solution as soon as it is prepared, unless it is immediately administered.

- Immediately discard any medication or solution found unlabeled.

- Remove all labeled containers on the sterile field and discard their contents at the conclusion of the procedure.

- All medications and solutions both on and off the sterile field and their labels are reviewed by entering and exiting staff responsible for the management of medications.

- NPSG 03.05.01: Reduce the likelihood of patient harm associated with use of anticoagulant therapy.

  - Use only oral unit-dose products, prefilled syringes, or premixed infusion bags when these types of products are available.

  - Use approved protocols for the initiation and maintenance of anticoagulant therapy.

  - Before starting a patient on warfarin, assess the patient's baseline coagulation status; for all patients receiving warfarin therapy, use a current international normalized ratio (INR) to adjust this therapy. The baseline status and current INR are documented in the medication record.

  - Use authoritative resources to manage potential food and drug interactions for patients receiving warfarin.

  - When heparin is administered intravenously and continuously, use programmable pumps to provide consistent and accurate dosing.

  - A written policy addresses baseline and ongoing laboratory tests that are required for anticoagulants.

  - Provide education regarding anticoagulant therapy to prescribers, staff, patients, and families. Patient/family education includes the following: the importance of follow-up monitoring, compliance, drug-food interactions, the potential for adverse drug reactions and interactions.

  - Evaluate anticoagulation safety practices, take action to improve practices, and measure the effectiveness of those actions in a time frame determined by the organization.

- NPSG 03.06.01: Maintain and communicate accurate patient medication information.
  - Obtain information on the medications the patient is currently taking when he or she is admitted to the hospital or is seen in an outpatient setting. This information is documented in a list or other format that is useful to those who manage medications.
  - Define the types of medication information to be collected in non-24-hour settings and different patient circumstances.
  - Compare the medication information by the patient brought to the hospital with the medications ordered for the patient by the hospital in order to identify and resolve discrepancies.
  - Provide the patient (or family as needed) with written information on the medications the patient should be taking when he or she is discharged from the hospital or at the end of an outpatient encounter.
  - Explain the importance of managing medication information to the patient when he or she is discharged from the hospital or at the end of an outpatient encounter.

MEDICATION THERAPY MANAGEMENT

Medication therapy management (MTM) is a process in which a health care professional monitors a patient's medications in order to improve the patient's therapeutic outcomes. MTM provides patient-specific services that promote the best outcomes for each individual and reduce medication related problems. MTM can be conducted in any setting, either in a face-to-face manner or electronically. Services can be provided by a pharmacist or health care provider and are covered under Medicare Part D.

MTM services may include the following:

- Assessment of the patient's health status
- Comprehensive medication review to identify medication-related problems
- Creation of a medication treatment program which may add new therapy or modify existing therapy
- Patient education and counseling resources to optimize therapeutic outcomes and patient adherence
- Medication monitoring for efficacy and safety parameters
- Documentation of services
- Coordination of services with other health care providers

LEARNING POINTS

- HIPAA was established to ensure patient privacy and regulate the electronic transmission of medical information.

- All pharmacies are considered covered entities and must comply with HIPAA regulations.

- To gain FDA approval of a drug, the sponsor must submit an NDA to the FDA for review.

- Information for an IND is collected from Phase I, II, and III trials.

- The Orphan Drug Act provides incentives for drug companies to create medications to treat rare diseases.

- MTM is the provision of patient-specific services to optimize pharmacotherapy outcomes.

- The Joint Commission national patient safety goals contain practices to ensure the safe provision of medications.

PRACTICE QUESTIONS

1. An orphan drug product might apply to which of the following disease states?

   (A) Asthma
   (B) Diabetes mellitus
   (C) Gaucher's disease
   (D) Hypertension
   (E) Hypertriglyceridemia

2. Which of the following statements regarding protected health information (PHI) is TRUE?

   (A) PHI applies only to current health conditions.
   (B) PHI excludes information about future treatment.
   (C) PHI excludes mental health diagnoses.
   (D) PHI includes de-identified information.
   (E) PHI includes the payment of health services.

3. Which of the following statements regarding medication therapy management (MTM) services is/are TRUE? (Select ALL that apply.)

   (A) MTM services must be performed in person.
   (B) MTM services must be performed electronically.
   (C) MTM services must be performed by pharmacists.
   (D) MTM services focus on patient-specific outcomes.
   (E) MTM services may include modification of medication therapy.

4. Which of the following is included in an investigational new drug application?

   (A) Clinical trial protocols
   (B) Manufacturing information
   (C) Pharmacology data
   (D) Toxicology data
   (E) All of the above

5. Which of the following phases of clinical trials would be conducted after a medication has been approved and is being used?

   (A) Phase I
   (B) Phase II
   (C) Phase III
   (D) Phase IV
   (E) None of the above

6. Which of the following investigational new drug (IND) applications should be submitted to allow an individual to use a clinical trial medication who would otherwise be excluded by exclusion criteria?

   (A) Emergency-use IND application
   (B) Investigator IND application
   (C) Treatment IND application
   (D) All of the above
   (E) None of the above

7. The Joint Commission does which of the following?

   (A) Accredits health care facilities
   (B) Approves investigational new drugs
   (C) Creates drug products for rare diseases
   (D) Ensures electronic patient privacy
   (E) Provides payments to health care facilities

ANSWERS AND EXPLANATIONS

1. **C**

Orphan drugs are those drugs that aid in the diagnosis or treatment of rare diseases. Gaucher's disease is a rare disease and would be eligible for the creation of a medication through the Orphan Drug Product Act. Disease states that affect millions of people, such as asthma (A), diabetes mellitus (B), hypertension (D), and hypertriglyceridemia (E), would not be granted orphan drug product status.

2. **E**

Protected health information (PHI) includes the payment of health services. PHI consists of any type of identifiable health information that pertains to a patient's past, present, and future medical or mental health conditions and treatments (A and B), and to both the provision and payment of health care services. Mental health diagnoses (C) are not excluded, and PHI does not apply to de-identified information (D).

3. **D, E**

Medication therapy management provides patient-specific services to improve pharmacotherapy outcomes. It may include a variety of services, such as assessment of patient health, comprehensive medication therapies, and optimization of pharmacotherapy regimens, which may include modification of drug therapy. Although MTM is often provided by pharmacists (C), it can be delivered by other health care professionals. While it can be done in person (A) or electronically (B), it can also be conducted via telephone.

4. **E**

An Investigational New Drug (IND) application is submitted to provide information that the new drug may be used safely in humans. An IND contains information about clinical trial protocols (A), manufacturing information (B) to ensure consistency and safety of the drug product, preclinical pharmacology data (C) from animal and toxicology trials (D), and investigator information.

5. **D**

Phase IV trials are conducted after a medication has been approved for clinical use. Phase IV trials are conducted to gain information about the use of medications in various populations and to determine the prevalence of rare side effects.

6. **A**

An emergency-use IND application can be submitted to allow individuals to use a study drug even though they are not participating in a clinical trial due to study criteria. An investigator IND application (B) is submitted upon initiation of a clinical trial studying a new compound. A treatment IND application (C) is submitted to distribute an investigational drug that has shown clinical promise for a serious condition while remaining clinical trials and FDA review are being conducted.

7. **A**

The Joint Commission accredits health care facilities, ensuring that they meet the standards of care to provide optimal patient care. Facilities undergo periodic visits to ensure standards are being consistently met.

Part Five

Practice Test

Practice Test

To mimic the conditions of the NAPLEX, allow yourself a total of **4 hours and 15 minutes** to complete all 185 questions. Take a 10-minute break at the 2-hour time point.

While every test-taker is different, the average candidate takes 2.5 to 3 hours to complete this practice exam. There are no bonus points for finishing early.

The computer-adaptive format of the exam requires that you **answer all questions in the order in which they are presented**. You cannot skip a question or return to a previous question to review your answer. Again, to use this practice test as effectively as possible, **do not** return to the previous question to change your answer.

ANSWER GRID

1. A B C D E	41. A B C D E	81. A B C D E
2. A B C D E	42. A B C D E	82. A B C D E
3. A B C D E	43. A B C D E	83. A B C D E
4. A B C D E	44. A B C D E	84. A B C D E
5. A B C D E	45. A B C D E	85. A B C D E
6. A B C D E	46. A B C D E	86. A B C D E
7. A B C D E	47. A B C D E	87. A B C D E
8. A B C D E	48. A B C D E	88. A B C D E
9. A B C D E	49. A B C D E	89. A B C D E
10. A B C D E	50. A B C D E	90. A B C D E
11. A B C D E	51. A B C D E	91. A B C D E
12. A B C D E	52. A B C D E	92. A B C D E
13. A B C D E	53. A B C D E	93. A B C D E
14. A B C D E	54. A B C D E	94. A B C D E
15. A B C D E	55. A B C D E	95. A B C D E
16. A B C D E	56. A B C D E	96. A B C D E
17. A B C D E	57. A B C D E	97. A B C D E
18. A B C D E	58. A B C D E	98. A B C D E
19. A B C D E	59. A B C D E	99. A B C D E
20. A B C D E	60. A B C D E	100. A B C D E
21. A B C D E	61. A B C D E	101. A B C D E
22. A B C D E	62. A B C D E	102. A B C D E
23. A B C D E	63. A B C D E	103. A B C D E
24. A B C D E	64. A B C D E	104. A B C D E
25. A B C D E	65. A B C D E	105. A B C D E
26. A B C D E	66. A B C D E	106. A B C D E
27. A B C D E	67. A B C D E	107. A B C D E
28. A B C D E	68. A B C D E	108. A B C D E
29. A B C D E	69. A B C D E	109. A B C D E
30. A B C D E	70. A B C D E	110. A B C D E
31. A B C D E	71. A B C D E	111. A B C D E
32. A B C D E	72. A B C D E	112. A B C D E
33. A B C D E	73. A B C D E	113. A B C D E
34. A B C D E	74. A B C D E	114. A B C D E
35. A B C D E	75. A B C D E	115. A B C D E
36. A B C D E	76. A B C D E	116. A B C D E
37. A B C D E	77. A B C D E	117. A B C D E
38. A B C D E	78. A B C D E	118. A B C D E
39. A B C D E	79. A B C D E	119. A B C D E
40. A B C D E	80. A B C D E	120. A B C D E

121. Ⓐ Ⓑ Ⓒ Ⓓ Ⓔ
122. Ⓐ Ⓑ Ⓒ Ⓓ Ⓔ
123. Ⓐ Ⓑ Ⓒ Ⓓ Ⓔ
124. Ⓐ Ⓑ Ⓒ Ⓓ Ⓔ
125. Ⓐ Ⓑ Ⓒ Ⓓ Ⓔ
126. Ⓐ Ⓑ Ⓒ Ⓓ Ⓔ
127. Ⓐ Ⓑ Ⓒ Ⓓ Ⓔ
128. Ⓐ Ⓑ Ⓒ Ⓓ Ⓔ
129. Ⓐ Ⓑ Ⓒ Ⓓ Ⓔ
130. Ⓐ Ⓑ Ⓒ Ⓓ Ⓔ
131. Ⓐ Ⓑ Ⓒ Ⓓ Ⓔ
132. Ⓐ Ⓑ Ⓒ Ⓓ Ⓔ
133. Ⓐ Ⓑ Ⓒ Ⓓ Ⓔ
134. Ⓐ Ⓑ Ⓒ Ⓓ Ⓔ
135. Ⓐ Ⓑ Ⓒ Ⓓ Ⓔ
136. Ⓐ Ⓑ Ⓒ Ⓓ Ⓔ
137. Ⓐ Ⓑ Ⓒ Ⓓ Ⓔ
138. Ⓐ Ⓑ Ⓒ Ⓓ Ⓔ
139. Ⓐ Ⓑ Ⓒ Ⓓ Ⓔ
140. Ⓐ Ⓑ Ⓒ Ⓓ Ⓔ
141. Ⓐ Ⓑ Ⓒ Ⓓ Ⓔ
142. Ⓐ Ⓑ Ⓒ Ⓓ Ⓔ
143. Ⓐ Ⓑ Ⓒ Ⓓ Ⓔ
144. Ⓐ Ⓑ Ⓒ Ⓓ Ⓔ
145. Ⓐ Ⓑ Ⓒ Ⓓ Ⓔ

146. Ⓐ Ⓑ Ⓒ Ⓓ Ⓔ
147. Ⓐ Ⓑ Ⓒ Ⓓ Ⓔ
148. Ⓐ Ⓑ Ⓒ Ⓓ Ⓔ
149. Ⓐ Ⓑ Ⓒ Ⓓ Ⓔ
150. Ⓐ Ⓑ Ⓒ Ⓓ Ⓔ
151. Ⓐ Ⓑ Ⓒ Ⓓ Ⓔ
152. Ⓐ Ⓑ Ⓒ Ⓓ Ⓔ
153. Ⓐ Ⓑ Ⓒ Ⓓ Ⓔ
154. Ⓐ Ⓑ Ⓒ Ⓓ Ⓔ
155. Ⓐ Ⓑ Ⓒ Ⓓ Ⓔ
156. Ⓐ Ⓑ Ⓒ Ⓓ Ⓔ
157. Ⓐ Ⓑ Ⓒ Ⓓ Ⓔ
158. Ⓐ Ⓑ Ⓒ Ⓓ Ⓔ
159. Ⓐ Ⓑ Ⓒ Ⓓ Ⓔ
160. Ⓐ Ⓑ Ⓒ Ⓓ Ⓔ
161. Ⓐ Ⓑ Ⓒ Ⓓ Ⓔ
162. Ⓐ Ⓑ Ⓒ Ⓓ Ⓔ
163. Ⓐ Ⓑ Ⓒ Ⓓ Ⓔ
164. Ⓐ Ⓑ Ⓒ Ⓓ Ⓔ
165. Ⓐ Ⓑ Ⓒ Ⓓ Ⓔ
166. Ⓐ Ⓑ Ⓒ Ⓓ Ⓔ
167. Ⓐ Ⓑ Ⓒ Ⓓ Ⓔ
168. Ⓐ Ⓑ Ⓒ Ⓓ Ⓔ
169. Ⓐ Ⓑ Ⓒ Ⓓ Ⓔ
170. Ⓐ Ⓑ Ⓒ Ⓓ Ⓔ

171. Ⓐ Ⓑ Ⓒ Ⓓ Ⓔ
172. Ⓐ Ⓑ Ⓒ Ⓓ Ⓔ
173. Ⓐ Ⓑ Ⓒ Ⓓ Ⓔ
174. Ⓐ Ⓑ Ⓒ Ⓓ Ⓔ
175. Ⓐ Ⓑ Ⓒ Ⓓ Ⓔ
176. Ⓐ Ⓑ Ⓒ Ⓓ Ⓔ
177. Ⓐ Ⓑ Ⓒ Ⓓ Ⓔ
178. Ⓐ Ⓑ Ⓒ Ⓓ Ⓔ
179. Ⓐ Ⓑ Ⓒ Ⓓ Ⓔ
180. Ⓐ Ⓑ Ⓒ Ⓓ Ⓔ
181. Ⓐ Ⓑ Ⓒ Ⓓ Ⓔ
182. Ⓐ Ⓑ Ⓒ Ⓓ Ⓔ
183. Ⓐ Ⓑ Ⓒ Ⓓ Ⓔ
184. Ⓐ Ⓑ Ⓒ Ⓓ Ⓔ
185. Ⓐ Ⓑ Ⓒ Ⓓ Ⓔ

Directions: Complete each of the following questions with the best possible answer.

1. Diarrhea is most common with which of the following medications?

   (A) Allopurinol
   (B) Probenecid
   (C) Indomethacin
   (D) Acetaminophen
   (E) Colchicine

2. Which of the following laboratory tests is used as a measure of coagulability?

   (A) A1c
   (B) AST
   (C) INR
   (D) BNP

3. Which of the following atypical antipsychotics requires rigorous monitoring of WBC and ANC?

   (A) Olanzapine
   (B) Risperidone
   (C) Quetiapine
   (D) Ziprasidone
   (E) Clozapine

4. Which recommendation is most appropriate when initiating Mirapex in a patient with Parkinson's disease?

   (A) Decrease the levodopa dose by 20–30% when initiating Mirapex.
   (B) Patient must wear patch for 24 hours for efficacy.
   (C) Monitor for serious cardiac side effects.
   (D) Dose adjustment required in hepatic disease.

5. A patient has been diagnosed with depression and will begin antidepressant therapy today. Which of the following treatment regimens is MOST appropriate, assuming the patient has no other health conditions?

   (A) Venlafaxine 37.5 mg PO BID
   (B) Lexapro 10 mg PO BID
   (C) Fluvoxamine 80 mg PO weekly
   (D) Nortriptyline 300 mg PO daily
   (E) Mirtazapine 10 mg PO q A.M.

6. Which of the following medications should be stored in the refrigerator prior to use?

   (A) Seasonale
   (B) NuvaRing
   (C) Ovrette
   (D) Xulane

7. Which of the following medications requires routine ocular exams?

   (A) Hydroxychloroquine
   (B) Metformin
   (C) Enbrel
   (D) Methotrexate

8. Which of the following statements regarding serum creatinine is TRUE?

   (A) Serum creatinine is most commonly used to assess hepatic disease.
   (B) Serum creatinine is dependent upon the amount of iron consumed in the diet.
   (C) Serum creatinine is a more accurate measure in the very elderly than in young adults.
   (D) Serum creatinine is used in the Cockroft-Gault equation.
   (E) Serum creatinine is synonymous with microalbumin.

9. Patients must enroll in the TOUCH REMS program to receive which of the following medications?

   (A) Mitoxantrone
   (B) Teriflunomide
   (C) Natalizumab
   (D) Fingolimod

10. Allopurinol is indicated for which of the following gout presentations?

   (A) Prophylaxis in patients with slightly elevated uric acid levels
   (B) Prophylaxis in patients with moderately elevated uric acid and uric acid overproduction
   (C) Prophylaxis in patients with uric acid excretion indicative of underexcretion
   (D) Treatment of acute gout
   (E) Treatment of asymptomatic hyperuricemia

11. Which of the following medications require(s) monitoring of serum drug concentrations? (Select ALL that apply.)

   (A) Lamotrigine
   (B) Valproic acid
   (C) Lithium
   (D) Levetiracetam

12. Which of the following is the correct generic name for Geodon?

   (A) Aripiprazole
   (B) Olanzapine
   (C) Quetiapine
   (D) Risperidone
   (E) Ziprasidone

13. Migraine prophylaxis could be achieved with which of the following medication classes?

   (A) ACE inhibitors
   (B) Acetaminophen
   (C) Antidepressants
   (D) H_2 antagonists
   (E) Anticholinergics

14. What is the MOST appropriate recommendation for a patient with osteoarthritis and stomach ulcers?

   (A) Aspirin 325 mg PO every 4–6 hours
   (B) Tramadol 50 mg PO every 4–6 hours
   (C) Diclofenac 50 mg PO BID
   (D) Daypro 600 mg PO daily
   (E) Mobic 7.5 mg PO daily

Questions 15–19 refer to the following patient profile.

Patient Name: Tamara Yates

Age: 40   **Height:** 5′2″
Sex: F   **Weight:** 90 lb

Allergies: Geodon

Diagnosis

  Primary:
    Hypertension
    Depression
    Schizophrenia
  Chief Complaint: tardive dyskinesia, dystonia

Lab/Diagnostic Tests

Date	Test/Result	
03/02	Sodium	133 mEq/L
(last week)	Potassium	3.5 mEq/L
	Serum creatinine	1.0 mg/dL
	Blood pressure	166/98 mmHg
	Heart rate	80 bpm

Medications

Date	Name and Strength	Route	Directions
02/20	HCTZ 25 mg	PO	1 tablet in the morning
	Citalopram 20 mg	PO	1 tablet daily
	Haloperidol 2 mg	PO	1 tablet BID

Additional Information

Date	Comment
03/02	Patient has been suspected of bulimia by her primary physician and dentist.

---

15. Which of the following is likely causing Ms. Yates's chief complaint?

(A) Hydrochlorothiazide
(B) Citalopram
(C) Haloperidol
(D) Hyponatremia
(E) Uncontrolled blood pressure

16. What additional monitoring is needed to evaluate haloperidol?

(A) Serum drug levels
(B) A1c
(C) Ejection fraction
(D) Bone mineral density
(E) CBC

17. Which of the following recommendations is appropriate to address Ms. Yates's chief complaint?

    (A) Switch to the liquid formulation of haloperidol.
    (B) Switch the haloperidol to ziprasidone.
    (C) Switch the haloperidol to risperidone.
    (D) Add vitamin E 400 IU daily.

18. What education should be provided to Ms. Yates concerning her antipsychotic medications?

    (A) Medications for schizophrenia are absorbed better in an acidic environment and should be taken with orange juice or vitamin C.
    (B) Medications for schizophrenia work quickly and should start to take effect within two to three doses.
    (C) If side effects are bothersome, stop taking the medication.
    (D) Alcohol should be avoided.
    (E) If side effects are bothersome, cut the dose in half.

19. Ms. Yates was told by a friend that her citalopram is bad for her. Although you have tried to talk with her about it, she wants another antidepressant. Which of the following is the MOST appropriate recommendation?

    (A) Bupropion 100 mg PO BID
    (B) Alprazolam 1 mg PO TID
    (C) Lexapro 10 mg PO daily
    (D) Venlafaxine 37.5 mg PO BID
    (E) Propranolol 80 mg PO daily

20. What is the purpose of adding carbidopa to levodopa in the treatment of Parkinson's disease?

    (A) It prevents the peripheral degradation of levodopa.
    (B) It allows for extended dosing intervals.
    (C) It prevents some of the CNS side effects of levodopa from occurring.
    (D) It provides anticholinergic properties.

21. Which of the following treatment regimens is considered first-line for acute gout?

    (A) Acetaminophen 1,000 mg PO PRN up to QID
    (B) Colchicine 2 mg PO PRN
    (C) Indomethacin 50 mg PO TID
    (D) Allopurinol 100 mg PO daily
    (E) Probenecid 250 mg PO BID

22. Which of the following medications has the lowest risk of erectile dysfunction?

    (A) Bupropion
    (B) Paroxetine
    (C) Venlafaxine
    (D) Sertraline

23. Which of the following medications, if taken in combination with phenytoin, would result in increased serum concentrations of phenytoin?

    (A) Carbamazepine
    (B) Valproic acid
    (C) Quinidine
    (D) Cimetidine

24. What is the role of NSAIDs in rheumatoid arthritis?

    (A) NSAIDs function as a disease-modifying antirheumatic drug (DMARD).
    (B) NSAIDs are used for PRN symptomatic relief.
    (C) NSAIDs are used as adjunctive therapy in patients with refractory symptoms.
    (D) NSAIDs can prevent the flushing associated with biological injections.
    (E) NSAIDs must be given in combination with infliximab.

25. What abortive therapy would be appropriate for a patient who experiences severe nausea and vomiting every time a migraine occurs?

    (A) Amerge oral tablets
    (B) Relpax oral tablets
    (C) Maxalt MLT
    (D) Topiramate tablets

26. Which of the following statements is TRUE?

    (A) Oxcarbazepine and lamotrigine both have a possibility of causing Stevens-Johnson syndrome.
    (B) Oxcarbazepine is the generic name for Tegretol.
    (C) Lithium has a significant drug interaction with beta-blockers.
    (D) Valproic acid is contraindicated in renal impairment.
    (E) Lithium works by increasing GABA concentrations in the brain.

27. Which of the following is a contraindication to using bupropion?

    (A) Current smoker
    (B) Erectile dysfunction
    (C) Seizure disorder
    (D) Hypertension

28. Which of the following medications is/are often used in combination with folic acid supplementation? (Select ALL that apply.)

    (A) Carbamazepine
    (B) Leflunomide
    (C) Sulfasalazine
    (D) Methotrexate

29. Dry mouth and dry eyes would MOST likely occur with which of the following medications?

    (A) Mirabegron
    (B) Doxazosin
    (C) Oxybutinin IR
    (D) Tolterodine ER

30. Which of the following medications can be used for both treatment and prevention of gout?

    (A) NSAIDs
    (B) Corticosteroids
    (C) Colchicine
    (D) Probenecid

Questions 31–35 apply to the following case.

Patient Name: Janelle Brown

Age: 21   **Height:** 5'2"
Sex: F   **Weight:** 120 lb

Allergies: Pollen

Diagnosis

   <u>Primary:</u>
      1. Acne vulgaris
      2. Migraine headaches

   <u>Chief Complaint:</u> Acne lesions and frequent migraine headaches

Lab/Diagnostic Tests

Date	Test/Result	
03/02	Sodium	134 mEq/L
(last week)	Potassium	3.5 mEq/L
	Serum creatinine	1.0 mg/dL
	Blood pressure	116/82 mmHg
	Heart rate	78 bpm

Medications

Date	Name and Strength	Route	Directions
02/20	Ovcon-50	PO	1 tablet daily
	Maxalt MLT 10 mg	PO	Take PRN

---

31. Which of the following side effects is MOST common with Ms. Brown's oral contraceptive?

    (A) Breast tenderness
    (B) Decreased libido
    (C) Dyspareunia
    (D) Hot flushes
    (E) Spotting

32. After talking with Ms. Brown, it seems she may be experiencing some side effects from her Ovcon-50. You call her physician, who provides you with a new prescription for Seasonale. Which is an appropriate counseling point for this medication?

    (A) The device will be inserted at your physician office.
    (B) Smoking while on this medication will increase your risk of serious side effects.
    (C) Apply one patch each week.
    (D) Store in refrigerator (36°F–46°F) prior to use.

33. Ms. Brown is prescribed amoxicillin 500 mg PO TID for 1 week. Which of the following is the MOST appropriate counseling information for her?

   (A) There is no drug interaction present. Take the antibiotic three times daily as prescribed.
   (B) There is a drug interaction between the antibiotic and oral contraceptive, which renders the antibiotic less effective. Hold the contraceptive until the antibiotic regimen is complete.
   (C) There is a drug interaction between the antibiotic and oral contraceptive, which renders the oral contraceptive less effective. Do not take the antibiotics.
   (D) There is a drug interaction between the antibiotic and oral contraceptive, which renders the oral contraceptive less effective. Take two extra Seasonale tablets daily during the week of antibiotic therapy.
   (E) There is a drug interaction between the antibiotic and oral contraceptive, which renders the oral contraceptive less effective. Take both medications as prescribed and use a backup method of contraception for at least 7 days after finishing the antibiotic therapy.

34. Ms. Brown has several noninflammatory comedones on her face. She states that she has never tried therapy for her acne and requests a recommendation for a medication. Which of the following would be the MOST appropriate initial recommendation?

   (A) Tetracycline 500 mg PO QID
   (B) Isotretinoin 20 mg PO daily
   (C) Benzoyl peroxide 5% topical cream daily
   (D) Benzoyl peroxide 5% topical cream and tretinoin 0.1% gel applied daily
   (E) Isotretinoin 20 mg PO daily and tretinoin 0.1% gel applied daily

35. Ms. Brown asks for information about prophylactic migraine medications. She states that she is currently experiencing about four migraine headaches per week. Which of the following would be the MOST appropriate recommendation for migraine prophylaxis for Ms. Brown?

   (A) She is not a good candidate for migraine prophylaxis because she does not have headaches frequently enough.
   (B) Hydrocodone
   (C) Imitrex
   (D) Propranolol
   (E) Topiramate

36. Which of the following medications has no known drug interaction with oral contraceptives?

   (A) Neurontin
   (B) Carbamazepine
   (C) Valproic acid
   (D) Rifampin
   (E) Phenobarbital

37. Which of the following trade names is correctly matched with its generic name?

   (A) Detrol – oxybutynin
   (B) Vesicare – tolterodine
   (C) Enablex – darifenacin
   (D) Ditropan – imipramine
   (E) Tofranil – solifenacin

38. When should biologics be initiated in rheumatoid arthritis?

   (A) Within 3 months of a diagnosis
   (B) For PRN symptom relief
   (C) When DMARDs have been ineffective
   (D) Upon radiologic confirmation of joint damage

39. Which of the following statements regarding tricyclic antidepressants is TRUE?

    (A) They often exhibit stimulating side effects.
    (B) They are very dangerous and often fatal in overdosage.
    (C) They have a significant drug–food interaction with aged cheese.
    (D) They can be discontinued abruptly with no withdrawal symptoms.

40. A patient was started on a selegiline patch 3 days ago for major depression. The family states that it is not working. Which of the following is the MOST appropriate action to take at this time?

    (A) Add fluoxetine if the selegiline is still not working in 2 weeks.
    (B) Add duloxetine if he/she is not feeling better in 6–8 weeks.
    (C) Have the patient start a high caffeine intake so that the selegiline will be absorbed better.
    (D) Inform the family that the selegiline has not had time to work yet and may take 1–2 months.
    (E) Switch the patient to oral selegiline for better efficacy.

41. Which of the following products contains aspirin with butalbital and caffeine?

    (A) Fiorinal
    (B) Fioricet
    (C) Excedrin Migraine
    (D) Migranal
    (E) Amerge

42. A 15-year-old female patient is given a new prescription for Retin-A. Which of the following would be an appropriate counseling point for this patient?

    (A) This medication works best if combined with an astringent or abrasive soap.
    (B) This medication should result in rapid improvement within 1–2 days.
    (C) This medication should be used only as a "spot treatment" for blemishes.
    (D) It is important to use sunblock prior to sun exposure due to the risk of photosensitivity.
    (E) It is important to apply this product to wet skin immediately after washing the face.

43. A postmenopausal woman has a history of multiple fractures and pulmonary embolism, and she cannot tolerate bisphosphonates due to osteonecrosis of the jaw. Which of the following options would be BEST for the treatment of osteoporosis in this patient?

    (A) Raloxifene
    (B) Zoledronic acid
    (C) Teriparatide
    (D) Calcitonin

44. Which of the following antianxiety medications takes 2–3 weeks to reach maximal efficacy?

    (A) Xanax
    (B) Librium
    (C) Buspar
    (D) Valium
    (E) Vistaril

45. Common side effects of oral isotretinoin include which of the following?

    (A) Cheilitis
    (B) Leukopenia
    (C) Hypertrichosis
    (D) Hypoglycemia

46. Which of the following is NOT a treatment option for psoriasis?

    (A) Methotrexate
    (B) Prednisone
    (C) Coal tar
    (D) Benzoyl peroxide
    (E) Anthralin

47. In the TNM classification of cancer staging, N represents which of the following?

    (A) The size of the tumor in centimeters
    (B) The number of tumors
    (C) The number of involved lymph nodes
    (D) The number of involved organs
    (E) The presence of distant metastases

48. Which of the following statements regarding neoadjuvant chemotherapy is TRUE?

    (A) It is given postsurgery.
    (B) The goal is to reduce tumor burden.
    (C) It is given to relieve symptoms and has no effect on survival.
    (D) It is given to reduce nausea and vomiting.

49. Leucovorin should be given as rescue therapy to patients receiving _____, but will increase both the toxicity and the chemotherapeutic activity of _____.

    (A) fluorouracil; methotrexate
    (B) doxorubicin; fluorouracil
    (C) fluorouracil; cytarabine
    (D) methotrexate; fluorouracil
    (E) methotrexate; doxorubicin

50. Which of the following statements regarding cytarabine is/are TRUE? (Select ALL that apply.)

    (A) The mechanism of action is inhibition of DNA polymerase.
    (B) Monitoring should include a neurological exam at each office visit.
    (C) Pre- and post-treatment corticosteroid eye drops should be given to prevent conjunctivitis.
    (D) The powder must be refrigerated before reconstitution and injection.

51. Which of the following is the MOST significant adverse effect of anthracyclines?

    (A) Ototoxicity
    (B) Infusion-related reactions
    (C) Folate deficiency
    (D) Cardiotoxicity
    (E) Hand and foot syndrome

52. Which of the following is the trade name for bevacizumab?

    (A) Gleevec
    (B) Herceptin
    (C) Avastin
    (D) Tarceva
    (E) Taxol

Questions 53–56 refer to the following patient profile.

Patient Name: Mary Jefferson

Age: 42   **Height:** 5′6″
Sex: F   **Weight:** 125 lb

Allergies: None known

Diagnosis

Primary:
1. Adenocarcinoma
2. Asthma

Lab/Diagnostic Tests

WBC 1×10^3 cells/mm^3; 50% segs
    10% bands 30% lymphs
    10% monos
Hgb: 14.5 g/dL
Blood pressure: 134/85 mmHg
Heart rate: 75 bpm

---

53. What is Ms. Jefferson's absolute neutrophil count?

    (A) 3,000 cells/mm^3
    (B) 750 cells/mm^3
    (C) 600 cells/mm^3
    (D) 300 cells/mm^3
    (E) 50 cells/mm^3

54. Ms. Jefferson's neutropenia would be considered

    (A) transient.
    (B) mild.
    (C) moderate.
    (D) severe.
    (E) absent. This patient is not neutropenic, as the ANC is within normal range.

55. Which of the following situations will put patients with neutropenia at risk for developing infection? (Select ALL that apply.)

    (A) Severe neutropenia
    (B) A rapid fall in ANC
    (C) Invasive procedures such as enemas, catheter placement, or dental procedures
    (D) Neutropenia lasting more than 7 days

56. Which of the following medications would be appropriate for Ms. Jefferson?

    (A) Neupogen
    (B) Epogen
    (C) Procrit
    (D) Aranesp

57. Gender and race are considered which of the following types of data?

    (A) Nominal
    (B) Ordinal
    (C) Interval
    (D) Ratio
    (E) Frequency

58. To increase the power of a study, the researchers could

    (A) decrease the sample size.
    (B) lengthen the duration of the study.
    (C) decrease the duration of the study.
    (D) increase the number of dependent variables being studied.
    (E) increase the sample size.

59. Which of the following statements regarding Type II errors is/are TRUE? (Select ALL that apply.)

   (A) A Type II error occurs when a study fails to detect a difference between study groups but in fact a difference does exist.
   (B) Not achieving power in a study may increase the likelihood of Type II errors.
   (C) A Type II error means that the null hypothesis was accepted when it actually is false.
   (D) A Type II error occurs when researchers find a difference between study groups when no difference actually exists.

60. A clinical trial is evaluating whether there is a difference in the mean LDL cholesterol levels between adults in three different treatment groups. The data collected follows a normal distribution. Which of the following would be the MOST appropriate statistical test for this analysis?

   (A) Student's t-test
   (B) Paired t-test
   (C) Chi-square test
   (D) ANOVA
   (E) Mann-Whitney U test

61. You need to make 30 g of 0.4% w/w hydrocortisone ointment. You have 2.5% w/w hydrocortisone ointment in stock. How much of the 2.5% ointment must you mix with white petrolatum to make the appropriate quantity of 0.4% ointment?

   (A) 2.4 g
   (B) 2.5 g
   (C) 4.8 g
   (D) 9.6 g
   (E) 30 g

62. The formula for hydrophilic petrolatum USP is given below. How much white wax do you need to weigh out to compound 70 g of hydrophilic petrolatum?

   Hydrophilic petrolatum:
   3% w/w cholesterol
   3% w/w stearyl alcohol
   8% w/w white wax
   86% w/w white petrolatum

   (A) 2.1 g
   (B) 8 g
   (C) 5.6 g
   (D) 60.2 g
   (E) 70 g

63. How many 4-mg tablets of chlorpheniramine maleate would be required to compound 4 fluid ounces of a syrup containing 2 mg of chlorpheniramine maleate in every tablespoonful dose?

   (A) 1
   (B) 2
   (C) 4
   (D) 8
   (E) 12

64. A 60-kg patient is to receive a constant IV infusion of dobutamine at a rate of 5 mcg/kg/min. The IV bag has a concentration of 0.5 mg/mL. For what rate should the infusion pump be set?

   (A) 0.6 mL/hr
   (B) 3.6 mL/hr
   (C) 18 mL/hr
   (D) 36 mL/hr
   (E) 600 mL/hr

65. A patient is given an IV bolus dose of 1 g of Drug A. The plasma level is measured shortly after administration and is found to be 0.2 mg/mL. The same patient is later given an IV bolus dose of Drug B. The plasma level of Drug B shortly after administration is 83 mcg/mL. On the basis of this data, which of the following statements is TRUE?

   (A) Drug A has a smaller volume of distribution than Drug B.
   (B) Drug A is better absorbed than Drug B.
   (C) Drug A induced the metabolism of Drug B.
   (D) Drug A is lipophilic.

66. To treat preeclampsia, a patient receives an IV infusion of 40 mL of a 10% w/v solution of magnesium sulfate for injection. How many mEq of magnesium did she receive?

   (MW $MgSO_4 \cdot (H_2O)_7 = 246.36$)

   (A) 8.63 mEq Mg^{2+}
   (B) 16.25 mEq Mg^{2+}
   (C) 32.5 mEq Mg^{2+}
   (D) 65 mEq Mg^{2+}
   (E) 130 mEq Mg^{2+}

67. You receive a prescription for 240 mL of a potassium citrate solution with a concentration of 15 mEq/15 mL. How much potassium citrate must you weigh out to compound this prescription?

   (MW $C_6H_5K_3O_7 = 306$)

   (A) 2.72 g
   (B) 8.16 g
   (C) 24.48 g
   (D) 73.44 g
   (E) 367.2 g

68. You are considering adding HgbA1c monitoring services to your clinical pharmacy offerings and are evaluating an HgbA1c monitor to decide if it sufficiently precise and accurate to be used in your clinic. Using a test solution that produces a value of 7.5% on standardized laboratory tests, you perform 10 sample tests on the monitor. The values you obtain are:

   7.9
   8.1
   7.9
   8.0
   7.9
   7.9
   8.0
   8.1
   7.9
   8.0

   You would say that the monitor being evaluated produces readings that are

   (A) accurate but not precise.
   (B) precise but not accurate.
   (C) both precise and accurate.
   (D) neither precise nor accurate.
   (E) You do not have enough information to answer this question.

69. How much sodium chloride must be added to the prescription to make the solution isotonic?

Rx: Tetracaine hydrochloride   0.5% w/v
    (E = 0.18)
    NaCl (0.9%)   qs
    Sterile water   add 30 mL

M et ft isotonic eye drops

(A) 0.027 g NaCl
(B) 0.243 g NaCl
(C) 0.27 g NaCl
(D) 0.83 g NaCl
(E) 0.9 g NaCl

70. Given the capsule recipe provided below, how much diphenhydramine must you weigh out to compound 60 capsules?

Diphenhydramine hydrochloride: 0.5 g
Acetaminophen: 6.5 g
Lactose qs: M et div caps #10

(A) 0.5 g
(B) 3 g
(C) 7 g
(D) 30 g
(E) 42 g

Questions 71–74 refer to the following patient information:

AJ is a 70-kg male with a creatinine clearance of 100 mL/min. You have the following information about the behavior of a particular drug in this patient:

CL = 400 mL/min;
CLr = 25 mL/min
V_d = 140 L
95% bound to plasma proteins

71. What is the filtration clearance of this drug?

(A) 0 mL/min
(B) 1.25 mL/min
(C) 5 mL/min
(D) 20 mL/min
(E) 95 mL/min

72. You can conclude that this drug is

(A) only filtered.
(B) both filtered and reabsorbed.
(C) both filtered and secreted.
(D) secreted and reabsorbed but not filtered.
(E) You do not have enough information to answer this question.

73. The half-life of this drug in this patient is

(A) 4 hours.
(B) 12 hours.
(C) 24 hours.
(D) 48 hours.
(E) 60 hours.

74. What blood level would you expect after a single IV bolus dose of 250 mg of this drug?

    (A) 0.1 mg/dL
    (B) 0.13 mg/dL
    (C) 0.15 mg/dL
    (D) 0.18 mg/dL
    (E) 0.2 mg/dL

75. MT is being treated for a serious infection caused by *Pseudomonas aeruginosa*. After obtaining culture and sensitivity data, her physician starts her on tobramycin 70 mg IV q8h. During her hospital stay, MT's serum creatinine increased from 0.8 to 1.6 mg/dL. What pharmacokinetic parameters have been affected, and what modification should be made to MT's tobramycin therapy?

    (A) The bioavailability for tobramycin is increased, resulting in kidney impairment. The tobramycin should be discontinued.
    (B) The clearance for tobramycin has decreased, resulting in a longer half-life. MT may experience drug accumulation, so the tobramycin dose should be decreased.
    (C) The clearance for tobramycin has increased, resulting in a shorter half-life. MT may experience subtherapeutic drug concentrations, so the tobramycin dose should be increased.
    (D) The clearance for tobramycin has decreased, resulting in a longer half-life. MT may experience subtherapeutic drug concentrations, so the tobramycin dose should be increased.
    (E) The V_d of tobramycin has increased, resulting in a longer half-life. MT may experience drug accumulation, so the tobramycin dose should be decreased.

76. Penicillin is a weakly acidic drug that is excreted by the kidney. Probenecid, also a weakly acidic drug, competes for the carrier system that is responsible for the excretion of penicillin. When penicillin and probenecid are administered together, what do you expect will happen to penicillin's clearance and steady-state plasma concentrations?

    (A) Clearance decreases and steady-state concentrations increase.
    (B) Clearance increases and steady-state concentrations increase.
    (C) Clearance increases and steady-state concentrations decrease.
    (D) Clearance decreases and steady-state concentrations decrease.
    (E) Clearance and steady-state concentrations are nearly unchanged.

77. Which of the following modifications to a drug will increase its aqueous solubility?

    (A) Convert anhydrous to trihydrate form.
    (B) Convert crystalline to amorphous form.
    (C) Add a lipophilic group.
    (D) Remove a hydroxyl group.

78. The pKa of a weak base is 8.4. What form will the drug be in at an intestinal pH of 7.4?

    (A) 75% un-ionized
    (B) Greater than 90% un-ionized
    (C) 75% ionized
    (D) Greater than 90% ionized
    (E) Approximately equal amounts ionized/un-ionized

79. Which dosage form would be the BEST option for a drug that is prone to first-pass metabolism?

    (A) Tablet
    (B) Syrup
    (C) Capsule
    (D) Rapid-dissolve strip
    (E) Transdermal patch

80. Structured vehicles form suspensions by what means?

    (A) Promoting loose aggregation of suspended particles
    (B) Increasing viscosity, thereby slowing sedimentation
    (C) Maximizing sedimentation volume
    (D) Reducing repulsive forces between particles

81. Phenytoin is formulated in a cosolvent system. IV administration of this drug should occur slowly because

    (A) the onset of drug action will be faster.
    (B) slow injection will prevent precipitation of the drug from solution.
    (C) rapid infusion will lead to hemolysis.
    (D) it will prevent the drug from being metabolized too quickly.
    (E) the cosolvent system is too viscous for rapid administration.

82. Which of the following ophthalmic products must contain a preservative?

    (A) Saline in a multiple-dose container
    (B) Saline in a single-dose container
    (C) Single-use rinse solution used in eye surgery
    (D) Carboxymethylcellulose in a single-use container

83. Medications may be administered rectally to provide local treatment for which of the following conditions?

    (A) Nausea
    (B) Chronic pain
    (C) Ulcerative colitis
    (D) Hormone replacement
    (E) Migraines

84. Metronidazole leads to a disulfiram reaction when taken with alcohol. Which of the following liquid dosage forms would be the MOST appropriate way of delivering metronidazole?

    (A) Spirit
    (B) Elixir USP
    (C) Tincture
    (D) Suspension
    (E) Fluid extract

85. A bottle of drug solution was left open in a dark room. After one day, the solution had changed from colorless to pink. An identical bottle, left capped, remained unchanged. The opened solution has undergone what type of degradation?

    (A) Hydrolysis
    (B) Photolysis
    (C) Oxidation
    (D) Sedimentation
    (E) Polymorphism

86. Calamine lotion remains thick when sitting on the shelf, yet pours easily when shaken. What type of flow is calamine lotion exhibiting?

    (A) Dilatant
    (B) Newtonian
    (C) Plastic
    (D) Pseudoplastic
    (E) Thixotropic

87. How many 50-mg phenytoin tablets should a 5-year-old child receive per day, given the following information?

   $V_{max} = 300$ mg/day
   $K_M = 6.5$ mg/L
   C_{SS} (desired) $= 14$ mg/L
   Salt factor for phenytoin tablets $= 1$

   (A) 1 tablet
   (B) 4 tablets
   (C) 5 tablets
   (D) 6 tablets
   (E) 7 tablets

88. Which of the following tablet excipients would be MOST expected to decrease product bioavailability?

   (A) Starch
   (B) Microcrystalline cellulose
   (C) Lactose
   (D) Magnesium stearate
   (E) Mannitol

89. Poor metabolizers of CYP2D6 are most likely to receive therapeutic benefit from which of the following opioids?

   (A) Codeine
   (B) Morphine
   (C) Hydrocodone
   (D) Oxycodone
   (E) Dextromethorphan

90. Patients taking protease inhibitors should avoid drinking grapefruit juice because it

   (A) inhibits CYP3A, leading to toxic levels of the drug.
   (B) inhibits CYP3A, leading to subtherapeutic levels of the drug.
   (C) induces CYP3A, leading to toxic levels of the drug.
   (D) induces CYP3A, leading to subtherapeutic levels of the drug.
   (E) binds to the drug, preventing absorption.

91. You receive an order for 10 mL of epinephrine 1:10,000 solution. What is another way to express this concentration?

   (A) 10% w/v
   (B) 1% w/v
   (C) 0.1% w/v
   (D) 0.01% w/v
   (E) 0.001% w/v

92. You need to measure out 100 g of methyl salicylate to use in a compound. The specific gravity of methyl salicylate is 1.18. How much methyl salicylate should you measure, by volume, to deliver the appropriate amount?

   (A) 69.5 mL
   (B) 84.75 mL
   (C) 100 mL
   (D) 115.25 mL
   (E) 130.5 mL

Questions 93–97 refer to the following patient profile.

Patient Name: John Marx

Age: 70   **Height:** 5′10″
Sex: M   **Weight:** 198 lb
Race: Black

Allergies: NKDA

Diagnosis

Primary:
1. Hypertension
2. Dyslipidemia
3. Heart failure

Secondary:
1. MI (5 years ago)

Chief Complaint: Swelling in legs

Medications

Date	Name and Strength	Route	Directions
10/25	Aspirin 81 mg	PO	1 tablet daily
	Digoxin 0.125 mg	PO	1 tablet daily
	Furosemide 20 mg	PO	1 tablet in the morning
	Lisinopril 20 mg	PO	1 tablet daily
	Toprol XL 25 mg	PO	1 tablet daily
	Vytorin 40/10 mg	PO	1 tablet at bedtime

Lab/Diagnostic Tests

Date	Test/Result	
11/10	Sodium	145 mEq/L
	Potassium	3.9 mEq/L
	Serum creatinine	1.1 mg/dL
	Digoxin	0.8 ng/mL
	Blood pressure	122/80 mmHg
	Heart rate	70 bpm
	LVEF	35%

Additional Information

Date	Comment
11/10	Patient has gained 3 lb in the past week.

93. Vytorin is the brand name for which of the following combinations?

   (A) Atorvastatin and amlodipine
   (B) Lovastatin and niacin
   (C) Simvastatin and ezetimibe
   (D) Simvastatin and lisinopril

94. Which of the following is/are appropriate nonpharmacological recommendations for Mr. Marx? (Select ALL that apply.)

   (A) Restrict fluid intake.
   (B) Restrict sodium intake.
   (C) Restrict vitamin K intake.
   (D) Restrict potassium intake.

95. Which of the following signs/symptoms is/are associated with digoxin toxicity? (Select ALL that apply.)

   (A) Anorexia
   (B) Arrhythmias
   (C) Visual disturbances
   (D) Hypokalemia

96. Which of the following medications is contraindicated in Mr. Marx?

   (A) Aldactone
   (B) BiDil
   (C) Diovan
   (D) Calan SR
   (E) Inspra

97. Mr. Marx's furosemide is increased to 40 mg PO BID. The pharmacist should counsel the patient on which of the following?

   (A) He should separate both doses of furosemide from other medications by 2 hours.
   (B) He should take the second dose of furosemide before 5 P.M. each day.
   (C) He should take both doses of furosemide with food or milk.
   (D) He should take the second dose of furosemide at bedtime.
   (E) He should take both doses of furosemide on an empty stomach.

Questions 98–101 refer to the following patient profile.

Patient Name: Susan Brown

Age: 42   **Height:** 5'4"

Sex: F   **Weight:** 162 lb

Allergies: NKDA

Diagnosis

   Primary:
     1. UTI
     2. DVT (secondary to oral contraceptive use)
     3. Hypertension

   Chief Complaint: Pain with urination

Medications

Date	Name and Strength	Route	Directions
3/3	Depo-Provera 150 mg	IM	Every 3 months
5/5	Coumadin 5 mg	PO	1 tablet daily
	HCTZ 25 mg	PO	1 tablet daily
	Lisinopril 10 mg	PO	1 tablet daily

Lab/Diagnostic Tests

Date	Test/Result	
5/22	Urinalysis	pyuria, nitrite (+)
	Sodium	145 mEq/L
	Potassium	3.9 mEq/L
	Serum creatinine	0.9 mg/dL
	INR	2.3
	Blood pressure	125/72 mmHg
	Heart rate	71 bpm

Additional Information

Date	Comment
5/5	Patient contemplating smoking cessation
5/22	Patient prescribed Bactrim DS 1 tablet PO BID × 3 days, #6

98. Bactrim DS is MOST likely being used to treat which of the following microorganisms?

  (A) *Chlamydia pneumoniae*
  (B) *Clostridium difficile*
  (C) *Enterococcus faecalis*
  (D) *Escherichia coli*
  (E) *Pseudomonas aeruginosa*

99. Which of the following lab alterations would you expect to see in Ms. Brown as a result of starting the Bactrim DS?

  (A) Increased INR
  (B) Decreased INR
  (C) Increased potassium
  (D) Decreased potassium
  (E) Increased sodium

100. Bactrim DS is the brand name for which of the following medications?

  (A) Amoxicillin and clavulanic acid
  (B) Ciprofloxacin and doxycycline
  (C) Imipenem and cilastatin
  (D) Isoniazid and rifampin
  (E) Trimethoprim and sulfamethoxazole

101. Lisinopril belongs to which of the following classes of drugs?

  (A) Angiotensin-converting enzyme inhibitor
  (B) Angiotensin II receptor blocker
  (C) Aldosterone receptor antagonist
  (D) Calcium channel blocker
  (E) Potassium-sparing diuretic

102. A patient recently moved to the United States from England. She brings in her prescription bottle and asks the pharmacist if he carries the antibiotic that she has been taking for a UTI. Which of the following references could be used by the pharmacist to determine if there is an equivalent antibiotic available in the United States?

  (A) Facts and Comparisons
  (B) Martindale
  (C) Merck Index
  (D) PDR
  (E) Red Book

103. A patient presents with a prescription for Xalatan. Xalatan is probably being used to treat which of the following disease states?

  (A) Anxiety
  (B) Asthma
  (C) Depression
  (D) Glaucoma
  (E) Sepsis

104. Which of the following medications is used for the treatment of type 2 diabetes?

  (A) Kadian
  (B) Keppra
  (C) Kazano
  (D) Ketoconazole

105. Patients taking sulfasalazine for inflammatory bowel disease should be counseled on which of the following? (Select ALL that apply.)

  (A) Take on an empty stomach.
  (B) It may cause orange bodily fluids.
  (C) Wear sunscreen and protective clothing.
  (D) Take once daily.

106. During a hospital stay for pneumonia, David Jones developed *Clostridium difficile*. Which of the following antibiotics would be the BEST treatment for Mr. Jones?

    (A) Amoxicillin
    (B) Azithromycin
    (C) Levofloxacin
    (D) Metronidazole
    (E) Tobramycin

107. A 22-year-old woman comes to the pharmacy to pick up her new prescription for an oral contraceptive. Which of the following references would be the MOST appropriate source of important counseling advice for this patient?

    (A) Harriet Lane Handbook
    (B) Index Nominum
    (C) Merck Index
    (D) USP-DI Volume I
    (E) USP-DI Volume II

108. Cytotec is the brand name of which of the following medications?

    (A) Cimetidine
    (B) Metoclopramide
    (C) Misoprostol
    (D) Olsalazine
    (E) Sucralfate

109. Which of the following medications would be an appropriate treatment for genital herpes?

    (A) Acyclovir
    (B) Indinavir
    (C) Lamivudine
    (D) Oseltamivir
    (E) Valganciclovir

110. Which of the following references is the BEST source for obtaining the cost information of medications?

    (A) Facts and Comparisons
    (B) The Harriet Lane Handbook
    (C) PDR
    (D) Red Book
    (E) USP-DI Volume I

111. Which of the following is/are potential side effects of niacin? (Select ALL that apply.)

    (A) Flushing
    (B) Hyperglycemia
    (C) Hyperuricemia
    (D) Hypertriglyceridemia

112. Cosopt is the brand name for which of the following combinations?

    (A) Timolol and brimonidine
    (B) Timolol and dorzolamide
    (C) Latanoprost and carbachol
    (D) Pilocarpine and brinzolamide
    (E) Pilocarpine and carbachol

113. Which of the following medications could be used intravenously to treat an invasive *Aspergillus* infection?

    (A) Voriconazole
    (B) Linezolid
    (C) Miconazole
    (D) Meropenem

114. Which of the following statements about omeprazole is TRUE? (Select ALL that apply.)

    (A) It is available without a prescription.
    (B) It is most effective when taken on an empty stomach.
    (C) Its tablet formulation can be crushed or chewed.
    (D) It interacts significantly with clopidogrel, and the combination should be avoided.

115. Which of the following IV medications should be protected from light?

   (A) Enalaprilat
   (B) Esmolol
   (C) Fenoldopam
   (D) Nitroglycerin
   (E) Nitroprusside

116. A patient presents to the pharmacy with prescriptions for Biaxin, Amoxil, and Nexium. The patient is probably being treated for which of the following infections?

   (A) *Helicobacter pylori*
   (B) *Haemophilus influenzae*
   (C) *Klebsiella pneumoniae*
   (D) *Moraxella catarrhalis*
   (E) *Neisseria meningitidis*

117. Trusopt belongs to which of the following classes of drugs?

   (A) Antihistamine
   (B) Beta-blocker
   (C) Carbonic anhydrase inhibitor
   (D) Cholinergic agonist
   (E) Prostaglandin analog

118. The Commission E Monographs provide information on which of the following?

   (A) Dietary supplements
   (B) Foreign drugs
   (C) Herbal products
   (D) Homeopathic products
   (E) Nonprescription drugs

119. Clotrimazole is available in which of the following dosage forms? (Select ALL that apply.)

   (A) Troche
   (B) Capsule
   (C) Powder
   (D) Cream

120. Which of the following is the MOST appropriate monitoring recommendation for a patient receiving amiodarone?

   (A) Chest x-ray should be performed every 6 months.
   (B) Thyroid function tests should be performed annually.
   (C) Liver function tests should be performed every 6 months.
   (D) Ophthalmic exams should be performed every 3 months.

121. A patient using ophthalmic preparations should be given which of the following counseling information?

   (A) The preparations can be used safely with contact lenses.
   (B) The dropper tip should be placed on the edge of the lower eyelid.
   (C) The upper eyelid should be pulled outward to form a pocket in which the medication can be placed.
   (D) The eyes should be rubbed after the eye drops are administered.
   (E) The administration of different medications should be separated by intervals of at least 10 minutes.

122. Information on IV medication compatibility can be found in which of the following references?

   (A) Facts and Comparisons
   (B) Physician's Desk Reference
   (C) Trissel's Handbook on Injectable Drugs
   (D) USP-DI Volume I

123. Tagamet belongs to which of the following classes of drugs?

   (A) Aminosalicylate
   (B) H$_2$ receptor antagonist
   (C) Immunosuppressant
   (D) Prostaglandin analog
   (E) Proton pump inhibitor

124. A patient brings in a prescription for methotrexate for the treatment of Crohn's disease. Which of the following tests should be monitored in this patient? (Select ALL that apply.)

    (A) Electrocardiogram
    (B) Complete blood count
    (C) Liver function tests
    (D) TSH

125. Which of the following medications may result in hyperkalemia? (Select ALL that apply.)

    (A) Candesartan
    (B) Eplerenone
    (C) Triamterene
    (D) Metolazone

126. Which of the following medications can be administered via a nasogastric tube? (Select ALL that apply.)

    (A) Esomeprazole
    (B) Lansoprazole
    (C) Pantoprazole
    (D) Rabeprazole

127. A patient is prescribed felodipine for her hypertension. She should be counseled to do which of the following?

    (A) Avoid drinking grapefruit juice.
    (B) Avoid foods with tyramine.
    (C) Take the felodipine with folic acid.
    (D) Take the felodipine on an empty stomach.
    (E) Take the felodipine 2 hours before taking other medications.

128. An otherwise healthy patient develops community-acquired pneumonia. The patient has NKDA. Which of the following antibiotics would be the MOST appropriate empiric treatment option for this patient?

    (A) Azithromycin
    (B) Metronidazole
    (C) Penicillin
    (D) Rifampin
    (E) Vancomycin

129. Amoxicillin is available in which of the following dosage forms? (Select ALL that apply.)

    (A) IV injection
    (B) Oral suspension
    (C) Capsule
    (D) Chewable tablet

130. Which of the following medications would be MOST appropriate to use for the treatment of hypertension in a pregnant patient?

    (A) Doxazosin
    (B) Lisinopril
    (C) Methyldopa
    (D) Metolazone
    (E) Valsartan

131. A patient is prescribed Prevacid for his peptic ulcer disease. He should be counseled to take it

    (A) 15 to 30 minutes before breakfast.
    (B) 30 minutes after breakfast.
    (C) 2 hours before taking other medications.
    (D) with the first bite of a meal.
    (E) with a high-fat meal.

132. Sporanox is the brand name for which of the following medications?

(A) Aripiprazole
(B) Fluconazole
(C) Itraconazole
(D) Lansoprazole
(E) Rabeprazole

133. A patient presents to the pharmacy with a prescription for simvastatin 40 mg PO at bedtime and gemfibrozil 600 mg PO BID. Which of the following adverse reactions is this patient likely to experience?

(A) Dyspnea
(B) Edema
(C) Headache
(D) Insomnia
(E) Myopathy

134. A patient presents with a new prescription for Synthroid. Which of the following medications might have contributed to her recent diagnosis of hypothyroidism?

(A) Amiodarone
(B) Bisoprolol
(C) Dofetilide
(D) Hydralazine
(E) Propafenone

135. Levaquin belongs to which of the following classes of drugs?

(A) Aminoglycosides
(B) Cephalosporins
(C) Fluoroquinolones
(D) Macrolides
(E) Tetracyclines

136. Which of the following statements regarding amiodarone is TRUE?

(A) It is only effective for the treatment of atrial arrhythmias.
(B) It does not undergo cytochrome P450 metabolism by the liver.
(C) If pulmonary fibrosis develops, the amiodarone should be discontinued.
(D) It is contraindicated in patients with heart failure.

137. Which of the following drug classes is/ are used in the treatment of inflammatory bowel disease? (Select ALL that apply.)

(A) Aminosalicylates
(B) Corticosteroids
(C) Immunosuppressants
(D) Chloride channel activators

138. Which of the following regimens would be appropriate for the treatment of *H. pylori* infection? (Select ALL that apply.)

(A) Omeprazole, clarithromycin, and metronidazole
(B) Esomeprazole, clarithromycin, and amoxicillin
(C) Pantoprazole, bismuth subsalicylate, and metronidazole
(D) Lansoprazole, bismuth subsalicylate, and tetracycline

Questions 139–143 refer to the following patient profile.

Patient Name: William Boyd

Age: 56   **Height:** 5′8″
Sex: M   **Weight:** 148 lb

Allergies: Codeine, PCN, Sulfa

Diagnosis

Primary
1. Hypertension
2. Hypothyroidism
3. Type 2 diabetes mellitus × 5 years

Secondary
1. Heartburn

Chief Complaint: Fatigue, tiredness, cold fingers, feeling down

Medications

Date	Name and Strength	Route	Directions
7/10	Prilosec OTC 10 mg	PO	3 tablets daily
	Synthroid 100 mcg	PO	1 tablet daily
	Metformin 1,000 mg	PO	1 tablet TID
	Lisinopril 10 mg	PO	1 tablet daily
	Ferrous sulfate 325 mg	PO	1 tablet daily

Lab/Diagnostic Tests

Date	Test/Result	
7/9	Sodium	141 mEq/L
	Potassium	3.5 mEq/L
	Serum creatinine	0.9 mg/dL
	TSH	10 mIU/L
	AST	18 IU/L
	ALT	16 IU/L
	A1c	5.5%
	Blood pressure	139/80 mmHg
	Heart rate	90 bpm
	GDS	4

Additional Information

Date	Comment
7/10	Patient complains of fatigue and lack of energy.
3/9	Pharmacist advised patient to start taking Prilosec OTC.
3/9	Pharmacist counseled patient to check blood sugars.

139. Which of the following statements regarding the metformin is TRUE?

    (A) It should be discontinued due to the patient's A1c level.
    (B) The pharmacist should contact the patient's physician because the dose is too high.
    (C) The pharmacist should recommend increasing the dose.
    (D) It is not indicated in this patient.
    (E) There is a significant drug interaction with lisinopril.

140. Which of the following is an appropriate recommendation for Mr. Boyd?

    (A) Continue taking all medications as prescribed.
    (B) Start taking a multivitamin for energy.
    (C) Call the doctor regarding the patient's heartburn.
    (D) Eat a low-potassium diet.

141. Which of the following is the MOST likely etiology of Mr. Boyd's chief complaints?

    (A) Undertreated hypothyroidism
    (B) Hypoglycemia
    (C) Untreated depression
    (D) Uncontrolled hypertension

142. Lisinopril helps to do which of the following for this patient?

    (A) Improve blood sugars by inhibiting ACE
    (B) Block renin to lower blood pressure
    (C) Inhibit ACE, which blocks the angiotensin II receptor
    (D) Block ACE to vasodilate
    (E) Protect his kidneys by lowering bradykinin

143. Mr. Boyd's Synthroid was increased to 125 mcg PO daily by the medical resident. The pharmacist should counsel Mr. Boyd to

    (A) monitor his blood sugar, as the Synthroid may cause hypoglycemia.
    (B) avoid taking the Synthroid with ferrous sulfate at the same time.
    (C) take the Synthroid only in the evening.
    (D) avoid taking the Synthroid with metformin.
    (E) take the Synthroid with milk.

144. Nevirapine is the generic name of which brand drug, and belongs in which drug class?

    (A) Viramune; non-nucleoside reverse transcriptase inhibitors
    (B) Ziagen; non-nucleoside reverse transcriptase inhibitors
    (C) Kaletra; protease inhibitors
    (D) Videx; nucleoside reverse transcriptase inhibitors
    (E) Fuzeon; fusion inhibitors

145. When should antiviral therapy for HIV be initiated? (Select ALL that apply.)

    (A) When diagnosis is confirmed by Western blot
    (B) When the CD4 cell count is less than 500 cells/mm^3
    (C) When the patient has a history of an opportunistic infection
    (D) When HIV RNA exceeds 50,000 copies/mL

Questions 146–151 refer to the following patient profile.

Patient Name: Mary Christensen

Age: 75 **Height:** 5′4″
Sex: F **Weight:** 183 lb

Allergies: NKDA

Diagnosis

Primary
1. Asthma
2. Hypertension
3. Osteoarthritis

Chief Complaint: Thrush, dizziness, tachycardia,
nausea, and vomiting

Lab/Diagnostic Tests

Date	Test/Result	
7/9	Sodium	140 mEq/L
	Potassium	3.5 mEq/L
	Serum creatinine	0.9 mg/dL
	Personal best FEV_1	325 L/sec
	FEV1	300 L/sec
	Blood pressure	90/70 mmHg
	Heart rate	110 bpm
	Theophylline level	23 mcg/mL

Medications

Date	Name and Strength	Route	Directions
7/20	Advair	PO	1 puff BID
	Theophylline XR 600 mg	PO	1 tablet daily
	Albuterol MDI	PO	1–2 puffs TID PRN
	Metoprolol 50 mg	PO	1 tablet BID
	Aspirin 325 mg	PO	1 tablet daily
	Fish oil 1,000 mg	PO	1 capsule daily
	Hydrocodone/ APAP 5/325 mg	PO	1–2 tablets q6h for pain
	Tylenol Arthritis 325 mg	PO	2 tablets TID

Additional Orders

Date	Comment
5/10	Pharmacist counseled patient on swish and spit after Advair use.
6/15	Pharmacist counseled patient on use of peak flow meter.
7/2	Patient stated she got a new cat.

146. The patient's chief complaint of thrush is most likely caused by which of the following?

    (A) Theophylline toxicity
    (B) Lack of swishing and spitting after Advair use
    (C) Excessive metoprolol dose
    (D) Adverse effects of fish oil

147. Which of the following medications would you recommend discontinuing in this patient?

    (A) Advair because of thrush
    (B) Aspirin because of nausea
    (C) Albuterol due to excessive use
    (D) Theophylline because of toxicity
    (E) Metoprolol because of tachycardia

148. What is/are the generic ingredient(s) of Advair?

    (A) Fluticasone
    (B) Salmeterol
    (C) Fluticasone and salmeterol
    (D) Flunisolide
    (E) Flunisolide and salmeterol

149. What is the most appropriate indication for this patient to take fish oil?

    (A) To reduce total cholesterol
    (B) To reduce LDL cholesterol
    (C) To increase HDL cholesterol
    (D) To reduce HDL cholesterol
    (E) To reduce triglycerides

150. Which of the following is the MOST appropriate action to take regarding the acetaminophen this patient is currently taking?

    (A) Call her doctor.
    (B) Discuss how much acetaminophen is appropriate per day.
    (C) Discontinue the hydrocodone/acetaminophen.
    (D) Discontinue the Tylenol Arthritis.
    (E) Consider switching the Tylenol Arthritis to an aspirin-containing product.

151. Which of the following medications is appropriately dosed once daily?

    (A) Atrovent
    (B) Spiriva
    (C) Combivent
    (D) Advair

152. Which of the following medications is an inhaled corticosteroid?

    (A) Pulmicort Respules
    (B) Singulair
    (C) Zyflo
    (D) Solu-Medrol

153. Which of the following is the mechanism of action of Zyban?

    (A) It inhibits reuptake of serotonin.
    (B) It inhibits reuptake of norepinephrine.
    (C) It inhibits reuptake of dopamine.
    (D) It inhibits reuptake of dopamine and norepinephrine.
    (E) It inhibits reuptake of serotonin, norepinephrine, and dopamine.

154. Which of the following drugs is NOT commonly used in the treatment of nonresistant tuberculosis?

(A) Isoniazid
(B) Rifampin
(C) Pyrazinamide
(D) Ethambutol
(E) Streptomycin

155. Vitamin K can be used to reverse the effects of which of the following drugs?

(A) Unfractionated heparin
(B) Dabigatran
(C) Enoxaparin
(D) Warfarin
(E) Clopidogrel

156. Flumazenil is used to treat an overdose of which of the following medications?

(A) Benzodiazepines
(B) Opioids
(C) Methanol
(D) Methotrexate
(E) Cisplatin

157. Cytomel is the brand name for which of the following active ingredients?

(A) Liothyronine
(B) Levothyroxine
(C) Dessicated thyroid
(D) T4
(E) TSH

158. Which of the following medications should be avoided in pregnancy? (Select ALL that apply.)

(A) Finasteride
(B) Isotretinoin
(C) Methyldopa
(D) Atorvastatin

159. In patients prescribed estrogen therapy for vasomotor symptoms associated with menopause, progestin therapy provides which of the following benefits?

(A) Decreased risk of venous thromboembolism
(B) Decreased risk of endometrial cancer
(C) Decreased risk of osteoporosis
(D) Decreased risk of weight gain

160. How long does it take for the fentanyl patch to begin working?

(A) 12 hours
(B) 24 hours
(C) 48 hours
(D) 72 hours
(E) 84 hours

161. A stimulant laxative is needed with which of the following pain medications?

(A) Ketorolac
(B) Gabapentin
(C) Morphine
(D) Desipramine

162. A woman comes into the pharmacy and requests an over-the-counter medication for pain in her knee, though she can't remember what her physician told her to purchase. She informs you that she has kidney problems. Which of the following medications would be MOST appropriate for this patient?

(A) Ibuprofen
(B) Ketoprofen
(C) Naproxen
(D) Acetaminophen
(E) Aspirin

163. A PPD should be performed on which of the following individuals? (Select ALL that apply.)

    (A) Healthcare worker
    (B) HIV-infected patient
    (C) Immigrant
    (D) 4-year-old entering preschool

164. The doses of which of the following pain medications must be adjusted in patients with renal impairment? (Select ALL that apply.)

    (A) Morphine
    (B) Codeine
    (C) Oxycodone
    (D) Tramadol

165. Which NSAID has a maximum dose of 1,500 mg per day?

    (A) Naprosyn
    (B) Ibuprofen
    (C) Relafen
    (D) Ketoprofen
    (E) Daypro

166. Which of the following is a warning symptom of stroke? (Select ALL that apply.)

    (A) Numbness or weakness of the face, arm, or leg
    (B) Sudden confusion, trouble speaking or understanding
    (C) Sudden trouble seeing in one or both eyes
    (D) Sudden seizure for no known reason
    (E) Sudden difficulty walking, dizziness, loss of balance

167. Folic acid is important in which of the following scenarios? (Select ALL that apply.)

    (A) Methotrexate treatment
    (B) Pregnancy
    (C) Iron deficiency anemia
    (D) Chronic kidney disease (CKD)

168. Which of the following is an appropriate indication for epoetin-alfa?

    (A) Male patient with stage 3 CKD and Hgb of 12 g/dL
    (B) Female patient with stage 4 CKD and Hgb of 12 g/dL
    (C) Patient with chemotherapy-induced anemia from chemotherapy being used with curative intent
    (D) Patient with chemotherapy-induced anemia from chemotherapy being used with palliative intent

169. A patient with osteomalacia would BEST be given a nutritional supplement high in

    (A) pyridoxine.
    (B) ascorbic acid.
    (C) beta-carotene.
    (D) nicotinic acid.
    (E) cholecalciferol.

170. Iron deficiency anemia requires a minimum of how many months of treatment?

    (A) 1 month
    (B) 3 months
    (C) 6 months
    (D) 9 months
    (E) 12 months

171. What is the mechanism of action of epoetin alfa?

(A) It induces reticulocytes to create more iron stores.
(B) It induces erythropoiesis and the release of reticulocytes.
(C) It stimulates granulocyte colony-stimulating factor to generate more reticulocytes.
(D) It is a thrombopoietic growth factor, which stimulates iron absorption in the gut.
(E) It stimulates colony-stimulating factor to generate more iron absorption.

172. A patient taking chronic doses of isoniazid should be supplemented with which of the following?

(A) Beta-carotene
(B) Ascorbic acid
(C) Cyanocobalamin
(D) Thiamine
(E) Pyridoxine

173. Which of the following organizations is responsible for the enforcement of controlled substances?

(A) Federal Drug Association
(B) Food and Drug Administration
(C) Drug Enforcement Administration
(D) National Provider Indicators
(E) State Patrol

174. Which of the following statements regarding lifestyle modifications is/are TRUE? (Select ALL that apply.)

(A) Smoking cessation for more than a year can lead to an improvement in lung function.
(B) Avoidance of asthma triggers such as mold, pollen, dust, cockroaches, grass, and smoke can replace the need for a short-acting beta-2 agonist bronchodilator.
(C) Six months of lifestyle modifications should be followed prior to starting cholesterol-lowering medications for the treatment of dyslipidemia in most cases.
(D) Patients with heartburn may raise the head of the bed by 2–3 inches to relieve symptoms during sleeping hours.
(E) Patients with hypertension should limit their salt intake to less than 2.4 g/day.

175. Which of the following statements regarding the Dietary Supplement Health and Education Act of 1994 is/are TRUE? (Select ALL that apply.)

(A) Manufacturers are not required to demonstrate safety, purity, or efficacy of supplements.
(B) Labeling must include the FDA statement: "This drug is not evaluated by the FDA, and not intended to diagnose, treat, cure, or prevent disease."
(C) Products cannot have specific claims on their labels or use phrases such as "helps boost/support/enhance."
(D) The FDA requires certain standards for manufacturing practices.

176. Which of the following herbal products has/have the potential to interact with anticoagulant/antiplatelet agents? (Select ALL that apply.)

    (A) Ginkgo biloba
    (B) Ginseng
    (C) Garlic
    (D) Saw palmetto
    (E) Feverfew

177. Which of the following organisms would MOST likely be present in a patient with a community-acquired skin and soft tissue infection?

    (A) *Haemophilus influenzae*
    (B) *Escherichia coli*
    (C) *Staphylococcus aureus*
    (D) *Streptococcus pneumoniae*
    (E) *Pseudomonas aeruginosa*

178. Which of the following insulin types has the shortest duration of action?

    (A) Regular insulin
    (B) Detemir insulin
    (C) NPH insulin
    (D) Glulisine insulin

179. Which of the following medications should be used cautiously in patients with a history of pancreatitis?

    (A) Exenatide
    (B) Detemir insulin
    (C) Dapagliflozin
    (D) Acarbose

180. Compilations of information concerning parenteral drug solutions are found in

    (A) Goodman and Gilman.
    (B) Martindale.
    (C) Merck Index.
    (D) Remington.
    (E) Trissel's Handbook on Injectable Drugs.

181. Which of the following supplements is used for the treatment of insomnia?

    (A) Black cohosh
    (B) Melatonin
    (C) St. John's wort
    (D) Saw palmetto

182. _____ are currently available on the market.

    (A) Metformin 1,250-mg tablets
    (B) Ferrous sulfate 5-grain tablets
    (C) Synthroid 212-mcg tablets
    (D) Coumadin 15-mg tablets
    (E) Lisinopril 80-mg tablets

183. Which statin is equivalent to Lipitor 10 mg?

    (A) Rosuvastatin 10 mg
    (B) Simvastatin 20 mg
    (C) Pravastatin 20 mg
    (D) Simvastatin 80 mg

184. St. John's wort interacts with which of the following medications? (Select ALL that apply.)

    (A) Pravachol
    (B) Sertraline
    (C) Warfarin
    (D) Aspirin

185. A patient who is experiencing a runny nose, sneezing, and watery eyes should be counseled to take which of the following OTC agents?

    (A) Diphenhydramine
    (B) Acetaminophen
    (C) Pseudoephedrine
    (D) Guaifenesin

Practice Test
Answers & Explanations

1. E

Diarrhea is a possible side effect of nearly any medication including approximately 1–10% of patients taking allopurinol (A), indomethacin (C), and acetaminophen (D); and <5% of patients taking probenecid (B). However, up to 25% of patients taking colchicine will experience this common, limiting side effect.

2. C

The international normalized ratio (INR) is a measure of coagulability and is the gold standard for monitoring anticoagulation therapy (vitamin K antagonists). A1c (A) is used to monitor the degree of glycemic control over the last 3 months in patients with diabetes. AST (B) is a transaminase used to monitor liver function, and brain natriuretic peptide (D) is a measure of cardiac muscle stretching and is used to assess whether patients have acutely decompensated heart failure.

3. E

Clozapine requires rigorous monitoring of white blood cell (WBC) count and absolute neutrophil count (ANC) due to the possibility of clozapine-induced agranulocytosis or severe granulocytopenia. Counts for both parameters should be obtained at baseline and at least weekly for the first 6 months of treatment with clozapine. If counts remain stable, then the WBC

and ANC can be monitored every other week for the next 6 months and monthly thereafter. Due to these frequent monitoring requirements, clozapine is used less than other atypical antipsychotics and is often used for refractory cases of schizophrenia. Agranulocytosis is not associated with olanzapine (A), risperidone (B), quetiapine (C), or ziprasidone (D).

4. A

When initiating a dopamine agonist such as Mirapex (pramipexole), the levodopa dose should be decreased by 20–30%. B is incorrect because Mirapex is not available as a patch. The ergot-derivative bromocriptine must be monitored for cardiac side effects (C), which is why the nonergot derivatives such as Mirapex are much more commonly used. (D) Dose adjustment of Mirapex is not required in hepatic disease because Mirapex undergoes minimal hepatic metabolism. However, the dose of Mirapex should be adjusted in patients with renal impairment.

5. A

Venlafaxine is an appropriate antidepressant medication to initiate and the initial dose should be 37.5 mg PO twice daily. Lexapro (escitalopram) is dosed once daily (B). Fluvoxamine should be dosed once daily and is indicated for the treatment of obsessive-compulsive disorder (C); fluoxetine can be dosed weekly. The maximum dose of nortriptyline is 150 mg/day (D). Mirtazapine does not come in a 10-mg formulation and should be dosed at bedtime due to somnolence (E).

6. B

NuvaRing should be stored in the refrigerator prior to use. Seasonale (A) and Ovrette (C) are oral contraceptives and do not require refrigeration. Xulane (D) is a transdermal patch and also does not require refrigeration.

7. A

Hydroxychloroquine may cause macular damage, corneal deposits, or retinopathy; therefore, patients receiving hydroxychloroquine therapy must have routine ocular exams. Metformin (B), Enbrel (etanercept; C), and methotrexate (D) are not known to cause ocular adverse effects and do not require ocular monitoring.

8. D

Serum creatinine is most commonly used to assess renal function, not hepatic function (A). Serum creatinine is not dependent upon the amount of iron in the diet and is sometimes an inaccurate representation of renal function in the very elderly (B, C). Serum creatinine is commonly used in the Cockroft-Gault equation to calculate creatinine clearance (CrCl) (D). Microalbumin, a microscopic protein, is measured in the urine and is not synonymous with serum creatinine (E).

9. C

Patients who are prescribed natalizumab must enroll in the TOUCH program before they can receive this medication. Mitoxantrone (A) and teriflunomide (B) do not have REMS programs. While fingolimod (D) does have a REMS program, enrollment is not required.

10. B

Allopurinol is indicated for prophylaxis of gout exacerbations in patients with moderately elevated serum uric acid levels and a history of nephrolithiasis, tophi, serum creatinine >2 mg/dL, or urinary uric acid excretion indicative of overproduction (B). If the serum uric acid levels are only slightly elevated, colchicine is used for prophylaxis (A). In patients who have urinary uric acid excretion levels indicative of underexcretion, uricosuric drugs (e.g., probenecid) are used for prophylaxis (C). Allopurinol should never be used to treat acute gout because it can actually worsen the symptoms (D). Asymptomatic hyperuricemia does not require therapy (E).

11. B, C

Valproic acid (B) should be monitored to achieve serum drug concentrations of 50–100 mcg/mL. Therapeutic serum drug concentrations of lithium (C) are 0.6–1.5 mEq/L. Lamotrigine (A) and levetiractam (D) do not require monitoring of serum drug concentrations.

12. E

Geodon is the trade name for ziprasidone. Aripiprazole (A) is the generic name for Abilify, olanzapine (B) is the generic name for Zyprexa, quetiapine (C) is the generic for Seroquel, and risperidone (D) is the generic for Risperdal.

13. C

Available prophylactic agents for migraines include beta-blockers (such as propranolol, atenolol, metoprolol), antidepressants (such as amitriptyline, paroxetine, fluoxetine, sertraline), and anticonvulsants (such as valproic acid, gabapentin, tiagabine, topiramate). Acetaminophen (B) is considered abortive treatment for migraines and is not taken for prophylaxis.

Angiotensin-converting enzyme inhibitors (ACEIs) (A), H_2 antagonists (D), and anticholinergics (E) have no role in the prevention of migraines.

14. B

Tramadol (B) is an oral analgesic that does not cause GI upset or bleeding. Aspirin (A) is a nonsteroidal anti-inflammatory drug (NSAID) that may cause GI bleeding. Diclofenac (C) and Daypro (oxaprozin; D) are both NSAIDs that may cause GI upset and bleeding. Although Mobic (meloxicam; E) is more COX-2–selective than traditional NSAIDs, it still possesses the potential to cause GI upset and stomach bleeding.

15. C

Haloperidol (C) is a first-generation antipsychotic. First-generation antipsychotics are known for their potential to cause extrapyramidal symptoms (EPS) such as tardive dyskinesia and dystonia. Hydrochlorothiazide (A) is a common antihypertensive that does not cause EPS. Citalopram (B) is a common antidepressant that does not cause EPS. Although low sodium (D) can be dangerous, it does not cause EPS. Uncontrolled blood pressure (E) may lead to organ damage but does not cause EPS.

16. E

Haloperidol (E) requires periodic monitoring of a CBC because of its potential to cause agranulocytosis. Serum drug levels (A) are not measured with haloperidol. Although a baseline electrocardiogram is recommended upon haloperidol initiation, monitoring of ejection fraction (C) is not necessary. A1c (B) could be monitored with atypical antipsychotics (such as olanzapine or ziprasidone) due to their likelihood of causing metabolic syndrome. Bone mineral density (D) does not need to be routinely monitored for any antipsychotic.

17. C

Changing the patient to an atypical antipsychotic would be the best option since atypicals have fewer extrapyramidal side effects. The atypical antipsychotic risperidone would be an appropriate option. Switching between formulations of haloperidol (A) would not provide any improvement of EPS. This patient is allergic to Geodon (ziprasidone; B) so this option would not be appropriate. Vitamin E (D) has no evidence to support use in tardive dyskinesia.

18. D

Alcohol should be avoided in combination with antipsychotics due to the excessive central nervous system (CNS) depression it may cause. An acidic environment is not required with antipsychotic medications and patients may take most of the medications with food if GI upset occurs (A). Medications for schizophrenia may take 2–4 weeks to work, so (B) is not correct. It is also important that antipsychotics not be abruptly stopped (C) or self-adjusted (E). If bothersome side effects occur, Ms. Yates should contact her provider so that appropriate adjustments and changes in the medications can be made.

19. C

Alprazolam (B) is not used for depression but may be used in anxiety disorders. Propranolol (E) is a beta-blocker that may actually worsen depression. Although not contraindicated, venlafaxine (D) may not be the best option for this patient considering her uncontrolled blood pressure. Venlafaxine can increase blood pressure and should be monitored closely. Bupropion (A) is contraindicated if the patient actually has an eating disorder. Since this woman is suspected of having an eating disorder, bupropion is not the most appropriate recommendation. Lexapro (escitalopram; C) is a selective serotonin reuptake inhibitor (SSRI) similar to her current citalopram and would be an appropriate substitution.

20. **A**

Carbidopa is a dopa-decarboxylase inhibitor, which must be combined with levodopa to prevent the peripheral degradation of levodopa (A). If the levodopa is degraded in the periphery, it does not enter into the blood-brain barrier for site of action. The carbidopa does not extend the dosing interval (B) or prevent CNS side effects of levodopa from occurring (C). Carbidopa does not provide (D) anticholinergic properties.

21. **C**

NSAIDs such as indomethacin are the first-line treatment for acute gout. If the patient is unable to take NSAIDs, the time course of the event must be evaluated. If the symptoms have been present for less than 48 hours, colchicine (B) is recommended. If the symptoms have been present for >48 hours, a corticosteroid is recommended. Allopurinol (D) is not effective for the treatment of acute gout and can worsen the symptoms. Probenecid (E) is not useful in an acute exacerbation of gout and should be avoided as it may precipitate attacks. Acetaminophen (A) plays no role in the treatment of acute gout.

22. **A**

All antidepressants carry some risk of erectile dysfunction (ED); however, the risk is significantly lower with bupropion, so this medication is often used in place of antidepressants for patients who experience ED.

23. **D**

The combination of phenytoin and cimetidine (D) results in increased serum concentration of phenytoin via inhibition of phenytoin metabolism. Phenytoin is a substrate of the cytochrome P450 (CYP) 2C19 isoenzymes. Cimetidine is a moderate inhibitor of CYP2C19. Quinidine (C) is a CYP2D6 inhibitor and would not affect serum phenytoin concentrations. Carbamazepine (A) and valproic acid (B) result in enzyme induction and subsequent decreases in serum phenytoin concentrations.

24. **B**

NSAIDs are used as needed for symptomatic relief during the onset of disease-modifying antirheumatic drug (DMARD) therapy (B). NSAIDs do not alter the disease progression of rheumatoid arthritis; therefore, they are not considered DMARDs (A). Although NSAIDs can be given along with DMARDs for symptoms, they are not considered adjunctive therapy for patients with refractory symptoms (C); that is the role of corticosteroids. The biologics are not known to cause flushing, (D) although NSAIDs could be used for PRN symptom relief with the biologics. Methotrexate, not NSAIDs, must be given in combination with infliximab in patients with rheumatoid arthritis (E).

25. **C**

If a patient is experiencing severe nausea and vomiting whenever a migraine occurs, most likely he/she will not receive maximum benefit from a regular oral tablet (A and B) due to the emesis. Many other dosage forms are available within the triptan class of abortive therapies. Maxalt MLT (rizatriptan) (C) is a rapidly disintegrating tablet that is one possible option for treatment in these patients. Other triptan options for patients experiencing severe nausea and vomiting include Imitrex (sumatriptan) injection or nasal spray and Zomig (zolmitriptan) orally disintegrating tablet or nasal spray. Topiramate tablets are also oral and topiramate is not effective as abortive therapy.

26. A

Oxcarbazepine and lamotrigine both have the potential to cause Stevens-Johnson syndrome (A), especially when lamotrigine is used in combination with valproic acid. Oxcarbazepine is the generic name for Trileptal (B). Lithium does not interact with beta-blockers (C); however, it does have significant drug interactions with ACEIs and diuretics. Lithium works by altering the sodium transport (E), which helps in understanding the interaction with ACEIs and diuretics; while valproic acid is thought to affect GABA. Valproic acid is contraindicated in hepatic impairment and requires baseline and periodic liver function tests (D).

27. C

Bupropion is contraindicated in patients with seizure disorders due to an increased risk of seizures. Bupropion is also contraindicated in patients with eating disorders such as bulimia or anorexia. Bupropion can be used for smoking cessation (A). Bupropion is not contraindicated in hypertension (D) or erectile dysfunction (B), and it has a lower incidence of ED than other antidepressants.

28. C, D

Sulfasalazine (C) impairs folate absorption; therefore, folic acid supplementation is often required. Because methotrexate (D) works by antagonism of folate synthesis, supplementing folic acid decreases the risk of side effects, and the two are often coprescribed. Carbamazepine (A) and leflunomide (B) do not affect folate levels.

29. C

Anticholinergic side effects are most common with oxybutynin and tolterodine, however, the extended release tolterodine exhibits side effects less commonly than the immediate release oxybutynin. Mirabegron (A) is a newer medication for the treatment of urge incontinence that exhibits fewer anticholinergic side effects than older anticholinergic medications. Doxazosin (B) is an alpha antagonist used for overflow incontinence causes by prostatic hyperplasia and dose not result in anticholinergic side effects other than orthostasis.

30. C

Colchicine can be used both for prophylaxis and treatment of gout. NSAIDs are used only for acute symptoms and do not prevent gout from occurring (A). Corticosteroids are used during acute gouty attacks when symptoms have been present for >48 hours (B). Probenecid (D) is used for gout prevention in patients unable to take uricosuric agents.

31. A

Decreased libido (B), dyspareunia (C), hot flushes (D), and spotting (E) are all common side effects of estrogen deficiency. Since Ovcon-50 is a high estrogen-containing oral contraceptive, side effects of estrogen excess (such as breast tenderness) would be more common.

32. B

Seasonale is an oral contraceptive and does not require insertion by a healthcare professional (A). Smoking while on any oral contraceptive will increase the risk of thromboembolic events (B). Seasonale is not available in a transdermal patch formulation (C). Unlike NuvaRing, Seasonale does not require refrigeration (D).

33. E

Oral antibiotics may inhibit the efficacy of oral contraceptive medications, so (A) is inaccurate.

It would be inappropriate to advise a patient not to take their oral contraceptive (B) or antibiotic (C), and it would also be inappropriate to advise a patient to double the dose of oral contraceptive during the use of the antibiotics (D); the safety and efficacy of this practice have not been established and this could pose harm to the patient. During the use of interacting antibiotics, it is important to advise a patient to adhere to a backup method of contraception during, for at least 7 days, and up to a full cycle after the completion of the antibiotic (E).

34. C

First-line therapy for comedonal acne is topical benzoyl peroxide (C). The use of oral antibiotics (A) would be recommended in pustular acne or in cases that were not responsive to topical therapy. Also, tetracycline would interact with Ms. Brown's oral contraceptive medication and would not be ideal. Isotretinoin (B and E) is reserved for severe cystic or refractory acne. Topical retinoid agents should not be initially combined with topical benzoyl peroxide (D) due to an increased risk of drying of the skin.

35. D

Propanolol is commonly used for migraine prophylaxis and would be the most appropriate of these options. Ms. Brown's headaches are quite frequent, making her a candidate for prophylactic therapy (A). Hydrocodone (B), an opioid analgesic, is used for the treatment of pain and would be inappropriate for migraine prophylaxis. Imitrex (sumatriptan; C) is an abortive therapy medication and is not appropriate for prophylaxis. Topiramate (E) is used as prophylactic therapy but would have a drug interaction with her oral contraceptive (may decrease efficacy).

36. A

Patients taking oral contraceptives should be educated to consult their pharmacist or physician when starting any new medication because of the strong possibility of multiple drug interactions. Neurontin (gabapentin; A) does not induce or inhibit CYP isoenzymes. Carbamazepine (B), rifampin (C), phenytoin (D), and phenobarbital (E) are strong inducers of CYP3A4, decreasing the effectiveness of oral contraceptives.

37. C

Tolterodine is the generic name for Detrol, oxybutynin is the generic name for Ditropan, solifenacin is the generic name for Vesicare, and imipramine is the generic name for Tofranil.

38. C

When a diagnosis of rheumatoid arthritis is made, DMARDs should be initiated within 3 months to slow the progression of the disease. Biologics should be initiated when methotrexate monotherapy has been ineffective and possibly other DMARDs have been tried and ineffective as well, not within the first 3 months after diagnosis (A). Biologics would not provide PRN relief (B), as they are given by injection at weekly or longer intervals, with the exception of anakinra, which is a daily injection; NSAIDs are used for PRN symptom relief. Therapy should target prevention of joint damage, not await confirmation of joint damage (D), and should be adjusted based upon patient response.

39. B

In overdose situations, tricyclic antidepressants (TCAs) are very dangerous and often fatal (B); therefore, in patients with high suicidality, they should be used with caution. TCAs often exhibit side effects of somnolence, not stimulatory side effects (A). There is no drug–food interaction between aged cheese and TCAs; this interaction is with the monoamine oxidase inhibitors (MAOIs; C). Abrupt discontinuation of TCAs generally results in withdrawal symptoms (D).

40. D

Antidepressants may take several weeks to show maximum efficacy. Neither SSRIs such as fluoxetine (A) nor serotonin norepinephrine reuptake inhibitors (SNRIs) such as duloxetine (B) should be used in combination with MAOIs (selegiline). Caffeine should be avoided in combination with MAOIs because of the risk of hypertensive crisis (C). Although there is an oral formulation of selegiline (E), it is not indicated for depression (used for Parkinson's disease) and would not increase efficacy.

41. A

Fiorinal contains aspirin with butalbital and caffeine. Fioricet (B) contains acetaminophen with butalbital and caffeine. Excedrin Migraine (C) contains acetaminophen and aspirin with caffeine. Migranal (D) is a dihydroergotamine nasal spray. Amerge (E) is naratriptan.

42. D

Photosensitivity is a common side effect with Retin-A (tretinoin), and the use of sunblock prior to sun exposure is very important. Retinoids such as Retin-A should not be used with astringents or abrasive soaps due to the increased risk of excessive drying of the skin (A). Topical retinoids take significantly longer than 1–2 days to result in a benefit (B). Topical retinoids are not used as spot treatment (C) and should be applied sparingly over the face after the face has been allowed to dry fully after cleansing (E).

43. C

Teriparatide is indicated as second-line therapy in patients with a history of osteoporosis who cannot tolerate bisphosphonate therapy. This patient's history of pulmonary embolism contraindicates raloxifene (A), which increases the risk of thromboembolism. Zoledronic acid (B), a bisphosphonate, would be inappropriate in a patient with a history of intolerance due to osteonecrosis of the jaw. Calcitonin (D) is reserved for third-line therapy due to its limited efficacy compared with other available therapies.

44. C

The benzodiazepines including Xanax (alprazolam; A), Librium (chlordiazepoxide; B), and Valium (diazepam; D) vary in their peak activity and duration of action, but all have an onset of effect of minutes to hours. Vistaril (hydroxyzine; E) also works within minutes to hours, while Buspar (buspirone; C) takes up to 2–3 weeks to reach maximal efficacy.

45. A

Cheilitis (chapped lips; A) is the most common side effect of isotretinoin therapy. Leukopenia (B), hypoglycemia (D), and hypertrichosis, or excessive hair growth (C), are not known side effects of this medication.

46. D

Topical agents such as coal tar (C) and anthralin (E) are commonly used in the treatment of psoriasis. Systemic agents such as antimetabolites (methotrexate; A) and corticosteroids (prednisone; B) are often used in combination with topical agents in the treatment of psoriasis. Benzoyl peroxide (D) is not an effective treatment option for psoriasis.

47. C

In the TNM classification, T represents the severity of the primary tumor, N represents the severity of lymph node involvement, and M represents the severity of distant metastases. Generally, N0 and M0 mean no nodal involvement and no metastases, respectively.

48. B

Neoadjuvant chemotherapy is given to provide an initial decrease in tumor burden. It is given prior to surgery, not postsurgery (A); adjuvant chemotherapy is the therapy given postsurgery to further reduce tumor burden. Both adjuvant and neoadjuvant chemotherapy are expected to increase survival (C). Neoadjuvant chemotherapy is not given to reduce nausea and vomiting (D); rather, these are possible side effects.

49. D

Methotrexate inhibits dihydrofolate reductase. When administered at the appropriate time in a chemotherapy cycle, leucovorin permits healthy cells to continue DNA replication and RNA transcription by providing a folic acid source that is not dependent on the action of dihydrofolate reductase. 5-fluorouracil inhibits thymidylate synthase, as does leucovorin. The two agents therefore have a synergistic effect. Doxorubicin is an anthracycline that works as an intercalating agent, interrupting DNA synthesis. Cytarabine inhibits DNA polymerase. Leucovorin does not interact with the mechanism of action of doxorubicin or cytarabine.

50. A, B, C

The primary mechanism of action of cytarabine is inhibition of DNA polymerase (A). Common side effects of treatment include conjunctivitis and neurotoxicity; thus, neurological monitoring at each office visit is recommended (B) as well as pre- and post-treatment with corticosteroid eye drops (C). Powder within vials prior to injection can be stored at room temperature and does not require refrigeration (D).

51. D

The most clinically important side effect of anthracyclines is cardiac damage, including acute arrhythmias and cardiomyopathy following prolonged exposure. The risk of cardiotoxicity increases with cumulative lifetime dose. Hand and foot syndrome (E), or palmar-plantar erythrodysesthesia, is more common with 5-fluorouracil. Ototoxicity (A) is rarely seen with anthracyclines, and is more commonly a side effect of platinum compounds and nitrogen mustards. Methotrexate can cause symptoms of folate deficiency (C). Infusion reactions (B) are more common with etoposide, platinum compounds, and mustard compounds.

52. C

Avastin is the brand name for bevacizumab (C). Gleevec (A) is imatinib, Herceptin (B) is trastuzumab, Tarceva (D) is erlotinib, and Taxol (E) is paclitaxel.

53. C

ANC = white blood cells × (% segs + % bands).

54. B

The ANC range for mild neutropenia is 500–1,000/mm³. Moderate neutropenia (C) is 100–500/mm³, while severe (D) is less than 100/mm³. A normal ANC is 3,000–7,000/mm³ (E).

55. A, B, C, D

Severe (A) or prolonged neutropenia (D) or a sudden drop in ANC (B) are all risk factors for infection. Invasive procedures, including dental procedures, catheter placement, and enemas, also increase the risk of infection (C).

56. A

Neupogen (filgrastim), a colony-stimulating factor, can be used to increase this patient's ANC. Erythropoiesis-stimulating agents (ESAs) such as Epogen (B), Procrit (C), and Aranesp (D) are not indicated in this patient, as her hemoglobin level is normal at 14.5 g/dL.

57. A

Nominal or categorical data are qualitative and have no implied order among the categories. These data can be answered by "yes" or "no" responses. Gender and race are considered nominal data. Ordinal data (B) are ordered categories where the differences between categories cannot be considered equal. Satisfaction surveys and pain scales are examples of ordinal data. With interval data (C), there is an equal distance between the numeric values; however, there is an arbitrary zero point. The Celsius temperature scale is an example of interval data. With ratio data (such as weight or blood pressure; D), there is an equal distance between values and the zero point is meaningful. Frequency (E) refers to a proportion and not a type of data.

58. E

Power depends on sample size and variation within groups. The easiest way to increase power is to increase the sample size of a study. Altering the duration of the study (B, C) or decreasing the sample size (A) will not increase power. Increasing the number of dependent variables being studied (D) will also not increase the power of the study.

59. A, B, C

Type II errors occur when it is stated that there is no difference when a difference actually exists. The null hypothesis is the hypothesis that there is no difference between study groups; not detecting a true difference between groups will lead to a Type II error. Insufficient study power may mean that a difference between groups will not be discovered or will not be found to be statistically significant. Therefore, choices (A), (B), and (C) are all true statements about Type II errors. Type I errors occur when a difference between groups is detected that does not actually exist (D).

60. D

ANOVA is the only test listed that is appropriate for such data (D). A student's *t*-test (A) and a paired *t*-test (B) are appropriate only when studying two groups. The Mann-Whitney U (E) is a nonparametric test appropriate for ordinal data. Chi-square tests (C) are used on nominal data.

61. C

$$30\,g\,ung \times \frac{0.4\,g\,HC}{100\,g\,ung} = 0.12\,g\,HC\,required$$

$$0.12\,g \times \frac{100\,g\,ung}{2.5\,g\,HC} = 4.8\,g\,ung$$

4.8 g of the 2.5% ointment is required to deliver the correct amount of hydrocortisone.

62. C

$$70\,g\,HPet \times \frac{8\,g\,WW}{100\,g\,HPet} = 5.6\,g\,WW$$

63. C

$$4\,fl\,oz \times \frac{30\,mL}{1\,fl\,oz} \times \frac{1\,tbsp}{15\,mL} \times \frac{2\,mg}{1\,tbsp} \times \frac{1\,tab}{4\,mg} = 4\,tabs$$

64. D

$$60\,kg \times \frac{5\,mcg}{kg\,x\,min} \times \frac{1\,mg}{1000\,mcg}$$

$$\frac{1\,mL}{0.5\,mg} \times \frac{60\,min}{1\,hr} = 36\,\frac{mL}{hr}$$

65. A

The initial concentration (C_0) will be obtained by drawing blood very soon after administration. Using the equation $V_d = \dfrac{dose}{C_0}$, we can see that for equal doses, V_d will vary inversely with C_0. Drug A has a higher C_0 than Drug B (0.2 mg/mL > 83 mcg/mL); therefore, Drug A has a smaller volume of distribution.

66. C

$$40\,\text{mL soln} \times \frac{10\,\text{g MgSO}_4}{100\,\text{mL soln}} \times \frac{1000\,\text{mg}}{1\,\text{g}} \times$$

$$\frac{1\,\text{mmol MgSO}_4}{246.36\,\text{mg MgSO}_4} \times \frac{1\,\text{mmol Mg}^{2+}}{1\,\text{mmol MgSO}_4} \times$$

$$\frac{2\,\text{mEq Mg}^{2+}}{1\,\text{mmol Mg}^{2+}} = 32.5\,\text{mEq Mg}^{2+}$$

67. C

$$240\,\text{mL} \times \frac{15\,\text{mEq}}{15\,\text{mL}} \times \frac{1\,\text{mmol K}^+}{1\,\text{mEq K}^+} \times$$

$$\frac{1\,\text{mmol C}_6\text{H}_5\text{K}_3\text{O}_7}{3\,\text{mmol K}^+} \times \frac{1\,\text{mol}}{1000\,\text{mmol}} \times$$

$$\frac{306\,\text{g C}_6\text{H}_5\text{K}_3\text{O}_7}{1\,\text{mol C}_6\text{H}_5\text{K}_3\text{O}_7} = 24.48\,\text{g C}_6\text{H}_5\text{K}_3\text{O}_7$$

68. B

Accuracy refers to how closely test values approach the true value. Precision refers to how closely test values approach each other. Because the test values given are tightly grouped (8.0 ± 0.1) but differ significantly from the true value given (7.5), it can be said the values are precise but not accurate.

69. B

$$\frac{0.9\,\text{g NaCl}}{100\,\text{mL}} \times 30\,\text{mL} = 0.27\,\text{g NaCl}$$

needed to make volume isotonic

$$30\,\text{mL} \times \frac{0.5\,\text{g TetHCl}}{100\,\text{mL}} \times \frac{0.18\,\text{g NaCl(Eq)}}{1\,\text{g TetHCl}} = 0.027\,\text{g}$$

NaCl equivalent present

0.27 g – 0.027 g = 0.243 g NaCl needed to make the solution isotonic

70. B

The recipe makes 10 capsules (M et div caps #10). Therefore each capsule contains (0.5/10) or 0.05 g diphenhydramine. Then, 0.05 × 60 = 3 g.

71. C

fup = 1 – (fraction bound to proteins) = 0.05

Filtration clearance = fup × CLcr = 0.05 × 100 mL/min = 5 mL/min

72. C

CLr = amount filtered + amount secreted – amount reabsorbed

All molecules small enough to pass through the glomerular membrane, which includes most nonprotein-bound small molecule drugs, are filtered.

If CLr > filtration clearance, some drug must be secreted. (Some reabsorption may also occur, but less is reabsorbed than secreted.)

If CLr < filtration clearance, some drug must be reabsorbed. (Some secretion may also occur, but less is secreted than is reabsorbed.)

Because CLr = 25 mL/min, while filtration clearance is only 5 mL/min, the drug must be secreted as well as filtered.

73. A

$$k = \frac{CL}{V_d} = \frac{400\,\text{mL}/\text{min}}{140\,\text{L}} \times \frac{1\,\text{L}}{1000\,\text{mL}} \times$$

$$\frac{60\,\text{min}}{\text{hr}} = 0.171\,hr^{-1}$$

$$t_{1/2} = \frac{0.693}{k} = \frac{0.693}{0.171\,\text{hr}^{-1}} = 4.04\,\text{hr}$$

74. D

$$C_{peak} = \frac{\text{dose}}{V_d} = \frac{250\,\text{mg}}{140\,\text{L}} = 1.79\,\text{mg/L}$$

$$= 0.179\,\text{mg/dL}$$

75. B

Tobramycin is predominantly cleared by the kidneys. The increase in serum creatinine concentration indicates a decrease in CrCl, which in turn implies a decrease in tobramycin clearance. Therefore, choices (C) and (E) are wrong. The bioavailability of any drug given IV is 1; therefore, choice (A) is wrong. When clearance decreases, the half-life and serum concentration will increase, leading to drug accumulation. Therefore, choice (D) is wrong and (B) is correct.

76. A

Because penicillin and probenecid compete for the same saturable excretion pathway, administration of probenecid will decrease the excretion and therefore the overall clearance of penicillin. Choices (B), (C), and (E) are incorrect. When clearance decreases, the steady-state plasma concentration of the drug will increase, so choice (D) is incorrect and (A) is the right answer.

77. B

Amorphous compounds are more soluble in water than their crystalline counterparts. Hydrates are less soluble in water than anhydrous drugs

(A). Adding lipophilic groups (C) and removing hydroxyl groups (D) will also decrease water solubility.

78. D

For weak bases, when pH < pKa the drug will be mostly ionized.

79. E

All medication given by mouth is subject to first-pass metabolism. Only medications given by routes that bypass the GI tract can escape first-pass metabolism. Syrups (B), tablets (A), and capsules (C) are all swallowed, and their contents undergo first-pass metabolism. The rapid-dissolve strip (D) is also an oral product; the strip dissolves in the mouth, and the resultant solution is swallowed. Do not confuse a rapid-dissolve strip with a sublingual or buccal tablet—in these latter two dosage forms, the drug is absorbed across the oral mucosa, escaping the first-pass effect. Of the choices listed, only the transdermal patch is given by a nonoral route. Therefore (E) is the only choice that is not subject to first-pass metabolism.

80. B

Maximizing sediment volume (C) and promoting loose aggregation of suspended particles (A) are functions of controlled flocculation, not structured vehicles. Reducing repulsion between particles (D) will lead to increased sediment density, causing caking. Only slowing sedimentation by increasing viscosity is a behavior of structured vehicles, so (B) is correct.

81. B

The cosolvent system for phenytoin injection contains water, propylene glycol, and alcohol. The cosolvent system is necessary to keep phenytoin in solution, as phenytoin has only limited aqueous solubility. Rapid infusion would dilute the cosolvents, creating a super-saturated concentration of drug in a primarily aqueous environment, leading to precipitation. Onset of action will not be faster as a result of slow injection (A). Rapid injection is unlikely to lead to hemolysis (C); this is a complication of hypertonic solutions. The cosolvent system would have no effect on drug metabolism (D). The viscosity of the solution is not high enough to prevent rapid injection (E).

82. A

Ophthalmic products must contain preservative if they are in multiple-use containers to limit the possibility of severe eye infections. They do not require preservative when packaged in single-dose containers (B and D) or when being used as rinse solutions in eye surgery or trauma (C).

83. C

Ulcerative colitis is a local condition of the intestinal tract; medications administered rectally are providing treatment at the site of action. Nausea (A), chronic pain (B), hormone deficiency (D), and migraines (E) may be treated with medications administered rectally; however, these drugs are absorbed into the systemic circulation to act at distant sites of action.

84. D

The disulfiram reaction results from the inhibition of acetaldehyde dehydrogenase. Ethanol consumption leads to the buildup of acetaldehyde, causing nausea, vomiting, and severe discomfort. Tinctures (C), spirits (A), fluid extracts (E), and Elixir USP (B) all contain ethanol, and will trigger this reaction if taken in combination

with metronidazole. Suspensions (D) do not customarily contain ethanol and would be an appropriate way to deliver metronidazole.

85. C

Hydrolysis (A) results when the drug reacts with water in the dosage form. Because the reaction occurred in only one of the two bottles, this is unlikely. Photolysis (B) is chemical breakdown caused by light exposure; however, the drug was stored in a dark room. Sedimentation (D) and polymorphism (E) are physical changes, rather than chemical changes, and there was no difference in conditions between the capped and uncapped bottles that would explain a difference in the occurrence of these changes. Because only the open bottle was affected, while the capped bottle did not change color, the oxygen in the atmosphere likely caused the degradation (C).

86. E

Dilatant substances (A) become more viscous on agitation, and thin at rest. Newtonian substances (B) do not change viscosity when stirred or agitated. Plastic flow (C) occurs when a substance is thick at rest and remains thick until it receives sufficiently vigorous agitation, after which it behaves in a Newtonian manner. Pseudoplastic flow (D) is similar to plastic flow, but the material continues to thin if agitated more vigorously. Thixotropy is the property where a suspension remains thick until agitated, and then becomes easily pourable.

87. B

$$DR = \frac{V_{max}\, Css}{Km + Css} = \frac{(300)(14)}{6.5 + 14} =$$

205 mg/day = 4 tablets

88. D

Magnesium stearate is a lubricant, and at high concentration has a tendency to waterproof particles, preventing them from dissolving. Starch (A), microcrystalline cellulose (B), lactose (C), and mannitol (E) would not be expected to affect bioavailability.

89. B

Morphine is the only one of these products not metabolized by CYP2D6. Codeine (A), hydrocodone (C), and oxycodone (D) require metabolism by CYP2D6 in order to be activated to a therapeutically useful form. While structurally related to codeine, dextromethorphan (E) is not considered an opioid. This cough suppressant also requires metabolism via CYP2D6 to produce its active form.

90. A

Grapefruit juice inhibits CYP3A, the enzyme that metabolizes protease inhibitors. Therefore, choices (C), (D), and (E) can be eliminated. Inhibition of CYP3A will decrease clearance of drugs metabolized by that enzyme, leading to increased serum concentrations. Increased serum concentration will lead to toxic, rather than subtherapeutic (B), levels.

91. D

$$1:10,000 = \frac{1\,g}{10,000\,mL} = \frac{0.01\,g}{100\,mL} = 0.01\%\,w/v$$

92. B

$$SG = \frac{\text{density}_{\text{substance}}}{\text{density}_{\text{water}}}$$

$$SG \times \text{density}_{\text{water}} = \text{density}_{\text{substance}}$$

$$1.18 \times 1\,g/mL = 1.18\,g/mL$$

$$100\,g \times \frac{1\,mL}{1.18\,g} = 84.75\,mL$$

93. C

Simvastatin and ezetimibe combined are called Vytorin. The combination of atorvastatin and amlodipine (A) is called Caduet. The combination of lovastatin and niacin (B) is called Advicor. There is no combination of simvastatin and lisinopril (D).

94. A, B

Nonpharmacological therapies that can be recommended to patients with heart failure include restricting fluid intake (<2 L/day) (A) and restricting sodium intake (≤3 g/day) (B). There is no specific reason why a patient with heart failure needs to restrict vitamin K (C) or potassium (D) in the diet; this patient's potassium is within normal limits.

95. A, B, C

Anorexia (A), arrhythmias (B), and visual disturbances (C) are all associated with digoxin toxicity. Although hypokalemia (D) would predispose a patient to digoxin toxicity, it is not a consequence.

96. D

Calan SR (verapamil) is a nondihydropyridine calcium channel blocker that is contraindicated in patients with heart failure with reduced ejection fraction (HFrEF) (left vertricular ejection fraction [LVEF] ≤40%). Aldactone (spironolactone; A) and Inspra (eplerenone; E), which are both aldosterone receptor antagonists, as well as the angiotensin receptor blocke (ARB), Diovan (valsartan; C), would be safe to use in a patient with heart failure. In addition, BiDil (B), the combination of hydralazine and isosorbide dinitrate, would also be appropriate to use in a patient with heart failure.

97. B

The second dose of furosemide should be taken before 5 P.M. to minimize nocturia. Furosemide does not need to be separated from other medications (A), does not need to be taken with food or milk (C), and does not need to be taken on an empty stomach (E). The second dose should not be taken at bedtime, as this will likely result in increased nocturia (D).

98. D

Bactrim DS (sulfamethoxazole/trimethoprim) is most likely being used to treat *Escherichia coli*, a common cause of urinary tract infections (UTIs). Bactrim DS does not cover the other bacteria listed.

99. A

The combination of Bactrim DS and Coumadin (warfarin) may lead to a significant drug interaction that would result in an increase in Ms. Brown's INR. Bactrim DS has no effect on plasma sodium or potassium concentrations.

100. E

The combination of trimethoprim and sulfamethoxazole is called Bactrim DS. The combination of amoxicillin and clavulanic acid (A) is called Augmentin, and the combination of imipenem and cilastatin (C) is called Primaxin. There are no combinations of ciprofloxacin and doxycycline (B), or of isoniazid and rifampin (D).

101. A

Lisinopril is an ACEI.

102. B

Martindale is the only reference that contains foreign drug information.

103. D

Xalatan (latanoprost) is an ophthalmic prostaglandin analog used to treat glaucoma.

104. C

Kazano is a combination of alogliptin (PPP-4 inhibitor) and metformin. Kadian (extended-release morphine sulfate; (A) is an opioid anaglesic, Keppra (levetiracetam; B) is an anticonvulsant, and ketoconazole (D) is an antifungal.

105. B, C

Sulfasalazine may cause bodily fluids (e.g., urine, tears) to turn orange (B) and may cause photosensitivity (C). Sulfasalazine should be taken with food rather than on an empty stomach (A) and is taken in 2–3 divided closes rather than once daily (D).

106. D

Metronidazole is the only option listed that can be used to treat *Clostridium difficile*.

107. E

USP-DI Volume II contains information for the patient in lay language. The other choices are all references for the healthcare professional.

108. C

Cytotec is the brand name for misoprostol. Cimetidine (A) is Tagamet. Metoclopramide (B) is Reglan. Olsalazine (D) is Dipentum. Sucralfate (E) is Carafate.

109. A

Acyclovir is an appropriate treatment for genital herpes. Indinavir (B) and lamivudine (C) are used to treat human immunodeficiency virus (HIV). Oseltamivir (D) is used to treat influenza. Valganciclovir (E) is used to treat cytomegalovirus.

110. D

The Red Book is the only choice listed that contains cost information.

111. A, B, C

Potential side effects of niacin include flushing (A), hyperglycemia (B), and hyperuricemia (C). Hypertriglyceridemia (D) is possible with bile sequestrants, but not niacin.

112. B

The combination of timolol and dorzolamide is called Cosopt. The combination of timolol and brimonidine (A) is called Combigan. There are no combinations of latanoprost and carbachol (C), pilocarpine and brinzolamide (D), or pilocarpine and carbachol (E).

113. A

Voriconazole is an antifungal that could be used to treat an invasive *Aspergillus* infection. Voriconazole can be administered either IV or orally. While miconazole (C) is also an antifungal drug, it is available only in topical formulations and as a buccal tablet and is used to treat superficial fungal infections. Linezolid (B) and meropenem (D) are used to treat bacterial infections.

114. A, B, D

Omeprazole is available in the 20 mg strength without a prescription (A). It works most effectively when taken on an empty stomach to allow time for proton pump inhibition to occur prior to eating (B). There is a significant drug interaction between omeprazole and clopidogrel (D), whereby omeprazole may inhibit the efficacy of clopidogrel; this combination should be avoided. The tablet formulation of omeprazole (C) is an extended-release product that should not be crushed or chewed.

115. E

Nitroprusside should be protected from light. None of the other IV medications listed need to be protected from light.

116. A

The three-drug combination regimen of Biaxin (clarithromycin), Amoxil (amoxicillin), and Nexium (esomeprazole) would be used to treat a *Helicobacter pylori* infection.

117. C

Trusopt (dorzolamide) is an ophthalmic carbonic anhydrase inhibitor used in treating glaucoma.

118. C

The Commission E monographs provide information on herbal products.

119. A, D

Clotrimazole is available as a troche (A), topical cream (D), vaginal cream, and topical solution. It is not available as a capsule (B) or powder (C).

120. C

In patients receiving amiodarone, liver function tests should be performed every 6 months to monitor for potential hepatotoxicity. A chest x-ray should be performed every 12 months, not every 6 months (A), to monitor for pulmonary toxicity. Thyroid function tests should be performed every 6 months, not every 12 months (B), to monitor for hyper- or hypothyroidism. Ophthalmic exams should be performed at baseline and then if symptoms develop, not every 3 months (D).

121. E

Patients should separate the administration of different ophthalmic preparations by intervals of at least 10 minutes. Contact lenses should be removed before using ophthalmic products (A). Patients should not touch the tip of the dropper to any part of the eye (B). Patients should pull out the lower eyelid (not the upper eyelid) to form a pocket for the medication to be placed (C). Patients should not rub their eyes after administration of ophthalmic preparations (D).

122. C

Trissel's (C) contains information on IV drug compatibility. Facts and Comparisons (A), the Physician's Desk Reference (B), and USP DI Volume I (D), contain general drug information and do not contain IV drug compatibility information.

123. B

Tagamet (cimetidine) is an H_2 receptor antagonist.

124. B, C

Patients taking methotrexate should have a CBC (B) monitored for potential bone marrow suppression, and their liver function tests (C) monitored for potential hepatotoxicity. It is not necessary to have an electrocardiogram (A) or to measure TSH (D) while taking methotrexate.

125. A, B, C

Candesartan (ARB; A), eplerenone (aldosterone receptor antagonist; B), and triamterene (potassium-sparing diuretic; C) may all result in hyperkalemia. Metolazone (D), a thiazide-like diuretic, may cause hypokalemia.

126. A, B, C

For esomeprazole (A), the capsules can be opened and mixed with water in a syringe or the granules for oral suspension can be mixed with water in a syringe prior to administration via nasogastric tube. For lansoprazole (B), the capsules can be opened and mixed with apple juice or the orally disintegrating tablets can be mixed with water in a syringe prior to administration via nasogastric tube. The pantoprazole (C) granules for suspension can be mixed with apple juice in a syringe prior to administration via nasogastric tube. Neither rabeprazole tablets nor the sprinkle capsules can be administered via nasogastric tube (D).

127. A

A patient who is taking felodipine should avoid drinking grapefruit juice because grapefruit juice inhibits CYP3A4, which would result in increased concentrations of felodipine. Tyramine-containing foods (B) should be avoided in patients taking MAOIs. Felodipine does not cause folate deficiency, and therefore does not to be administered with folic acid (C). Felodipine does not need to be taken on an empty stomach (D), and does not need to be separated from other medications (E).

128. A

Azithromycin is the best option, as it will cover the most likely bacteria that would cause community-acquired pneumonia in this patient, including the atypical organisms (*Streptococcus pneumoniae, Mycoplasma pneumoniae, Haemophilus influenzae*). The other antibiotic choices would not cover the appropriate bacteria.

129. B, C, D

Amoxicillin is available as an oral suspension (B), capsule (C), or chewable tablet (D) but not as an IV injection (A). A related antibiotic, ampicillin, can be administered IV.

130. C

Antihypertensives that can be used safely in pregnancy are methyldopa, a calcium channel blocker, and labetalol. ACEIs (such as lisinopril; B) and ARBs (such as valsartan; E) are contraindicated in pregnancy. Diuretics (such as metolazone; D) and α_1-receptor antagonists (such as doxazosin; A) are not recommended in pregnant patients.

131. A

Proton pump inhibitors (PPIs) should be taken 15–30 minutes before breakfast.

132. C

Sporanox is the brand name for itraconazole. Abilify is the brand name of aripiprazole (A). Diflucan is the brand name of fluconazole (B). Prevacid is the brand name of lansoprazole (D). Aciphex is the brand name of rabeprazole (E).

133. E

Simvastatin plus gemfibrozil is likely to result in myopathy (and possibly rhabdomyolysis). In fact, if a fibric acid derivative must be used with a statin, gemfibrozil should be avoided and fenofibrate should be used alternatively.

134. A

Amiodarone contains iodine and may potentially cause hyper- or hypothyroidism. The other listed medications do not cause hypothyroidism.

135. C

Levaquin (levofloxacin) is a fluoroquinolone.

136. C

Amiodarone-induced pulmonary fibrosis is a potentially life-threatening condition. Therefore, if this adverse effect occurs in a patient taking amiodarone, this antiarrhythmic must be discontinued. Amiodarone undergoes significant CYP450 metabolism (B) and is a substrate of the CYP2C8 and CYP3A4 isoenzymes. It is also an inhibitor of the CYP1A2, CYP2C9, CYP2D6, and CYP3A4 isoenzymes. Amiodarone is effective for the treatment of both ventricular and atrial arrhythmias (A) and is indicated for arrhythmias in patient with heart failure (D). In fact, amiodarone and dofelitide are the only antiarrhythmics that are safe to use in patients with heart failure.

137. A, B, C

Aminosalicylates (A), corticosteroids (B), and immunosuppressants (C) can all be used to treat inflammatory bowel disease. The chloride channel activator (D) lubiprostone is indicated for irritable bowel syndrome.

138. A, B

Eradication of *H. pylori* requires either triple therapy with a PPI, clarithromycin, and amoxicillin (or metronidazole for penicillin-allergic patients) or quadruple therapy with PPI, bismuth subsalicylate, metronidazole, and tetracycline. Regimens (A) and (B) include the PPI, clarithromycin, and either amoxicillin or metronidazole. Regimens (C) and (D) would require a fourth agent in order to effectively eradicate the infection.

139. **B**

The maximum dose of metformin is 2,550 mg/day. This patient's dose (3,000 mg/day) exceeds this, so the doctor should be contacted. Choice (A) is incorrect because this patient has controlled blood sugars based on an A1c less than 7%. The dose of metformin should not be increased (C), because it already exceeds the maximum recommended daily dose. Choice (D) is incorrect because the American Diabetes Association recommends metformin as the drug of choice in newly diagnosed patients with type 2 diabetes and this patient has no contraindications such as heart failure, renal impairment, or age greater than 80 years. Lisinopril does not interact with metformin (E). In fact, there truly are no major drug interactions with metformin.

140. **C**

Encouraging Mr. Boyd to call his doctor is the best answer, because he is taking more than the recommended daily dose of Prilosec OTC: 20 mg daily × 14 days, which can be repeated in 4 months. Mr. Boyd has continued the treatment longer than the recommended 14 days for Prilosec OTC. Mr. Boyd should not continue taking all medications as prescribed, because his metformin dose is currently too high and he is taking more than the recommended dose of Prilosec OTC (A). A multivitamin (B) is not a bad option for any patient in any circumstances; however, Mr. Boyd's complaint of fatigue that he is experiencing is likely due to the symptoms of hypothyroidism. The patient's potassium is normal and doesn't warrant a recommendation to restrict intake (D).

141. **A**

Hypothyroidism is the best answer because Mr. Boyd's thyroid-stimulating hormone (TSH) con-

centration is well out of the normal range (0.3–6 mIU/L). His symptoms are very consistent with hypothyroidism: weakness, fatigue, depression, cold feeling, weight gain. Hypoglycemia (B) is incorrect because he is taking metformin only, which does not cause hypoglycemia in monotherapy. Depression (C) is incorrect because his general depression score (GDS) was not greater than 7 and the hypothyroidism must be ruled out first. Uncontrolled hypertension (D) would more likely cause symptoms such as headache and blurred vision, and his blood pressure is currently at goal.

142. **D**

Inhibition of ACE blocks the conversion of angiotensin I to angiotensin II. Angiotensin II is the most potent vasoconstrictor in the body; therefore, decreasing concentrations of angiotensin II results in vasodilation (D). Based on current literature, ACEIs do not lower blood glucose (A). ACEIs do not inhibit renin (B); this would be the mechanism of aliskiren. ARBs, not ACEIs, block the angiotensin II receptor (C). ACEIs lead to increased, not decreased, concentrations of bradykinin by preventing its breakdown (E).

143. **B**

Mr. Boyd should avoid taking the Synthroid (levothyroxine) at the same time as the ferrous sulfate, which will bind to the levothyroxine and prevent it from being absorbed. This interaction can be avoided by taking these medications at least 4 hours apart. Synthroid does not cause hypoglycemia (A). Taking Synthroid only in the evening (C) is possible, but the patient must be informed not to take it with the ferrous sulfate, so (B) is still the best option. There is no drug interaction with metformin (D), so Mr. Boyd could take the Synthroid at the same time as the metformin. Synthroid should not be taken with dairy products, as the calcium will bind to levothyroxine and prevent it from being absorbed (E).

144. A

There are only four drugs in the nonnucleoside reverse transcriptase inhibitor class, nevirapine, efavirenz, etravirine, and rilpivirine. The brand name of nevirapine is Viramune. Ziagen (abacavir) is a nucleoside reverse transcriptase inhibitor (NRTI; B). Kaletra (lopinavir/ritonavir) is a protease inhibitor (C). Videx (didanosine) is an NRTI (D). Fuzeon (enfuvirtide) is a fusion inhibitor (E).

145. B, C

Patients diagnosed with HIV will need to have a Western blot performed (A); however, starting highly active antiretroviral therapy is not always recommended upon initial diagnosis because of the long-term side effects and because some patients' viral load and CD4 cell count rise and drop differently. However, when the CD4 cell count drops to less than 500 cells/mm^3 (B), it is recommended to start antiviral therapy. In addition, if patients have a history of an opportunistic infection regardless of their CD4 cell count (C), antiviral therapy and treatment for the opportunistic infection should be initiated. Treatment initiation is unrelated to viral load (D).

146. B

Thrush is a common side effect of inhaled corticosteroids; it is most likely due to this patient not swishing and spitting, as directed, after using Advair (B). The classic toxicity symptoms for theophylline include tachycardia, nausea, and vomiting, along with a theophylline level that exceeds the normal range of 5–15 mcg/mL (A). The metoprolol dose is well within the normal range, and this patient has tachycardia (C); metoprolol would cause bradycardia. Thrush (D) is not a known side effect of fish oil.

147. D

The Advair does not need to be discontinued (A). Thrush must be treated with nystatin and the patient must be counseled to swish and spit after each use of Advair. The patient's nausea is likely due to the theophylline toxicity, and not the aspirin (B). There is not enough information to assess whether the patient is using the albuterol excessively (C). Theophylline should be discontinued due to toxicity symptoms. Metoprolol (E) does not cause tachycardia; it would cause bradycardia. This patient is currently tachycardic, which is most likely due to theophylline toxicity.

148. C

Fluticasone and salmeterol combined are called Advair. The brand names of fluticasone (A) oral inhalers are Flovent and Arnuity Ellipta. Salmeterol alone (B) is called Serevent Diskus and is available only as a dry powder inhaler. The brand name of flunisolide (D) oral inhaler is Aerospan. There are no combinations of flunisolide and salmeterol (E).

149. E

Fish oil targets triglyceride reduction. It is available over-the-counter and as a prescription product (Lovaza, Epanova, Omtryg, Vascepa). Fish oil is thought to inhibit acylCA:1,2 diacylglycerol acyltransferase and to increase hepatic beta-oxidation, causing a reduction in the hepatic synthesis of triglycerides or an increase in plasma lipoprotein lipase activity. Fish oils have only modest effects on the other lipid profiles, so choices (A), (B), (C), and (D) are incorrect.

150. B

The maximum daily dose of acetaminophen is 4,000 mg per day. The patient could potentially take 4,550 mg/day by taking 2 hydrocodone/acetaminophen tablets every 6 hours and the Tylenol Arthritis 650 mg 3 times daily. Choice (B) is the best option because the pharmacist can easily educate the patient on the 4,000-mg guideline and help develop a plan of administration. There is no need to call the doctor (A); and the patient can have the flexibility to decide if she needs over-the-counter acetaminophen or the combination product with hydrocodone for more severe pain, so choices (C) and (D) are also incorrect. Aspirin is not a good option because she is already taking 325 mg/day of aspirin and giving her more aspirin could increase her risk of bleeding (E).

151. B

Spiriva (tiotropium; B) is a long-acting anticholinergic agent and is appropriately dosed once daily. Atrovent (ipratropium; A) is a short-acting anticholinergic, and its duration of action requires dosing 3–4 times daily; this medication can be used PRN. Combivent (C) is a combination of ipratropium and albuterol; both agents require multiple daily dosing for consistent efficacy, although they can be dosed PRN for rescue therapy. Advair (D) is a combination of fluticasone and salmeterol; it requires twice daily dosing for efficacy.

152. A

Pulmicort Respules (budesonide; A) is the only nebulized inhaled corticosteroid available on the market. Singulair (montelukast; B) is a leukotriene receptor antagonist and Zyflo (zileuton; C) is a 5-lipoxygenase inhibitor; both medications are available orally. Solu-Medrol (methylprednisolone; D) is an injectable corticosteroid.

153. D

The active ingredient in Zyban is bupropion. Bupropion is indicated both as an antidepressant and smoking cessation agent. It is not a serotonergic inhibitor (A); as a result, bupropion does not cause sexual dysfunction like most serotonergic antidepressants. Bupropion inhibits the reuptake of norepinephrine and dopamine; therefore, choices (B) and (C) are incorrect. Effexor (venlafaxine) inhibits the reuptake of serotonin, norepinephrine, and dopamine (E).

154. E

Streptomycin is used only as a substitute for ethambutol and for drug-resistant tuberculosis. The other choices are commonly used in combination for treatment of tuberculosis.

155. D

Vitamin K is used to reverse the anticoagulant effects of warfarin. Protamine is used to reverse the effects of unfractionated heparin (A), and it may be used to partially reverse the effects of low molecular weight heparins, such as enoxaparin (C). Idarucizumab can be used to reverse the anticoagulant effects of dabigatran (B). Clopidogrel (E) is an antiplatelet agent and does not have an antidote.

156. A

Flumazenil is the antidote for benzodiazepines. Choice (B) is incorrect because there are several antidotes for opioids, including naloxone and naltrexone. The antidote for methanol (C) or ethylene glycol toxicity is fomepizole. The antidote for an overdose of methotrexate (D) is leucovorin. Amifostine is used to prevent nephrotoxicity associated with repeated administration of cisplatin (E).

157. A

Liothyronine is called Cytomel. Levothyroxine (B) has multiple brand name products, including Levoxyl, Synthroid, Tirosint, and Unithroid. Choice (C) is the natural animal thyroid which is desiccated from pig or cow and is called Armour Thyroid. T4 (D) is the abbreviated name for levothyroxine. TSH (E) is not an active ingredient in any drug.

158. A, B, D

Finasteride (A) causes abnormalities of external male genitalia. Isotretinoin (B) causes major fetal abnormalities, both internal and external. Atorvastatin (D) causes congenital malformations. All of these medications should be avoided during pregnancy. Methyldopa (C) is actually the drug of first choice in pregnant women for the treatment of hypertension.

159. B

Progestin is indicated along with estrogen in women with an intact uterus in order to decrease the risk of endometrial cancer (B). Venous thromboembolism (A) and weight gain (D) are risks associated with progestin therapy. Estrogen therapy reduces the risk of osteoporosis (C), and progestin therapy does not affect this benefit.

160. B

During the initial application, the absorption of transdermal fentanyl requires 12 to 24 hours to reach plateau. Therefore, transdermal fentanyl is inappropriate for management of acute pain. Choice (D) is misleading, as the patch needs to be changed every 72 hours.

161. C

Morphine is an opioid analgesic. Because of the consistent incidence of constipation with opioid use, use of a stimulant laxative is recommended.

162. D

This question is designed to assess whether you know that choices (A), (B), (C), and (E) are all forms of NSAIDs. NSAIDs inhibit prostaglandins, which normally help to keep the afferent arterioles of the kidneys open. As a result, a recommendation other than acetaminophen (D) could compromise the patient's kidney function.

163. A, B, C

A PPD is a tuberculin test for tuberculosis. Tuberculosis results in individuals becoming sensitized to certain antigenic components of the *M. tuberculosis* organism. Healthcare workers (A) are at risk for being exposed to patients with tuberculosis. HIV-infected patients (B) are immunocompromised, which allows for easier inoculation and growth of the organism. Immigrant workers (C) have a higher rate of infection and lack of access to healthcare. A 4-year-old entering preschool does not need to have a PPD performed (D).

164. A, B, D

The doses of morphine (A) and codeine (B) should be reduced by 25% in patients with a CrCl of 10–50 mL/min. When the CrCl is less than 10 mL/min, the doses of these drugs should be reduced by 50%. Morphine has a metabolite, morphine-6-glucuronide, which can accumulate in renal impairment. The dose of oxycodone (C) should be adjusted in patients with hepatic impairment, not renal impairment. Tramadol (D) requires dose adjustment for CrCl less than 30 mL/minute.

165. A

Naprosyn's (naproxen's) maximum daily dose is 1,500 mg. Other maximum daily doses are: ibuprofen (B), 3,200 mg/day; Relafen (nabumetone; C), 2,000 mg/day; and ketoprofen (D), 300 mg/day.

Daypro's (oxaprozin; E) maximum daily dose is 1,200 mg/day in patients who weigh less than 50 kg and 1,800 mg/day in patients who weigh more than 50 kg.

166. **A, B, C, E**

There are four warning signs for stroke. Of the five answer choices, only sudden seizure for no reason (D) is not considered common with stroke. Regardless, a patient should be rushed to the emergency room for care if a seizure occurred. The four warning signs for stroke (choices A, B, C, and E) are important in helping patients to receive treatment as soon as possible.

167. **A, B**

Folic acid is used with methotrexate treatment (A) because methotrexate is a folate antimetabolite that inhibits DNA synthesis; methotrexate irreversibly binds to dihydrofolate reductase and inhibits the formation of reduced folates. Use of folic acid is important in preparation for pregnancy (B) to prevent neural tube defects. Iron deficiency anemia (IDA) (C) is a deficiency of iron; folate deficiency is found in megaloblastic (macrocytic) anemias. Anemia in chronic kidney disease (CKD) (D) is most commonly associated with a deficiency in enythropoietin and/or iron, not folic acid.

168. **D**

ESAs are indicated for patients with anemia of CKD, with a goal Hgb of 11–12 g/dL. Therapy would not be indicated in patients with a hemoglobin of 12 g/dL (A and B). ESAs are also indicated in patients with chemotherapy-induced anemia when the goal of the chemotherapy is palliative (D), not curative (C).

169. **E**

Cholecalciferol is vitamin D3 and can be used for the treatment of vitamin D deficiency. Pyridoxine (A) is used for vitamin B6 deficiency or acute toxicity from isoniazid. Ascorbic acid (B) is used for prevention and treatment of scurvy and to acidify the urine. Beta-carotene (C) is used for prophylaxis and treatment of polymorphous light eruption, and for erythropoietic protoporphyria. Nicotinic acid (D) is used for dyslipidemia.

170. **C**

One of the problems with treating IDA is the side effects associated with treatment. Patients are often unable to tolerate the side effects, which limits the length of therapy. The minimum length of therapy with the lowest rates of relapsing IDA is 6 months.

171. **B**

The mechanism of action of epoetin alfa is inducing erythropoiesis and releasing reticulocytes, which are immature red blood cells. Choices (A), (C), (D), and (E) are all combinations of other drug mechanisms of actions.

172. **E**

Pyridoxine is used to prevent neurological toxicities associated with isoniazid therapy. The other options are not used with isoniazid treatment.

173. **C**

The Drug Enforcement Administration is the organization that is ultimately responsible for controlling and regulating controlled substances. The Federal Drug Association (A) is not a known association. The Food and Drug Administration (FDA) (B) is in charge of approving drugs for particular indications. The National Provider Indicators (D) is a group that assigns a national provider number to all healthcare professionals. The State Patrol (E) is often called on to arrest or investigate persons involved in drug diversion.

174. A, B, D, E

Choices (A), (B), (D), and (E) are all correct lifestyle modifications for their respective diseases. Choice (C) is incorrect because the most recent cholesterol guidelines recommend that cholesterol-lowering medications be started at the same time as heart-healthy lifestyle modifications.

175. A, B, C

Choices (A), (B), and (C) are all correct statements within the Dietary Supplement Health and Education Act of 1994. Choice (D) is not written into that act and has created much debate and controversy; the FDA is considering making a change but, to date, has not.

176. A, B, C, E

Saw palmetto (D) has very few drug interactions. This is important because its prescription counterparts, finasteride and dutasteride, interact with warfarin. Choices (A), (B), (C), and (E) all interact with warfarin and can lead to an increased INR. These herbal products may also increase the risk of bleeding when used with antiplatelet drugs, such as aspirin.

177. C

The most common organisms causing community-acquired skin and soft tissue infections are the Gram-positive organisms, *Staphylococcus aureus* (especially methicillin-resistant strains) (C) and *Streptococcus pyogenes* (not *Streptococcus pneumoniae* [D]). Gram-negative organisms, such as *Escherichia coli* (B) and *Pseudomonas aeruginosa* (E), are more likely to be found in nosocomial skin and soft tissue infections. *Haemophilus influenzae* (A) does not cause skin and soft tissue infections.

178. D

Glulisine is a rapid-acting insulin with a short duration of action. Regular insulin (A) is a short-acting insulin whose duration is short, but longer than that of the rapid-acting insulin analogues glulisine, aspart, and lispro. Detemir insulin (B) is a long-acting insulin analogue, and NPH insulin (C) is an intermediate-acting insulin.

179. A

GLP-1 agonists including exenatide (A) are associated with acute pancreatitis and should, therefore, be used with caution in patients with a history of acute pancreatitis. Insulin products including detemir (B) are not known to increase the risk of pancreatitis. The SGLT2 inhibitors including dapagliflozin (C) and alpha glucosidase inhibitors such as acarbose (D) are also not associated with an increased risk of pancreatitis.

180. E

Trissel's provides a compilation of all currently available stability information on drugs in compounded oral, enteral, topical, and IV formulations. Goodman and Gilman (A) focuses on drug pharmacology. Martindale (B) contains foreign drug information. The Merck Index (C) focuses on precise, comprehensive information on chemicals, drugs, and biologicals, whereas the Merck Manual focuses on diseases. Remington (D) is considered the pharmacy encyclopedia for pharmacology, theoretical science, sterilization, and practical pharmacy practice.

181. **B**

Melatonin is used to treat insomnia. Black cohosh (A) is primarily used for vasomotor symptoms associated with menopause, St. John's wort (C) is used to treat depression, and saw palmetto (D) is used to treat prostate disorders.

182. **B**

Ferrous sulfate 5-grain tablets (B) are equivalent to 325 mg and are available on the market. Metformin tablets are available in 500-mg, 850-mg, and 1,000-mg, strengths; 1,250-mg tablets (A) are not available. The highest dosage form of Synthroid (levothyroxine) (C) is 300 mcg; however, a 212-mcg tablet is not available. The highest dosage form of Coumadin (warfarin) (D) is 10 mg; 15-mg tablets are not commercially available. Lisinopril's highest dosage form (E) is 40 mg.

183. **B**

Simvastatin is half as potent as Lipitor (atorvastatin), so simvastatin 20 mg is the correct answer. Rosuvastatin (A) is twice as potent as Lipitor. Pravastatin (C) is one-fourth as potent at atorvastatin and would require 40 mg to be equivalent.

184. **B, C**

St. John's wort can be used for the treatment of mild to moderate depression. However, it is associated with numerous drug interactions. It is a strong inducer of the CYP3A4 enzyme. Warfarin (C) is metabolized by CYP3A4; therefore, concomitant use with St. John's wort may lead to a reduction in warfarin concentrations, which may place a patient at risk for thromboembolic events. Sertraline (B) interacts with St. John's wort because both inhibit the reuptake of serotonin, which could result in serotonin syndrome. Pravachol (pravastatin; A) is the only statin not metabolized by CYP3A4; in fact, pravastatin is not metabolized at all via the CYP450 enzyme system. There is no interaction between St. John's wort and aspirin (D).

185. **A**

This is a classic NAPLEX question which guides you to assess each complaint of the patient. Diphenhydramine is used for the runny nose, sneezing, and watery eyes. Acetaminophen (B) is unnecessary but would be helpful if the patient had headaches or fever. There is no need to overtreat with an unneeded medication such as pseudoephedrine (C); the patient is not experiencing any congestion. Guaifenesin (D) is also unnecessary; it would be used for a productive cough or chest congestion.

INDEX